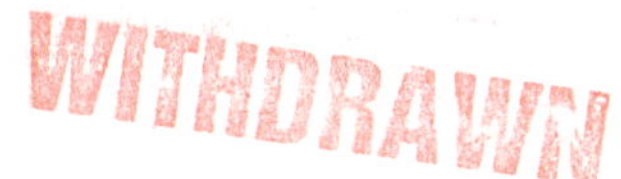

Wintrobe's
Atlas of Clinical Hematology

Wintrobe's Atlas of Clinical Hematology

EDITORS

Douglas C. Tkachuk, MD, FRCPC

Staff Pathologist
University Health Network
Associate Professor
Department of Laboratory Medicine and Pathobiology
University of Toronto
Toronto, Ontario

Jan V. Hirschmann, MD

Staff Physician
Seattle VA Medical Center
Professor
Department of Medicine
University of Washington
Seattle, Washington

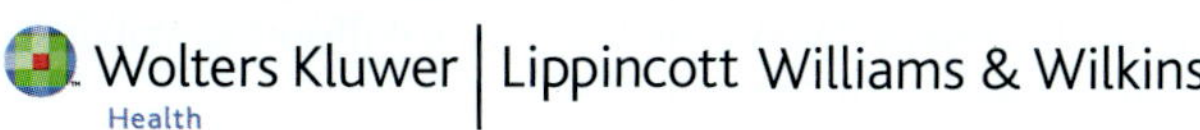

Wolters Kluwer | Lippincott Williams & Wilkins
Health

Philadelphia · Baltimore · New York · London
Buenos Aires · Hong Kong · Sydney · Tokyo

Acquisitions Editor: Jonathan W. Pine, Jr.
Managing Editor: Anne E. Jacobs
Associate Director of Marketing: Adam Glazer
Project Manager: David Murphy
Manufacturing Manager: Benjamin Rivera
Design Coordinator: Stephen Druding
Compositor: Techbooks
Printer: Walsworth

© 2007 by LIPPINCOTT WILLIAMS & WILKINS
530 Walnut Street
Philadelphia, PA 19106 USA
LWW.com

Printed in the USA

Library of Congress Cataloging-in-Publication Data

Wintrobe's atlas of clinical hematology/editors, Douglas C. Tkachuk,
    Jan V. Hirschmann.
      p. ; cm.
    Includes index.
    ISBN 978-0-7817-7023-1
    ISBN 0–7817–7023–8 (case)

    1. Hematology—Atlases. 2. Blood—Diseases—Atlases.
I. Tkachuk, Douglas C. II. Hirschmann, Jan V. III. Wintrobe,
Maxwell Myer, 1901–1986. IV. Title: Atlas of clinical hematology.
    [DNLM: 1. Hematologic Diseases—diagnosis—Atlases.
    2. Hematologic Diseases—pathology—
Atlases.   WH 17 W794 2007]
    RB145.W564 2007
    616.1′5—dc22
2006025285

9 8 7 6 5 4 3 2

Contents

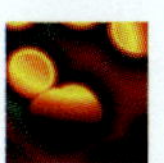

CHAPTER **1**
Anemia

DAVID BARTH, MD, FRCPC, AND JAN V. HIRSCHMANN, MD

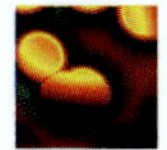

CHAPTER **2**
Acute Leukemias

DOUGLAS C. TKACHUK, MD, FRCPC, AND JAN V. HIRSCHMANN, MD

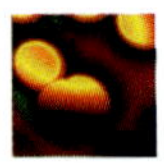

CHAPTER **3**
Myelodysplastic Syndromes   94

DOUGLAS C. TKACHUK, MD, FRCPC, KATHY CHUN, PhD, FCCMG, AND JAN V. HIRSCHMANN, MD

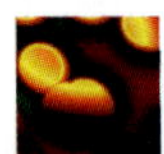

CHAPTER **4**
Chronic Myeloproliferative Syndromes   105

TRACY I. GEORGE, MD

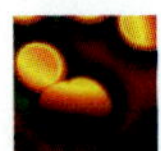

CHAPTER **5**
Lymphoproliferative Disorders   137

JAN V. HIRSCHMANN, MD, DENIS J. BAILEY, MD, FRCPC, AND DOUGLAS C. TKACHUK, MD, FRCPC

C H A P T E R 6

Flow Cytometry in the Diagnosis of Hematopoietic Diseases   212

STEVEN J. KUSSICK, MD, PhD

C H A P T E R 7

Cytology and Laser Scanning Cytometry   242

WILLIAM R. GEDDIE, MD, FRCPC

C H A P T E R 8

Approach to the Microscopic Evaluation of Blood and Bone Marrow   275

DOUGLAS C. TKACHUK, MD, FRCPC, AND JAN V. HIRSCHMANN, MD

Hematology is a very visual subspecialty of medicine. Examining the patient, evaluating bone marrow and other tissue specimens, scrutinizing blood films, and inspecting information derived from recently developed techniques, such as flow cytometry, all require careful observation. The purpose of this text-atlas is to provide clear, accurate, and detailed images to help the reader learn how to interpret these examinations both in normal people and in those with a wide variety of hematologic disorders. The book also provides brief descriptions of the relevant clinical, diagnostic, and pathophysiologic features of the diseases depicted. These accounts and the several accompanying tables contain the most important information, rather than being encyclopedic compilations. Those interested in more extensive coverage of the topics should refer to *Wintrobe's Clinical Hematology*. Because the major purpose of this text-atlas is to help the reader learn how to diagnose hematologic problems, it does not contain information about treatment, which, in any event, is rapidly changing for many of the diseases included. The proposed audience is anyone interested in blood disorders, including laboratory technicians, medical students, physicians in training, oncologists, and hematologists of all levels of experience. We hope that even experts will benefit, for education, as Samuel Johnson stated, is often more a matter of being reminded than informed.

Douglas C. Tkachuk, MD, FRCPC
Jan V. Hirschmann, MD

It has been my great privilege to study under Dr. M.M. Wintrobe's tutelage for three years and to be asked later, as one of five former fellows, to contribute as writer and editor of the seventh through twelfth editions of *Wintrobe's Clinical Hematology*. In the process, we taught a generation of medical students about the wonders and challenges inherent in the study of the blood and its diseases, as well as the application of the scientific method to clinical practice and research. One of my students was Douglas Tkachuk, now one of the editors and a driving force behind the creation of *Wintrobe's Atlas of Clinical Hematology*. The circle is almost complete.

Dr. Wintrobe was a tough taskmaster as clinician, scientist, and communicator of knowledge; the standards he set for himself and his students were high. He would have been proud of this book that honors his name and that emphasizes the three pillars on which he considered excellence in all of medicine to rest—critical apprehension of physical findings, astute laboratory testing of derived hypotheses, and informed decision-making based on the most up-to-date evidence provided by research in molecular and cellular biology. *Wintrobe's Atlas of Clinical Hematology* makes a superb contribution in these areas. The illustrations of physical findings are excellent and well described in the accompanying text; the reproductions of blood and marrow smears, as well as the histologic sections and other microscopic and submicroscopic illustrations, are among the best I have seen. Most important, wherever possible, clinical and laboratory findings are explained on the basis of the most up-to-date scientific insights available. All these features make the *Atlas* an excellent companion to *Wintrobe's Clinical Hematology* and, indeed, a growing number of textbooks dealing with the fascinating subject of hematology.

In the preface to an early edition of *Clinical Hematology*, Dr. Wintrobe quoted Leonardo da Vinci as saying that, "The love of anything is the fruit of our knowledge, and grows deeper as our knowledge becomes more certain." *Wintrobe's Atlas of Clinical Hematology* contributes to this process in significant measure.

John Foerster, MD
Professor of Medicine
University of Manitoba
Winnipeg, Manitoba

Acknowledgments

We wish to acknowledge the generosity of the many contributors who made this book possible. Special thanks is extended to our colleagues at Toronto Medical Laboratories, Dr. Mark Minden and the attending staff at the Princess Margaret Hospital's acute leukemia service, and Bryan Kautz, Keith Oxley, Allan Connor and Bruna Ariganello from Photographic services at University Health Network. The authors would like to thank the editorial and technical staff at Lippincott Williams & Wilkins, especially Jonathan W. Pine, Anne E. Jacobs, Adam Glazer, and David Murphy, and also Cindy Fullerton from Tech-Books.

This book is dedicated to Evy, Claire, Jean, and Jennifer.

Douglas C. Tkachuk, MD, FRCPC
Jan V. Hirschmann, MD

Denis J. Bailey, MD, FRCPC
Pathologist
University Health Network
Assistant Professor
Department of Laboratory Medicine and Pathobiology
University of Toronto
Toronto, Ontario

David Barth, MD, FRCPC
Hematologist and Hematopathologist
Assistant Professor
Departments of Laboratory Medicine and Pathobiology
  and Medicine
Hematology Division
University of Toronto
Toronto, Ontario

Kathy Chun, PhD, FCCMG
Director
Cytogenetics and Molecular Genetics
North York General Hospital
Genetics Program
Toronto, Ontario

William R. Geddie, MD, FRCPC
Cytopathologist
University Health Network
Assistant Professor
Department of Laboratory Medicine and Pathobiology
University of Toronto
Toronto, Ontario

Tracy I. George, MD
Associate Director
Hematology Laboratory
Stanford Hospital and Lucile Packard Children's Hospital
Assistant Professor of Pathology
Stanford University
Stanford, California

Franklin Goldberg, MD, FRCPC
Diagnostic Radiologist
St. Michaels Hospital
Assistant Professor
Department of Medical Imaging
University of Toronto
Toronto, Ontario

Jan V. Hirschmann, MD
Staff Physician
Seattle VA Medical Center
Professor
Department of Medicine
University of Washington
Seattle, Washington

Suzanne Kamel-Reid, PhD, ABMG
Director
Molecular Diagnostics
University Health Network
Professor
Department of Laboratory Medicine and Pathobiology
University of Toronto
Toronto, Ontario

Steven J. Kussick, MD, PhD
Director of Flow Cytometry
PhenoPath Laboratories
Seattle, Washington

Douglas C. Tkachuk, MD, FRCPC
Staff Pathologist
University Health Network
Associate Professor
Department of Laboratory Medicine
  and Pathobiology
University of Toronto
Toronto, Ontario

Anemia

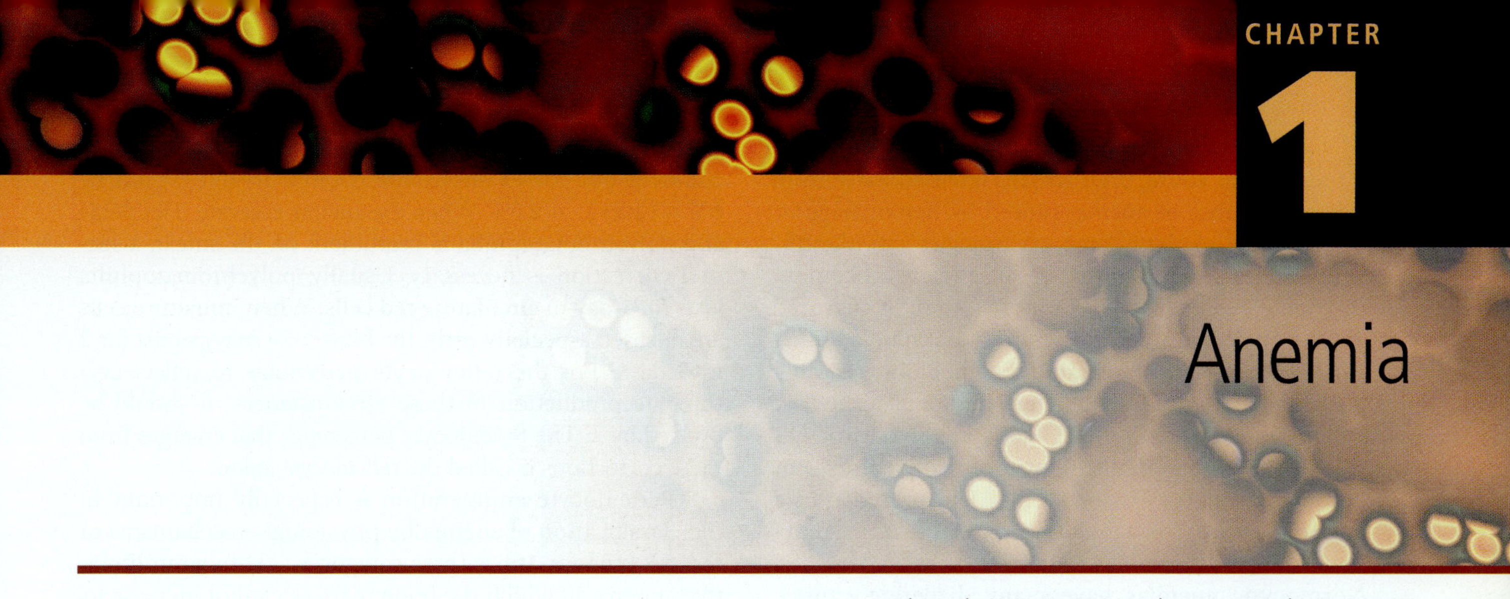

David Barth, MD, FRCPC, and Jan V. Hirschmann, MD

The World Health Organization (WHO) has defined anemia in adults as a hemoglobin of <13 g/dL in males (a hematocrit [Hct] of about 39) and <12 g/dL in females (Hct about 36). For African-Americans, the hemoglobin is about 0.5 g/dL less. Using these values, anemia is common in the elderly, primarily from the presence of more disease in this population, rather than as a phenomenon of normal aging.

Especially when mild and insidious in onset, anemia often causes no symptoms. When they occur, fatigue and listlessness are common. As the anemia worsens, dyspnea may occur because of the diminished oxygen supplied to the tissues or from high-output cardiac failure, which usually occurs only when the hematocrit drops below 20, unless the patient has underlying heart disease. In patients with coronary artery disease, angina may develop or worsen. When the anemia becomes severe, faintness, dizziness, and diminished concentration can occur from decreased oxygen delivery to the brain. Diminished tissue oxygenation may provoke the compensatory mechanisms of tachycardia and increased force of ventricular contraction, which patients sometimes detect as palpitations.

Physical examination may be unremarkable, but pallor is sometimes apparent in the conjunctiva, palms, and face. Systolic murmurs, usually in the pulmonic area, can develop, probably from a combination of decreased blood viscosity and increased flow across the valves. Retinal examination in severe anemia may reveal hemorrhages that are white-centered (Roth spots), flame-shaped, or round. Some may be pre-retinal. The retinal veins are sometimes tortuous, and cotton wool spots, representing infarction of the nerve fiber layer, may occur. Ischemia of the vessels can lead to leakage of proteinaceous material, causing "hard" exudates.

The classification systems for anemia emphasize either erythrocyte size or the mechanism that reduced the number of red cells. The morphologic scheme divides anemia into three groups, based on mean corpuscular volume (MCV): (1) normocytic (MCV 90–100); (2) macrocytic (MCV >100); and (3) microcytic (MCV <80). In some disorders, the red cells may vary considerably and can cause anemias of more than one category. In hypothyroidism, for example, the red cells may be normocytic or macrocytic. A valuable aspect of this classification is that the measurement of red cell size is immediately available from automated blood counts and that the differential diagnosis of microcytic and macrocytic anemias is small. The diseases causing normocytic, normochromic anemias, however, are more numerous and complex.

Microcytic anemias represent disordered hemoglobin synthesis from inadequate iron, abnormal globin formation, or deficiencies in heme and porphyrin synthesis that occur in some types of sideroblastic anemia, such as those due to lead poisoning and pyridoxine deficiency. The commonest cause of microcytic anemia is iron deficiency. The second most frequent type is the anemia of chronic disease, in which microcytosis occurs in about 30% of cases. One of the components of the pathophysiology of this disorder is reduced transfer of iron from the macrophages in bone marrow to the plasma. Abnormal globin formation causing microcytic anemia occurs in the thalassemias and some hemoglobinopathies, such as hemoglobin C and E.

Macrocytic anemias may occur from several mechanisms. One is abnormal DNA synthesis, most commonly produced by deficiencies of folic acid and vitamin B_{12}, causing abnormally large erythrocyte precursors (megaloblasts) in the bone marrow. Other etiologies are inherited disorders of DNA synthesis or medications that interfere with it. Macrocytic anemia also occurs frequently in the myelodysplastic syndromes because of altered erythrocyte maturation caused by a clonal expansion of abnormal hematopoietic stem cells. Macrocytosis, usually with an MCV of 100 to 110, but typically without anemia, is present in about 60% of alcoholics. The cause is not deficiency of folic acid or vitamin B_{12}, but a direct effect of ethanol itself on the bone marrow. Another source of macrocytosis is the presence of young erythrocytes released early from the marrow because of anemia caused by hemorrhage or hemolysis. Some of these large erythrocytes are identifiable on peripheral blood smears because they still contain nuclei (nucleated red cells). Others, although matured beyond the nucleated stage, possess residual blue-staining nuclear RNA, as well as red-staining hemoglobin, leading to a purplish color with the Romanowsky stains ordinarily used for peripheral blood films. These large erythrocytes are called polychromatophilic ("lover of many colors") or polychromatic ("many colors") cells. The presence of a few is common on normal smears, but numerous polychromatophilic cells can lead to macrocytosis.

Normocytic anemias have many disparate causes. With acute hemorrhage or hemolysis, the bone marrow responds maximally by increasing red cell production and releasing young erythrocytes prematurely. In the other forms of normocytic anemia, however, the bone marrow response is reduced because of intrinsic bone marrow disease, insufficient iron, or inadequate erythropoietin effect. Categories of intrinsic bone marrow disorders include: (1) diminished erythrocyte precursors, such as in aplastic anemia or following cancer chemotherapy; (2) infiltration of the marrow with abnormal tissue, such as with fibrosis or leukemia; and (3) myelodysplastic disorders, in which abnormal red cell maturation leads to erythrocyte death in the marrow. In iron deficiency a normocytic anemia typically occurs before further progression leads to a microcytic one. Inadequate erythropoietin effect can develop from: (1) impaired production in the kidney because of renal disease; (2) reduced stimulation, possibly the cause of anemia in some endocrine disorders, such as hypothyroidism and hypogonadism; or (3) interference with both production and its bone marrow effects, caused by the presence of inflammatory cytokines, which is part of the pathogenesis of the anemia of chronic disease. Other components include a diminished red cell life span and impaired iron utilization.

In assessing anemias, it is useful to know whether the bone marrow has responded with a robust increase in red cell production. One assessment is to get a marrow sample to detect hyperplasia of the red cell precursors. A simpler, indirect measure is to enumerate the immature red cells in the peripheral blood by finding those with residual ribosomal RNA. When mixed with certain dyes, such as new methylene blue, that stain RNA, such immature erythrocytes show at least two blue granules or a network of material (reticulum). These young red cells are, therefore, called *reticulocytes*. Automated counters use a chemical, such as acridine orange, which binds to RNA and fluoresces. The reticulocyte count is expressed as a total number per volume of blood or as a percentage of the red cells. When a percentage is used, it should be corrected for the severity of anemia by multiplying it by the patient's hemoglobin (or hematocrit) divided by the normal hemoglobin (hematocrit). With a hematocrit of 20 and a reticulocyte

count of 6%, for example, the corrected value would be 6% × (20/45) = 2.6%. When the anemia is severe (Hct ≤25) and polychromatophilia is prominent on the smear, a second correction is necessary. Usually, polychromatophilia lasts for 1 day in circulating red cells. When immature cells are released especially early, the blue color may persist for 2 to 3 days. For the reticulocyte percentage to reflect erythrocyte production in these circumstances, it should be divided by 2. The reticulocyte percentage that emerges from these corrections is called the *reticulocyte index*.

Reticulocyte enumeration is especially important in the classification of anemia by physiologic mechanisms or red cell kinetics. It has three categories: (1) hypoproliferative anemia, in which the bone marrow cannot increase its erythrocyte production; (2) maturation defects, in which bone marrow hyperplasia occurs, but many cells die in the marrow, a situation called *ineffective erythropoiesis*; and (3) acute hemorrhage or hemolysis, in which the red cell production increases and erythrocytes leave the marrow intact but die prematurely in the peripheral circulation.

Assigning an anemia to one of these categories utilizes the reticulocyte index and the results from a bone marrow sample. In the absence of anemia, the reticulocyte index is 1. With a moderately severe anemia (Hct <30) and a normal bone marrow, the reticulocyte index should exceed 3. This response typically occurs with hemolysis or acute hemorrhage. The reticulocyte index is less than 2 in hypoproliferative and maturation defect disorders. In a normal bone marrow sample, the ratio of erythroid to myeloid cells (E:M ratio) is about 1:3. With a moderately severe anemia, exuberant red cell production occurs and the E:M ratio should exceed 1:1. This kind of hyperplasia occurs with both maturation disorders and hemolysis. With the ineffective erythropoiesis of maturation defects, many red cells die within the bone marrow, whereas with hemolysis, the erythrocyte destruction is in the peripheral blood. In both cases, the serum lactate dehydrogenase (LDH) and indirect bilirubin levels may increase.

The reticulocyte index, the bone marrow findings, and these serum studies allow an accurate designation of the category of anemia. In hypoproliferative anemias, the erythrocytes are usually normocytic, the reticulocyte index is <2, the E:M ratio is <1:2, and the indirect bilirubin and LDH are normal. Early iron deficiency and the anemia of chronic disease are hypoproliferative disorders. Hypoproliferation also occurs when erythropoietin production (renal failure) or response (endocrine disorders) is diminished or when the bone marrow is damaged by injury to stem cells (e.g., cancer chemotherapy), by altered marrow structure (e.g., fibrosis), or by autoimmune or unknown mechanisms (e.g., pure red cell aplasia). Helping to distinguish among these possibilities is examining the blood smear for polychromatophilia, which is present in marrow damage and iron deficiency, but diminished in renal failure and the anemia of chronic disease.

In maturation defects, the reticulocyte index is <2, the E:M ratio is >1:1 with severe anemias, the serum LDH and indirect bilirubin are elevated (except in iron deficiency), and polychromasia is present. Examples of nuclear maturation defects, which cause macrocytosis, are vitamin B_{12} and folate deficiencies. Cytoplasmic maturation defects produce microcytic erythrocytes and include thalassemias, certain hemoglobinopathies, and some sideroblastic anemias.

In hemolysis, the reticulocyte index is >3, the E:M ratio is >1:1, serum LDH and indirect bilirubin are characteristically elevated, and polychromatophilia is prominent. In acute hemorrhage, the bone marrow takes 7 to 10 days to achieve a robust erythrocyte production. In the first few days, the anemia appears hypoproliferative. Later, the picture resembles ineffective erythropoiesis as bone marrow production increases, but the red cell precursors are not mature enough to leave the marrow. The reticulocyte index is <2; the E:M ratio is increased, yet still <1:1; and polychromatophilia is increased but not markedly. When the marrow finally achieves its maximal response, the findings are similar to those of hemolysis, with the reticulocyte index >3, the E:M ratio >1:1, and polychromasia prominent. Hemorrhage is distinguishable from hemolysis by the serum LDH and indirect bilirubin, which are normal because the red cells are not being destroyed, either in the bone marrow or in the peripheral blood.

For most clinicians, dividing anemia according to red cell size is the easiest approach, especially since the differential diagnosis of microcytic and macrocytic anemias is small. One use of the physiologic classification is in analyzing normocytic anemias, where the number of possibilities is large and that system of categorization provides a framework for distinguishing among them.

MICROCYTIC ANEMIA

The major diagnostic considerations in microcytic anemia are iron deficiency, anemia of chronic disease, and thalassemias. Less common causes include hemoglobinopathies and certain types of sideroblastic anemias. As discussed in the section on normocytic anemias, the anemia of chronic disease is microcytic in about 30% of cases, but usually with an MCV of 70 to 80 fl and unaccompanied by significant morphologic changes on peripheral smear. In iron deficiency, thalassemias, and hemoglobinopathies, the cell size is often smaller, and the blood film can disclose dramatic changes in red cell morphology.

Iron deficiency usually arises from chronic blood loss. The major cause in younger women is menstruation. In nonmenstruating women and in men, the most common source is gastrointestinal hemorrhage. Other less common reasons include hematuria, nosebleeds, hemoptysis, or intrapulmonary hemorrhage from such disorders as idiopathic pulmonary hemosiderosis, microscopic polyangiitis, or Goodpasture syndrome. A rare cause is intravascular hemolysis from such diseases as paroxysmal nocturnal hemoglobinuria or mechanical fragmentation of erythrocytes from prosthetic heart valves, in which destruction of red cells leads to excretion of iron in the urine in the form of ferritin, hemosiderin, or hemoglobin.

Iron deficiency occasionally develops from inadequate dietary intake or iron malabsorption. Little absorbable iron is present in the majority of foods, including most fruits and vegetables. Good sources are meat, poultry, fish, beans, and peas. Because daily iron loss is slight in adult males, primarily small amounts in the alimentary canal, they need little dietary iron, and deficiency from inadequate dietary intake is uncommon. When iron utilization is increased in infancy and during growth, or when concurrent blood loss occurs, as in menstruation, dietary intake may be insufficient, especially because women and children tend to consume less than the recommended minimal daily requirement. The problem increases during pregnancy, when some iron is diverted to the fetus for hematopoiesis, and with breast feeding, when iron is lost in the milk. Iron is absorbed throughout the gastrointestinal tract, but especially in the duodenum. With small intestinal disease, such as celiac sprue, or with gastric resection, which may accelerate the movement of intestinal materials through the duodenum and thereby diminish absorption time, iron deficiency may develop.

The clinical features of iron deficiency are generally similar to other anemias, but three uncommon but distinctive findings are pica, koilonychia, and blue sclera. Pica is the craving for, and ingestion of, certain unusual substances, such as starch, dirt, cardboard, and ice (pagophagia). Pagophagia is especially suggestive of iron deficiency. Virtually pathognomonic of iron deficiency is koilonychia, in which the fingernails become thin, brittle, and concave (spoon-shaped) in the distal half. Thinning of the sclera from impaired epithelial growth causes a blue tint because of the more visible choroid beneath.

With mild and recent iron deficiency, the red cell indices (MCV, mean corpuscular hemoglobin [MCH], mean corpuscular hemoglobin concentration [MCHC]) and the blood film are normal, but with time and increasingly severe anemia, the MCV and MCHC diminish. An early change in the erythrocytes is anisocytosis, indicated on automated counters by an increase in red cell distribution width (RDW). Later morphologic changes include poikilocytosis, microcytosis, and hypochromia. Tiny microcytes, elongated pale elliptical red cells (pencil cells), and target cells may be visible, but many of the erythrocytes may appear normal. Often, thrombocytosis is apparent. In iron deficiency anemia, the serum iron is decreased, the total iron binding capacity is elevated, and the saturation is <20%. The serum ferritin is decreased. Usually, the diagnosis is established by these tests, but occasionally obtaining a bone marrow sample for iron staining or a trial of iron therapy may be necessary to confirm the presence of iron deficiency (see Microcytic Anemia Tables and Diagrams).

HEMOLYTIC ANEMIAS

In hemolytic anemias, red cell destruction significantly shortens the normal life span of the erythrocyte in the peripheral circulation, which is about 120 days. Classifications of hemolytic anemia emphasize either the site of destruction—intravascular versus extravascular—or the site of the abnormality provoking it—as intrinsic or extrinsic to the red cell. In intravascular hemolysis, the red cells are destroyed within the bloodstream, whereas extravascular hemolysis indicates destruction within macrophages present in organs, such as the spleen, liver, or bone marrow.

Intravascular hemolysis is typically severe and arises from several mechanisms. One is mechanical damage to the red cell caused by: (1) fibrin present in the vessel lumen from such diseases as disseminated intravascular coagulation or vasculitis; (2) physical trauma from red cells passing through prosthetic valves or small vessels of the feet during hard marching; (3) thermal injury from burns. Intravascular hemolysis may also occur from infections, such as malaria, or from toxins, such as venom from some poisonous snakes. A third type is complement-mediated damage to erythrocytes caused by cold agglutinins, incompatible red cell transfusions, and paroxysmal nocturnal hemoglobinuria. Initially, the hemoglobin released into the circulation during intravascular hemolysis binds to haptoglobin, reducing its serum level. When the hemoglobin exceeds the binding capacity of haptoglobin, it makes the plasma appear pink. Free hemoglobin is filtered in the kidneys, and the urine may appear red. The dipstick testing for blood is positive, but the urine microscopy is negative for increased red cells. The renal tubular epithelium cells take up some of the hemoglobin, transforming it into hemosiderin, which is visible within these cells on iron stains of the urinary sediment. Evidence of recent or ongoing intravascular hemolysis, thus, includes a reduced serum haptoglobin level (which also occurs in extravascular hemolysis), the presence of plasma or urine hemoglobin, and detection of hemosiderin in renal tubular cells in the urinary sediment.

In most cases of hemolytic anemia, the red cell destruction is extravascular. The differential diagnosis includes: (1) an abnormal environment in the circulation because of infections, medications, or immunologic processes; (2) erythrocyte membrane abnormalities; (3) red cell metabolic defects; and (4) abnormalities in hemoglobin structure.

The other major classification system for hemolytic anemias differentiates disorders intrinsic to the red cell, which are typically hereditary, and those extrinsic to the red cell, usually acquired diseases. The intrinsic disorders include: (1) abnormal hemoglobins; (2) enzyme defects; (3) membrane abnormalities. The extrinsic disorders

are: (1) immunologic; (2) mechanical factors; (3) infections and toxins; (4) liver disease (spur cell anemia); and (5) hypersplenism.

Abnormalities in red cell morphology may be apparent on peripheral smear, such as sickle cells, bite cells, schistocytes, and spherocytes. Other findings may include red cell agglutination from the presence of increased Igm, organisms such as malarial parasites, and ingestion of erythrocytes by macrophages (erythrophagocytosis), which especially suggests immune hemolytic anemias, but also can occur with infections or toxins. The peripheral smear in hemolytic anemia should reveal substantial polychromatophilia caused by the increased release of immature red cells from the bone marrow. The reticulocyte index is >3 and the absolute reticulocyte count is >100,000/mm^3. The indirect bilirubin is elevated and represents >80% of the total bilirubin. The serum LDH may be increased and the serum haptoglobin diminished. With suspected intravascular hemolysis, helpful tests include urine and plasma hemoglobin measurements, as well as iron stains of urinary sediment. With extravascular hemolysis, Coombs tests detect immunoglobulin and complement on the red cell surface, indicating an immune hemolysis. A hemoglobin electrophoresis is indicated for suspected hemoglobinopathies.

HEMOGLOBINOPATHIES AND THALASSEMIAS

Hemoglobin A (HbA), which constitutes more than 90% of the adult hemoglobin, consists of four polypeptide chains, two α and two β ($\alpha_2 \beta_2$). Hemoglobin A_2, composed of two α and two δ ($\alpha_2\delta_2$), is present in small quantities. Hemoglobin F ($\alpha_2\gamma_2$) constitutes <1% of the normal adult's hemoglobin, but is the main hemoglobin during fetal life. As β-chain production begins just before birth, the level of HbF decreases and represents about 75% of the hemoglobin at delivery. By 6 months of age, it has diminished to 5%. The thalassemias are inherited disorders with reduced or absent synthesis of one or more globin chains. Two major consequences occur: reduced production of functioning hemoglobin, leading to hypochromic, microcytic erythrocytes; and continued production of the unaffected chains, which have decreased solubility or diminished oxygen-carrying capacity that causes damage to the red cell or its precursors, leading to ineffective erythropoiesis and hemolytic anemia. The thalassemias are labeled according to the chain with impaired production. With β-thalassemia, β-chains are absent or diminished; with α-thalassemia, α-chains are affected. These are the two most important thalassemias, although others exist.

The β-thalassemias are common in the Mediterranean area (thalassemia in Greek means "sea in the blood"), India, Southeast Asia, and the Middle East. The clinical spectrum includes severe (thalassemia major), moderate (thalassemia intermedia), and mild (thalassemia minor) cases.

β-Thalassemia major, or homozygous disease, is caused by the inheritance of two β-thalassemia alleles, resulting in little or no β-chain production although α-chain synthesis remains normal. Because of diminished HbA synthesis, anemia is severe, and the red cells produced contain diminished hemoglobin, making them very hypochromic. The accumulation of free α-chains leads to their deposition in red cell precursors, causing erythrocyte destruction in the bone marrow (ineffective erythropoiesis). Red cells containing these precipitates that do reach the peripheral blood are prematurely destroyed by macrophages in the liver, spleen, and bone marrow. Because HbF is present in substantial quantities at birth, anemia emerges only when γ-chain synthesis diminishes. Adequately transfused children grow and thrive until iron overload problems begin to develop. In untreated or insufficiently transfused patients, growth is subnormal. Increased erythropoiesis in response to the anemia leads to expanded marrow cavities that can eventuate in long-bone fractures and expansion of skull and maxillary areas, causing abnormal contours of the face and head. Increased erythrocyte destruction in the spleen causes splenomegaly, which can lead to hypersplenism with thrombocytopenia and leukopenia. On blood smear, the erythrocytes demonstrate anisocytosis and poikilocytosis, with elliptocytes, teardrop cells, and other bizarrely shaped red cells. Hypochromia is pronounced, and microcytosis is apparent, although the cells are flat and they spread out on drying, giving them a diameter larger than expected, based on the MCV. Target cells and nucleated red cells are typically numerous, and basophilic stippling is common. Red cell inclusions, representing excess α-chains, may be apparent. Findings on bone marrow examination include erythroid hyperplasia, basophilic stippling, and diminished hemoglobin in the red cell precursors, which also show inclusions. Iron content is increased.

Thalassemia intermedia is usually the result of the inheritance of two β-thalassemia mutations: both mild or one mild, one severe. The anemia is typically moderately severe, but transfusions may not always be necessary. The blood smear is similar to that of thalassemia major.

Thalassemia minor occurs from the inheritance of a single β-thalassemia mutation and a normal β-globin gene on the other chromosome. No clinical problems emerge, and anemia is mild or absent. The smear, however, is abnormal, with microcytic, hypochromic red cells. The MCV is 50 to 70 fl. Poikilocytosis, target cells, and basophilic stippling are typically present. Hemoglobin electrophoresis demonstrates HbA_2 that is about twice normal and an HbA_2:HbA ratio of 1:20, rather than the normal 1:40. HbF is increased in many patients.

Production of α-globin chains is regulated by four gene loci. Four α-thalassemia types occur, depending on how many gene foci are affected. No hematologic abnormalities develop with α-thalassemia-2, in which one focus fails to function. In α-thalassemia-1, two foci are affected, and the condition is mild, with slight or absent anemia. The blood smear shows microcytosis, hypochromia, and slight anisocytosis and poikilocytosis.

When three gene foci are defective, α-chain synthesis is substantially decreased, and excess β-chains form tetramers called HbH, which are soluble and do not precipitate in the marrow to cause damage of erythrocyte precursors. They are present in the circulating red cells, but precipitate as they age, forming inclusion bodies. The spleen, which enlarges in this disorder, prematurely destroys these cells, causing hemolytic anemia. This disease most commonly occurs in Asians, and the anemia is usually moderate, with hematocrits of 20 to 30. The blood smear shows substantial hypochromia, microcytosis, basophilic stippling, and polychromasia. Abnormal erythrocytes apparent on blood smear include target cells, teardrop cells, and nucleated and fragmented cells. Heinz-body preparations disclose precipitated HbH, visible as multiple small erythrocyte inclusions. On hemoglobin electrophoresis, about 3% to 30% of the total is HbH.

When four genes are defective, α-chains are absent, and tetramers of γ-chains called Hb Bart, form in the fetus. This hemoglobin oxygenates poorly, producing tissue hypoxia, and they are unstable, resulting in hemolysis and anemia. The fetus develops heart and liver failure, resulting in massive edema (hydrops fetalis) and intrauterine death. The disease almost always occurs in Southeast Asians.

NORMOCYTIC ANEMIAS

Many of the causes of normocytic anemia, such as hemolysis, iron deficiency, leukemia, and myelodysplastic syndromes, are discussed and illustrated in other sections. The main causes considered here are pure red cell aplasia, aplastic anemia, the anemias caused by renal disease and endocrine disorders, and the anemia of chronic disease.

Pure Red Cell Aplasia

In this disorder, a normocytic anemia occurs with diminished reticulocytes (<1%), absence of polychromasia on the peripheral blood smear, and almost no erythroblasts in the bone marrow (<0.5% of the marrow differential count), despite normal megakaryocytes and white cell precursors. It may develop without apparent cause or be associated with a wide variety of systemic diseases. It occurs in about 5% of patients with thymoma, and this tumor accounts for approximately 10% of cases of pure red cell aplasia. Hematologic malignancies, especially chronic lymphocytic and large granular lymphocytic leukemias, have been associated, as have some solid tumors, rheumatic diseases (such as Sjögren syndrome and systemic lupus erythematosus [SLE]), and infections, primarily parvovirus B19. Numerous medications have been implicated, including phenytoin, azathioprine, and isoniazid. Sometimes, pure red cell aplasia occurs during pregnancy without any apparent explanation and typically disappears following delivery. In many patients, no cause is found. Often, in these cases, an IgG that inhibits erythropoiesis is present in the serum.

Aplastic Anemia

In aplastic anemia, a reduction in red cells occurs in the setting of pancytopenia in the peripheral blood and hypocellularity of the bone marrow. Certain forms, such as Fanconi anemia, are hereditary, whereas some acquired types have identifiable causes, such as medications, benzene exposure, or infections with certain viruses. Transfusion-associated graft-versus-host disease consists of fever, pancytopenia, and a generalized morbilliform eruption a few days to weeks following receipt of blood products containing competent lymphocytes. Aplastic anemia may develop in patients with paroxysmal nocturnal hemoglobinuria or as a complication of certain rheumatic diseases, such as eosinophilic fasciitis, SLE, or Sjögren syndrome. In the hemophagocytic syndrome, most commonly associated with viral infections or certain malignancies, pancytopenia, fever, hepatosplenomegaly, and lymph node enlargement occur, and the bone marrow, often hypocellular, shows macrophages ingesting erythrocytes.

Despite the many causes identified, most cases of aplastic anemia are unexplained. Many probably originate from immunologic damage to the bone marrow. Whether a cause is identified or not, the usual presentation is anemia and/or bleeding because of thrombocytopenia; infections are uncommon initially.

Anemia of Chronic Renal Disease

Anemia typically occurs with chronic renal disease only after the creatinine clearance decreases below 40 mL/min, which corresponds to a serum creatinine of about 2.5 mg/mL. The anemia tends to worsen as the renal function decreases, but it usually stabilizes at a hematocrit of 15 to 30. The cause of the kidney disease is not usually important in determining the severity of anemia, but it is typically less severe with polycystic kidney disease. Several factors cause the decrease in red cells, the most important, however, being inadequate renal production of erythropoietin, a glycoprotein hormone synthesized in the kidney and responsible for the proliferation, maturation, and differentiation of erythrocytes in the bone marrow. In addition, the red cell survival is shortened in uremia, and various toxins ordinarily excreted by the kidney accumulate in the serum and appear to depress erythropoiesis. The processes involved in the anemia of chronic disease, discussed later in this section, may also contribute.

The anemia is normochromic, normocytic, and most red cells are unremarkable on the peripheral smear. Burr cells (echinocytes), however, may form via unknown mechanisms, and sometimes schistocytes appear.

Anemia of Endocrine Disorders

Anemia, usually normocytic, occurs in several endocrine disorders. About 30% of patients with hypothyroidism have anemia, and about one-third of these are macrocytic. The anemia, usually mild, seems to be from the hormone deficiency itself, and its severity is related to the duration and degree of the hypothyroidism. Approximately 10% to 25% of patients with hyperthyroidism, usually with severe, prolonged disease, are anemic. The mechanism is uncertain.

Most patients with adrenal insufficiency have anemia, usually normocytic, normochromic. In those with autoimmune causes, pernicious anemia, producing a macrocytic anemia, is present in about 10%. Androgen deficiency also is a cause of normochromic, normocytic anemia. Hypopituitarism causes anemia through deficiencies of the previously mentioned thyroid, adrenal, and androgenic hormones.

A small number of patients with hyperparathyroidism have a normocytic, normochromic anemia, with bone marrow examinations typically demonstrating fibrosis. The increased parathyroid hormone may also decrease erythropoiesis.

Anemia of Chronic Disease

Anemia of chronic disease is quite common among certain illnesses lasting longer than 1 to 2 months, especially those with infection, noninfectious inflammation, or malignancy. In about 25% of cases, however, the only chronic diseases present in the patient, such as congestive heart failure or diabetes mellitus, have none of these features. Usually, the anemia is mild to moderate, with a hematocrit of >25 but, in about 20% of patients, it is more severe. Although the red cells are typically normocytic, normochromic, in about 30% they are microcytic (usually 70–79 fl), and in about 50% they are hypochromic (MCHC 26–32). The red cells on peripheral smear may display mild poikilocytosis and anisocytosis, but markedly small and thin cells, often seen in iron deficiency, are absent.

As in iron deficiency, the serum iron is reduced, but so is the iron-binding capacity, which is typically elevated in iron deficiency. As in iron deficiency, the saturation may be <10%. The serum ferritin, which is characteristically <15 µg/L in iron deficiency, is at least 30 µg/L and usually much higher in anemia of chronic disease. When the two disorders coexist in an individual patient, the serum ferritin is usually <30 µg/L. In ambiguous circumstances, definitive evidence to determine whether the patient has iron deficiency, anemia of chronic disease, or both simultaneously requires bone marrow samples stained for iron. A trial of oral iron therapy is an alternative; supplemental iron has no effect on a pure case of the anemia of chronic disease.

The main pathogenesis of the anemia of chronic disease appears to be the effects of cytokines on erythropoiesis. They impair the proliferation and differentiation of erythroid precursors, diminish erythropoietin production, and decrease the bone marrow response to erythropoietin. They also affect iron metabolism by increasing the retention of it in the bone marrow stores and by decreasing its availability for erythroid precursors. An additional contribution to the anemia is a mild to moderate decrease in erythrocyte lifespan.

MACROCYTIC ANEMIAS

The differential diagnosis of macrocytic anemias is primarily between those whose cause is impaired DNA synthesis in the bone marrow, leading to megaloblastic changes in the red cell precursors, and those whose macrocytosis originates from other mechanisms. Among the latter are alcoholism, liver disease, hypothyroidism, and hemolysis or hemorrhage that causes the release of immature, enlarged red cells. In general, the macrocytosis in these disorders is mild (MCV 100–110 fl) and the enlarged red cells are round, rather than oval, as occurs with megaloblastic anemias. Many of the immature red cells released by the bone marrow in response to hemolysis or hemorrhage are easily recognizable by being polychromatic. Hypersegmented neutrophils, a feature of megaloblastic anemias, are not present in the nonmegaloblastic macrocytic anemias, except with myelodysplastic disorders.

The megaloblastic anemias arise from deficiencies in folic acid or vitamin B_{12} or from medications that impair DNA synthesis, such as cytotoxic agents used in cancer chemotherapy or immunosuppression (e.g., cyclophosphamide, azathioprine, hydroxyurea) and drugs that interfere with folic acid metabolism (e.g., methotrexate, trimethoprim). The result is defective nuclear maturation of hematopoietic cells in the bone marrow, in which nuclear division diminishes, but cytoplasmic growth, regulated by RNA, continues unabated. As a consequence, an erythrocytic megaloblast forms—a large cell with greater cytoplasm than normal and a relatively immature nucleus having a decreased condensation of the chromatin, leading to a lacy pattern. The discrepancy between maturation of the nucleus and cytoplasm is called *nuclear–cytoplasmic asynchrony*. Granulocyte precursors are enlarged as well, especially the metamyelocytes and bands, which are two to three times normal in size and have poorly condensed chromatin. Megakaryocytes are hypersegmented and also have lacy chromatin. The bone marrow is hypercellular, but many erythrocytes are destroyed there rather than reaching the systemic circulation, a process known as *ineffective erythropoiesis*. This intramedullary hemolysis causes increased levels of serum iron, unconjugated bilirubin, and LDH.

Early in the course of disease, the only finding in the peripheral blood may be mild macrocytosis (usually >110 fl). As anemia emerges, other abnormalities become apparent on the peripheral blood smear, including anisocytosis, poikilocytosis, teardrop cells, schistocytes, and basophilic stippling. Polychromasia is sparse, and the reticulocyte count is inappropriately low. Leukopenia and thrombocytopenia may occur. The presence of oval-shaped macrocytes and hypersegmented neutrophils (>5% of cells with five lobes or any with six or more lobes) strongly suggests a megaloblastic process.

Vitamin B_{12} is cyanocobalamin, one of a group of molecules called *cobalamins* that contain a central cobalt atom and are important in DNA synthesis. Cyanocobalamin is not found in the human body, but the term *vitamin B_{12}* often is used to apply to all cobalamins, which microbes in the soil, water, or intestinal tract synthesize. They are not found in plants, unless contaminated by microbes, and the main human source is meat, poultry, seafood, and dairy products. The recommended daily allowance of cobalamins is 5 µg, and the total body content is about 2 to 5 mg, about 1 mg being present in the liver. Because the daily losses are minute, cobalamin deficiency from diet alone takes years and occurs almost exclusively in strict vegetarians. In adults, the main cause of vitamin B_{12} deficiency is impaired absorption. Cobalamin binds to a substance in the gastric juice called R protein (haptocorrin) and is released by pancreatic enzymes when it reaches the second portion of duodenum. It then binds to *intrinsic factor*, a glycoprotein produced by the parietal cells in the fundus and cardia of the stomach. Intrinsic factor receptors are present on the ileal mucosa, especially in its terminal area, where cobalamin absorption occurs.

Disorders of the ileum, such as Crohn disease or lymphoma, can cause cobalamin deficiency because of malabsorption. Malabsorption of cobalamin also can occur with pancreatic insufficiency, when inadequate pancreatic enzymes are present to release cobalamin from the R proteins. Another cause of cobalamin deficiency is its consumption in the small intestine by a fish tapeworm, *Diphyllobothrium latum*, found mostly in fish from Canada, Alaska, and the Baltic Sea and acquired by eating undercooked fish or fish roe. Excessive intestinal bacteria in diseases associated with impaired motility or intestinal stasis, such as systemic sclerosis, extensive diverticula, or surgical blind loops, also can consume enough cobalamin to cause disease.

A major cause of cobalamin deficiency is from reduced intrinsic factor because of elimination of parietal cells from gastric resection or from chronic inflammation due to autoimmune mechanisms that lead to mucosal atrophy in the stomach's fundus and body. The latter disorder, pernicious anemia, occurs primarily in older adults, often with a family history of the disease; northern European descent; or concurrent autoimmune disorders, such as Graves disease, vitiligo, or Hashimoto thyroiditis. About 90% of patients have antibodies to parietal cells, compared with 5% in the general population, and approximately 60% have antibodies to intrinsic factor, which is rare in healthy people.

The clinical features of cobalamin deficiency include those from the anemia, but also gastrointestinal complaints, such as diarrhea and weight loss, and episodes of glossitis, leading to erythema and soreness, and, eventually, to loss of papillae, causing a smooth surface. Most importantly, cobalamin deficiency impairs nerve myelination, leading to degeneration of white matter in the brain and in both the dorsal and lateral columns of the spinal cord (subacute combined degeneration). Dorsal column involvement causes diminished vibratory sensation, creating numbness and tingling in the feet and hands (stocking–glove distribution), and decreased proprioception, producing gait difficulties and a positive Romberg sign. Lateral column damage causes limb weakness, spasticity, hyperactive reflexes, and a positive Babinski sign. Evidence of cerebral involvement includes depression, dementia, confusion, delusions, and hallucinations.

Folic acid deficiency usually is caused by an inadequate diet. Rich sources are fruits, vegetables, and animal protein, but cooking easily destroys folate. Furthermore, the body stores of folate are small, and only a few months of poor intake, caused by food fads, ignorance, poverty, or alcoholism, are necessary before anemia develops. Alcohol intake compounds the problem by increasing urinary folate excretion, impeding liver storage, and decreasing absorption, which occurs primarily in the duodenum and jejunum. Disorders affecting these portions of the intestine, such as sprue, lymphoma, amyloidosis, and Crohn's disease, can cause folate malabsorption. Folic acid deficiency also can occur when the body's demand for it increases, as in pregnancy and conditions associated with increased cell turnover, such as acute exacerbations of hemolytic anemia, leukemia, and exfoliative dermatitis. Some medications, such as methotrexate and trimethoprim, cause folate deficiency by altering its metabolism.

The diagnosis of folate and vitamin B_{12} deficiencies may be confusing. With cobalamin deficiency, serum cobalamin levels are usually low, but many are normal. The serum folate level is very sensitive to folate intake, and a recent folate-rich meal can normalize it. Red cell folate measurements, which can better reflect tissue levels, have several problems and are not generally helpful. Nevertheless, ordering serum levels of folate and cobalamin is a reasonable approach to a megaloblastic anemia. An alternate, or complementary, tactic to diagnosing these deficiencies is to measure homocysteine, which increases in both disorders because methionine synthesis is impaired by deficiency of either, and this laboratory finding typically precedes decreases in serum levels of folate and cobalamin. A cobalamin-dependent, but folate-independent, enzymatic reaction leads to increased serum levels of methylmalonic acid (MMA) with cobalamin deficiency. This finding also tends to precede changes in serum cobalamin. Accordingly, measurement of both homocysteine and MMA can reliably detect, and distinguish between, folate and cobalamin deficiencies. When both are elevated, cobalamin deficiency is confirmed, although concurrent folate deficiency is possible. If homocysteine is elevated and MMA is normal, folate deficiency is likely. If both are normal, deficiency of either is highly improbable. If cobalamin deficiency is present, the presence of antibody against intrinsic factor confirms the diagnosis of pernicious anemia.

A Schilling test can help distinguish among the causes of cobalamin deficiency. In normal people, oral radioactive cobalamin is absorbed from the alimentary tract and much of the dose will be excreted in the urine within 24 hours. With pernicious anemia, the absorption and urinary excretion are both decreased, but will normalize if the patient receives intrinsic factor along with the cobalamin. With other forms of intestinal malabsorption, urinary excretion of cobalamin remains low despite intrinsic factor. With bacterial overgrowth, the Schilling test may normalize after a course of antibiotics, and with pancreatic insufficiency, it should become normal with ingestion of pancreatic enzymes.

Diagram 1.1

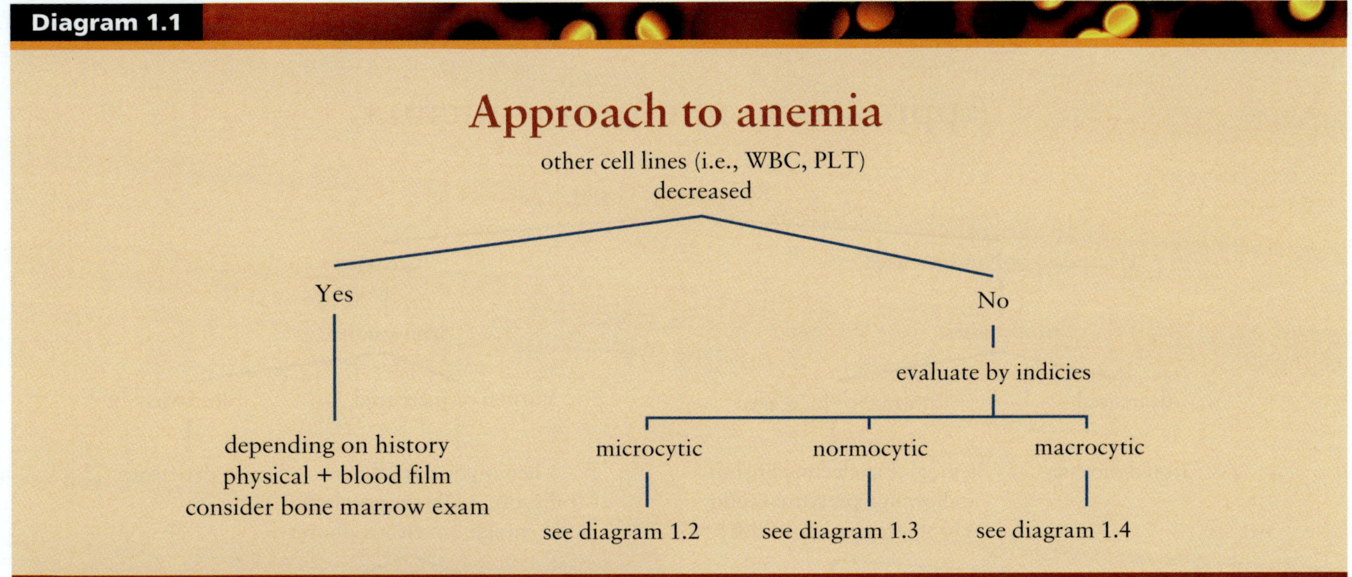

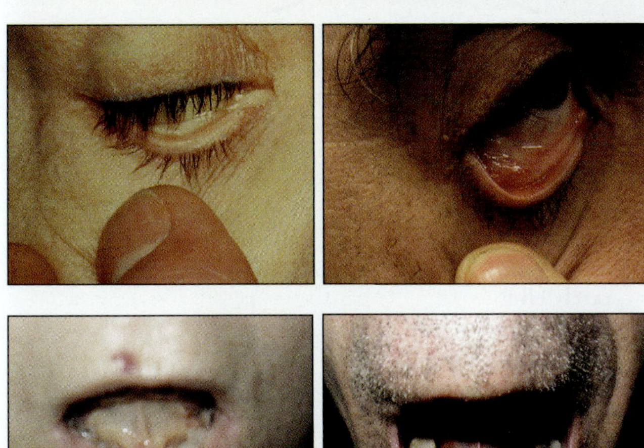

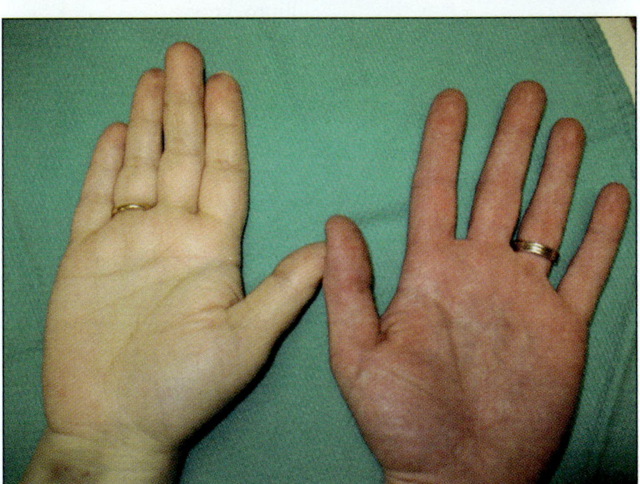

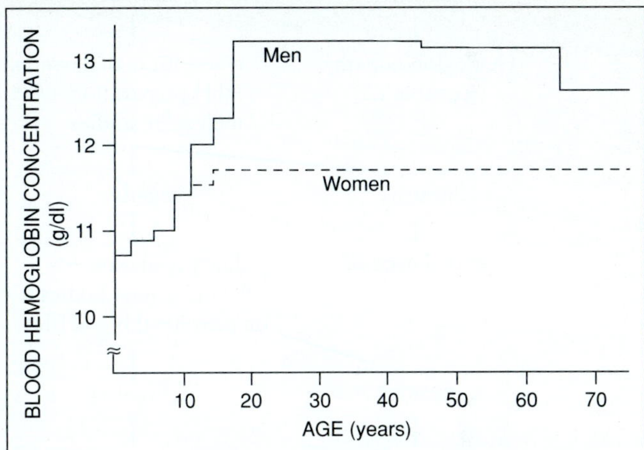

Figure 1.2 Curve of normal ranges of Hb in population studies. The lower limit of normal Hb concentration in men and women of various ages. Values were calculated from 11,547 subjects from the United States. (From Dallman PR, et al. *Am J Clin Nutr* 1984;39(4):437–445, with permission).

Figure 1.1 Pallor from anemia. *Top to bottom panels:* The conjunctiva, sublingual area, and hand on the left demonstrate pallor from anemia (hemoglobin of 5 g/dL) compared with the normal controls on the right.

Diagram 1.2

Approach to microcytic anemia

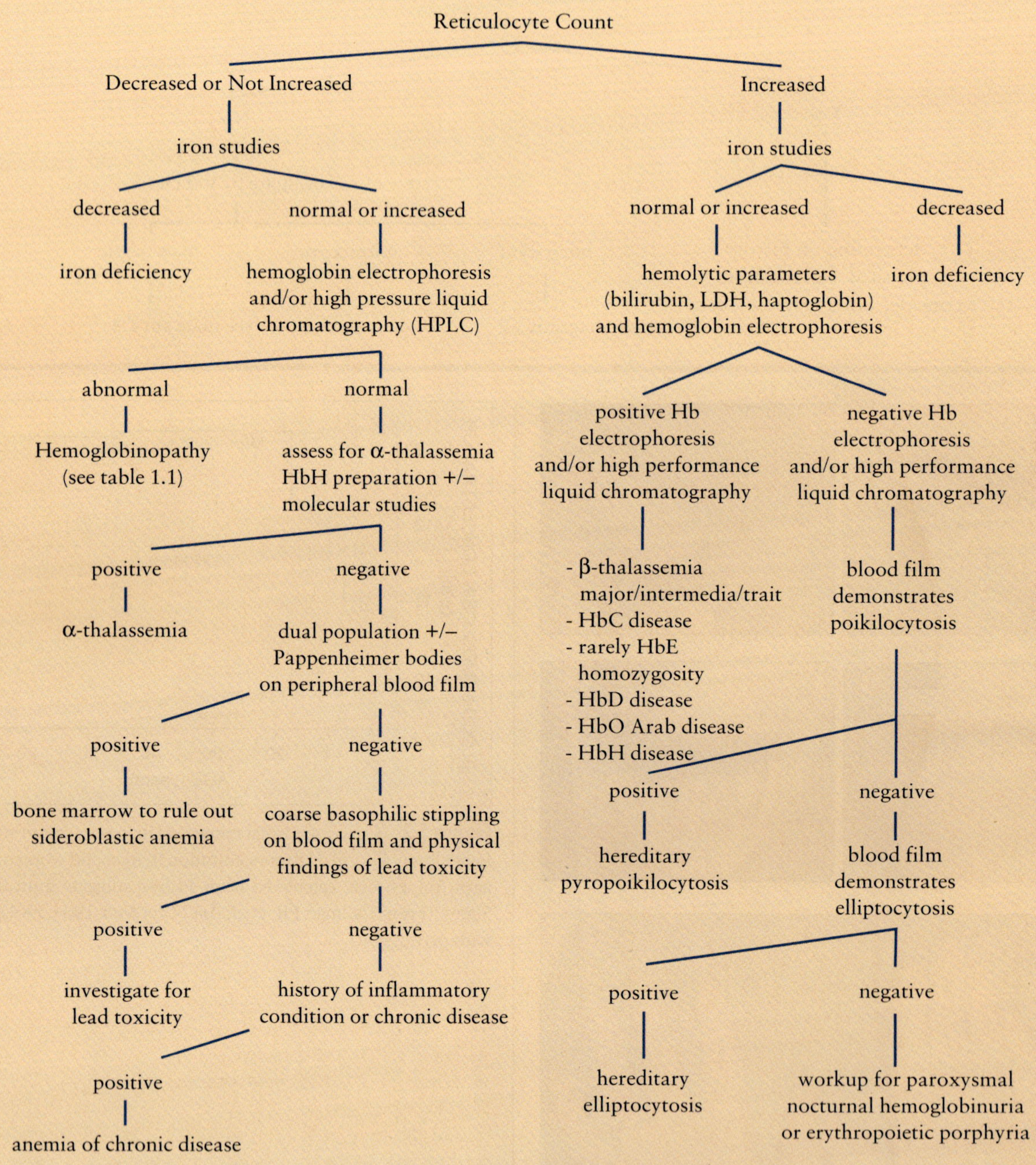

Reticulocyte Count

- **Decreased or Not Increased**
  - iron studies
    - **decreased**
      - iron deficiency
    - **normal or increased**
      - hemoglobin electrophoresis and/or high pressure liquid chromatography (HPLC)
        - **abnormal**
          - Hemoglobinopathy (see table 1.1)
            - **positive**
              - α-thalassemia
            - **negative**
        - **normal**
          - assess for α-thalassemia HbH preparation +/− molecular studies
            - **positive**
            - **negative**
              - dual population +/− Pappenheimer bodies on peripheral blood film
                - **positive**
                  - bone marrow to rule out sideroblastic anemia
                    - **positive**
                      - investigate for lead toxicity
                    - **negative**
                - **negative**
                  - coarse basophilic stippling on blood film and physical findings of lead toxicity
                    - **negative**
                      - history of inflammatory condition or chronic disease
                        - **positive**
                          - anemia of chronic disease

- **Increased**
  - iron studies
    - **normal or increased**
      - hemolytic parameters (bilirubin, LDH, haptoglobin) and hemoglobin electrophoresis
        - **positive Hb electrophoresis and/or high performance liquid chromatography**
          - β-thalassemia major/intermedia/trait
          - HbC disease
          - rarely HbE homozygosity
          - HbD disease
          - HbO Arab disease
          - HbH disease
            - **positive**
              - hereditary pyropoikilocytosis
        - **negative Hb electrophoresis and/or high performance liquid chromatography**
          - blood film demonstrates poikilocytosis
            - **negative**
              - blood film demonstrates elliptocytosis
                - **positive**
                  - hereditary elliptocytosis
                - **negative**
                  - workup for paroxysmal nocturnal hemoglobinuria or erythropoietic porphyria
    - **decreased**
      - iron deficiency

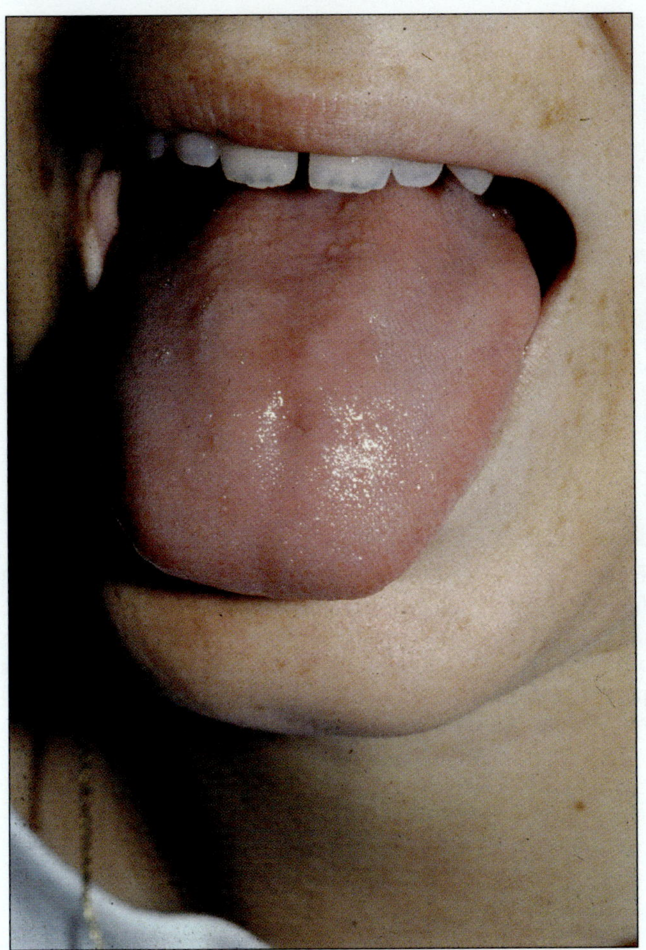

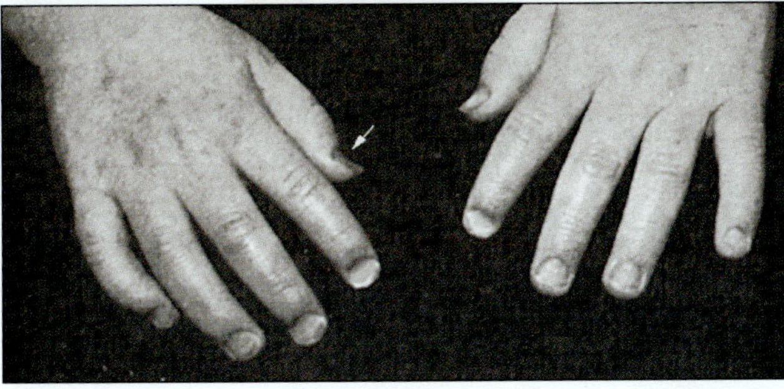

Figure 1.3   Smooth tongue and koilonychia in iron deficiency. *Top panel*: Iron deficiency can result in a painless, smooth, shiny, and reddened tongue (courtesy Dr. P. Galbraith). *Bottom panel*: Koilonychia, a condition also referred to as "spoon-shaped nails," is associated with iron deficiency in which the fingernails are thin, brittle, and concave with raised edges.

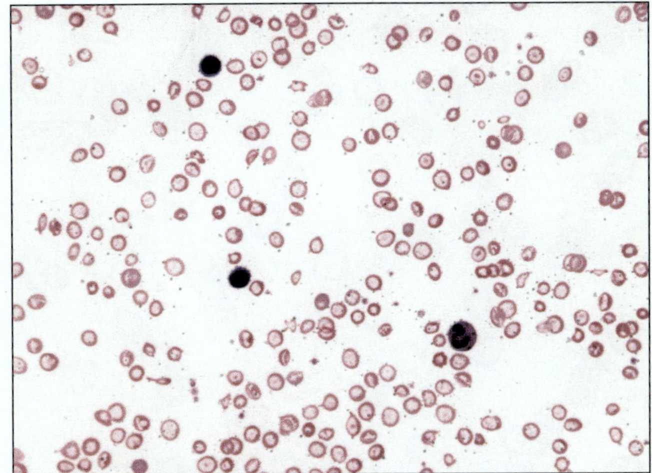

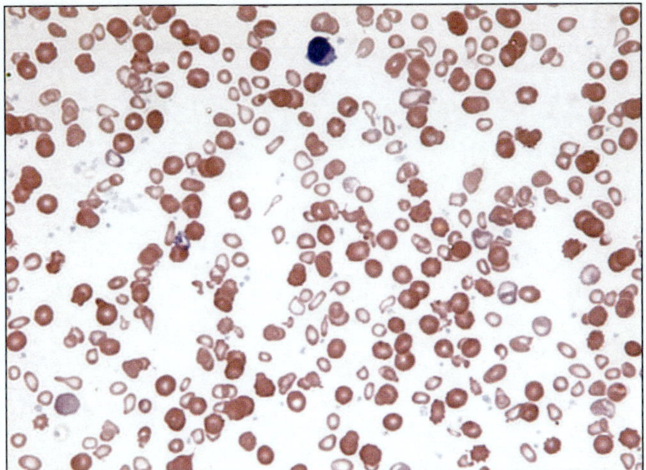

Figure 1.4   Iron deficiency blood films. *Top panel:* This peripheral blood film demonstrates severe iron deficiency with microcytosis, hypochromasia, and multiple morphologic changes: pencil cells, target cells, teardrops, and rare fragments. Early iron deficiency may be normocytic with no significant morphologic changes. Once the hemoglobin drops below 10–11 g/dL, red blood cell changes appear. Thrombocytosis may occur, but thrombocytopenia occasionally develops in severe iron deficiency. The morphologic changes in iron deficiency may be indistinguishable from α- or β-thalassemia trait, and iron studies, hemoglobin electrophoresis, and α-thalassemia testing may be required to differentiate these processes accurately. Red blood cell indices may be helpful: a mild, moderate, or severe decrease in hemoglobin, low MCV/MCH, and high RDW suggest iron deficiency. *Bottom panel:* Peripheral blood film of dual population in transfused iron deficiency. Most of the erythrocytes are hypochromic microcytic cells, (native iron deficient cells) with a minority of interspersed normocytic red blood cells (transfused red blood cells). This combination occurs in partially treated iron deficiency. It differs from sideroblastic anemia with a dual population in which most red cells are normochromic and the minority hypochromic.

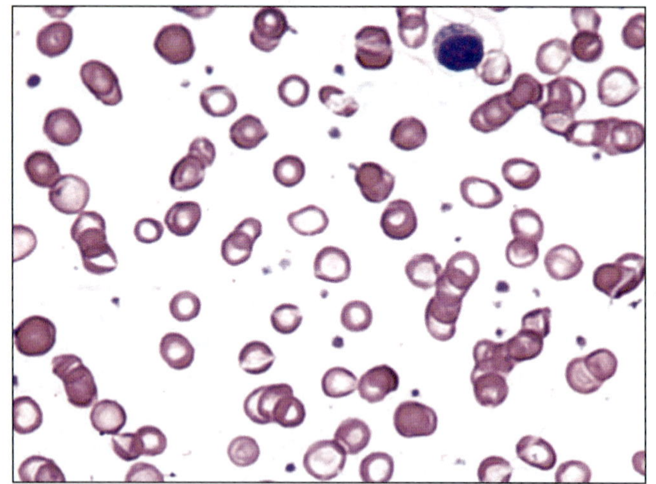

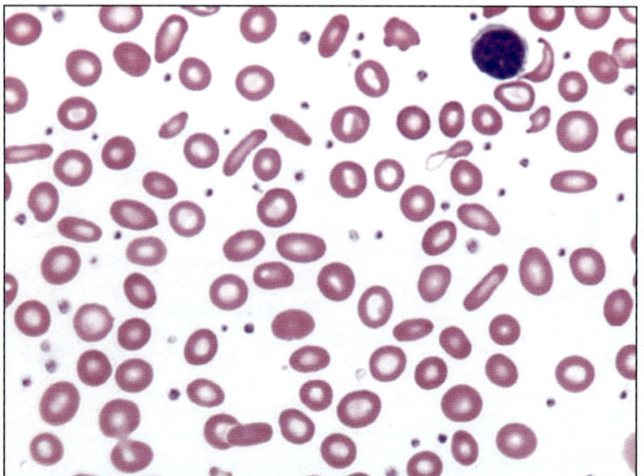

Figure 1.5 Iron deficiency blood films. *Top panel:* Microcytic blood film. This peripheral blood film demonstrates microcytosis. Red blood cell size can be visually estimated by comparing with the size of a small mature lymphocyte nucleus. Microcytic red blood cells should be smaller than the condensed nucleus of a mature lymphocyte. *Bottom panel:* Poikilocytosis and microcytosis that include numerous pencil cells are shown in this iron deficiency blood film. The degree of poikilocytosis has been observed to correlate with the degree of iron deficiency anemia.

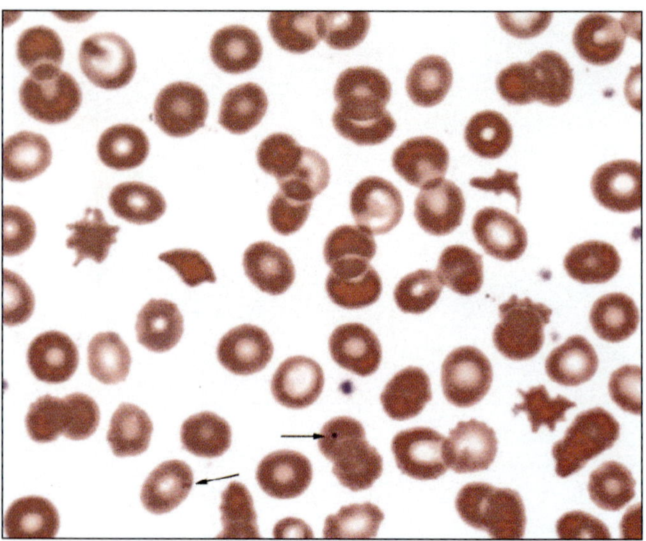

Figure 1.6 Iron deficiency and malabsorption. Peripheral blood film demonstrating hyposplenic changes in a patient with celiac disease causing iron deficiency due to malabsorption. Target cells, acanthocytes, and Howell-Jolly bodies (*arrows*) are seen. This patient has not had splenectomy, but this disease is a cause of functional hyposplenism.

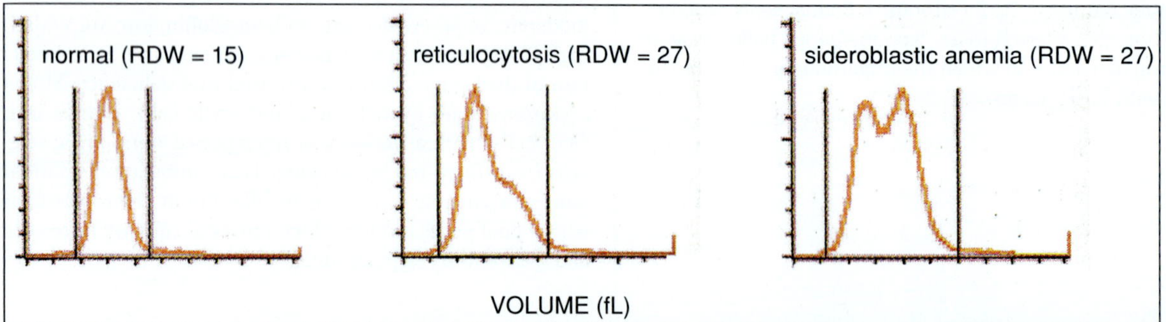

Figure 1.7 Automated hemocytometer report. Red blood cell volume curves demonstrating, from left to right: normal, unimodal RBC population; a small macrocytic population from a reactive increase in reticulocytes following therapy in iron deficiency; and a dual population of red blood cells in sideroblastic anemia.

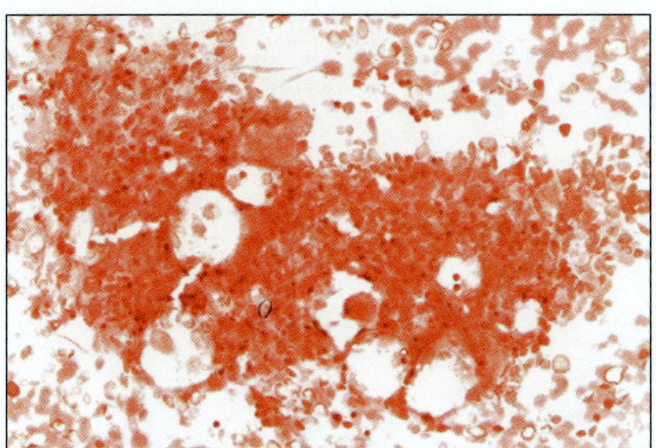

Figure 1.8 Bone marrow iron stores. Bone marrow aspirate stained with Prussian blue that shows absent iron stores with no visible blue staining, consistent with iron deficiency. Absence of bone marrow iron is one of the earliest findings in iron deficiency.

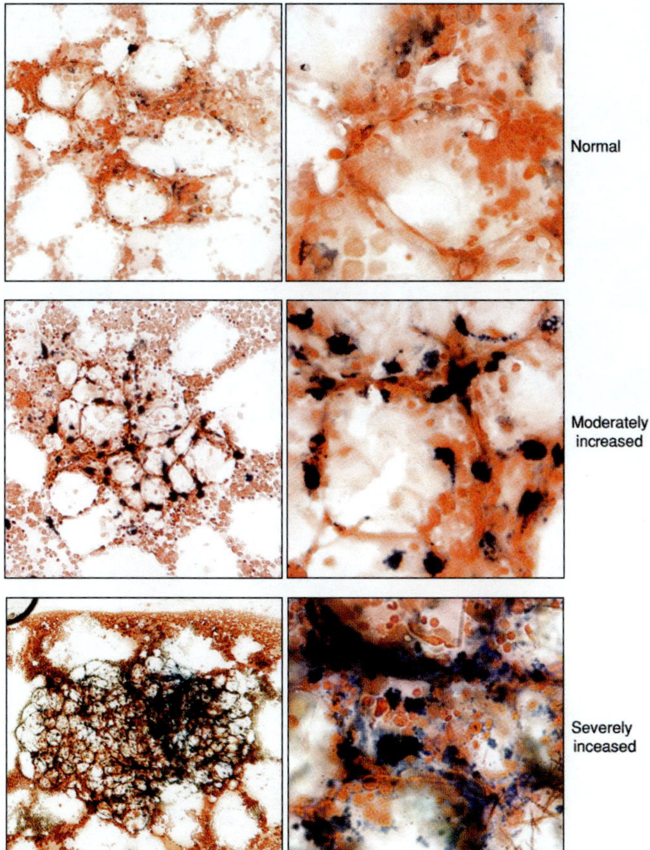

Figure 1.9 Bone marrow iron stores. Low and higher magnification views (*left* and *right*, respectively) of bone marrow aspirate smears stained with Prussian blue showing varying degrees of iron staining in histiocytes.

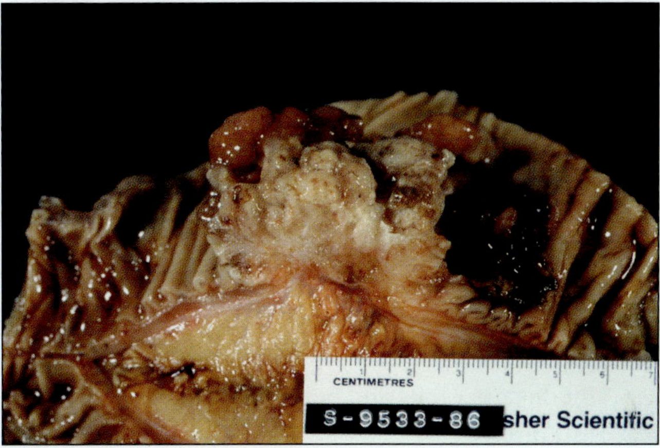

Figure 1.10 Iron deficiency from adenocarcinoma of the large bowel. A large polypoid adenocarcinoma is shown that is penetrating through the wall of the large intestine. Patients with bowel tumors often present with signs and symptoms of iron-deficiency anemia related to chronic blood loss.

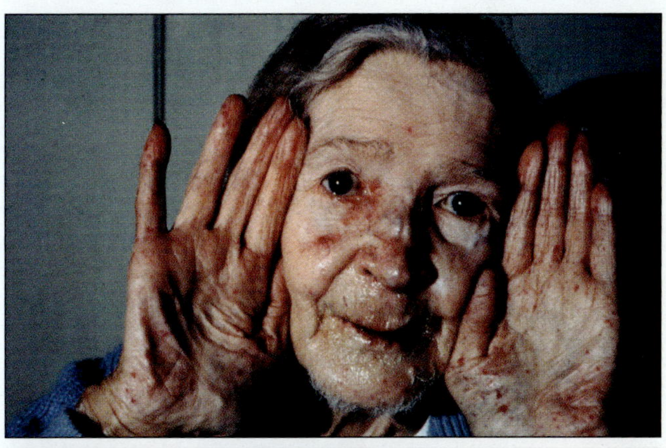

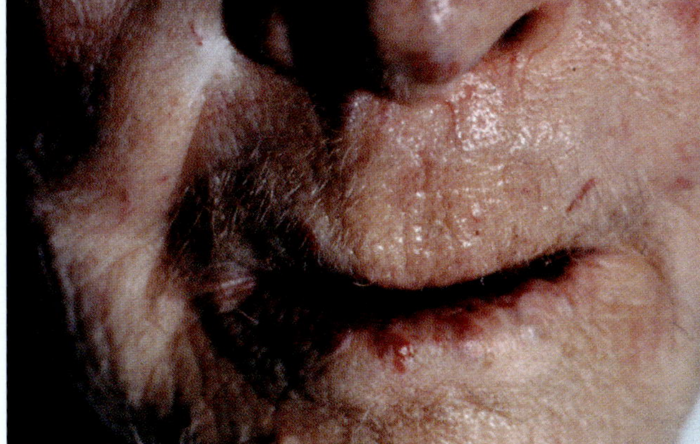

Figure 1.11 Hereditary telangiectasia. Vascular malformations are present on the face, lips, and hands in this patient with hereditary telangiectasia. This patient presented with iron-deficiency anemia caused by recurrent GI bleeding from gastrointestinal tract telangiectasia. (Courtesy Dr. J. Crookston.)

Table 1.1

Hemoglobinopathies associated with microcytosis

- β-Thalassemia trait (heterozygous)
- β-Thalassemia major (homozygous)
- α-Thalassemia trait
- HbH disease
- α-Thalassemia trait and hemoglobin constant spring
- HbC heterozygous and homozygous
- HbE heterozygous and homozygous
- HbD disease
- HbO Arab disease
- Hb Lepore heterozygous and homozygous
- δβ-Thalassemia heterozygous and homozygous
- γδβ-Thalassemia heterozygous and homozygous
- Hereditary persistence of fetal hemoglobin homozygous
- Hereditary persistence of fetal hemoglobin (HPFH); specific types of heterozygous HPFH

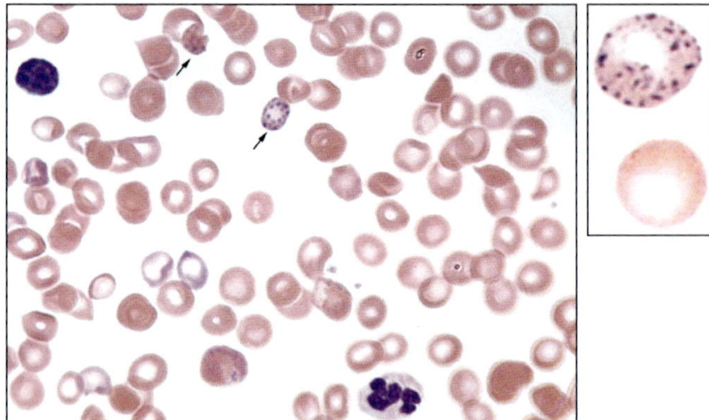

Figure 1.13 Basophilic stippling in thalassemia. Peripheral blood film demonstrating microcytic hypochromic RBCs and basophilic stippling (*arrows*). Basophilic stippling occurs in thalassemia as well as in other hematologic disorders.

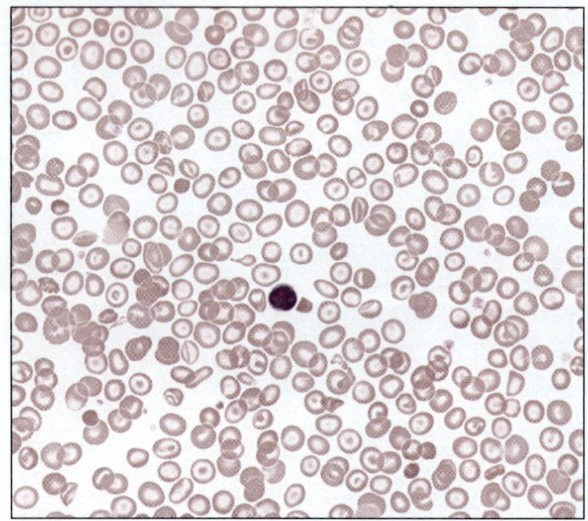

Figure 1.12 Thalassemia trait blood film. Peripheral blood films in β-thalassemia trait may demonstrate microcytosis and possibly hypochromasia. Multiple morphologic changes including target cells, teardrop cells, and rare fragments may occur. These features can appear identical to the morphologic picture of iron deficiency. Basophilic stippling can occur in Mediterranean populations with β-thalassemia trait and is less common in other populations with this disorder. Basophilic stippling may help distinguish β-thalassemia trait from iron deficiency, but is not always present in patients with β-thalassemia trait. Red blood cell indices may help: a normal or slightly decreased hemoglobin with a low MCV/MCH and a low or mildly increased RDW suggests thalassemia. Red blood cell indices may not always distinguish iron deficiency from thalassemia trait, however. Patients also may have combined iron deficiency and β-thalassemia trait and therefore require further testing to exclude the former.

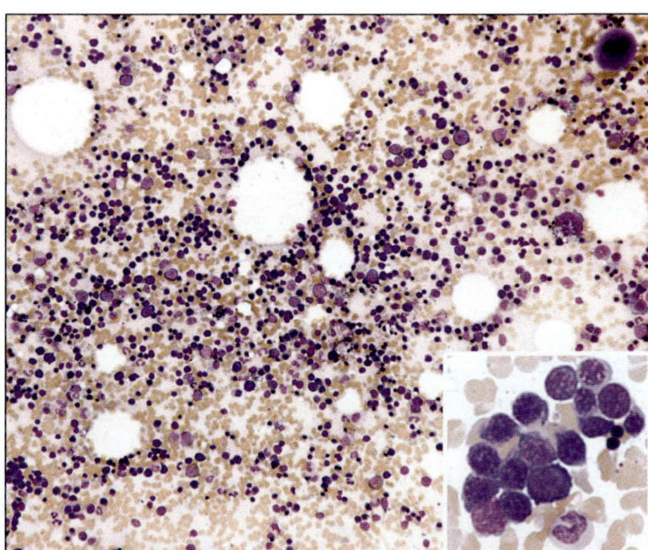

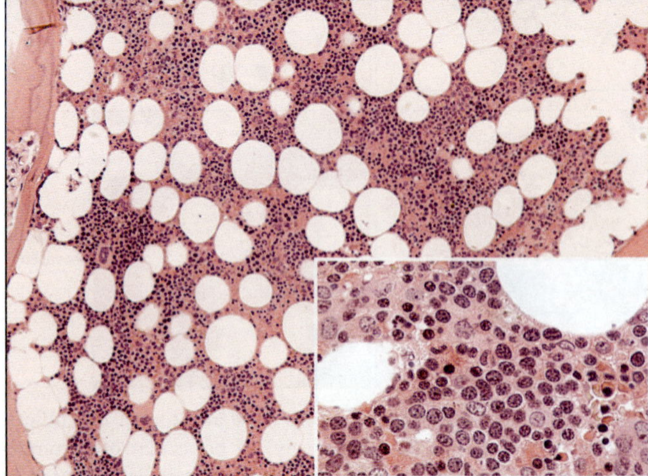

Figure 1.14 Bone marrow in thalassemia. Top and bottom panels show bone marrow aspirate and biopsy, respectively, from a case of thalassemia trait. The bone marrow has increased numbers of erythroid precursors (a low myeloid to erythroid ratio) related to the increased peripheral RBC destruction in this disease.

Table 1.2

Basophilic stippling

- Thalassemia trait and major
- Hemolytic anemia
- Myelodysplastic syndrome/sideroblastic anemia
- Megaloblastic anemia
- Pyrimidine 5′ nucleotidase deficiency
- Heavy metal poisoning (coarse basophilic stippling)
  - Lead, zinc, arsenic, silver, mercury

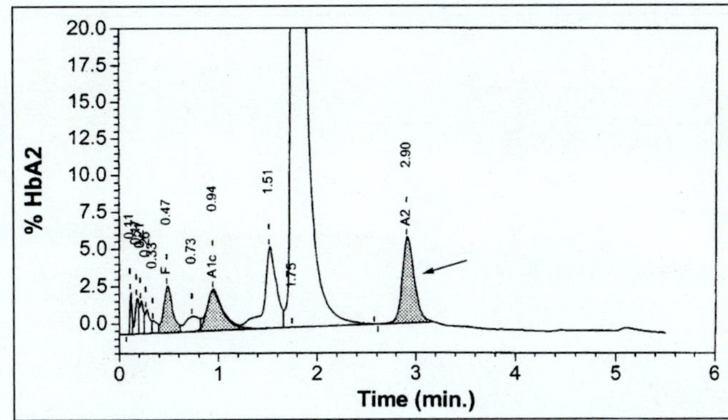

Figure 1.15 High-performance liquid chromatography (HPLC) sample demonstrating increased hemoglobin A_2 (*arrow*) in a case of β-thalassemia trait. HPLC is an automated way of separating and identifying variant hemoglobins and is more accurate at quantifying hemoglobin A_2 than is Hb electrophoresis. It can separate HbA_2 from certain hemoglobins, which is not possible using hemoglobin electrophoresis alone.

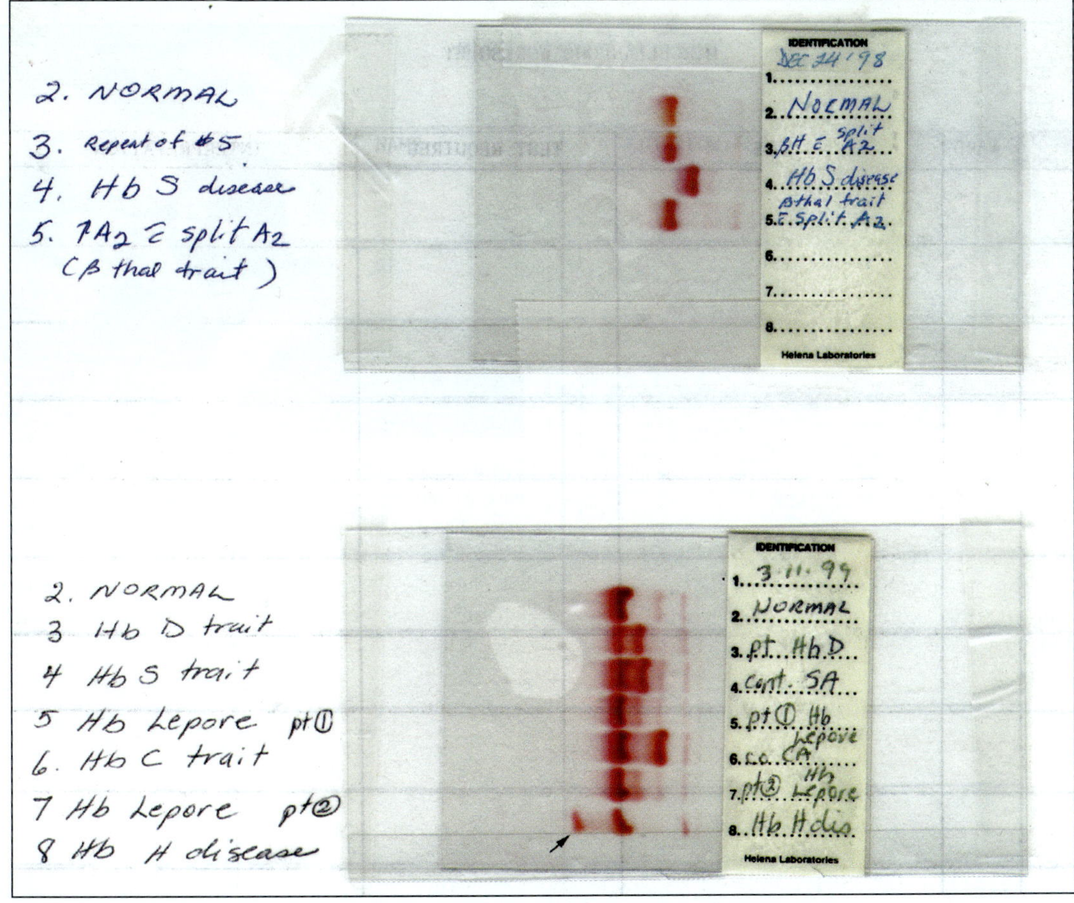

Figure 1.16 Alkaline hemoglobin (Hb) electrophoresis. *Top panel:* Lane 2: Normal. Lanes 3 and 5: β-thalassemia trait. Lane 4: HbS disease. *Bottom panel:* Lane 2: Normal. Lane 3: Hb D trait. Lane 4: HbS trait. Lanes 5 and 7: Hb Lepore trait (faint band around HbS band area). Lane 6: HbC trait. Lane 8: HbH disease (note fast-moving Hb band, *arrow*). Hemoglobins that move with HbS on alkaline include D/G/Lepore, and hemoglobins that move with HbC on alkaline include E/O/A_2.

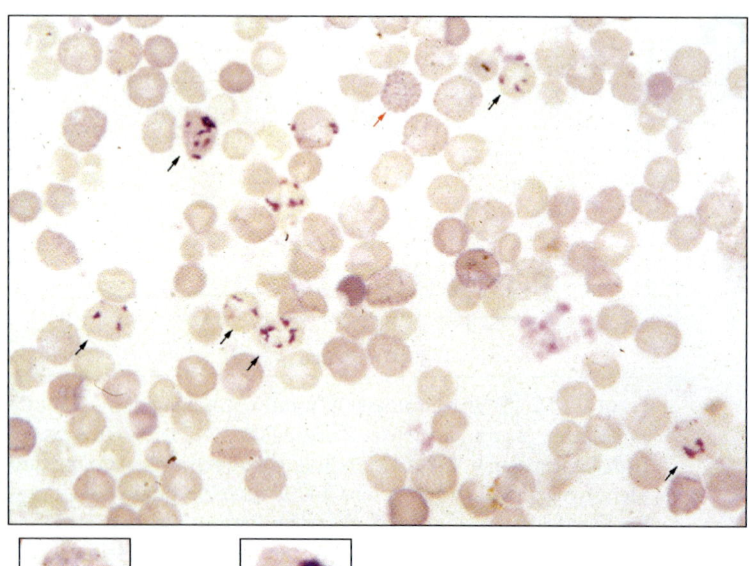

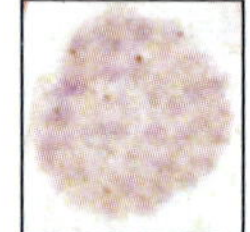

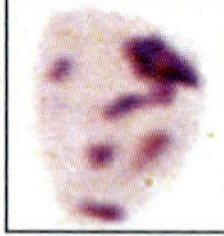

Figure 1.17 HbH inclusions. Peripheral blood stained with supravital stain brilliant cresyl blue. The red blood cell near the top central area (*red arrow*) demonstrates numerous inclusions in an evenly diffuse distribution, creating a "golf ball" pattern. This cell is an HbH inclusion body seen in α-thalassemia. The difference between the HbH bodies that appear like dimpled golf balls with diffuse even involvement can be seen from reticulocytes with uneven reticulin deposits (*black arrows*). The HbH inclusions are precipitated β-globin tetramers. Reticulocytes, Heinz bodies, and Howell-Jolly bodies stain positive with brilliant cresyl blue. Reticulocytes are darker, more reticular, clumped, and uneven in distribution. Heinz bodies are larger and not so numerous. Howell-Jolly bodies are usually single inclusions. These inclusions appear after 10 minutes of incubation at room temperature, whereas HbH inclusions require incubation at 37°C for 1 to 2 hours. Rare HbH inclusion bodies may be seen in one or two α-gene deletions in α-thalassemia trait, but there the absence of identifying these inclusion bodies does not exclude the disorder, which may require molecular studies for definitive diagnosis. In HbH disease (three α-gene deletion), HbH bodies are frequent and easily identifiable. (Courtesy Dr. D. Amato.)

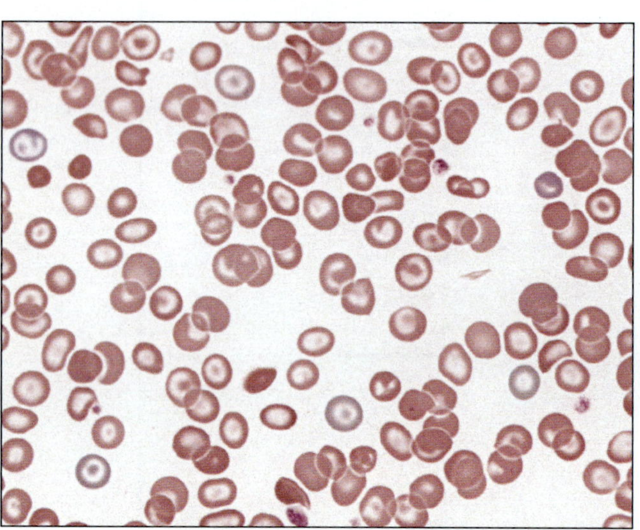

Figure 1.18 Hemoglobin H disease. This blood film demonstrates microcytosis, hypochromasia, and numerous morphologic abnormalities, including target cells, microspherocytes, and fragments. Basophilic stippling may occur. Polychromasia is present.

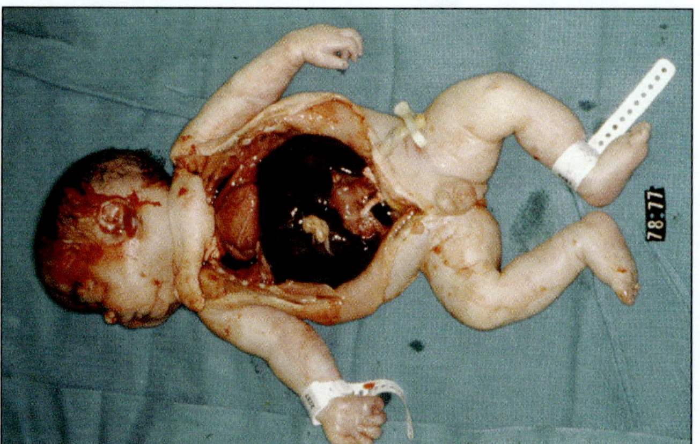

Figure 1.19 Hydrops fetalis at autopsy in hemoglobin Bart disease. Hepatosplenomegaly in a newborn with hemoglobin Bart disease. The loss of all four α-globin genes results in severe anemia, high-output heart failure, splenomegaly, edema, and intrauterine or immediately postpartum death for the affected fetus. Dystocia, eclampsia, and hemorrhage can occur in the mother carrying the affected fetus. (Courtesy Dr. D. Amato.)

Table 1.3

HbH inclusions

- HbH disease
- Acquired HbH disease (myeloproliferative, myelodysplastic, AML syndromes)
- Erythroleukemia
- Refractory sideroblastic anemia

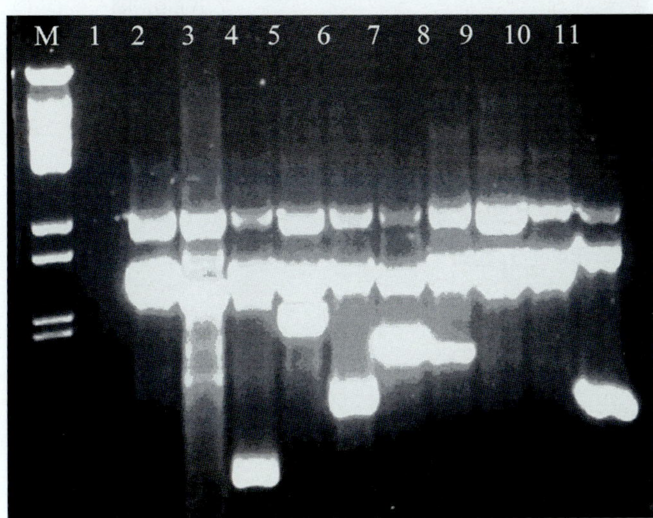

Figure 1.20 α-Thalassemia diagnosis by polymerase chain reaction (PCR) amplification of DNA. Multiplex PCR results for the seven most common deletional mutations of the α-globulin gene cluster. The LIS1 gene at 17p13.3 was included as an amplification control. Using genomic DNA from known genotypes for the following mutant alleles: –α 3.7, –α 4.2, – –FIL, – –MED, and –Sea. Plasmid controls for –THAI and –(α)20.5 were mixed with normal genomic DNA to mimic the heterozygous state. M represents the γ-BstE II molecular weight marker. Lane 1, blank; lane 2, αα/αα ; lane 3, –3.7/–4.2; lane 4, αα/– –FIL; lane 5, αα/– –SEA; lane 6, αα/ – –MED; lane 7, αα/– –THAI; lane 8, αα/–(α)20.5; lane 9, αα/αα ; lane 10, αα /αα ; lane 11, – –MED/–α .7. (Courtesy C. Wei.)

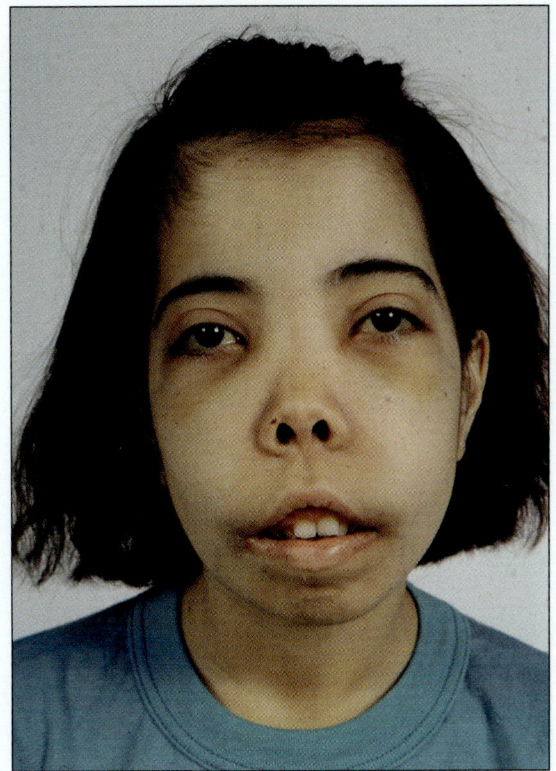

Figure 1.21 β-Thalassemia facial bone abnormalities. These changes include bossing of the skull; hypertrophy of the maxilla, exposing the upper teeth; depression of nasal bridge; and periorbital puffiness. (Courtesy Dr. N.F. Olivieri.)

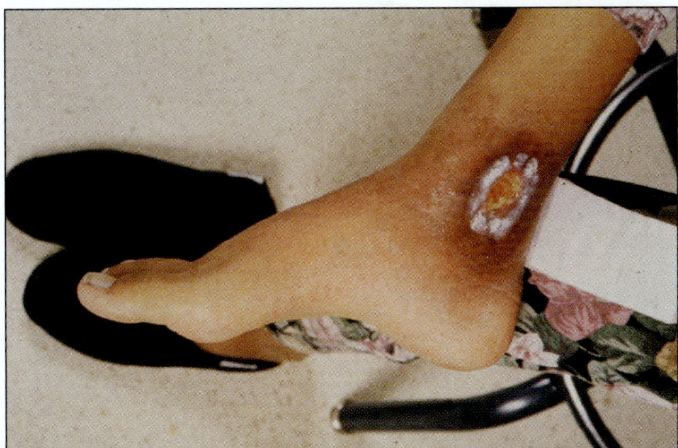

Figure 1.22 β-Thalassemia major leg ulcer. Leg ulcers can occur in all types of hereditary hemolytic anemias, including sickle cell disease and hereditary spherocytosis. (Courtesy Dr. N.F. Olivieri.)

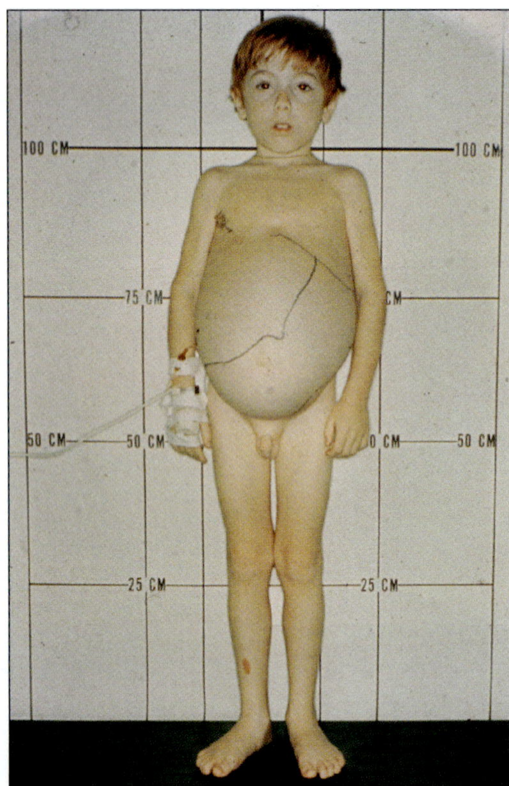

Figure 1.23 β-Thalassemia major. Note the pallor, short stature, massive hepatosplenomegaly, and wasted limbs in this undertransfused case of β-thalassemia major. (Courtesy Dr. N.F. Olivieri.)

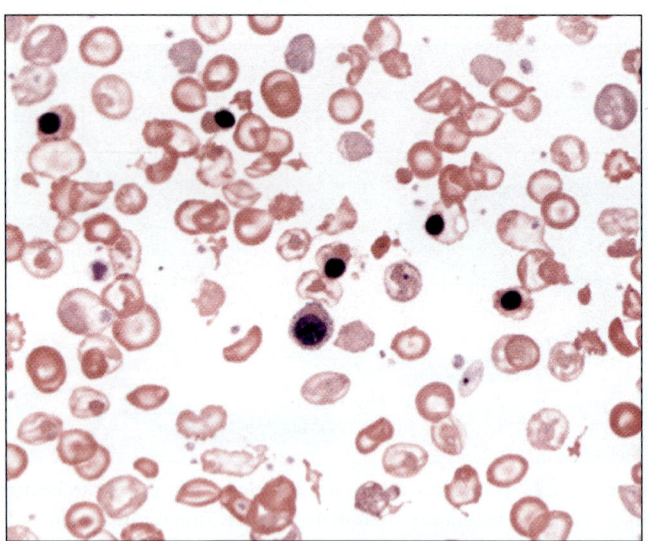

Figure 1.24 β-Thalassemia major. Unless they have had transfusions, patients with this disease usually have severe anemia. This peripheral blood film demonstrates many nucleated red blood cells, microcytosis, and hypochromasia with multiple morphologic changes: target cells, teardrop cells, fragments, basophilic stippling, and Pappenheimer bodies. The nucleated red blood cells may be dysplastic or show abnormal hemoglobinization. Neutrophilia and thrombocytosis may occur. This patient has undergone splenectomy for hypersplenism and increased transfusion requirements. Howell-Jolly bodies are present.

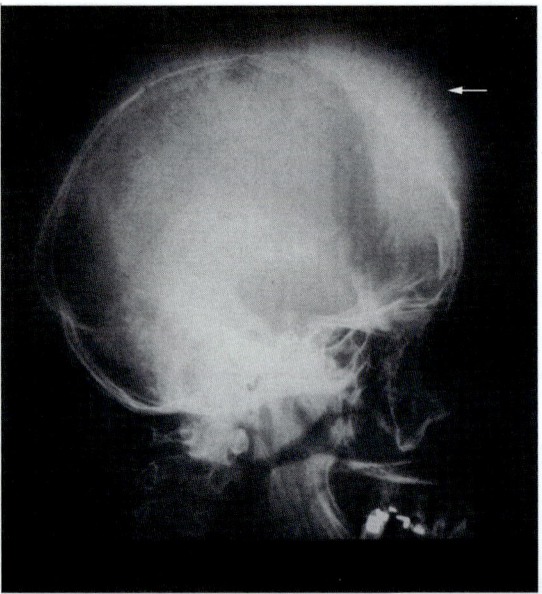

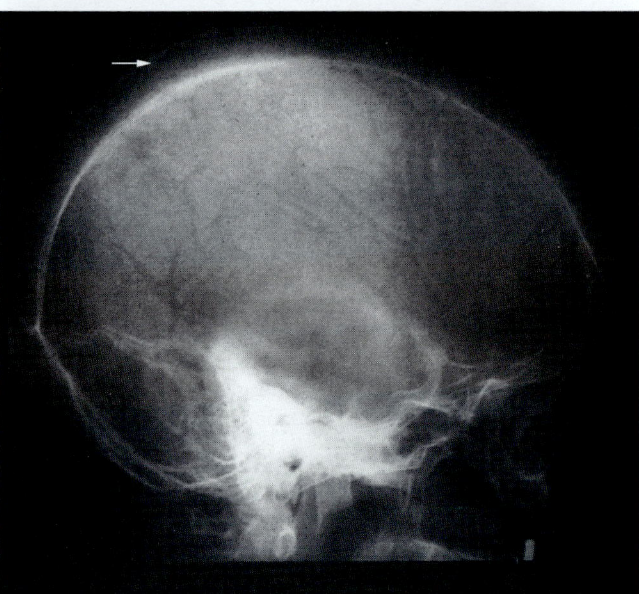

Figure 1.25 β-Thalassemia bone abnormalities. Note the "hair on end" appearance of the cortical bone caused by expansion of the bone marrow (*arrows*). The subperiosteal bone grows in radiating striations, which appears as "hairs." (Courtesy Dr. N.F. Olivieri.)

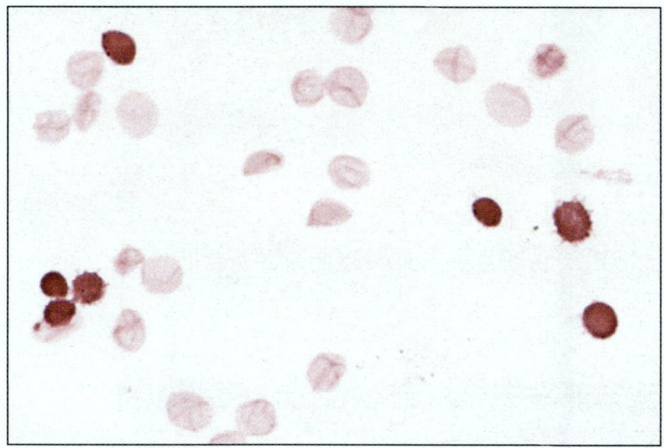

Figure 1.26 Kleihauer Betke test. This peripheral blood from a postpartum woman with fetomaternal hemorrhage demonstrates HbF containing fetal cells (*dark red*) in a background of maternal cells (ghost-like cells). HbF cells are resistant to acid elution of hemoglobin. Aside from detecting fetal cells in the mother's blood in a fetomaternal hemorrhage, it can be used to detect HbF–containing cells in β-thalassemia, hereditary persistence of hemoglobin F (some types have homogeneous distribution of HbF in the cells), sickle cell disease, δβ-thalassemia, and myelodysplastic syndrome.

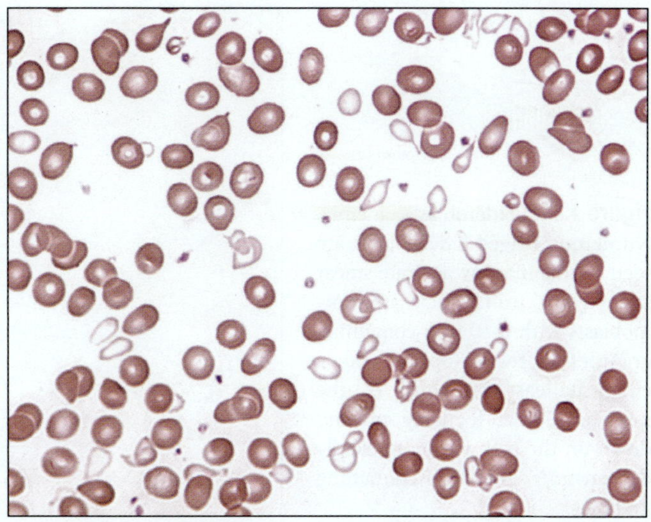

Figure 1.27 Sideroblastic anemia. Peripheral blood film of dual population and sideroblastic anemia. Normocytic cells are present, along with a minor population of microcytic, hypochromic erythrocytes possessing a thin rim of cytoplasm. Occasional teardrop cells are visible. Pappenheimer bodies, target cells, and basophilic stippling occur in some cases.

Figure 1.28 RBC inclusions. In Wright-stained blood, Pappenheimer bodies are usually multiple and vary in size and Howell-Jolly bodies are typically round, smooth, and single.

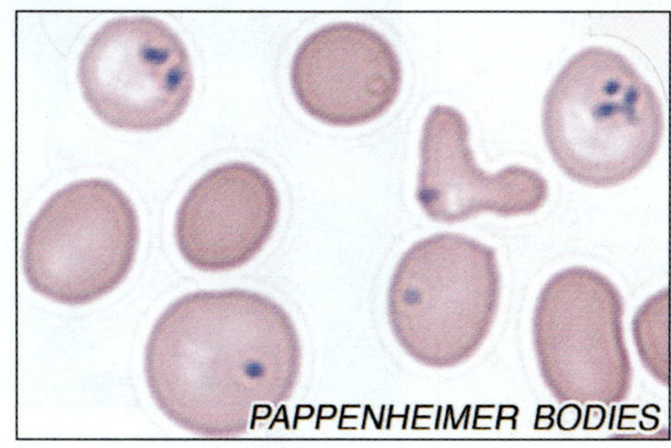

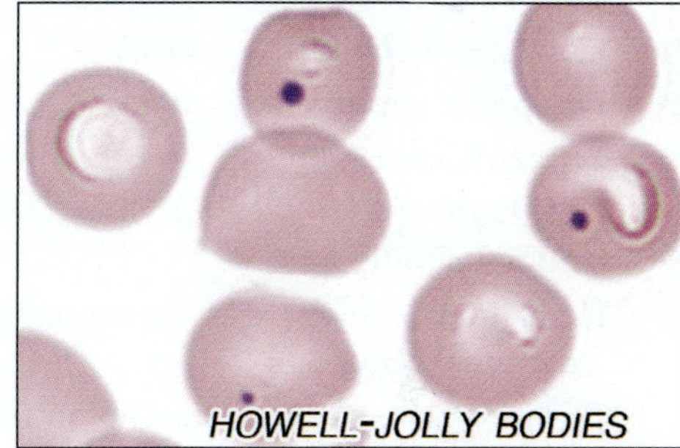

Figure 1.29 Pappenheimer bodies. Pappenheimer bodies are single or multiple blue, small, and angular inclusions within the erythrocyte. By contrast, Howell-Jolly bodies are usually single inclusions that are larger and round, not angular. Basophilic stippling is evenly distributed over the whole cell. Pappenheimer bodies are positive when stained for iron.

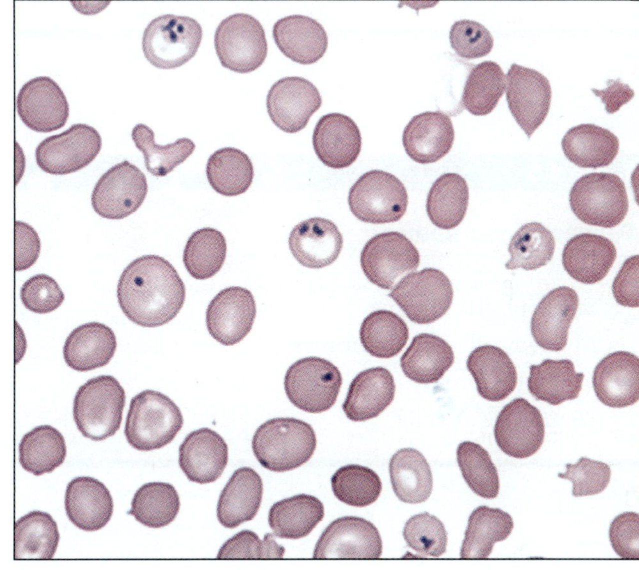

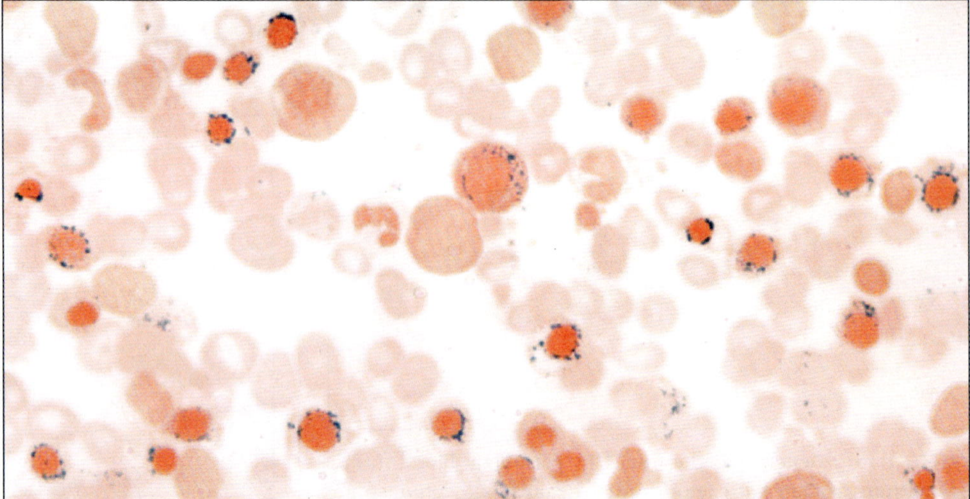

Figure 1.30 Sideroblastic anemia. Numerous ringed sideroblasts are seen in this marrow aspirate smear stained for iron. They are normoblasts with ≥10 iron-containing granules in the cytoplasm encircling at least one-third of the nucleus. Often, focusing up and down on the cell will more clearly demonstrate the iron-containing granules.

Table 1.4

Red blood cell inclusions

Name of Inclusion	Content
• Howell-Jolly body	DNA
• Basophilic stippling	RNA
• Pappenheimer body	Iron
• HbH body (supravital only)	β-Globin tetramers (β^4)
• Heinz body (supravital only)	Denatured hemoglobin
• Fessus body (supravital only)	α-Globin tetramers (α^4)
• Crystals	Hemoglobin-C
• Cabot rings	Mitotic spindle remnants
• Nucleus	DNA

Table 1.5

Pappenheimer bodies

- Sideroblastic anemia
- Myelodysplastic syndromes
- Postsplenectomy
- Hemolytic anemia

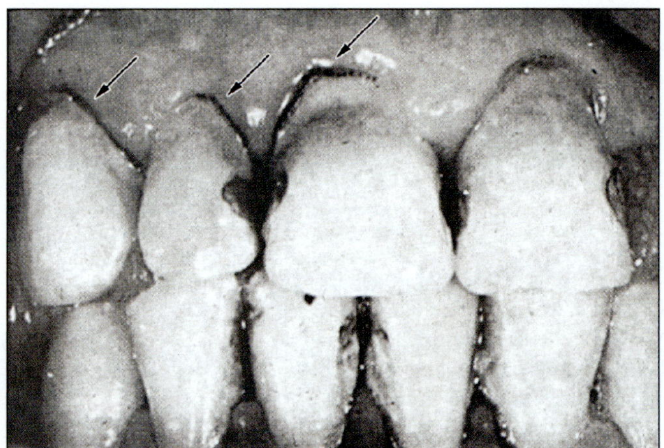

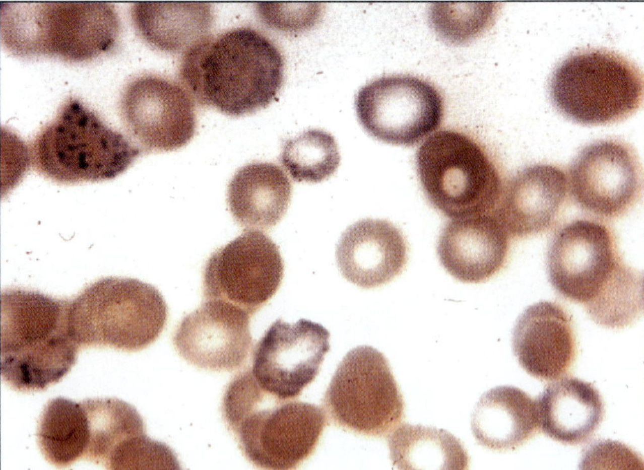

Figure 1.31 *Top panel:* Gums in lead poisoning. Lead lines are shown in gums of this patient suffering from lead poisoning. *Bottom panel:* Peripheral blood film demonstrating coarse basophilic stippling. Normocytic or microcytic anemia may be present.

Diagram 1.3

Approach to normocytic anemia

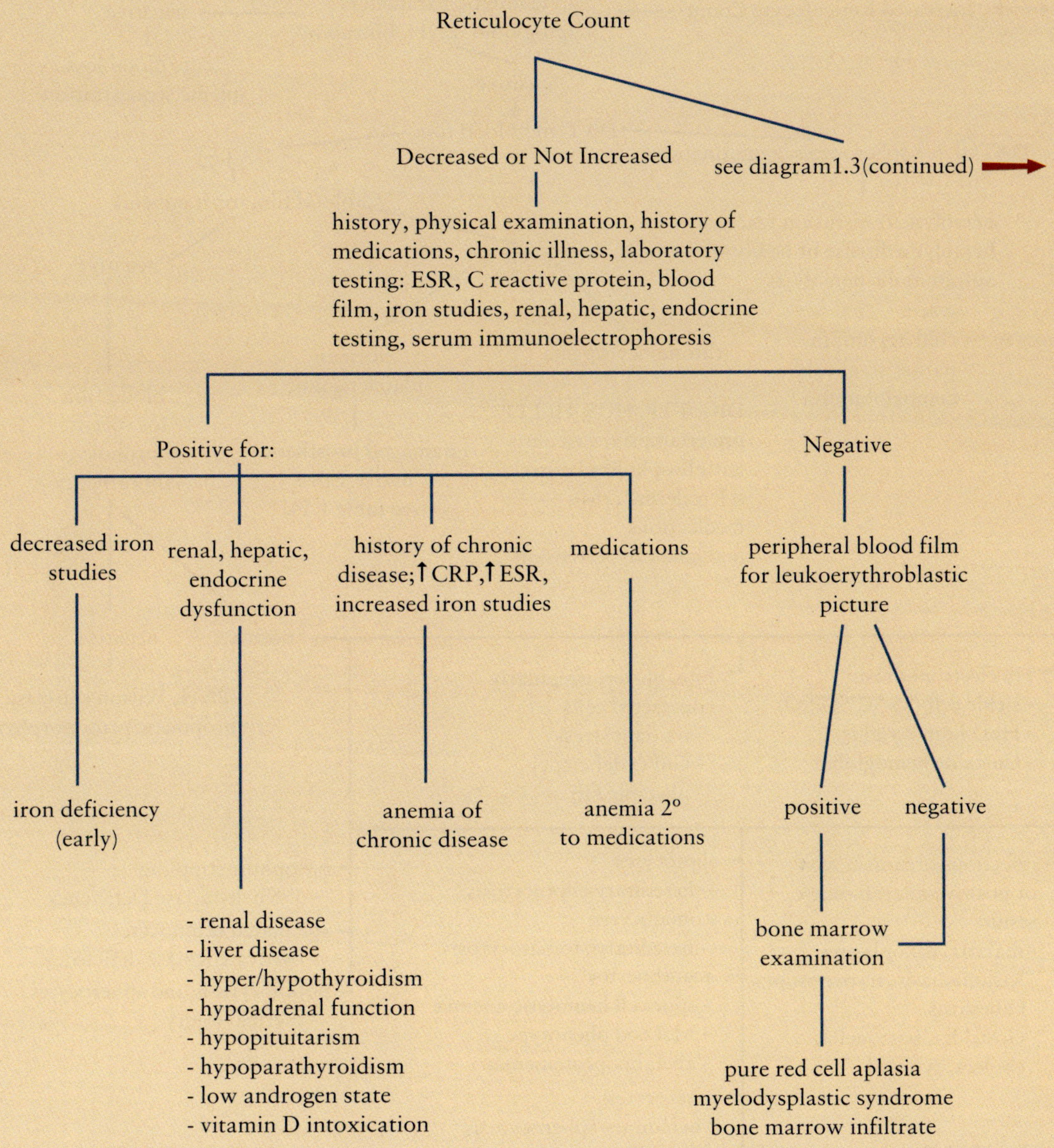

Reticulocyte Count

Decreased or Not Increased

see diagram1.3(continued) ➡

history, physical examination, history of medications, chronic illness, laboratory testing: ESR, C reactive protein, blood film, iron studies, renal, hepatic, endocrine testing, serum immunoelectrophoresis

Positive for:

Negative

decreased iron studies

renal, hepatic, endocrine dysfunction

history of chronic disease; ↑ CRP, ↑ ESR, increased iron studies

medications

peripheral blood film for leukoerythroblastic picture

iron deficiency (early)

anemia of chronic disease

anemia 2° to medications

positive   negative

- renal disease
- liver disease
- hyper/hypothyroidism
- hypoadrenal function
- hypopituitarism
- hypoparathyroidism
- low androgen state
- vitamin D intoxication

bone marrow examination

pure red cell aplasia
myelodysplastic syndrome
bone marrow infiltrate

(continued)

Diagram 1.3 (continued)

Approach to normocytic anemia

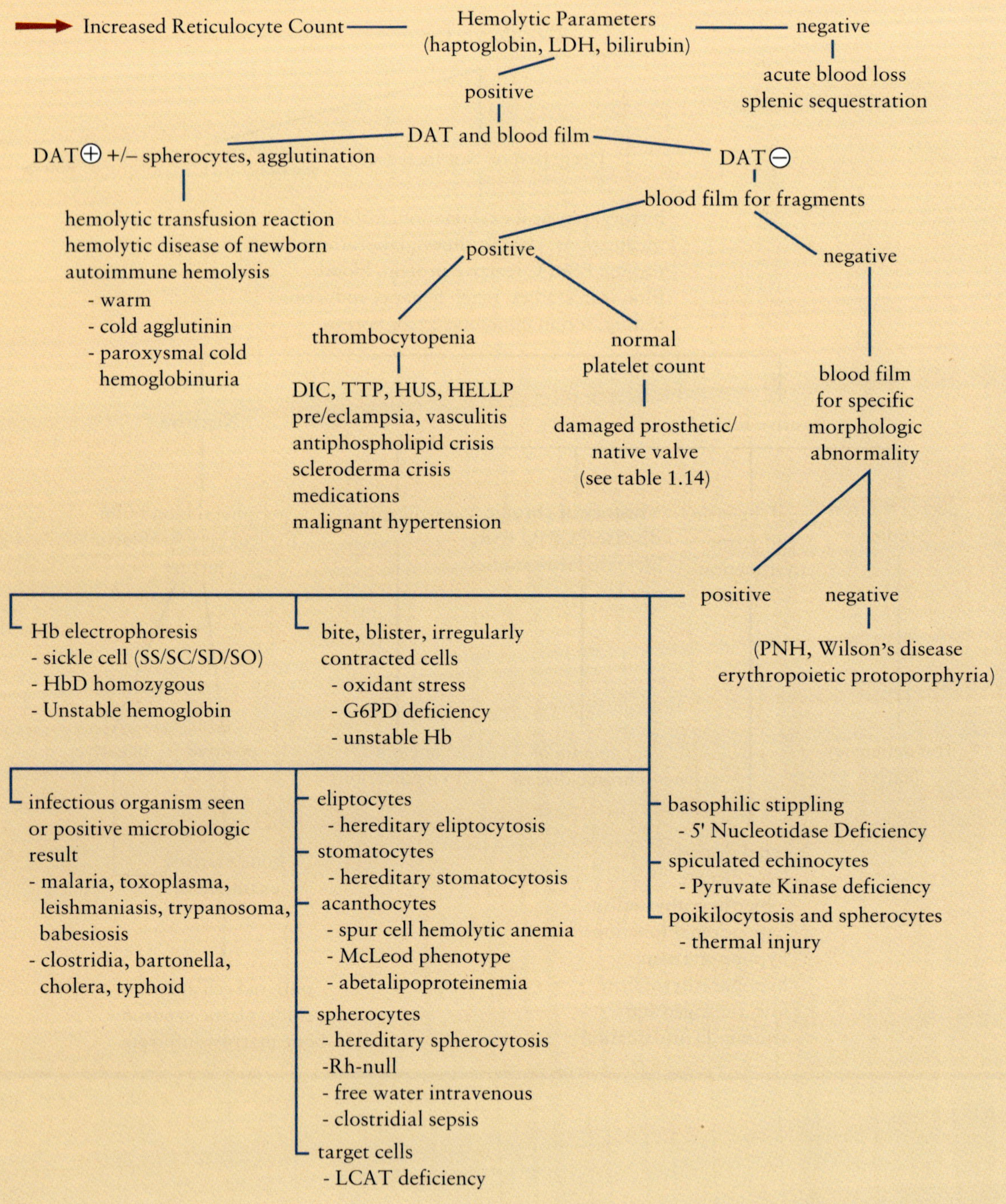

→ Increased Reticulocyte Count —— Hemolytic Parameters —— negative
(haptoglobin, LDH, bilirubin)

acute blood loss
splenic sequestration

positive

DAT and blood film

DAT⊕ +/− spherocytes, agglutination   DAT⊖

blood film for fragments

hemolytic transfusion reaction
hemolytic disease of newborn   positive   negative
autoimmune hemolysis
 - warm
 - cold agglutinin
 - paroxysmal cold   thrombocytopenia   normal
   hemoglobinuria   platelet count   blood film
                          DIC, TTP, HUS, HELLP   for specific
                          pre/eclampsia, vasculitis   damaged prosthetic/ morphologic
                          antiphospholipid crisis   native valve   abnormality
                          scleroderma crisis   (see table 1.14)
                          medications
                          malignant hypertension

                                                              positive   negative

Hb electrophoresis   bite, blister, irregularly   (PNH, Wilson's disease
- sickle cell (SS/SC/SD/SO)   contracted cells   erythropoietic protoporphyria)
- HbD homozygous   - oxidant stress
- Unstable hemoglobin   - G6PD deficiency
                         - unstable Hb

infectious organism seen   eliptocytes   basophilic stippling
or positive microbiologic   - hereditary eliptocytosis   - 5' Nucleotidase Deficiency
result   stomatocytes   spiculated echinocytes
- malaria, toxoplasma,   - hereditary stomatocytosis   - Pyruvate Kinase deficiency
  leishmaniasis, trypanosoma, acanthocytes   poikilocytosis and spherocytes
  babesiosis   - spur cell hemolytic anemia   - thermal injury
- clostridia, bartonella,   - McLeod phenotype
  cholera, typhoid   - abetalipoproteinemia

                             spherocytes
                              - hereditary spherocytosis
                              -Rh-null
                              - free water intravenous
                              - clostridial sepsis
                             target cells
                              - LCAT deficiency

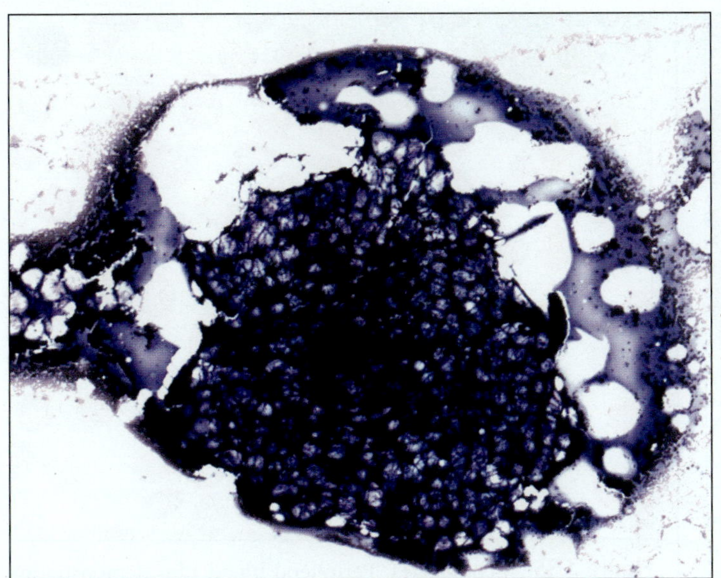

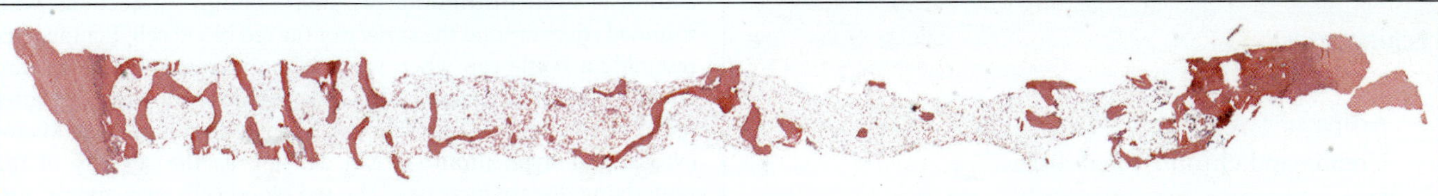

Figure 1.32   *Top panel:* Bone marrow aspirate demonstrating a hypocellular fragment from a patient with aplastic anemia. Although bone marrow cellularity can be estimated from fragments on the aspirate, the bone marrow biopsy is a better sample to estimate cellularity. *Bottom panel:* Aplastic bone marrow biopsy showing <10% cellularity.

Figure 1.33   Parvovirus B19-induced pure red cell aplasia. *Left panel:* Bone marrow aspirate smear shows a giant erythroblast with intranuclear viral inclusion. This inclusion can resemble a large nucleolus, and the cytoplasm may be dark blue and contain vacuoles. *Right panel:* Bone marrow biopsy with early erythroid precursors showing "glassy" intranuclear inclusions (so-called lantern cells; *arrows*).

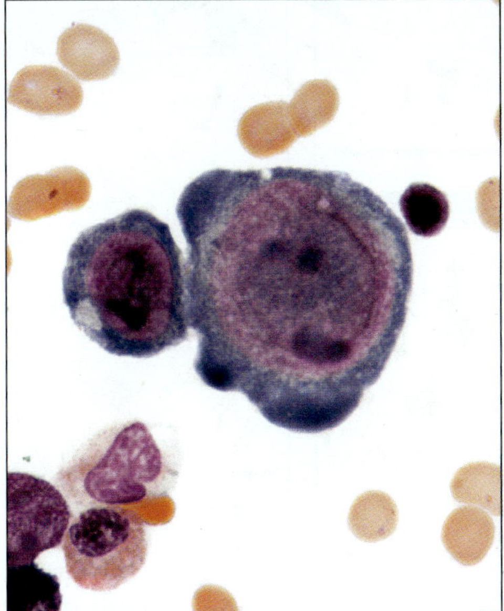

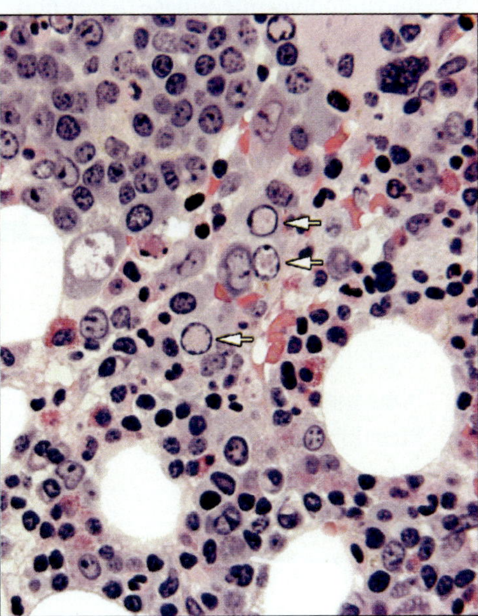

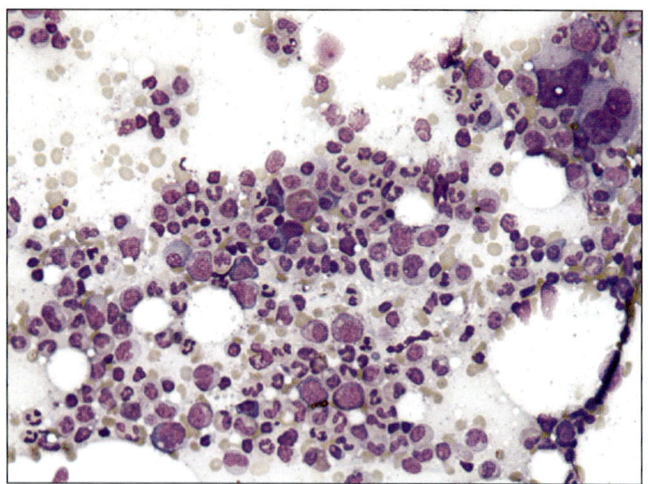

Figure 1.34   Pure red cell aplasia. Bone marrow aspirate smear showing absence of erythroid precursors in PRCA.

Table 1.6

Echinocytes

- Artifact
- Uremia and chronic renal disease
- Hypophosphatemia
- Disseminated malignancy
- Liver disease
- Vitamin E deficiency
- Pyruvate kinase deficiency
- Phosphoglycerate kinase deficiency
- Early posttransfusion of RBC
- Hyperlipidemia
- Myeloproliferative disorders

Table 1.7

Teardrop cells

- Myelofibrosis
- Bone marrow infiltration
- Megaloblastic anemia
- Hemolytic anemia
- Thalassemia major

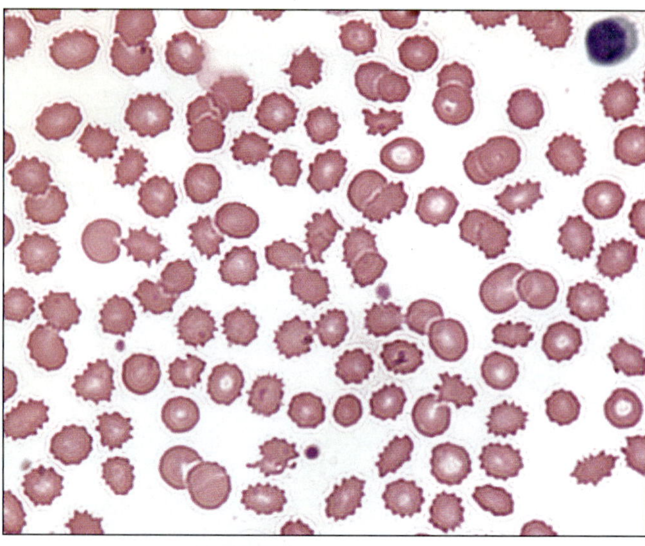

Figure 1.35   Echinocytes. Peripheral blood film demonstrating echinocytes, also called *burr cells*. The cells have central pallor and a diffuse, even distribution of short, bumpy projections with rounded edges around the surface of the red blood cell. Echinocytes resemble a bottle cap when viewed from above. This blood film could represent an example of anemia of chronic disease. The latter usually demonstrates a normocytic, normochromic anemia. Microcytosis and hypochromasia can develop as the severity of the underlying disease increases. The red blood cells may appear normal, demonstrate nonspecific changes, or display features secondary to the underlying cause (e.g., rouleaux due to inflammatory protein or hyperfibrinogenemia). Neutrophilia and thrombocytosis may occur.

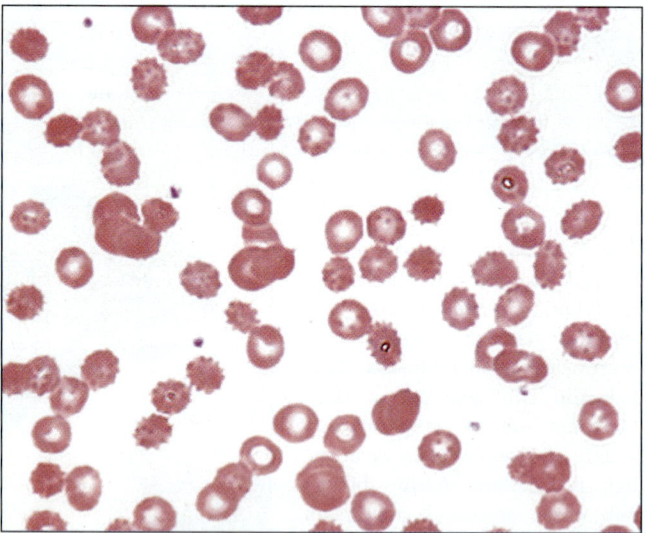

Figure 1.36   Peripheral blood film of patient recently transfused with red blood cells. Note a small population of echinocytes, which represent the recently transfused red blood cells.

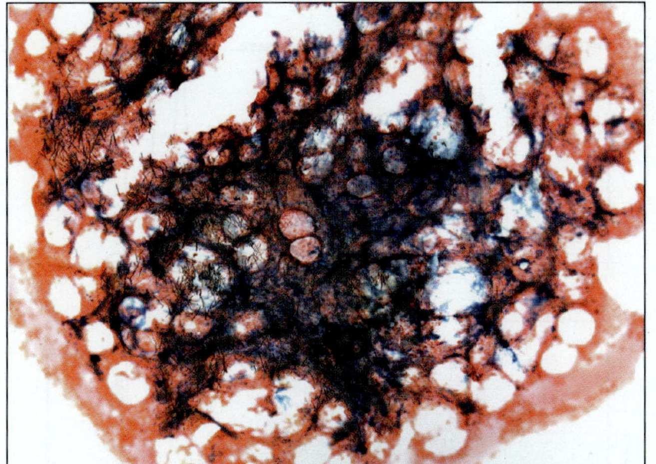

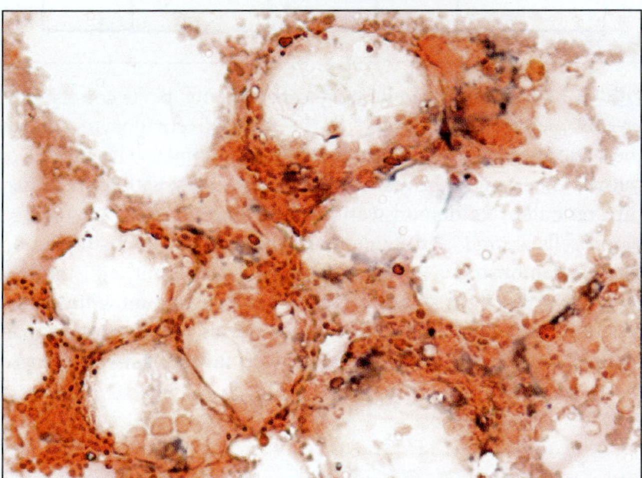

Figure 1.37 Increased marrow iron stores. *Top panel:* Bone marrow aspirate demonstrating increased iron staining in a fragment. This finding is present in a patient with anemia of chronic disease. Increased iron stores also occur in frequently transfused patients. *Bottom panel:* Normal iron staining in histiocytes is shown for comparison.

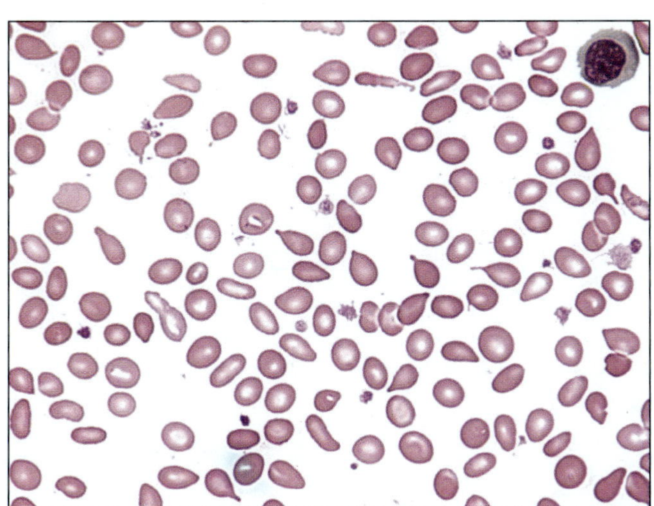

Figure 1.38 Peripheral blood film demonstrating teardrop cells in myelofibrosis. One side of the cell is tapered and ends in a blunt tip.

Table 1.8

Leukoerythroblastic picture

Increased Demand
- Hemorrhage
- Hemolysis
- Severe infection
- Recovery from bone marrow failure or suppression
- Sickle cell crisis
- Thalassemia major
- Systemic lupus erythematosus

Bone Marrow Infiltration
- Myelofibrosis
- Other causes of bone marrow fibrosis
- Hematologic malignancies
  - CML, AML, ALL, Hodgkin disease, non-Hodgkin lymphoma, myeloma
- Nonhematologic malignancies
  - Metastatic to bone marrow
- Granuloma
- Bone marrow infarction
- Storage disease
- Severe megaloblastic anemia
- Severe rickets

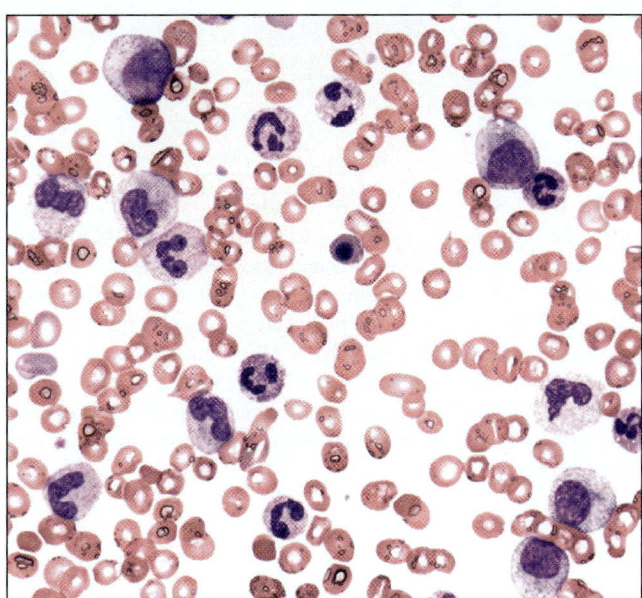

Figure 1.39 Leukoerythroblastic picture. Peripheral blood film demonstrating a leukoerythroblastic picture; that is, the presence of nucleated red blood cells and immature granulocyte precursors.

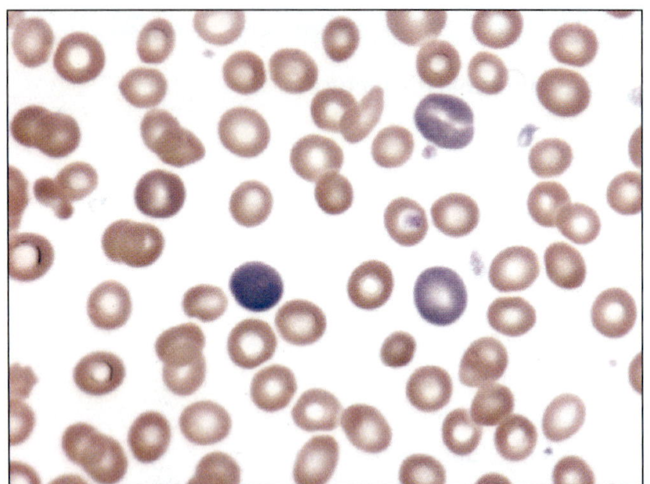

Figure 1.40 Peripheral blood film with Romanowsky stain demonstrating polychromatophilic cells. The polychromatophilic cells are basophilic because of increased RNA content. Not all reticulocytes are polychromatophilic on Romanowsky stains, and assigning the number of polychromatophilic cells alone as a surrogate marker for reticulocytosis underestimates the reticulocyte count. The cells are usually larger than normocytic red blood cells.

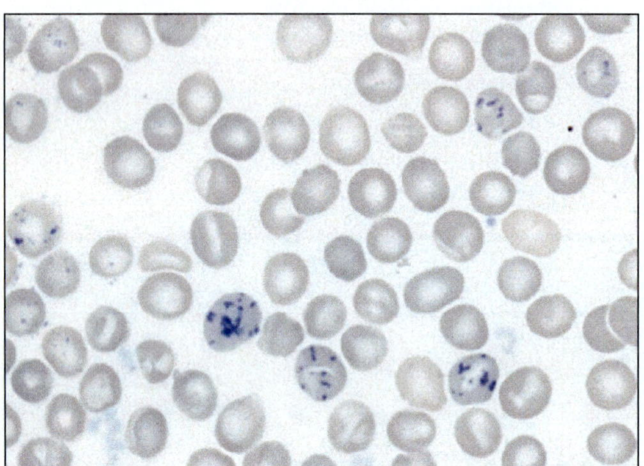

Figure 1.41 Supravital stain of reticulocytes with brilliant cresyl blue. The blue-stained reticular inclusions in the red blood cells represent ribosomes that are precipitated when exposed to brilliant cresyl blue. The National Committee for Clinical Laboratory Standards (NCCLS) definition of reticulocyte is "any non-nucleated red blood cell containing ≥ 2 particles of blue-staining material corresponding to ribosomal RNA." Howell-Jolly bodies, Pappenheimer bodies, and Heinz bodies can be mistaken for reticulin precipitation. The more immature the reticulocyte, the more reticulin precipitation occurs.

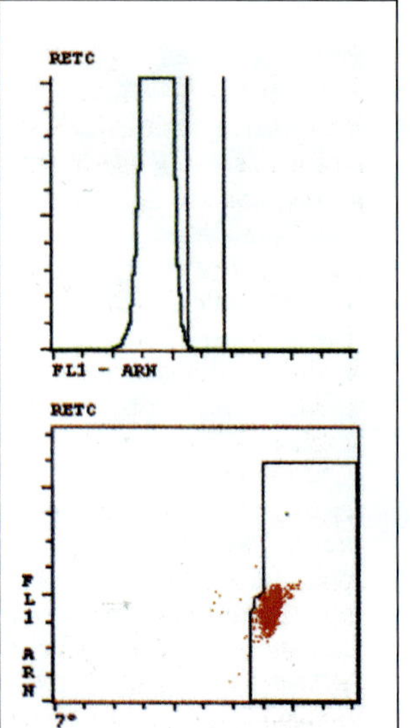
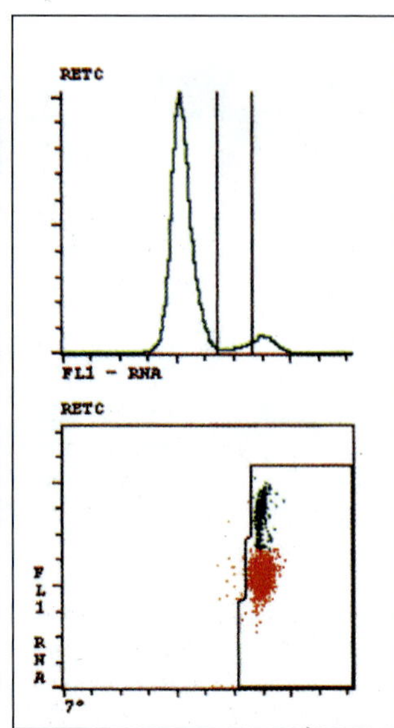

Figure 1.42 Automated hemocytometer reticulocyte counts. Fluorochromes are used to bind to the RNA of reticulocytes, which then fluoresce and can be counted by flow cytometry. The degree of fluorescence gauges the maturity of reticulocytes, with more immature reticulocytes demonstrating more fluorescence. Mature red blood cells are red, and reticulocytes are green. The histogram on the left demonstrates a very low reticulocyte count, and the histogram on the right shows a high reticulocyte count. Automated reticulocyte counts allow more reticulocytes to be counted than manual reticulocyte counts and provide more precise and rapid measurement.

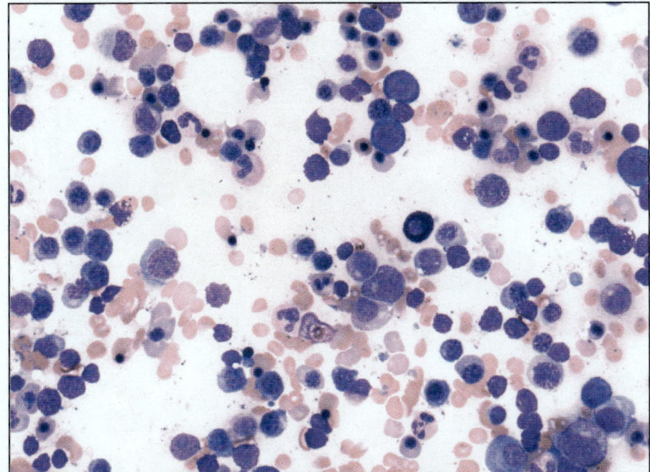

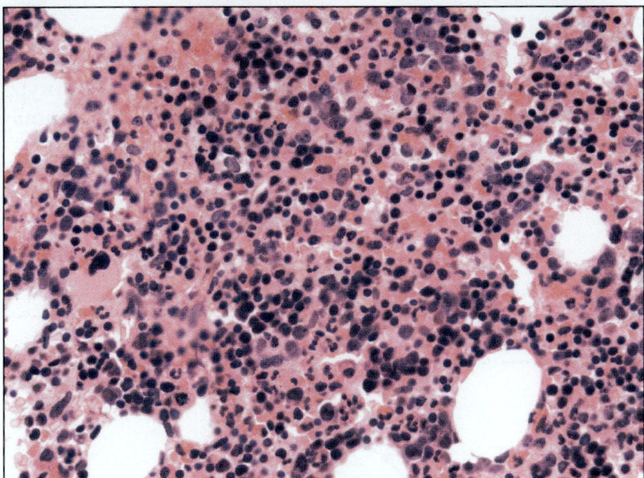

Figure 1.43 Bone marrow findings in hemolytic anemia. *Top panel:* Erythroid hyperplasia is present with a predominance of erythroid precursors. The normal myeloid to erythroid ratio in a bone marrow aspirate is 3 to 5:1. In this case, there occurs a reversal of the myeloid to erythroid ratio of 1:4. A similar picture occurs in acute hemorrhage. Occasional mild dysplastic erythroid precursors may be presenting these cases. *Bottom panel:* Bone marrow biopsy in a patient with hemolytic anemia. Erythroid hyperplasia is seen with a predominance of erythroid precursors.

Table 1.9

Spherocytosis

- Warm autoimmune hemolytic anemia
- Acute and delayed hemolytic transfusion reactions
- ABO hemolytic disease of newborn/Rh hemolytic disease of newborn
- Hereditary spherocytosis
- Clostridium sepsis
- Intravenous water infusion or drowning (fresh water)
- Hypophosphatemia
- Bartonellosis
- Snake bite
- Cold autoimmune hemolytic anemia/paroxysmal cold hemoglobinuria
- Hyposplenism
- Rh-null phenotype

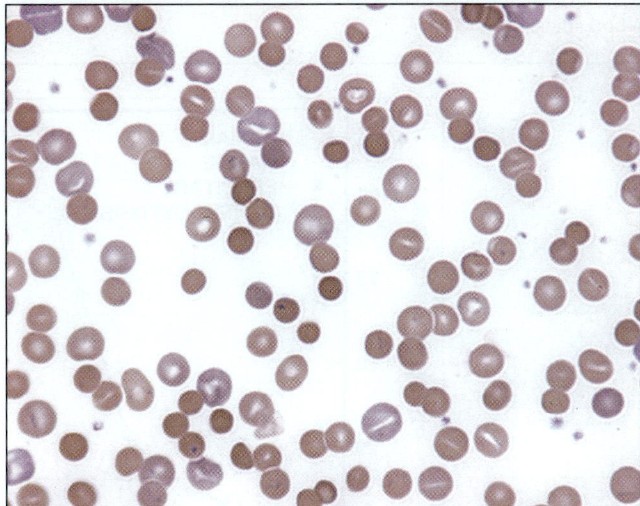

Figure 1.44 Autoimmune hemolytic anemia. Numerous spherocytes, small round RBCs lacking central pallor, are shown in this blood smear from a case of Coombs-positive hemolytic anemia.

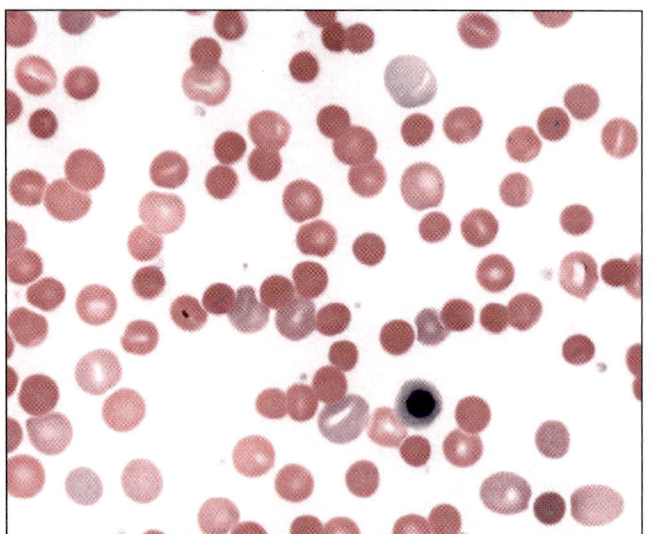

Figure 1.45 Hereditary spherocytosis. Peripheral blood film of spherocytic hemolysis. Spherocytes are round, are slightly smaller than normal red blood cells, and lack central pallor. Note the nucleated red blood cells and polychromatophilic cells. It is important to look in the area of the slide where red blood cells are nearly touching each other to properly identify spherocytes. Red blood cells normally have a spherical appearance at the tail (thin) end of the blood smear.

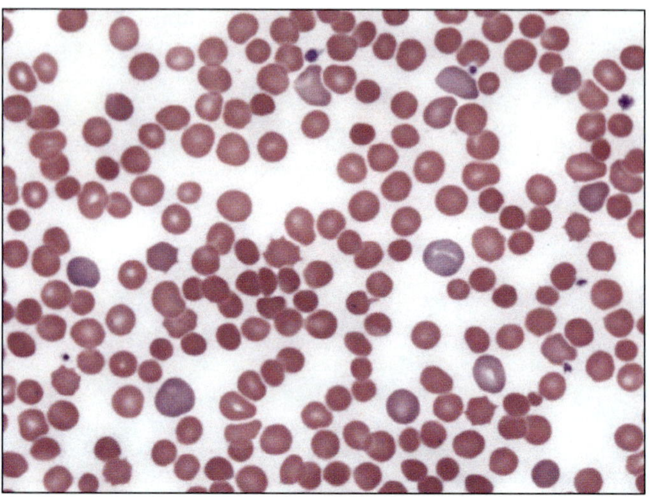

Figure 1.47 Peripheral blood film of microspherocytes seen in *Clostridium perfringens* sepsis. Although regular spherocytes are usually smaller than normocytic red blood cells, microspherocytes are even smaller than that. This finding is usually seen in critically ill, septic patients with severe *C. perfringens* infection.

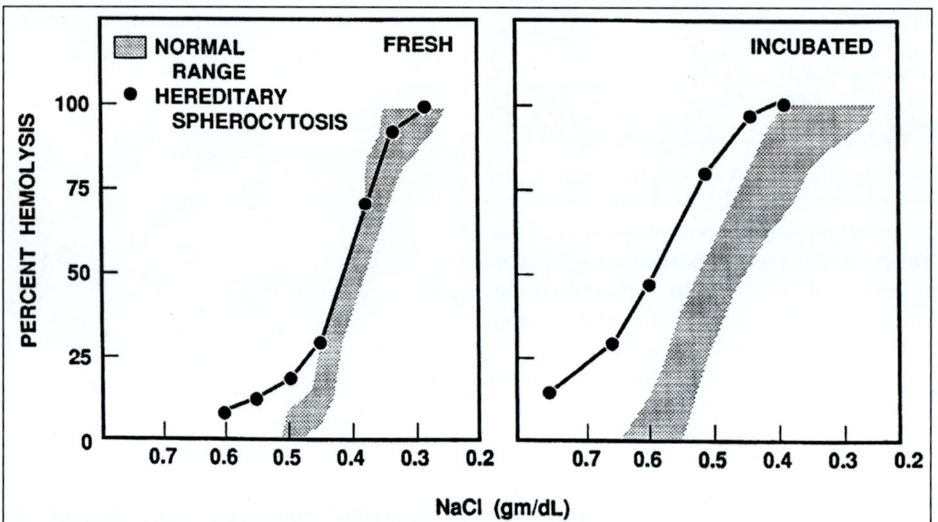

Figure 1.46 Osmotic fragility curves of normal and hereditary spherocytosis red blood cells. RBCs are exposed to decreasing strengths of hypotonic saline solutions, and the degree of hemolysis (%) is measured. Increased fragility is indicated by a shift of the curve to the left, and is seen in conditions associated with spherocytosis. In the fresh sample on the left, a tail of HS cells occurs with increased sensitivity. Incubation of the sample for 24 hours prior (graph on the right) accentuates the osmotic fragility of spherocytes, whereas normal cells only become more slightly fragile. The osmotic fragility of unincubated blood may be normal in some patients with HS; therefore, incubated testing should be performed as well.

Table 1.10

Red blood cell agglutination

- Cold agglutinins
- Cold autoimmune hemolytic anemia
- Paroxysmal cold hemoglobinuria
- IgM paraproteinemias

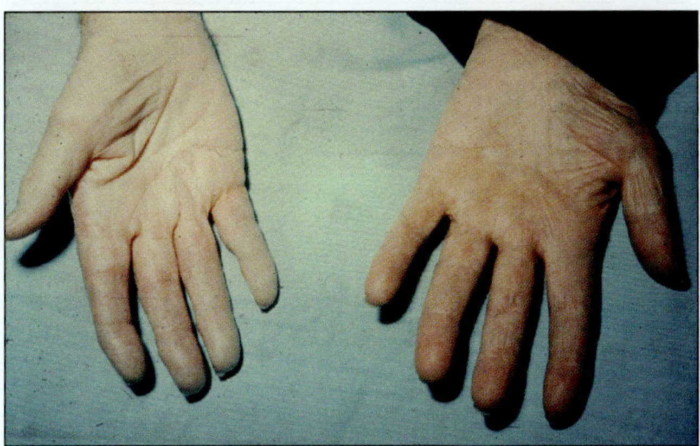

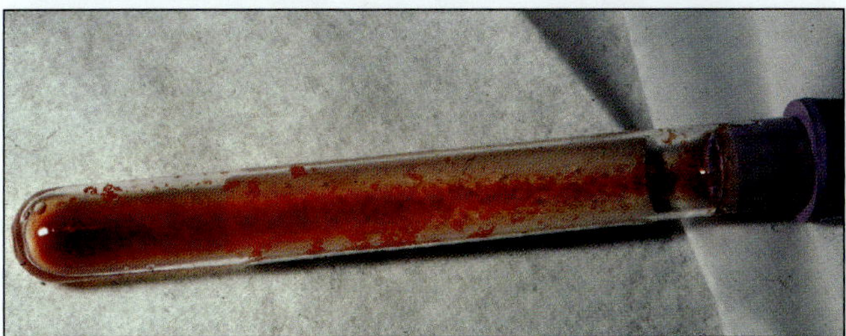

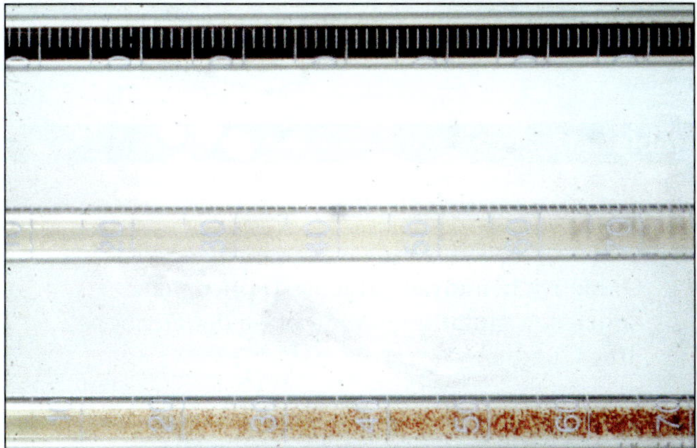

Figure 1.48 Chronic cold agglutinin disease. The hand on the right in this picture is warmed in a patient with chronic cold agglutinin disease. *Middle panel:* Macroscopic appearance of red blood cell agglutination at 37°C in a tube of blood from a patient with cold-agglutinin hemolytic anemia secondary to infection with *Mycoplasma pneumoniae*. *Bottom panel:* Serum in capillary tubes from a cold agglutinin specimen at room temperature (*top*) and 4°C (*bottom*) illustrating RBC agglutination at cold temperature. (Courtesy Dr. I. Quirt.)

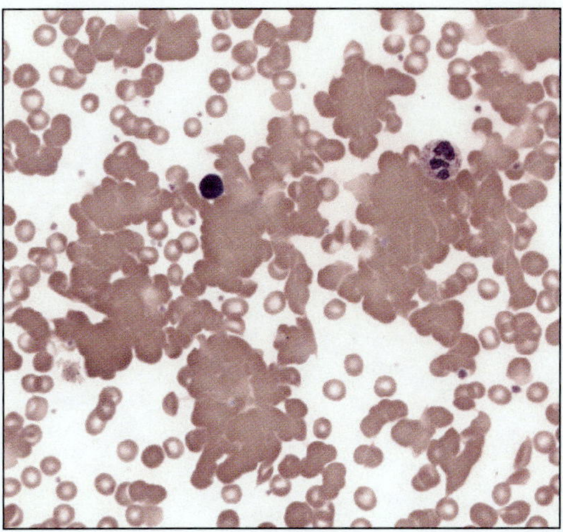

Figure 1.49 Cold agglutinin. Peripheral blood film of red blood cell aggregates and cold agglutinin disorder. The red blood cells form clumps in which distinguishing the borders of individual erythrocytes is difficult. In cold autoimmune hemolysis, polychromasia, nucleated red blood cells, and spherocytes also may be present. The width and length of the red blood cell agglutinates are approximately equal, unlike rouleaux, in which red blood cells are arranged linearly in chains. The borders of erythrocytes are more easily distinguishable in rouleaux.

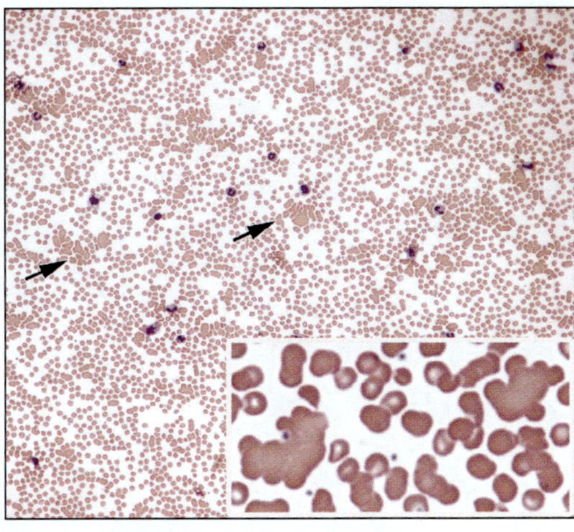

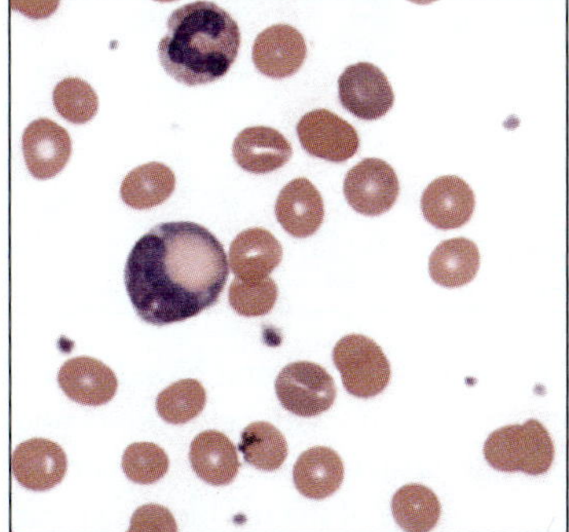

Figure 1.50 Paroxysmal cold hemoglobinuria. *Top panel:* Blood film demonstrates small red blood cell agglutinates in a patient with paroxysmal cold hemoglobinuria. The bottom panel discloses erythrophagocytosis by a neutrophil in a patient with this disorder.

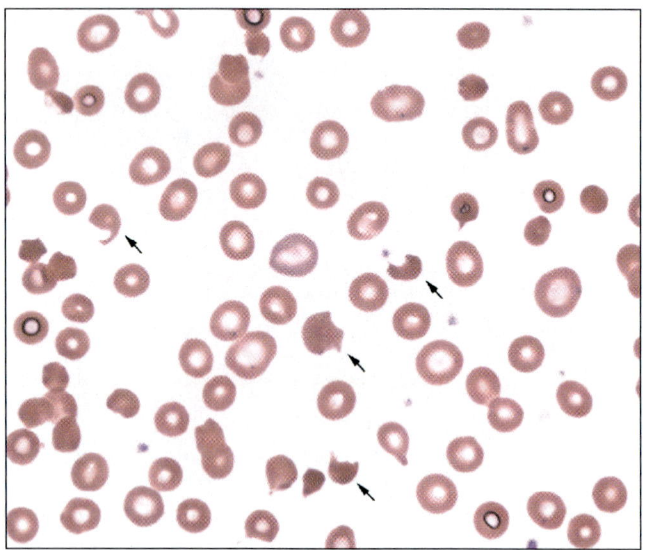

Figure 1.51 Bite cells. The red blood cells in this peripheral smear appear bitten. The erythrocyte may retain or lose central pallor, depending on the size and numbers of bites. In some cases, the bite cell may be mistaken for *helmet cells*, a type of fragmented erythrocyte. The examiner, therefore, should consider the company that this cell keeps (i.e., the predominant morphology of the surrounding red blood cells) before deciding if the process is one of oxidation or fragmentation. A double bite cell is displayed in the center of the figure.

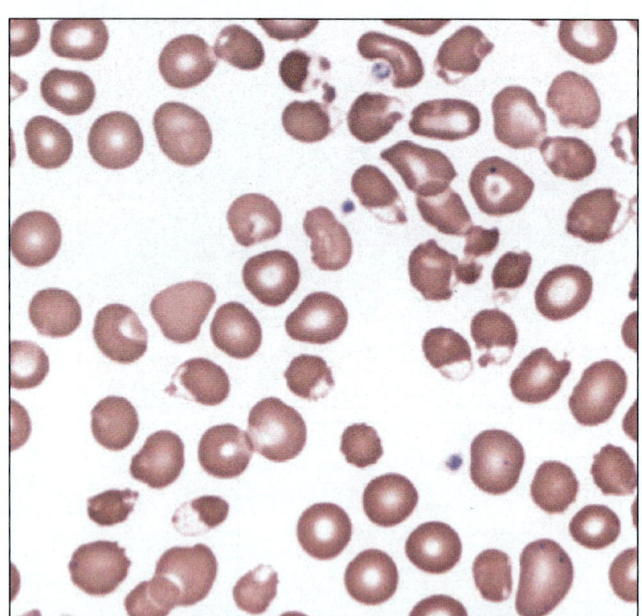

Figure 1.52 Oxidative hemolysis. Peripheral blood film demonstrating blister cells in a patient with glucose-6-phosphate dehydrogenase deficiency. The blister appears as a vacuole in the erythrocyte's hemoglobin at the edge of the red blood cell surface. A thin rim of cytoplasm seems to enclose this vacuole. This cell is usually a precursor to a bite cell.

Table 1.11

Bite cells/blister cells

- Oxidative hemolysis (glucose-6-phosphate dehydrogenase deficiency, glutathione synthetase deficiency, drugs, toxins)
- Unstable hemoglobins

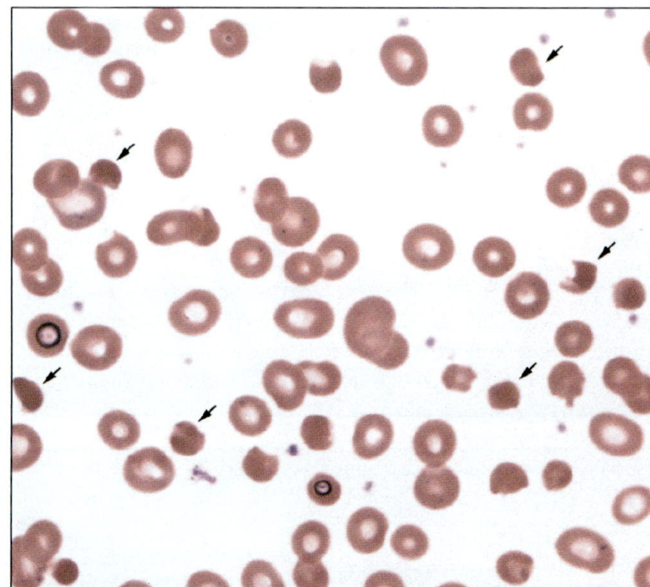

Figure 1.53 Oxidative hemolysis. Irregularly contracted cells are smaller than normocytic red blood cells in this blood film from a case of oxidative hemolysis. They do not have central pallor but, in contrast to spherocytes, they are irregular in shape and not spherical. The increased density of the irregularly contracted cells may give the hemoglobin a dark copper color. Occasional bite cells are present.

Table 1.12

Irregularly contracted cells

- Oxidative hemolysis (glucose-6-phosphate deficiency, glutathione synthetase deficiency, drugs, toxins)
- Unstable hemoglobins
- Hemoglobin C homozygous
- Hemoglobin SC disease
- Wilson's disease
- Zieve's syndrome

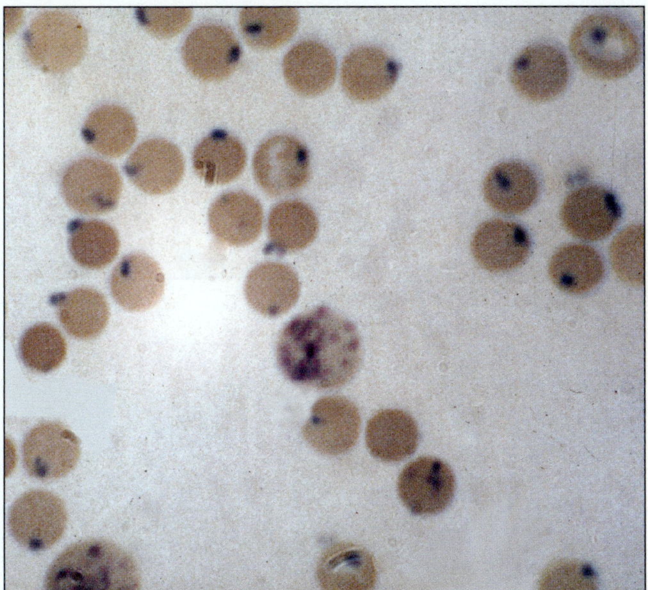

Figure 1.54 Heinz bodies. Peripheral blood stained with crystal violet supravital stain demonstrating Heinz-body inclusions, which are not visible with Romanowsky stains alone. Heinz bodies are purple-blue, large, single or multiple inclusions attached to the inner surface of the red blood cell membrane. They represent precipitated normal or unstable hemoglobins. Heinz bodies are more frequently seen postsplenectomy, and testing should be done within 1 hour after blood is collected. Reticulocytes do not stain with crystal violet.

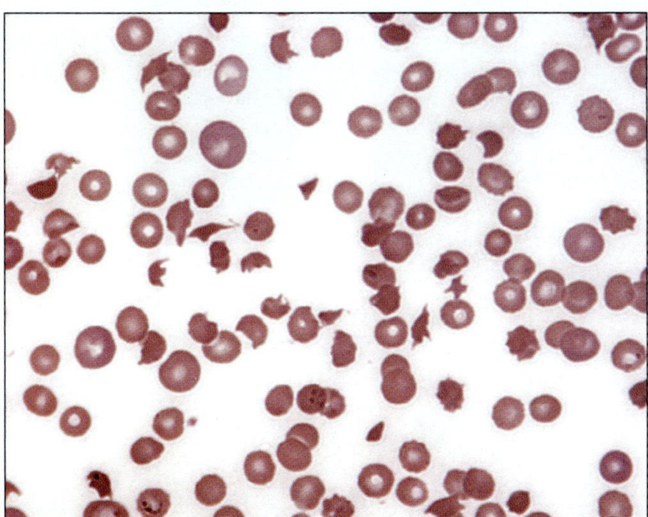

Figure 1.55 Microangiopathic hemolytic anemia. RBC fragments of variable shapes and sizes that lack central pallor are seen in this blood smear. RBC fragments have received specific names because of their shape; for example, comet cell, triangular cell, and schistocyte. The presence or absence of any of these cells does not have an impact on diagnosis or prognosis. In the process of red cell fragmentation, an occasional irregularly contracted erythrocyte, a bite cell, or spherocytes can be seen, but the diagnosis of microangiopathic hemolytic anemia should be made by the morphology of the majority of cells, which in this case are fragments. Note the severe thrombocytopenia.

Table 1.13

Heinz bodies

- Oxidative stress
  - glucose-6-phosphate dehydrogenase deficiency, glutathione synthetase deficiency
  - Drugs
  - Toxins
- Unstable hemoglobins

Table 1.14

Fragmentation

With thrombocytopenia
- Disseminated intravascular coagulopathy (DIC)
- Thrombotic thrombocytopenic purpura (TTP)
- Hemolytic uremic syndrome (HUS)
- HELLP syndrome
- Preeclampsia/eclampsia
- Malignant hypertension
- Systemic lupus erythematosus (SLE)
- Vasculitis
- Scleroderma crisis
- Antiphospholipid antibody crisis
- Drugs (cyclosporine, tacrolimus, mitomycin C, gemcitabine)
- Sepsis
- Disseminated carcinoma (mucin secreting)
- Extracorporeal circulation devices
- Vascular malformations

Without thrombocytopenia
- Damaged native and prosthetic heart valves
- Malignant hypertension
- Acute glomerulonephritis
- Rejection of transplanted kidney
- Renal cortical necrosis
- Drugs (cyclosporine, tacrolimus)
- Vasculitis
- Systemic lupus erythematosus (SLE)

Table 1.15

Causes of intravascular hemolysis

- Fragments
- Hemolytic transfusion reaction
- Paroxysmal nocturnal hemoglobinuria
- Paroxysmal cold hemoglobinuria
- Infection: malaria, clostridia
- Chemical: arsine, intravascular distilled water, venom
- Thermal injury
- glucose-6-phosphate dehydrogenase deficiency
- Occasional overwhelming autoimmune hemolytic anemia

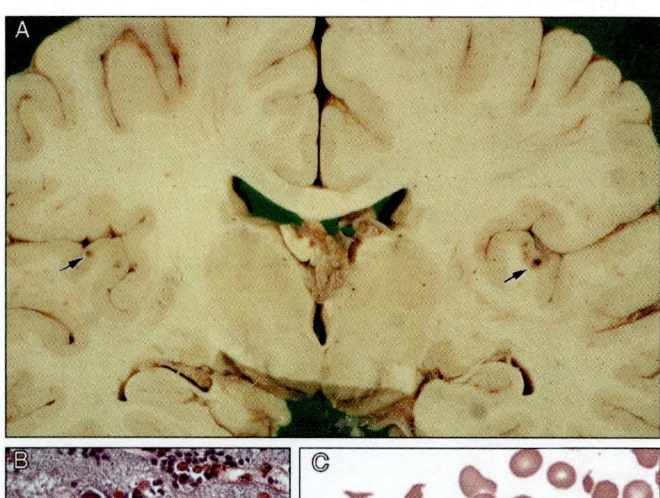

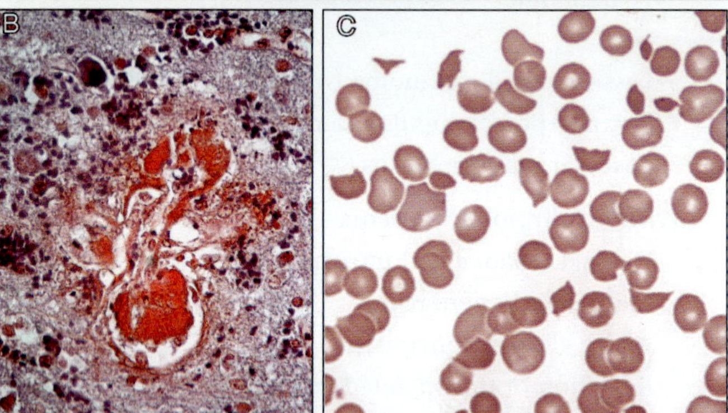

Figure 1.56 Thrombotic thrombocytopenic purpura (TTP). **A.** Coronal section through autopsy brain showing multiple small hemorrhages (*arrows*) from diffuse microvascular occlusion of arterioles and capillaries (**B**). Part **C** is the blood smear from the same patient, displaying a microhemangiopathic picture with RBC fragments and profound thrombocytopenia. (Courtesy Dr. J. Bilbao.)

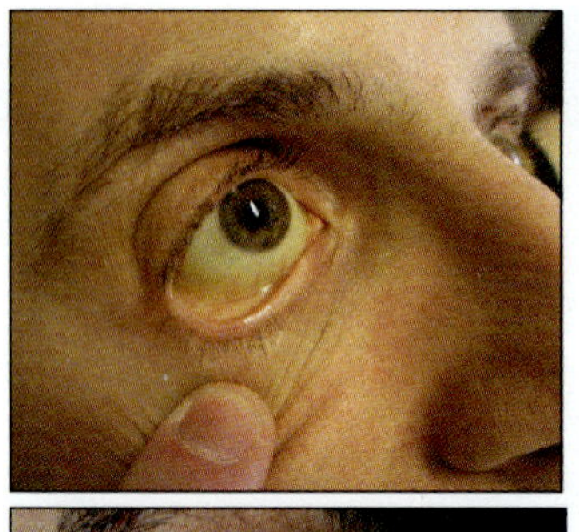
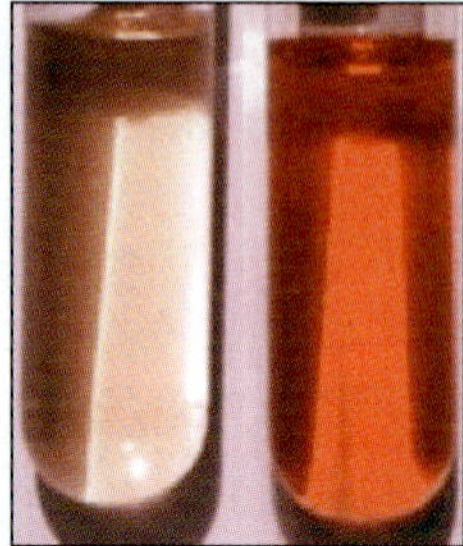
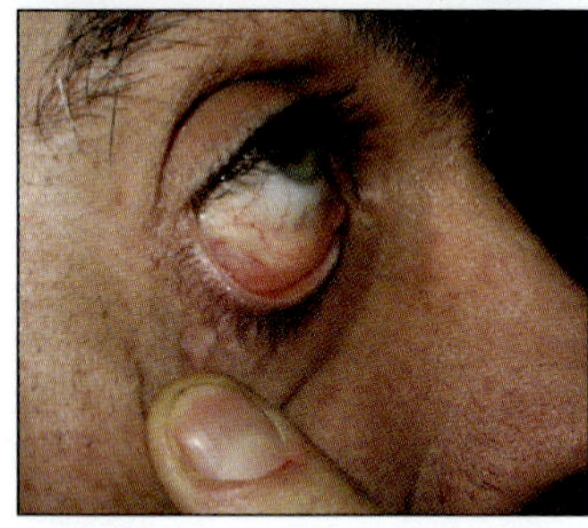

Figure 1.57 Jaundice, anemia, and hemoglobinemia from intravascular hemolysis. *Top panels:* Scleral icterus and pallor from autoimmune hemolysis is shown in the left upper panel. The right upper panel shows serum samples: The clear sample on the left is normal and the sample on the right is from a patient with hemolysis. The red color is from free hemoglobin released from lysed red blood cells in the serum. *Lower panel:* Normal control without scleral icterus and pallor.

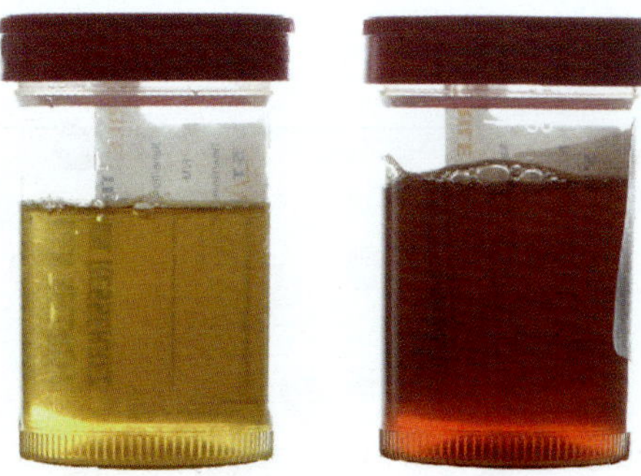

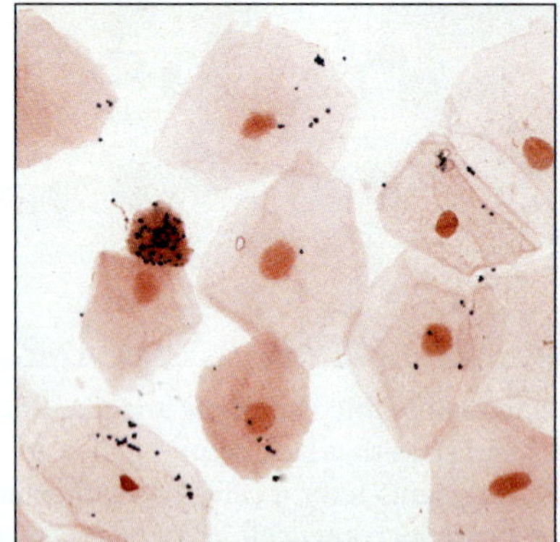

Figure 1.58 Hemoglobinuria from intravascular hemolysis. *Top panel:* The urine sample on the left is normal. The sample to the right demonstrates the red appearance of urine due to hemoglobinuria during acute hemolysis. *Bottom panel:* Urine positive for hemosiderin in a patient with intravascular hemolysis. This urine sample is stained for iron with Perl stain. Hemosiderin deposition (*blue*) in sloughed epithelial cells of renal tubules occurs in patients who have had intravascular hemolysis within the last 7 days. This test may be useful in detecting a recent episode of hemolysis that has resolved.

Figure 1.59 *Top panel:* Hemoglobinuria in paroxysmal nocturnal hemoglobinuria (PNH). Urine taken over the course of days in a patient with PNH. The varying color depends on the degree of hemolysis at any one time. First morning urines tend to be darker, as well as urines taken during intercurrent illnesses, due to increased intravascular hemolysis. (Courtesy Dr. J. Crookston.) *Bottom panel:* Flow cytometry histogram of granulocytes marked for CD59. CD59 is a protein anchored by a GPI anchor that is deficient in individuals with PNH. This histogram demonstrates a population of negative CD59 granulocytes (PNH cells; PNH type I cells) and positive CD59 granulocytes (normal cells; PNH type III cells) in a patient with PNH. No population exists in the middle with weak CD59 expression (PNH type II cells). (Courtesy J. Davidson and R. Sutherland)

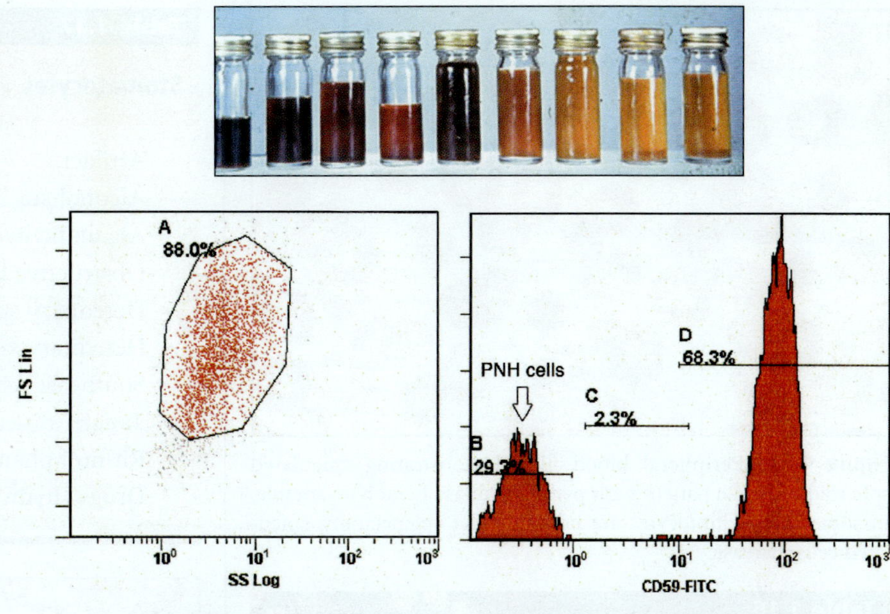

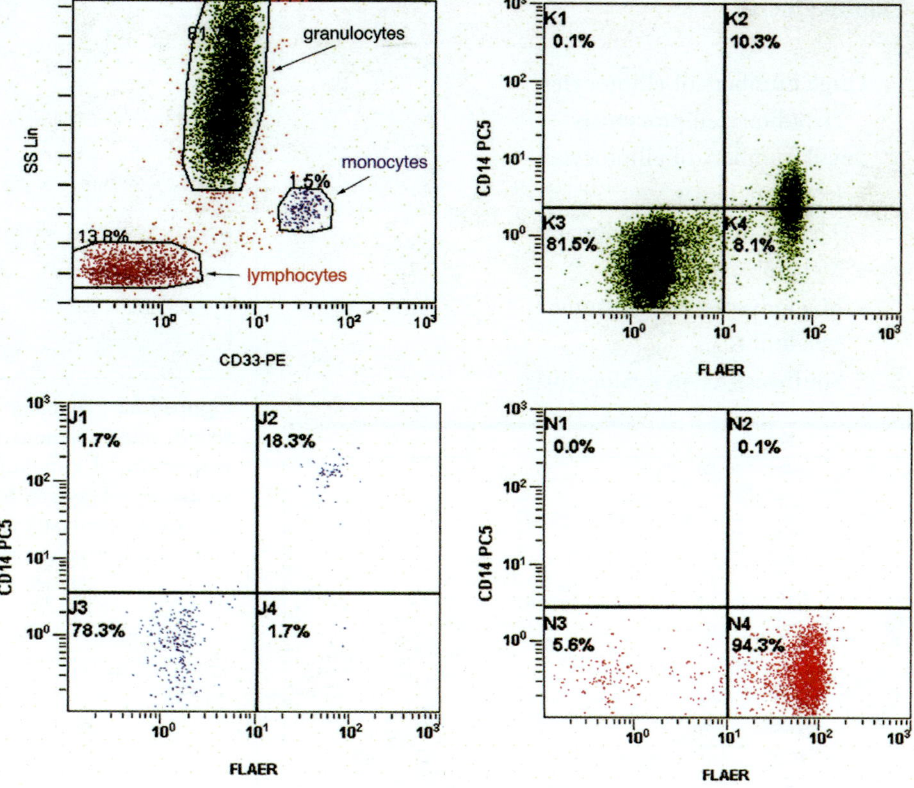

Figure 1.60 Flow cytometry histogram of WBC marked for fluorescent aerolysin (FLAER). The aerolysin stains positive those cells that have a GPI anchor. PNH cells do not have this and will stain negative. The green cells are granulocytes, the blue cells monocytes, and the red cells lymphocytes. A large population of granulocytes and monocytes stain negative for FLAER, consistent with PNH cells. (Courtesy J. Davidson and R. Sutherland.)

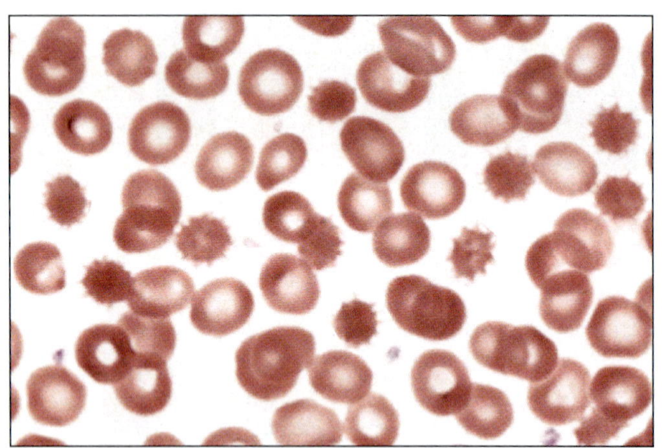

Figure 1.61 Peripheral blood film demonstrating spiculated spheroid cells in a patient with pyruvate kinase hemolytic anemia. In some cases, elliptocytes are present. After splenectomy, spiculated cells increase.

Table 1.16

Elliptocytosis

- Large numbers of elliptocytes
  - Hereditary elliptocytosis
- Small numbers of elliptocytes
  - Iron deficiency
  - Thalassemia trait and major
  - Megaloblastic anemia
  - Myelodysplastic syndrome
  - Myelofibrosis
  - Southeast Asian ovalocytosis

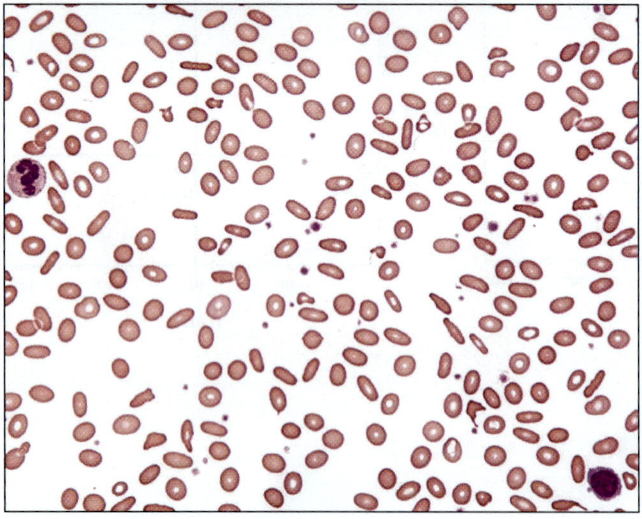

Figure 1.62 Hereditary elliptocytosis. Elliptocytes and ovalocytes are present in this blood film from a case of hereditary elliptocytosis. Elliptocytes are elongated with rounded edges (as opposed to sharp edges in sickle cells).

Table 1.17

Stomatocytes

- Artifact
- Alcoholism
- Alcoholic liver disease
- Obstructive liver disease
- Hereditary stomatocytosis
- Hereditary xerocytosis
- Southeast Asian ovalocytosis
- Tangier disease
- Rh-null phenotype
- Drugs (hydroxyurea)

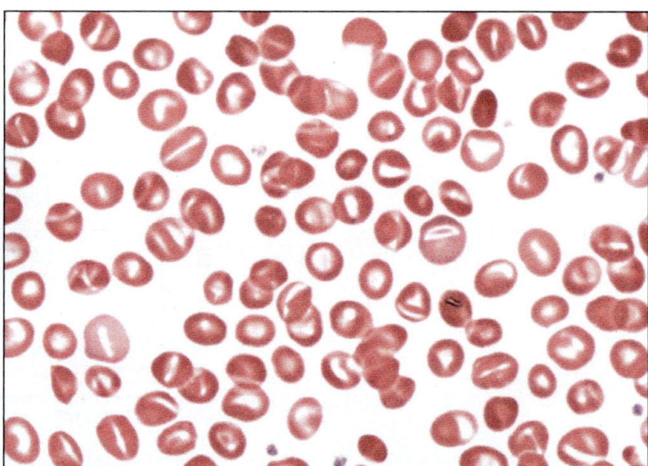

Figure 1.63 Hereditary stomatocytosis. The red blood cells in this blood smear demonstrate slit-like central pallor, creating the appearance of a mouth (*stoma* in Greek), from which the name stomatocytes derives. Hereditary stomatocytosis may demonstrate 10% to 50% stomatocytes on the peripheral blood film. Ovalocytes and macrocytes also may be present.

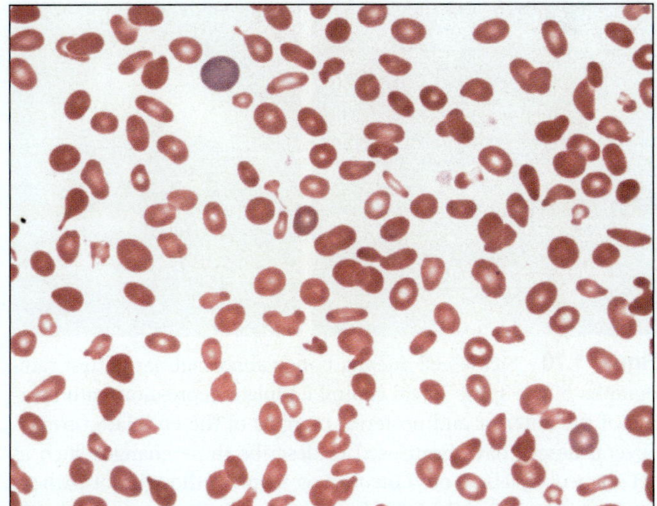

Figure 1.64 Hereditary pyropoikilocytosis. Peripheral blood film in patient with hereditary pyropoikilocytosis. Significant variations in size and shape are present: teardrops, fragments, microspherocytes, elliptocytes, and small pieces and buds of red blood cells. Heating the specimen increases this effect. These morphologic changes occur at a lower temperature than with samples from people without this disorder.

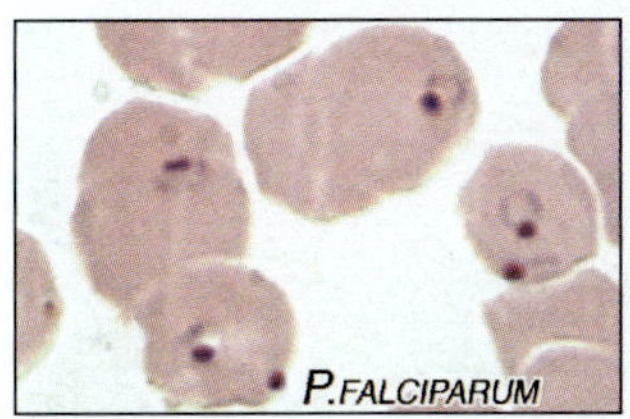

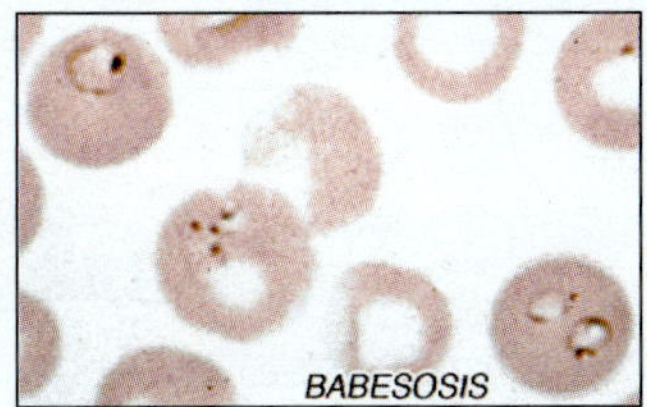

Figure 1.65 Infectious organisms in the peripheral blood that can cause hemolysis: On the left red blood cell inclusions of *Falciparum malaria* are seen. On the right *Babesiosis* is seen within the red blood cells. *Bartonellosis* causes hemolytic anemia as well.

Table 1.18
Sickling disorders

- HBSS
- HBSC
- HbSβ-thalassemia
- HbSD
- HbSO-Arab
- HbS/C Harlem
- HbS/S Antilles
- HbS/Lepore
- HbC/C Harlem
- HbS Antilles (heterozygous)
- HbS Oman (heterozygous)

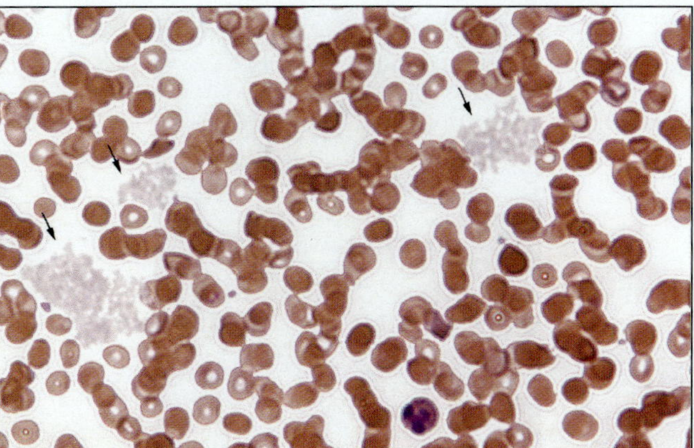

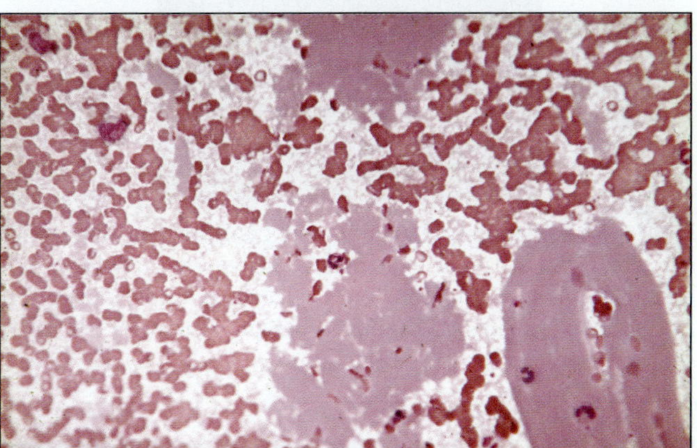

Figure 1.66 Cryoglobulinemia. Precipitated cryoglobulins (*arrows, top panel*) may appear as white spots on top of red blood cells, usually at the edges of the erythrocyte, and can be easily mistaken for bite cells and blister cells. Purplish clouds of precipitated cryoglobulins overlapping onto the red blood cells are displayed in both of these blood smears.

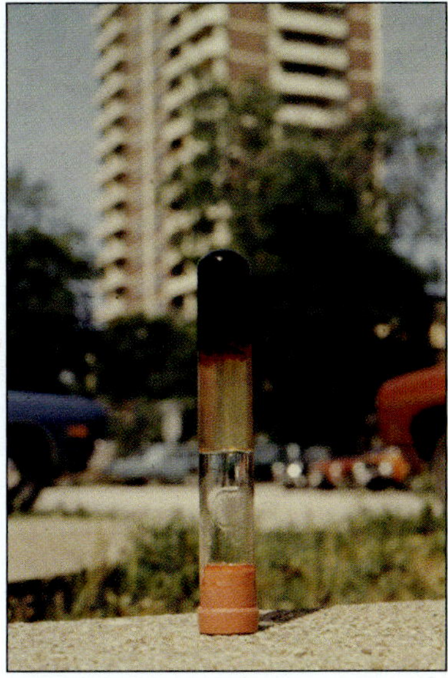

Figure 1.67 Picture of centrifuged blood from a patient with a high IgA paraprotein. The IgA paraprotein has crosslinked and become hyperviscous so that the red blood cells at the bottom of the tube are not able to pass through the plasma despite the tube being inverted. (Courtesy Dr. I. Quirt.)

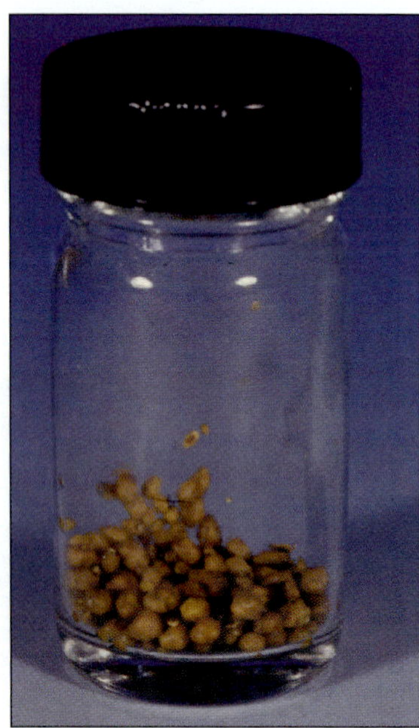

Figure 1.68 Sickle cell anemia and cholelithiasis. Gallstones extracted from a patient with chronic hemolysis from sickle cell disease. These stones may provoke cholecystitis. Cholelithiasis also can occur in patients with other hereditary hemolytic disorders, such as hereditary spherocytosis. (Courtesy Dr. N.F. Olivieri.)

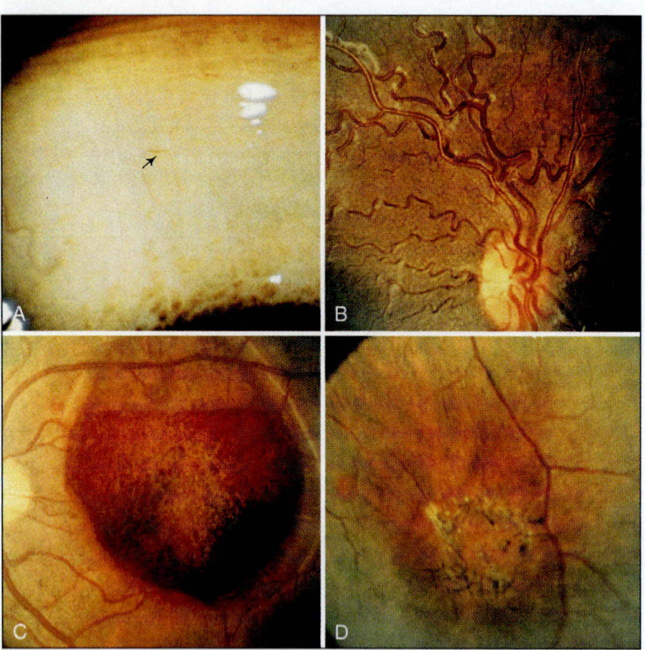

Figure 1.69 Sickle cell retinal changes. **A.** "Comma" vascular sign: superficial conjunctival vessel that contains densely packed sickle cells (*arrow*). **B.** Widened veins and tortuous large retinal vessels. **C.** Large preretinal hemorrhage of approximately 2 weeks' duration. **D.** Old pigmented chorioretinal scar.

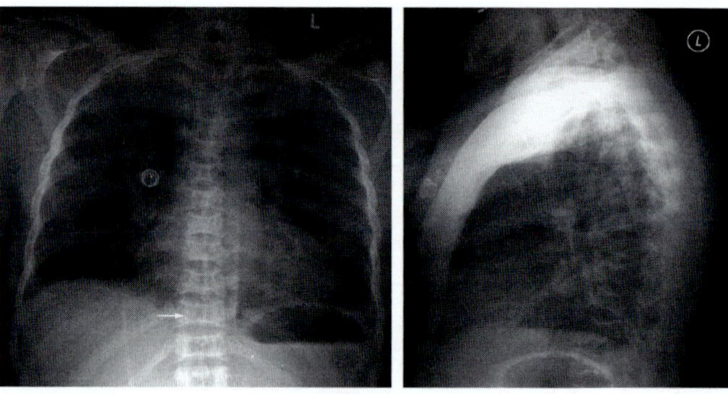

Figure 1.70 Sickle cell anemia boney abnormalities. Chest radiographs of the spine reveal central endplate depression with sparing of the anterior and posterior margins of the endplate (*arrow*). Several names have been used to describe these changes such as "H-shaped vertebra" or "Lincoln-Log Sign." Although not pathognomonic, these radiologic findings are seen most often in sickle cell disease. In addition, the gastric air bubble occupies most of the region under the left hemidiaphragm extending to the left lateral thoracic cage, suggesting the absence of a spleen.

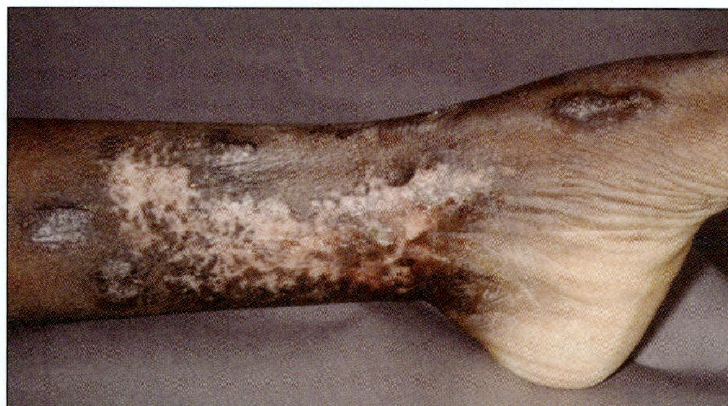

Figure 1.71 Sickle cell anemia skin ulcers. The most common site of skin ulcers in sickle cell anemia is the lower limb, often over bony prominences. The ulcerations often have no antecedent trauma and can progress over time to extend into the dermis and subcutaneous tissue. (Courtesy Dr. N.F. Olivieri.)

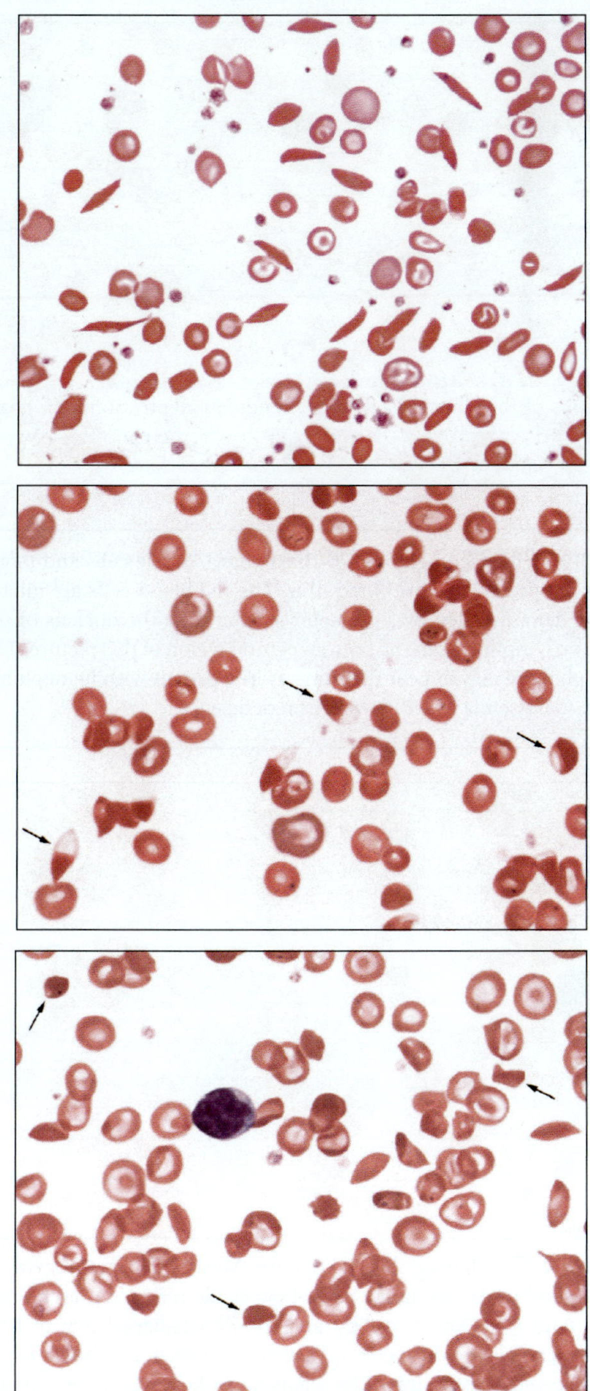

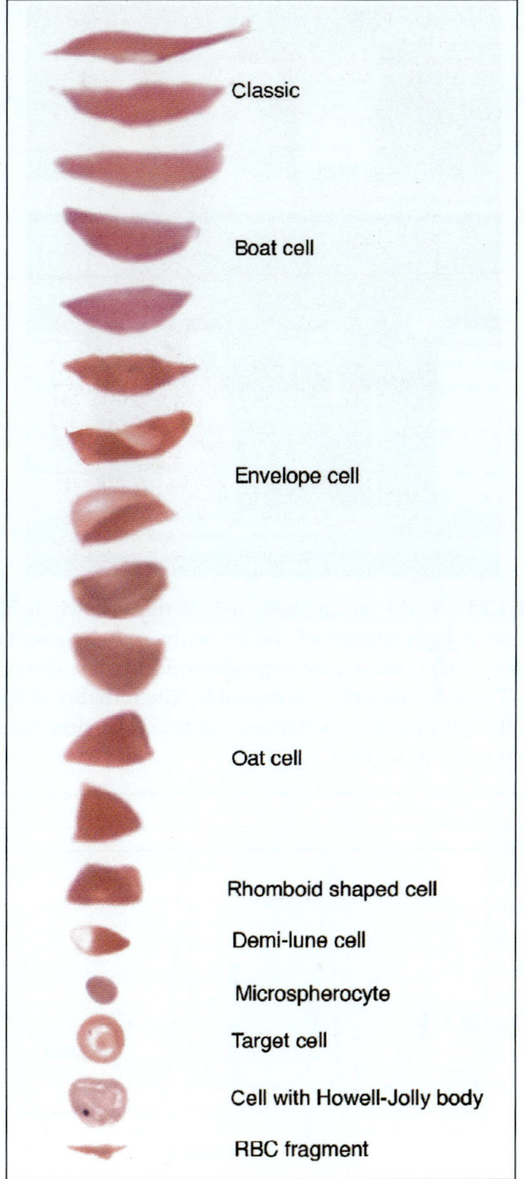

Figure 1.73   Sickle cells. A composite figure taken from different sickle cell anemia cases showing various types of sickle cells.

Figure 1.72   Sickle cell anemia. *Top panel:* Peripheral blood film of hemoglobin SS (HbS disease). The numerous elongated erythrocytes with sharp points are classic sickle cells. Sickle cells that appear folded over are called *envelope cells.* Target cells are present, in this case because of hyposplenism from the splenic infarction that occurs in HbSS patients. Howell-Jolly bodies may be seen as well. *Middle panel:* Peripheral blood film in patient with HbSS, demonstrating sickle cells with Hb concentrated at one end and absent at the other, called hemi-lunes (*arrows*), a finding seen in HbSS or HbSC. *Bottom panel:* Peripheral blood film in patient with HbSS, demonstrating short, stubby, and rhomboid-shaped sickle cells called oat and boat cells (*arrows*).

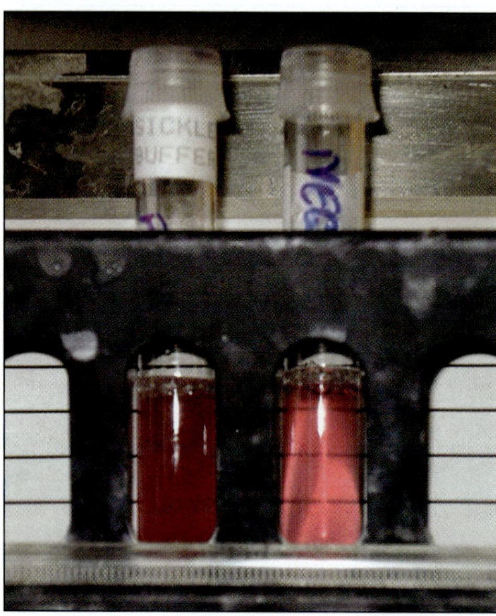

Figure 1.74 Sickle cell solubility test. In this test, whole blood is added to a high phosphate buffer with saponin and sodium dithionite, which causes the hemoglobin to become deoxyhemoglobin. Deoxyhemoglobin S is insoluble. The turbidity of the sample on the left indicates the presence of HbS. The clear sample on the right contains no HbS.

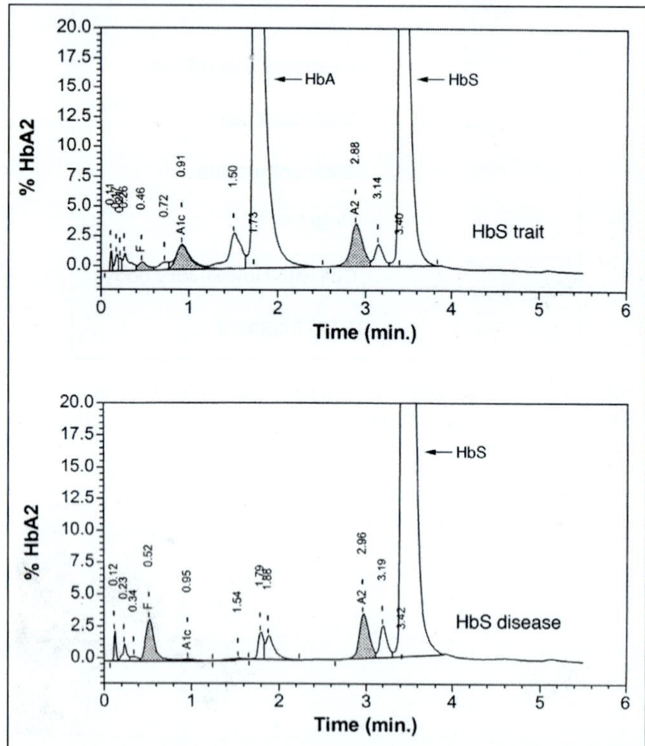

Figure 1.75 *Top panel:* High-performance liquid chromatography (HPLC) sample demonstrating hemoglobin S trait (HbA = 60%, HbS = 40%). HPLC can separate HbS from HbD/G/Lepore, which are seen in the same band on alkaline Hb electrophoresis. *Lower panel:* HPLC sample demonstrating hemoglobin S disease (HbS = 90%). Note the absence of hemoglobin A.

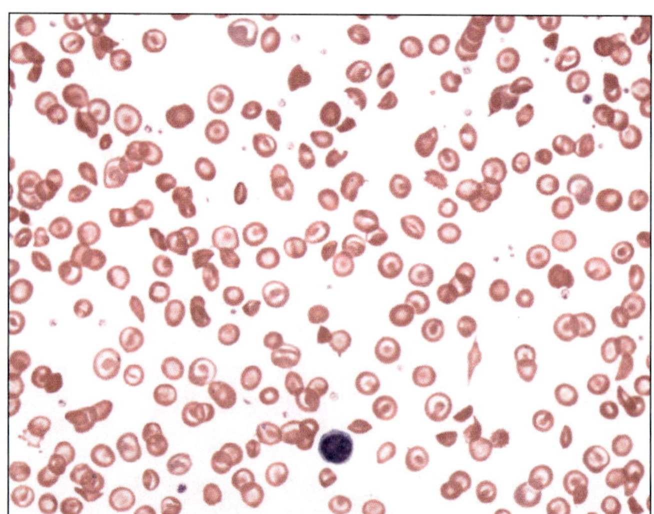

Figure 1.76 Hemoglobin S/β-thalassemia. Sickle cells and target cells are present in this blood film. The red blood cells are microcytic, demonstrated by a diameter smaller than the nucleus of the mature lymphocyte in the bottom central region of this picture. The morphology may appear the same as in a patient with hemoglobin SS/α-thalassemia or HBSS with iron deficiency.

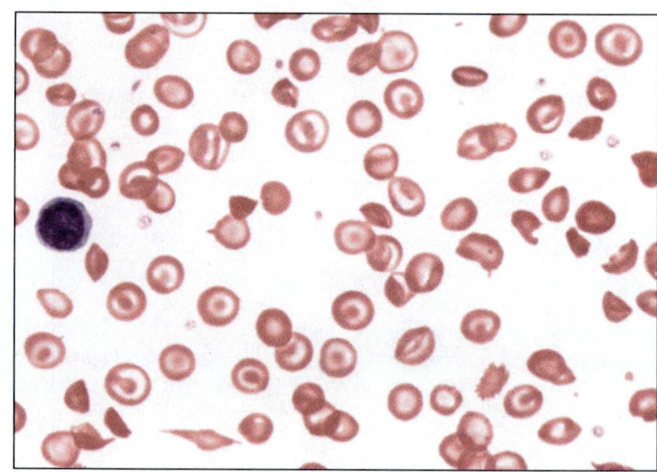

Figure 1.77 Hemoglobin SC disease. Most of the erythrocytes in this blood smear are target cells. Few sickle cells are present, and they tend to be short, stubby, and rhomboid-shaped (oat or boat cells). Irregularly contracted cells also are present. Rarely, hemoglobin C crystals are visible. The diagnosis of hemoglobin SC disease can be difficult using peripheral blood films alone because few sickle cells are present. It may appear very similar to HbC disease. These patients may not demonstrate hyposplenic changes and may have fewer nucleated red cells than do HbSS patients.

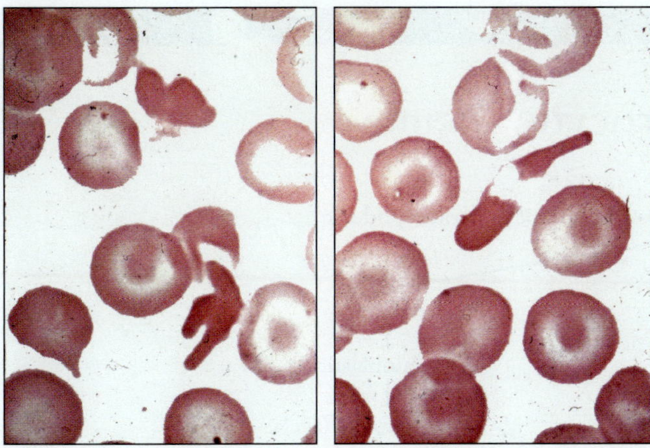

Figure 1.78 HbSC disease. The condensation of Hb crystals in this blood film produces dark, blunt protuberances and other distortions. (From Diggs LW, Bell A. 1965. Intraerythrocytic crystals in sickle cell-hemoglobin C disease, American Society of Hematology, with permission.)

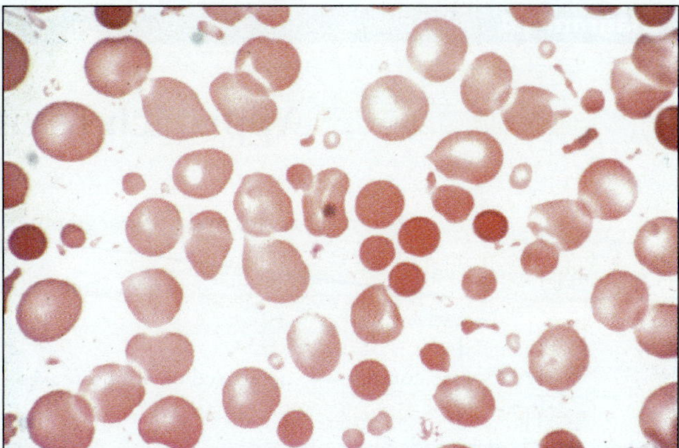

Figure 1.80 Peripheral blood film of thermal injury. This slide, from a patient with severe burns, demonstrates microspherocytes and pieces of red blood cells that can appear as barbell shapes, rod-like cells, or budding erythrocytes. Even these small pieces may retain a central pallor. Similar morphologic changes occur in hereditary pyropoikilocytosis. Clinical history will differentiate these two processes.

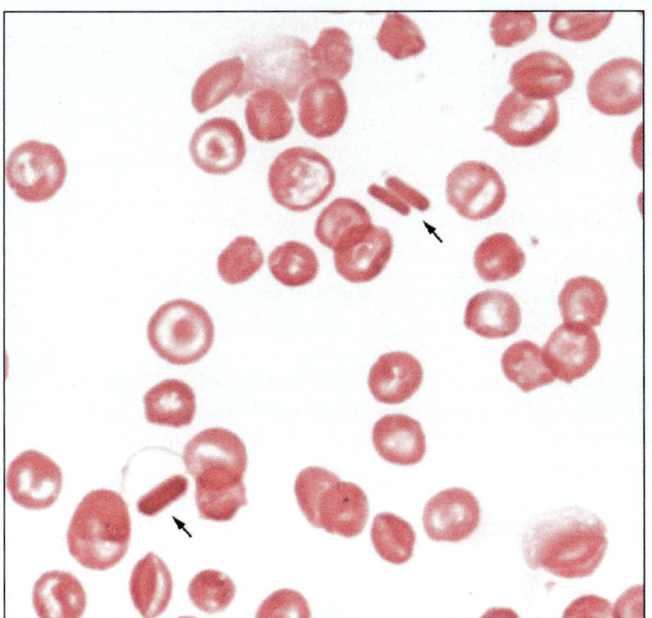

Figure 1.79 Hemoglobin C disease. Target cells, irregularly contracted cells, and hemoglobin C crystals are present with microcytosis in this blood smear. Hemoglobin C crystals (*arrows*) are seen in cells that are otherwise empty of hemoglobin. Hemoglobin C crystals are an uncommon finding. More frequent are target cells, irregularly contracted erythrocytes, and microcytosis. (Courtesy Dr. A. Chesney.)

Diagram 1.4

Approach to macrocytic anemia

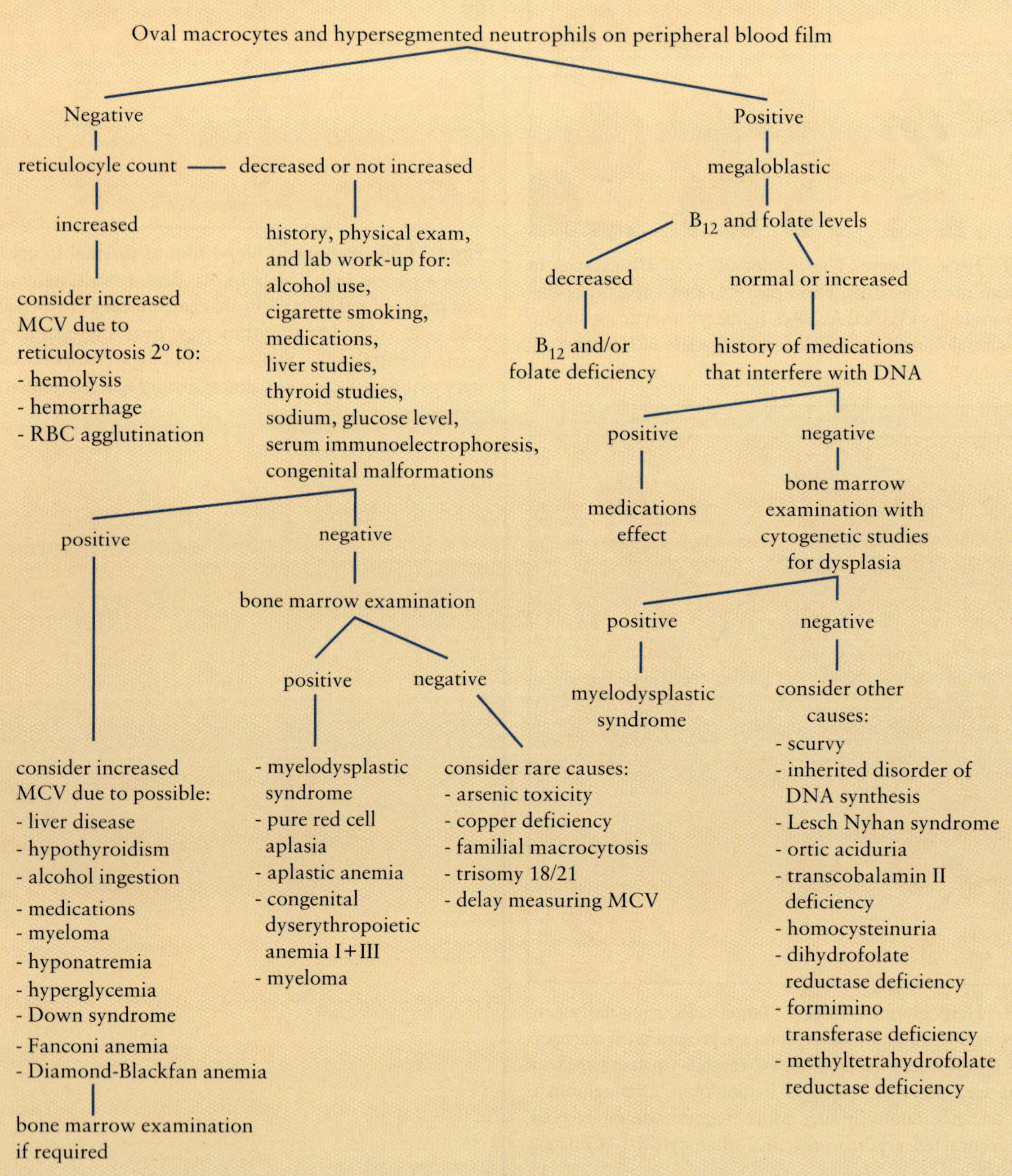

Oval macrocytes and hypersegmented neutrophils on peripheral blood film

Negative
- reticulocyle count ——— decreased or not increased
- increased
  - consider increased MCV due to reticulocytosis 2° to:
    - hemolysis
    - hemorrhage
    - RBC agglutination

history, physical exam, and lab work-up for: alcohol use, cigarette smoking, medications, liver studies, thyroid studies, sodium, glucose level, serum immunoelectrophoresis, congenital malformations

- **positive**
  - consider increased MCV due to possible:
    - liver disease
    - hypothyroidism
    - alcohol ingestion
    - medications
    - myeloma
    - hyponatremia
    - hyperglycemia
    - Down syndrome
    - Fanconi anemia
    - Diamond-Blackfan anemia

    bone marrow examination if required

- **negative**
  - bone marrow examination
    - **positive**
      - myelodysplastic syndrome
      - pure red cell aplasia
      - aplastic anemia
      - congenital dyserythropoietic anemia I+III
      - myeloma
    - **negative**
      - consider rare causes:
        - arsenic toxicity
        - copper deficiency
        - familial macrocytosis
        - trisomy 18/21
        - delay measuring MCV

Positive
- megaloblastic
  - B_{12} and folate levels
    - **decreased**
      - B_{12} and/or folate deficiency
    - **normal or increased**
      - history of medications that interfere with DNA
        - **positive**
          - medications effect
        - **negative**
          - bone marrow examination with cytogenetic studies for dysplasia
            - **positive**
              - myelodysplastic syndrome
            - **negative**
              - consider other causes:
                - scurvy
                - inherited disorder of DNA synthesis
                - Lesch Nyhan syndrome
                - ortic aciduria
                - transcobalamin II deficiency
                - homocysteinuria
                - dihydrofolate reductase deficiency
                - formimino transferase deficiency
                - methyltetrahydrofolate reductase deficiency

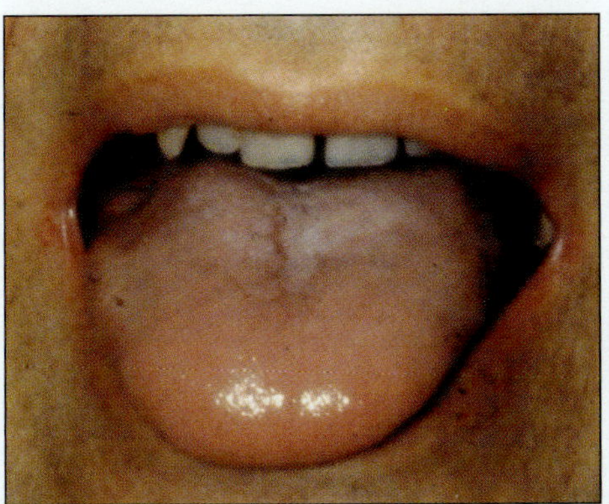

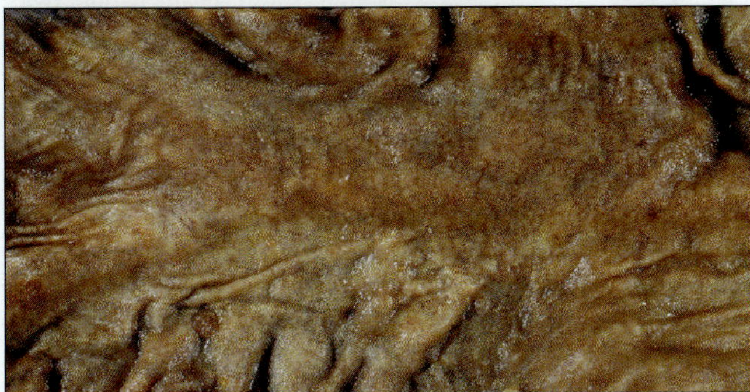

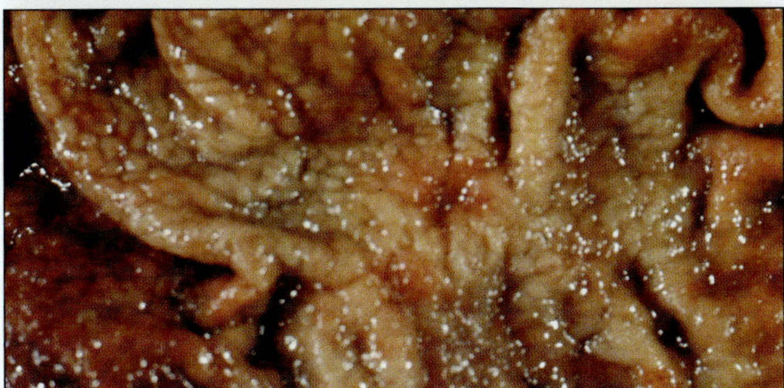

Figure 1.81　Smooth tongue of pernicious anemia. *Top panel:* The loss of papillae in pernicious anemia causes the tongue to be smooth, usually most marked along the edges. The tongue also may be red and painful. Occasionally, red patches are observed on the edges of the dorsum of the tongue. *Middle panel:* Atrophic gastritis of pernicious anemia. Gross pathologic sample of stomach from a patient with pernicious anemia and vitamin B_{12} deficiency. Atrophy of the fundus is present. Classic pernicious anemia is caused by the failure of gastric parietal cells to produce intrinsic factor to permit the absorption of vitamin B_{12}. This disease is associated with gastric atrophy and achlorhydria. Coexistent iron deficiency is common because achlorhydria decreases iron absorption. Pernicious anemia is associated with an increased incidence of gastric carcinoma. *Lower panel:* normal gastric mucosa for comparison.

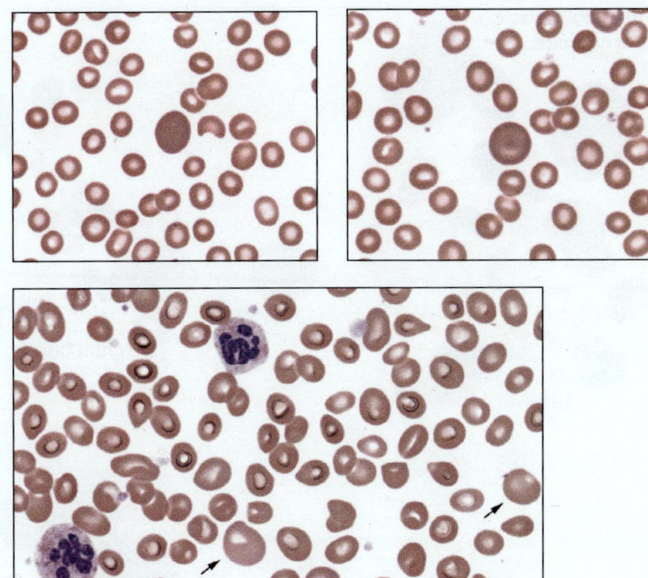

Figure 1.82　Macrocytic RBCs and hypersegmented neutrophils. *Top left panel:* Peripheral blood film demonstrating oval macrocytes. The cells are larger than normocytic red blood cells (MCV >100 fl). The rule of thumb is that oval macrocytes are larger than the condensed nucleus of a mature lymphocyte. The cells should not be polychromatophilic (blue/purple staining), which differentiates them from reticulocytes. Oval macrocytes usually occur in megaloblastic states. Because the MCV is an average of cell size, macrocytes can be present in the peripheral blood film with a normocytic MCV (< 100 fl). Accordingly, the finding of oval macrocytes on the peripheral blood film with a normal MCV still may be clinically significant. When oval macrocytes are present, the examiner should search for neutrophil abnormalities, including hyper- and hyposegmented nuclei or hypogranulated cytoplasm. The rule of thumb is that round macrocytes are larger than the condensed nucleus of a mature lymphocyte. The cells should not be polychromatophilic (blue/purple staining), which differentiates them from reticulocytes. *Right upper panel:* Blood film displaying a round macrocyte. Round macrocytes occur in several disorders. *Lower panel:* Peripheral blood film demonstrating hypersegmented neutrophils with oval macrocytes (*arrows*) in a patient with vitamin B_{12} deficiency. Neutrophils are hypersegmented when >5% of neutrophils have five lobes or more, or occasional neutrophils have six lobes or more.

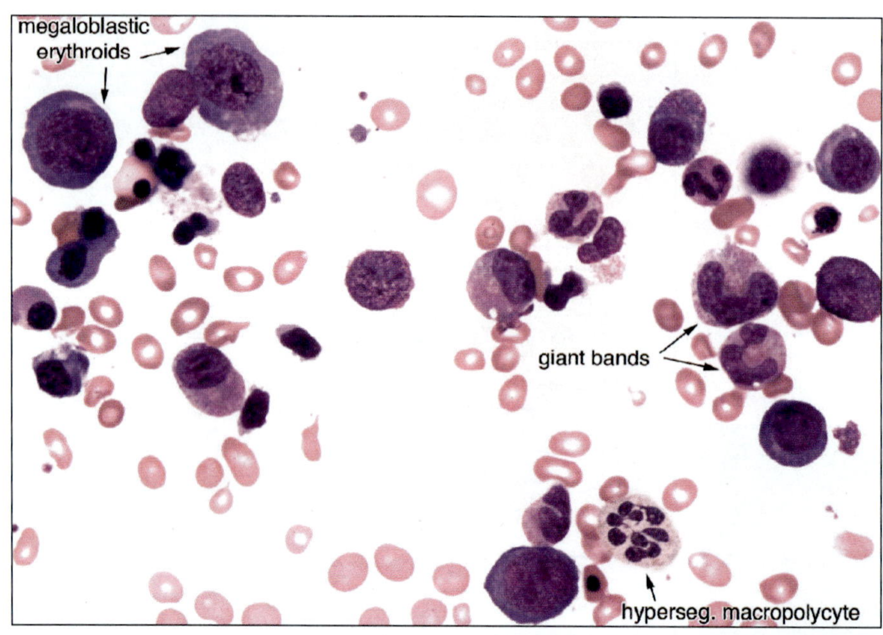

Figure 1.83 Bone marrow in megaloblastic anemia. Megaloblastic erythroid and granulocytic precursors are demonstrated in this marrow aspirate smear. Giant bands, twice the size of a normal counterpart and a hypersegmented macropolycyte are shown. Hypersegmented macropolycytes may be seen in megaloblastic states, myeloproliferative disorders, granulocyte colony-stimulating factor (G-CSF) administration, and chronic infections.

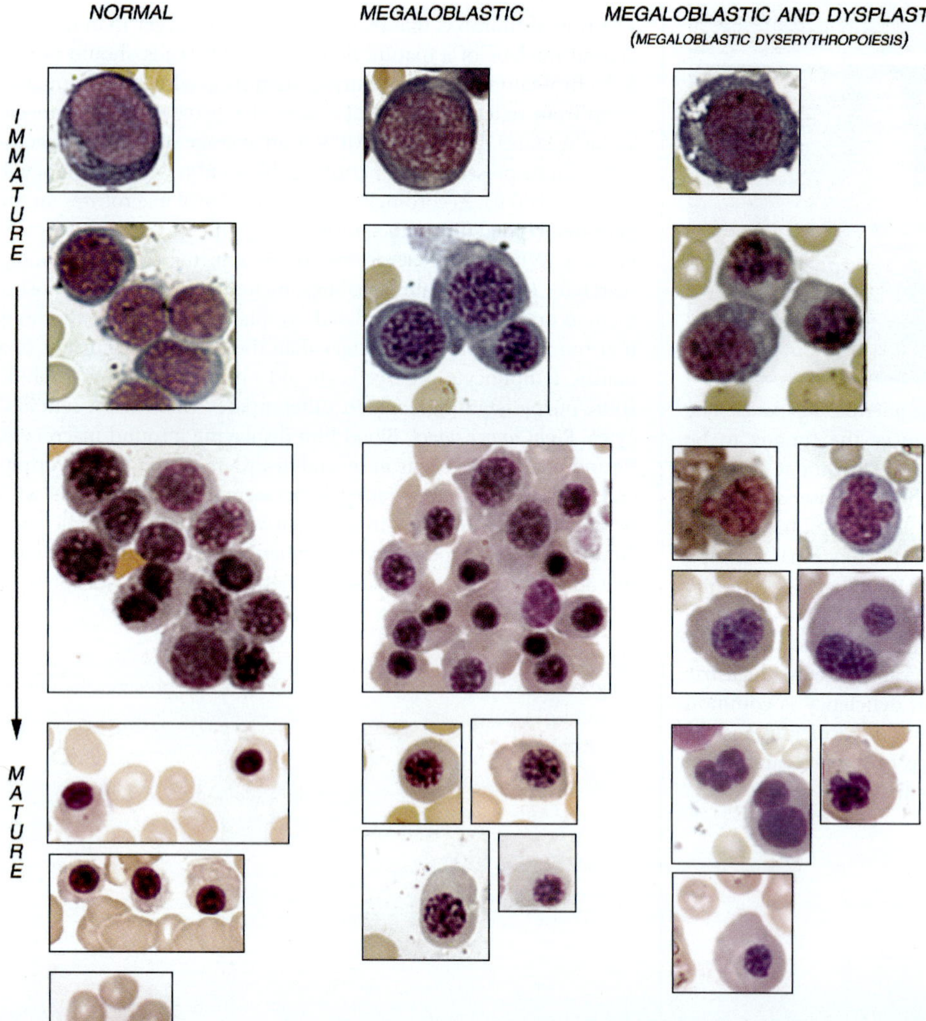

Figure 1.84 Megaloblastic versus dysplastic changes in marrow precursors. Composite figure from several cases comparing normal, megaloblastic and dysplastic findings in various stages of differentiation of the three major marrow cell lineages.

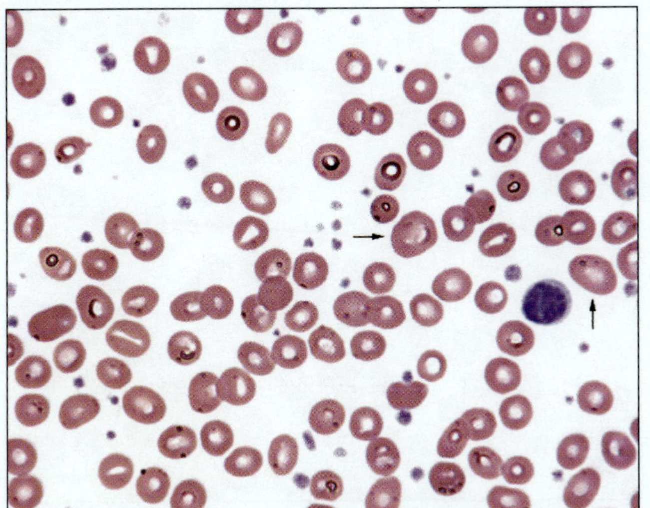

Figure 1.85 Macrocytic anemia in MDS. Macrocytic anemia and thrombocytosis are seen in this case of isolated del(5q) chromosome abnormality. Macrocytic RBCs (*arrows*) are larger than the nucleus of small mature lymphocytes, as shown here.

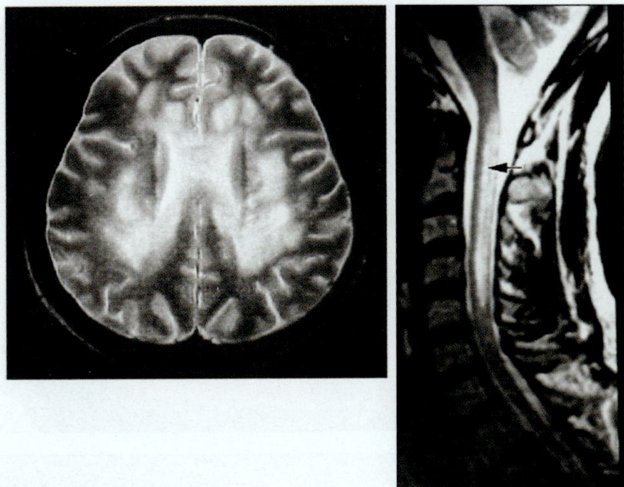

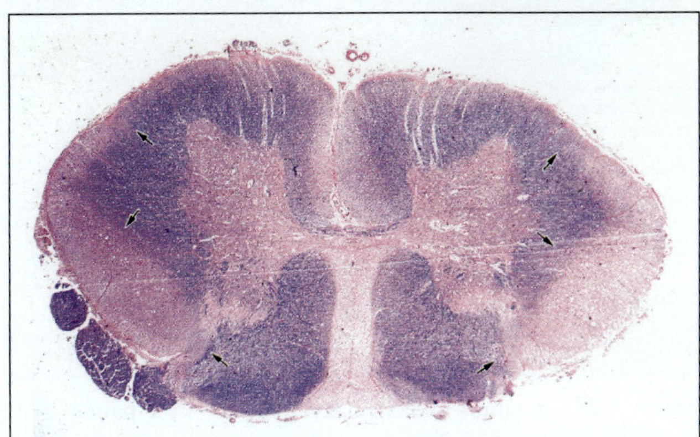

Figure 1.86 Demyelination in pernicious anemia. *Top left panel:* Head magnetic resonance imaging (MRI) showing a T2-weighted image with multiple high signal foci in the periventricular white matter. This is nonspecific but compatible with demyelination associated with vitamin B_{12} deficiency. *Top right panel:* T2-weighted image of the cervical spine displaying high signal in the posterior aspect of the cervical cord (*arrow*). This appearance is consistent with demyelination. *Bottom panel:* Subacute combined degeneration of spinal cord in vitamin B_{12} deficiency. Cross-section of autopsy spinal cord showing spongiform changes and myelin and axonal destruction in the posterior and lateral columns (*arrows*). This neurologic complication of vitamin B_{12} deficiency may precede any hematologic abnormality. Elevated serum or urinary levels of methylmalonic acid and homocysteine are sensitive for the diagnosis of vitamin B_{12} deficiency and usually precede the development of hematologic abnormalities and reductions in the serum vitamin B_{12} level. (Courtesy Dr. J. Bilbao.)

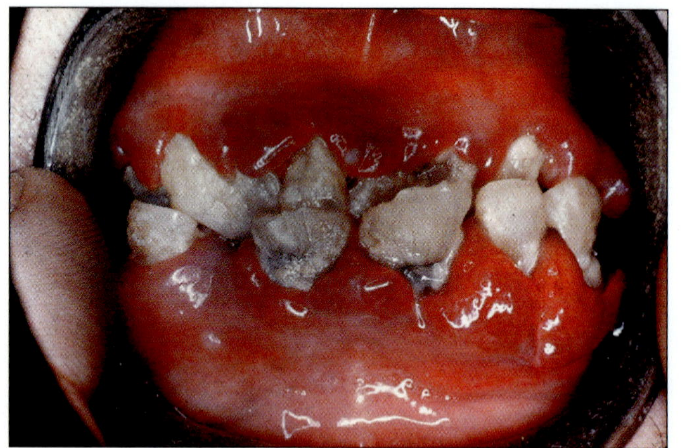

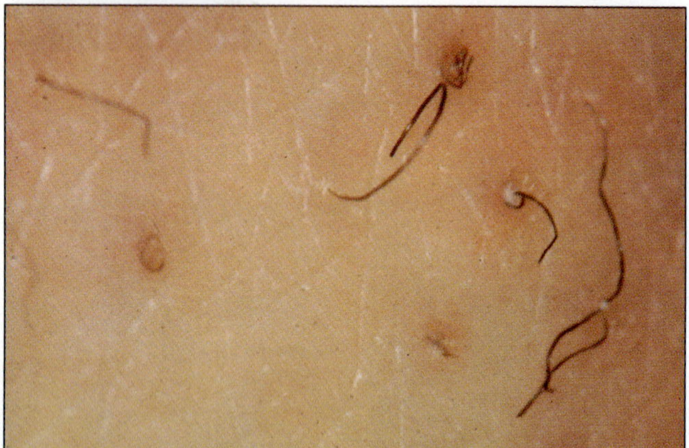

Figure 1.87   Vitamin C deficiency (scurvy) in a patient with megaloblastic anemia. The gums demonstrate gingival hemorrhage; corkscrew hairs with perifollicular hemorrhages are visible on a close-up view of skin in this patient suffering from vitamin C deficiency. (Courtesy Drs. J. Crookston and D. Amato.)

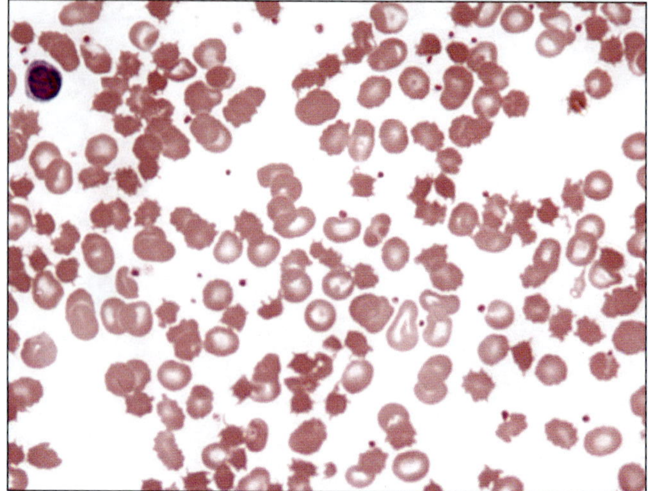

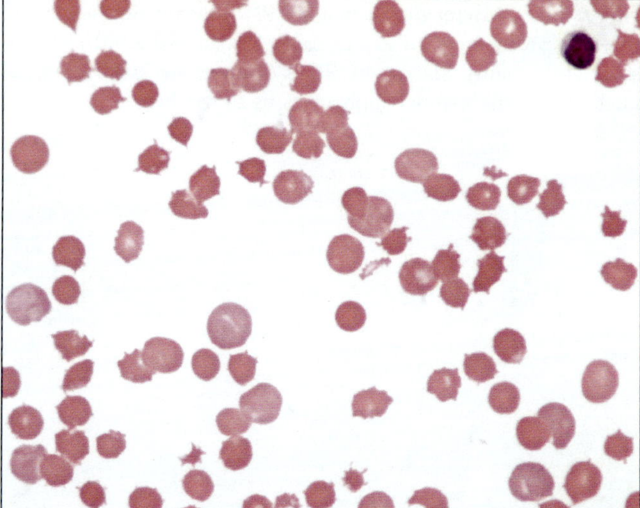

Figure 1.88   Acanthocytes and liver disease. *Top panel:* Peripheral blood film demonstrating acanthocytes, alternatively called *spur cells.* The acanthocytes do not have central pallor and are smaller than the normocytic red blood cell. They have long thin projections, some with bulbous or pointy edges, which are unevenly distributed around the surface of the red blood cell. Note target cells as well. *Bottom panel:* This peripheral blood film demonstrates many acanthocytes in a patient with severe liver disease and hemolysis. This disorder is known as *spur-cell hemolytic anemia.*

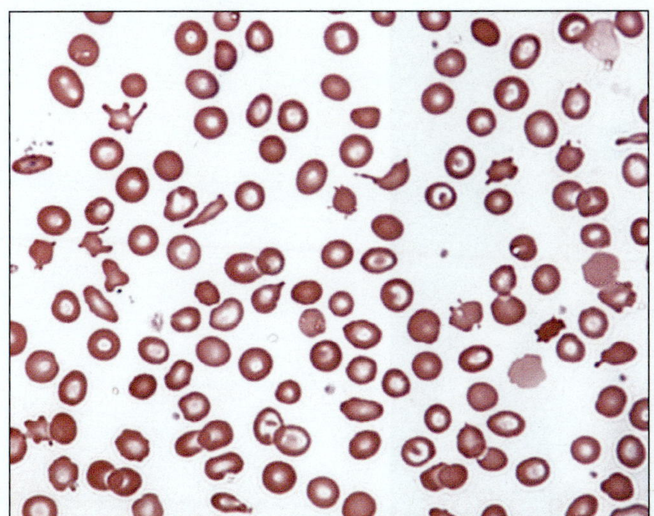

Figure 1.89 Obstructive jaundice and acanthocytes. Peripheral blood film of target cells in a patient with obstructive jaundice. A central area of hemoglobin is surrounded by a clear area and then encircled by an outside hemoglobinated ring, creating a target-like appearance.

Table 1.19

Acanthocytes

Large numbers of acanthocytes
- Advanced liver disease
- Spur cell hemolytic anemia
- Abetalipoproteinemia
- Hypobetalipoproteinemia, homozygous
- McLeod phenotype
- In(Lu) phenotype
- Choreoacanthycytosis

Small numbers of acanthocytes
- Postsplenectomy
- Hypothyroidism
- Panhypopituitarism
- Vitamin E deficiency
- Malnutrition
- Thalassemia
- Iron deficiency
- Psoriasis

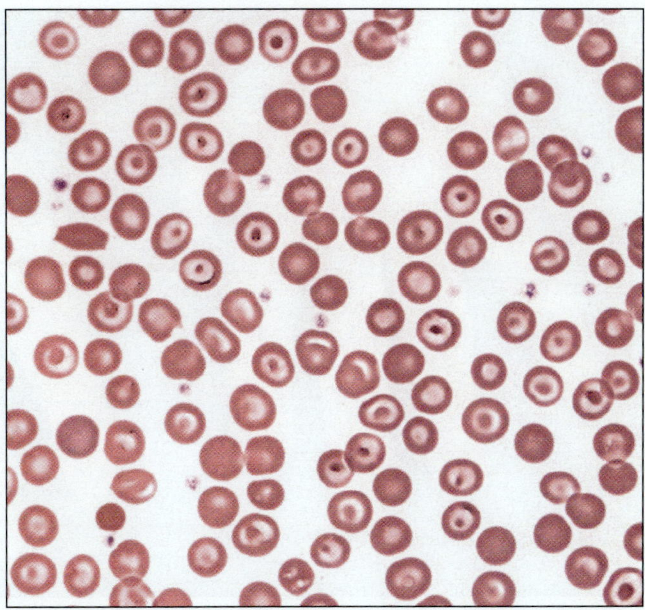

Figure 1.90 Liver disease. Patients with liver disease and obstructive jaundice have macrocytosis and target cells caused from increased cholesterol and/or phospholipids deposition on red blood cell membranes. This blood smear, from a case of alcoholic liver disease, shows prominent numbers of macrocytic targets cells. The macrocytosis associated with alcoholism may be multifactorial and include poor nutrition with a resulting folate or vitamin B_{12} deficiency and direct toxicity of alcohol on the marrow.

Table 1.20

Target cells

Microcytic
- Hemoglobin E heterozygous + homozygous
- β-Thalassemia trait + major
- α-Thalassemia trait
- HbH disease
- HbC trait + disease
- Hb Lepore heterozygous + homozygous
- HbO Arab disease
- HbD disease
- Iron defciency
- Hb Lepore trait

Normocytic or macrocytic
- Obstructive jaundice
- Liver disease
- LCAT deficiency (Lecithin-cholesterol acyl transferase deficiency)
- HbSC disease
- Hyposplenic state
- HbO Arab disease

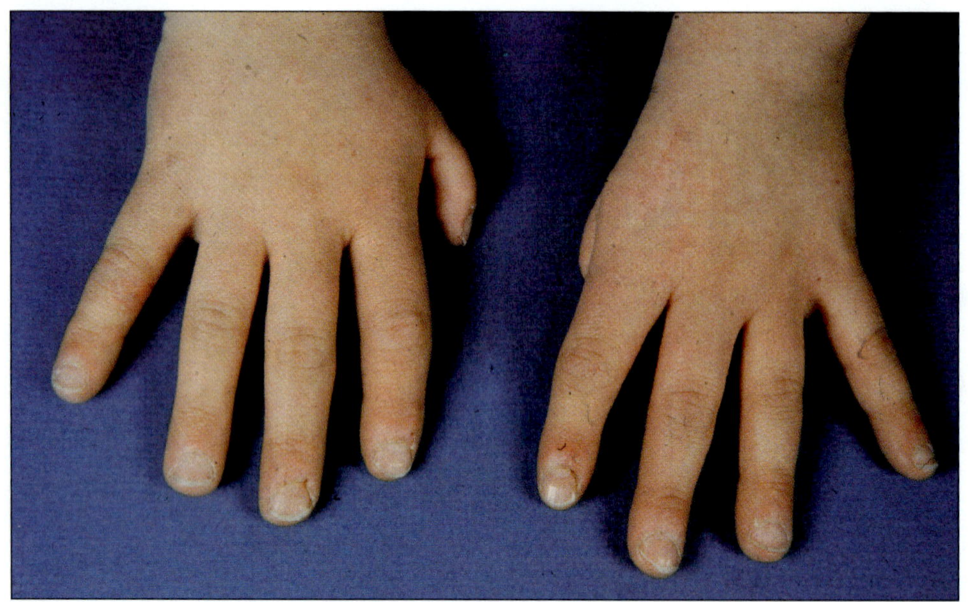

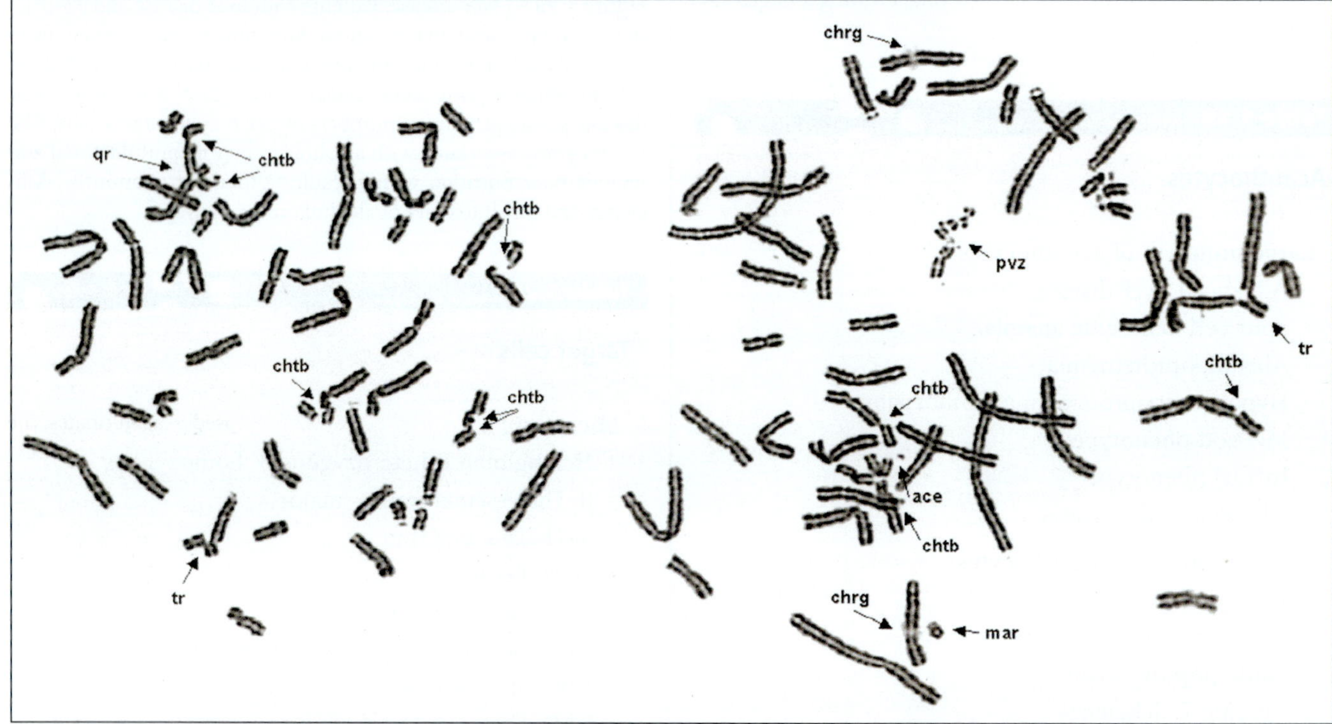

Figure 1.91 Fanconi syndrome. *Upper panel:* Hands in a patient with Fanconi syndrome. Bilateral thumb hypoplasia is present. Other congenital anomalies may occur: skin pigmentation changes, short stature, upper limb abnormalities, renal malformations, ophthalmologic problems, hypogonadism, and cardiac malformations. Thrombocytopenia and leukopenia precede macrocytic anemia. Eventually, aplastic anemia develops. (Courtesy Dr. I. Quirt.) *Lower panel:* Spontaneous chromosomal breakage in Fanconi syndrome. Chromosomal karyotyping of peripheral blood lymphocytes in a patient with Fanconi anemia. Increased spontaneous chromosomal breakage may be seen, but on exposure to mitomycin C or diepoxybutane (*right panel*) increased chromosomal breaks and radial chromosomal fusions occur. (Courtesy M. Chago.)

Table 1.21

Rouleaux

- Increased plasma proteins (polyclonal or other proteins)
  - Inflammatory state
  - Infection
- Increased plasma proteins (monoclonal)
  - MGUS (monoclonal gammopathy of unknown significance)
  - Myeloma
  - Amyloidosis
  - Lymphoma

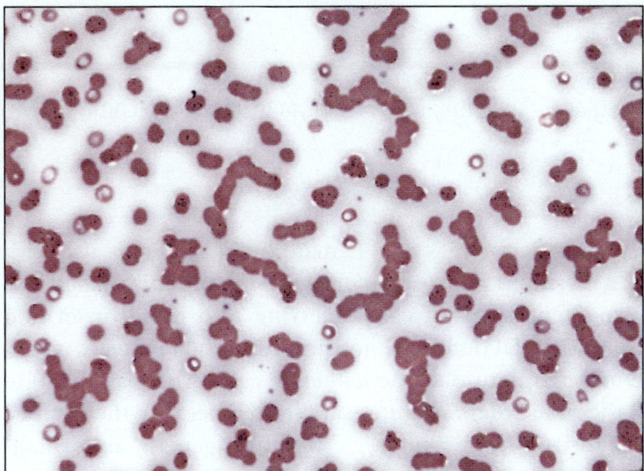

Figure 1.92 Peripheral blood film of rouleaux and background staining. Excessive amounts of acidic proteins (often immunoglobins produced by the myeloma cells) cause an increase in background bluish staining in blood smears (*upper panel:* Top slide is normal and bottom slide shows background staining). The abnormal proteins cause the RBCs to stick and arrange in columns (*lower panel*). Rouleaux have been defined as linear patterns of RBCs of at least four red blood cells. As opposed to agglutinates, the borders of the red blood cells still can be distinguished. It is important to look in the area of the slide (*middle*) where red blood cells nearly touch each other to identify rouleaux. Red blood cells normally have a rouleaux appearance in the thick, and sometimes thin ends of peripheral blood films.

Acute Leukemias

Douglas C. Tkachuk, MD, FRCPC, and Jan V. Hirschmann, MD

Acute leukemias are hematologic malignancies with increased numbers of myeloid or lymphoid blasts. The term "acute," historically referring to a rapid onset and promptly fatal outcome, now indicates the relatively undifferentiated nature of the leukemic cells. The classification of these disorders is quite complicated because they can be categorized by morphologic findings, genetic abnormalities, putative etiology, cell of origin, immunophenotypic qualities, and clinical characteristics. Two widely used classifications, one devised by a group of French, American, British (FAB) hematologists and the other by the World Health Organization (WHO), include these features in various ways, but both fundamentally divide acute leukemias into myeloid and lymphoid types, depending on the origin of the blast cell.

The overall annual incidence of these disorders in the general population is about 4 per 100,000, with approximately 70% of them being acute myeloid leukemia (AML). AML accounts for about 15% of childhood leukemias and for approximately 80% to 90% of acute leukemias in adults, with the median age at diagnosis being about 70 years. Acute lymphoblastic leukemia (ALL) is primarily a childhood disease, with the peak incidence between the ages of 2 to 3 years. It diminishes in frequency until it reaches a nadir from about the ages of 25 to 50, after which it increases to achieve a second, but minor, peak at ages older than 80.

The etiology of most cases is unknown, but a few patients have had previous exposure to ionizing radiation, cytotoxic chemotherapeutic agents, or benzene, which are considered causes. Several congenital diseases, such as Down syndrome, Bloom syndrome, and Turner syndrome, have an increased incidence of AML, as do certain types of bone marrow failure, such as Fanconi anemia and the Blackfan-Diamond syndrome. Patients with myelodysplastic and myeloproliferative disorders have varying, but elevated risks of developing AML. Heavy cigarette smoking also increases the incidence.

At the time of diagnosis, most patients with acute leukemia have nonspecific symptoms, such as fatigue, lethargy, and weight loss. Some complaints, such as dyspnea, angina, and dizziness arise from anemia. Fever from the disease itself or from an infection related to neutropenia can be the presenting manifestation. Bleeding, such as epistaxis or cutaneous ecchymoses, may occur from thrombocytopenia or from disseminated intravascular coagulation (DIC) in patients with acute promyelocytic leukemia. Bone pain and tenderness can develop from bone marrow expansion or direct periosteal involvement. Gums may swell from leukemic infiltration, especially in the monocytic types of AML.

On physical examination, lymph node enlargement and hepatosplenomegaly may be detectable, more commonly in ALL than in AML. Pallor from anemia and petechiae or ecchymoses from thrombocytopenia or DIC may be apparent. Approximately 5% to 20% of patients with AML and ALL have skin infiltration with leukemic cells (leukemia cutis) sometime during the course of their disease. In about 5% to 10% of these patients, the cutaneous lesions precede the diagnosis, in about 35% to 45% they are simultaneous, and in about 55% they appear afterwards, usually months later. They are typically erythematous or violaceous papules or nodules, but plaques, macules, palpable purpura, or ulcers also can occur. Patients with AML also may develop Sweet syndrome, characterized by an acute onset of fever and tender violaceous plaques that are often extensive, may affect the mucous membranes, and sometimes develop into blisters. Biopsies demonstrate mature neutrophils in the dermis. The fever and skin lesions disappear with systemic corticosteroid therapy, but recurrences are common with AML. Occasionally, prior to, or concurrent with, the diagnosis of AML, patients develop granulocytic sarcomas (also called chloromas), which are tumors of leukemic cells outside the bone marrow. These tumors can involve lymph nodes, skin, periosteum, extramedullary bone, and soft tissues.

They most often affect the subperiosteal bony structures of the skull, sternum, ribs, vertebrae, and pelvis.

At the time of presentation, the blood smear typically reveals decreased red cells and platelets, with the white count varying from leukopenia to very high numbers. A decrease in the number of mature neutrophils is common. Circulating blasts are usually detectable. *Aleukemic leukemia*, in which blasts are not apparent, is slightly more common in AML than ALL. With DIC, which occurs primarily with acute promyelocytic leukemia, microangiopathic features may be present, including red cell fragments, marked polychromatophilia, microcytes, and profound thrombocytopenia. In patients with preceding myelodysplastic syndromes, features of those disorders are typically apparent, such as hypolobulated and hypogranular neutrophils, giant and agranular platelets, and erythrocytic macrocytosis and poikilocytosis.

All patients with suspected leukemia should undergo bone marrow aspirate and biopsy, with cytogenetic analysis, histochemical analysis, and immunophenotyping done on the cells to delineate the proper classification of the leukemia. Usually, the presence of leukemia is obvious on bone marrow examination, which is typically hypercellular, with sheets of blasts replacing the normally maturing cells in the erythroid, myeloid, and megakaryocytic lines. The distinction between a myeloid or lymphoid origin of blasts is crucial to classifying acute leukemia. The presence in the cytoplasm of Auer rods—red, needle-like structures thought to be coalescences of primary granules—indicates a myeloblast. Otherwise, the distinction requires histochemical or phenotypic studies. The first step is to use stains specific for myeloperoxidase activity or for myeloid granules, such as Sudan black, and those that detect monocytic cells, such as α-naphthyl acetate or α-naphthyl butyrate. If fewer than 3% of blasts are positive using these stains, flow cytology is appropriate to distinguish between minimally differentiated AML and ALL, to detect megakaryoblastic leukemia, and to discriminate between B- and T-cell forms of ALL.

The criterion for the diagnosis of AML is that myeloblasts constitute at least 20% of the nucleated cells in the blood (based on counting 200 cells) or the bone marrow (counting 500 cells). The abnormal promyelocytes in acute promyelocytic leukemia and the promonocytes in AML with monocytic differentiation are considered blast equivalents.

ACUTE MYELOID LEUKEMIAS

These disorders are defined as clonal expansions of myeloid blasts, most commonly in the blood or bone marrow, but occasionally as tumor masses (myeloid or granulocytic sarcomas) in other tissues, such as skin and lymph nodes. The WHO classification (Table 2.1) separates AML into four general groups: (1) AML with recurrent genetic abnormalities; (2) AML with multilineage dysplasia; (3) AML and myelodysplastic syndromes, therapy-related; and (4) AML not otherwise categorized. A preceding classification developed by a collaboration among FAB hematologists (Table 2.2) divides AML into eight major subtypes, M0 through M7, defined by the nature of the blast cells and the degree of differentiation and maturation. In the WHO classification, the fourth group—AML not otherwise categorized—is a revision of the FAB types. The FAB classification recognizes three types of myeloid blasts: Type I lack cytoplasmic granules, but possess prominent nucleoli, a central nucleus, and uncondensed chromatin; type II are similar but have a few primary, azurophilic (reddish-purple) cytoplasmic granules; type III have >10 azurophilic cytoplasmic granules, but do not display a Golgi zone (perinuclear clear area), which is characteristic of promyelocytes.

AML with Recurrent Genetic Abnormalities

These disorders have genetic abnormalities, most commonly breaks in chromosomes in which the fragments join other chromosomes (translocations). These rearrangements create fusion genes that regulate the production of abnormal proteins.

AML with t(8;21)(q22;q22) constitutes about 5% to 10% of AML cases, predominantly in younger patients. Sometimes, granulocytic sarcoma is the presenting manifestation of the disease. The blasts are typically large, with abundant basophilic cytoplasm, often with Auer rods and numerous, sometimes very large, azurophilic granules. Dysplasia in the form of abnormal nuclear segmentation and cytoplasmic staining may be present in promyelocytes, myelocytes, and mature neutrophils.

AML with inv(16)(p13q22) or t(16;16)(p13;q22) is found in about 10% of cases of AML, primarily in younger patients. The bone marrow usually has elements of both granulocytic (including myeloblasts) and monocytic differentiation (including monoblasts, promonocytes, and monocytes), combined with abnormal eosinophils (acute myelomonocytic leukemia with abnormal eosinophils: M4eo in the FAB classification). Eosinophil precursors contain abnormally large, purple granules that can be sufficiently numerous to obscure the nuclei.

AML with t(15;17)(q22;q12) or acute promyelocytic leukemia constitutes about 5% of AML. Abnormal promyelocytes are present, either hypergranular or hypogranular (microgranular). These are equivalent to M3 and M3v in the FAB classification. DIC may occur in either form. In the hypergranular form, the cytoplasm is packed with pink, red, or purple granules that are usually large, but may be fine. Bundles of Auer rods are present in most cases. The nuclei, which may be bilobed, are irregular in size and variable in shape, and may be reniform (kidney-shaped).

AML with 11q23 abnormalities, which constitutes about 5% of AML, occurs at any age, but is more common in children. Some cases develop after treatment with topoisomerase

II inhibitors. Monocytic differentiation, with monoblasts and promonocytes predominating, is the most common morphologic pattern. Patients may have gum infiltration, leukemia cutis, and DIC. Monoblasts are large cells with round nuclei that usually contain lacy chromatin and large prominent nucleoli. The abundant basophilic and sometimes vacuolated cytoplasm may form pseudopods and contain scattered, fine azurophilic granules.

AML with Multilineage Dysplasia

This type of AML, which occurs primarily in older adults, has dysplasia in at least 50% of cells in two or more cell lines, including megakaryocytes. Abnormalities in granulopoiesis include hypogranular cytoplasm and hypolobulated or bizarrely segmented nuclei. Abnormal erythropoiesis is characterized by ringed sideroblasts, vacuolated cytoplasm, and nuclei that are multiple, fragmented, or megaloblastic. Abnormal megakaryocytes are small or have single-lobed or multiple, discrete nuclei.

AML and Myelodysplastic Syndromes, Therapy-Related

These occur as a consequence of cytotoxic drugs, radiation therapy, or both. One type follows alkylating agents or radiation therapy, most commonly about 5 years later. Myelodysplasia (MDS) usually occurs first, with evidence of bone marrow failure, to which many succumb without developing AML. About two-thirds have MDS with multilineage dysplasia, and about 25% have refractory anemia with excess blasts. Whether during the MDS phase or when it develops into an AML, these patients usually have dysplasia in all cell lines. Increased marrow basophils are present in about 25% of cases. When AML occurs, the type can be AML with maturation (M2 in the FAB classification) or, less commonly, acute myelomonocytic leukemia (M4), acute monocytic leukemia (M5), erythroleukemia (M6), or acute megakaryocytic leukemia (M7).

A second type occurs after therapy with topoisomerase II inhibitors, such as etoposide and doxorubicin. The average interval between treatment and AML is about 33 months, usually without an intervening MDS phase. Most cases are acute myelomonocytic (M4) or monoblastic (M5) leukemias.

AML Not Otherwise Categorized

This category is a revision of the older FAB classification, with some deletions and additions. The classification depends on the morphologic and cytochemical characteristics of the blasts and their degree of differentiation and maturation.

AML, minimally differentiated (M0 in the FAB classification) constitutes about 5% of AML and occurs mainly in adults. By morphology and light microscopic cytochemistry, the blasts show no myeloid differentiation. They are medium-sized, have an agranular basophilic cytoplasm,

round or slightly indented nuclei with one or two nucleoli, and dispersed chromatin. On cytochemical studies fewer than 3% of the blasts react to Sudan black, α-naphthyl acetate, or stains that detect myeloperoxidase.

AML, without maturation (M1 in the FAB classification) is responsible for about 10% of cases of AML, usually in adults. Azurophilic granules and Auer rods in the cytoplasm of the blasts may suggest their myeloid nature; in other cases the blasts resemble lymphoblasts, from which they are differentiated by positivity to myeloperoxidase stains or Sudan black in at least 3% of blast cells.

AML with maturation (M2 in the FAB classification) constitutes about 30% to 45% of cases of AML and may occur in all ages. Blasts may show azurophilic granules and Auer rods, and evidence of maturation is present, with >10% of the marrow cells being promyelocytes, myelocytes, and mature neutrophils and <20% being monocytes. The neutrophils may show abnormally increased or decreased segmentation and lobulation. Basophils, eosinophils, and mast cells may be increased.

Acute myelomonocytic leukemia (M4 in the FAB classification) accounts for about 15% to 25% of AML, usually in the elderly and sometimes in patients who have had preceding chronic myelomonocytic leukemia. Both neutrophilic and monocytic cells and their precursors are present, each constituting at least 20% of the marrow cells. Circulating monocytes may be numerous ($\geq$5 $\times$ 10^9/l). Monoblasts are large cells with round nuclei containing one or more prominent nucleoli and abundant basophilic cytoplasm, sometimes with fine azurophilic granules, vacuoles, and pseudopod formation. Promonocytes have a less basophilic and more granulated cytoplasm, containing occasional vacuoles and azurophilic granules. The nuclei are irregular and indented.

Acute monoblastic and acute monocytic leukemia (M5a, M5b in the FAB classification) each account for about 5% of AML, the former more common in children, the latter in adults. In both, at least 80% of the leukemic cells are in the monocytic line. In acute monoblastic leukemia, at least 80% of the monocytic cells are monoblasts; in acute monocytic leukemia, most of them are promonocytes. The monoblasts and promonocytes have the characteristics described in the previous paragraph.

Acute erythroid leukemias (M6a, M6b in the FAB classification) include two subtypes, *erythroleukemia (erythroid/myeloid)* and *pure erythroid leukemia.* The former constitutes about 5% of AML; the latter is very rare. In erythroleukemia at least 50% of the nucleated cells in the bone marrow are erythroid and at least 20% of the nonerythroid cells are myeloblasts. The erythroid cells are dysplastic, containing multiple and megaloblastoid nuclei, the cytoplasm often possessing poorly delineated, coalescing vacuoles. The myeloblasts are similar to those in AML with and without maturation. Some cases of erythroleukemia evolve from a myelodysplastic syndrome. In *pure erythroid leukemia,* >80% of the marrow cells are erythroid. The erythroblasts have deeply basophilic, often agranular, cytoplasm that may contain poorly delineated vacuoles. The round nuclei have fine chromatin and one or more nucleoli.

Acute megakaryoblastic leukemia (M7 in the FAB classification), which affects all ages, accounts for about 5% of AML. At least 50% of the blasts are from the megakaryocyte lineage. The megakaryoblasts are often pleomorphic and have a basophilic, often agranular, cytoplasm that may demonstrate pseudopod and bleb formation, indicating budding platelets. The nuclei have fine chromatin and one to three nucleoli. Dysplastic platelets may be visible in the blood, as may be circulating micromegakaryocytes and megakaryocyte fragments.

Acute Leukemias of Ambiguous Lineage

In less than 4% of cases of leukemia, tests currently available: (1) cannot determine whether the blasts have a myeloid or lymphoid origin (*acute undifferentiated leukemia*); (2) indicate two populations of cells, each having a distinct lineage from myeloid or T or B lymphocytes (*acute bilineal leukemia*); or (3) indicate that the blasts individually have markers of two or three lines of myeloid, T lymphocytes, and B lymphocytes (*acute biphenotypic leukemia*). In acute undifferentiated leukemia, the blasts lack any distinguishing characteristics, whereas in the bilineal and biphenotypic forms, the leukemic cells may resemble lymphoblasts, myeloblasts, or monoblasts.

ACUTE LYMPHOBLASTIC LEUKEMIAS

The WHO classification divides these leukemias into two forms, depending on whether the precursor cell is a T or B lymphocyte. The distinction between leukemia and lymphoma in these cases depends on whether the disease presents with abnormal cells in the blood and bone marrow or whether they appear primarily in lymph nodes or extranodal sites outside the bone marrow. Arbitrarily, if the patient has a mass lesion and fewer than 25% lymphoblasts in the bone marrow, the designation is lymphoma.

Precursor B-cell Acute Lymphoblastic Leukemia

About 75% of cases of this disease occur in children below the age of six. About 85% of ALL are this type. Enlarged lymph nodes, liver, and spleen are common. The leukocyte count is variable. Lymphoblasts are pleomorphic and vary from small to large, with nuclei having prominent or inconspicuous nucleoli, compact or dispersed chromatin. The blue or blue-gray cytoplasm is usually scant, but may be abundant. Coarse azurophilic granules may be present.

Precursor T-cell Acute Lymphoblastic Leukemia

This disorder accounts for about 15% of childhood ALL and about 25% of adult ALL. The leukocyte count is often markedly elevated, and a mediastinal mass is often present. The lymphoblasts are similar to those in precursor B-cell ALL, with a wide variation in morphology.

Table 2.1

WHO Classification of acute myeloid leukemia

Acute myeloid leukemia with recurrent genetic abnormalities
- AML with t(8;21)(q22;q22)
- AML with abnormal bone marrow eosinophils inv(16)p13q22) or t(16;16)(p13;q22)
- Acute promyelocytic leukemia—AML with t(15;17)(q22;q12) and variants
- AML with 11q23 abnormalities

Acute myeloid leukemia with multilineage dysplasia
- Following a myelodysplastic syndrome or myelodysplastic/myeloproliferative disorder
- Without antecedent myelodysplastic syndrome

Acute myeloid leukemia and myelodysplastic syndromes, therapy-related
- Alkylating agent–related
- Topoisomerase type II inhibitor–related (some may be lymphoid)
- Other types

Acute myeloid leukemia not otherwise categorized
- AML minimally differentiated
- AML without maturation
- AML with maturation
- Acute myelomonocytic leukemia
- Acute monoblastic and monocytic leukemia
- Acute erythroid leukemia
- Acute megakaryoblastic leukemia
- Acute basophilic leukemia
- Acute panmyelosis with myelofibrosis

Table 2.2

FAB classification of acute myeloid leukemia

M0	AML, minimally differentiated
M1	AML, without maturation
M2	AML, with maturation
M3	Acute promyelocytic leukemia, hypergranular
M3v	Acute promyelocytic leukemia, variant, microgranular
M4	Acute myelomonocytic leukemia
M4eo	Acute myelomonocytic leukemia with eosinophilia
M5a	Acute monoblastic leukemia, poorly differentiated
M5b	Acute monoblastic leukemia, differentiated
M6	Acute erythroleukemia
M7	Acute megakaryoblastic leukemia

Diagram 2.1

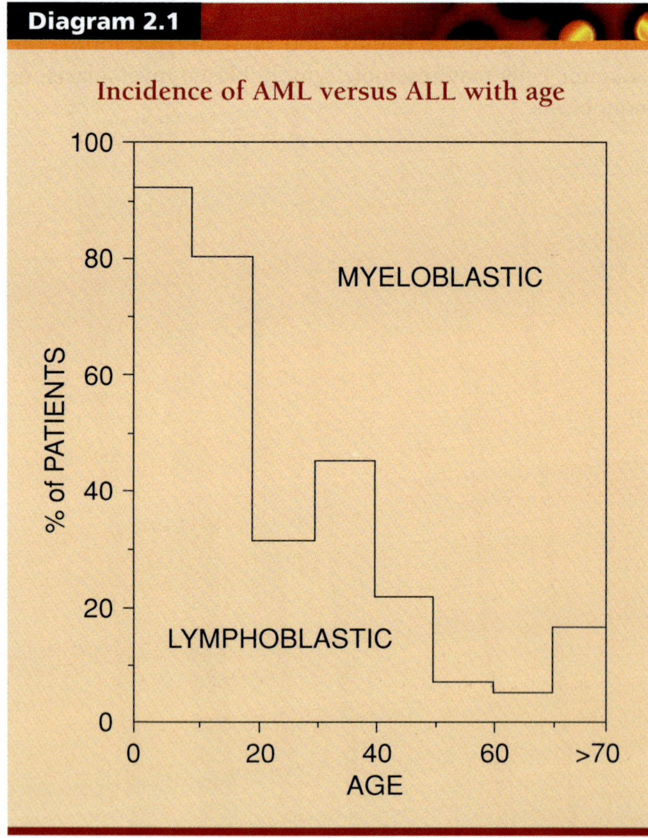

Reprinted with permission from *Wintrobe's Clinical Hematology*, 11th Edition, page 2064.

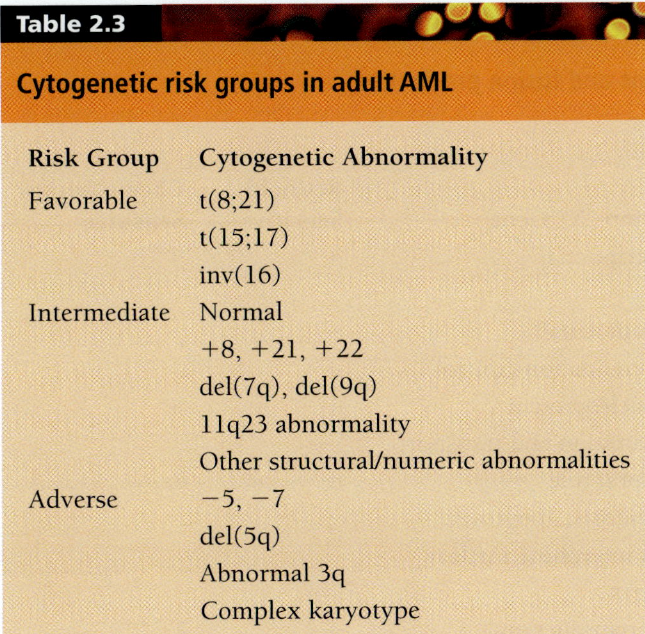

Table 2.3

Cytogenetic risk groups in adult AML

Risk Group	Cytogenetic Abnormality
Favorable	t(8;21)
	t(15;17)
	inv(16)
Intermediate	Normal
	+8, +21, +22
	del(7q), del(9q)
	11q23 abnormality
	Other structural/numeric abnormalities
Adverse	−5, −7
	del(5q)
	Abnormal 3q
	Complex karyotype

From Grimwade D, Walker H, Oliver F, et al. The importance of diagnostic cytogenetics on outcome in AML: analysis of 1,612 patients entered into the MRC AML 10 trial. *Blood* 1998;92:2322–2333, with permission.

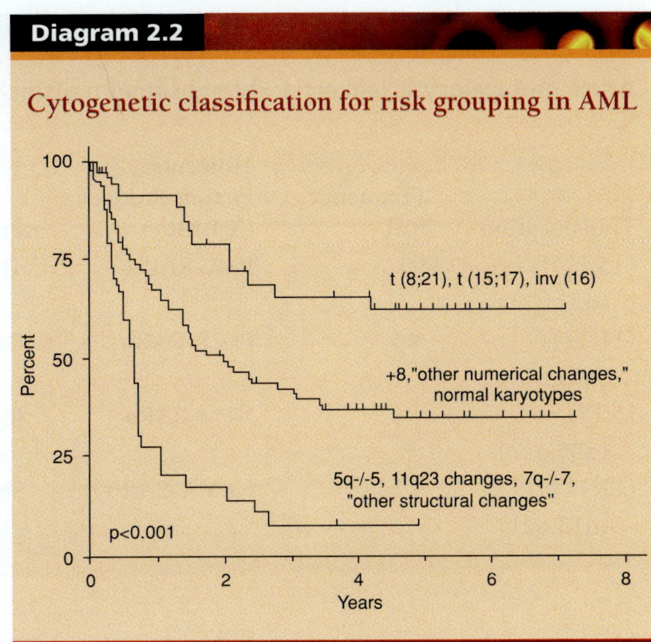

Diagram 2.2

Cytogenetic classification for risk grouping in AML

Reprinted with permission from *Wintrobe's Clinical Hematology,* 11th Edition, page 2115.

Diagram 2.3

AML diagnosis requires a multiparameter approach: morphology, flow cytometry, cytogenetics, and molecular analysis

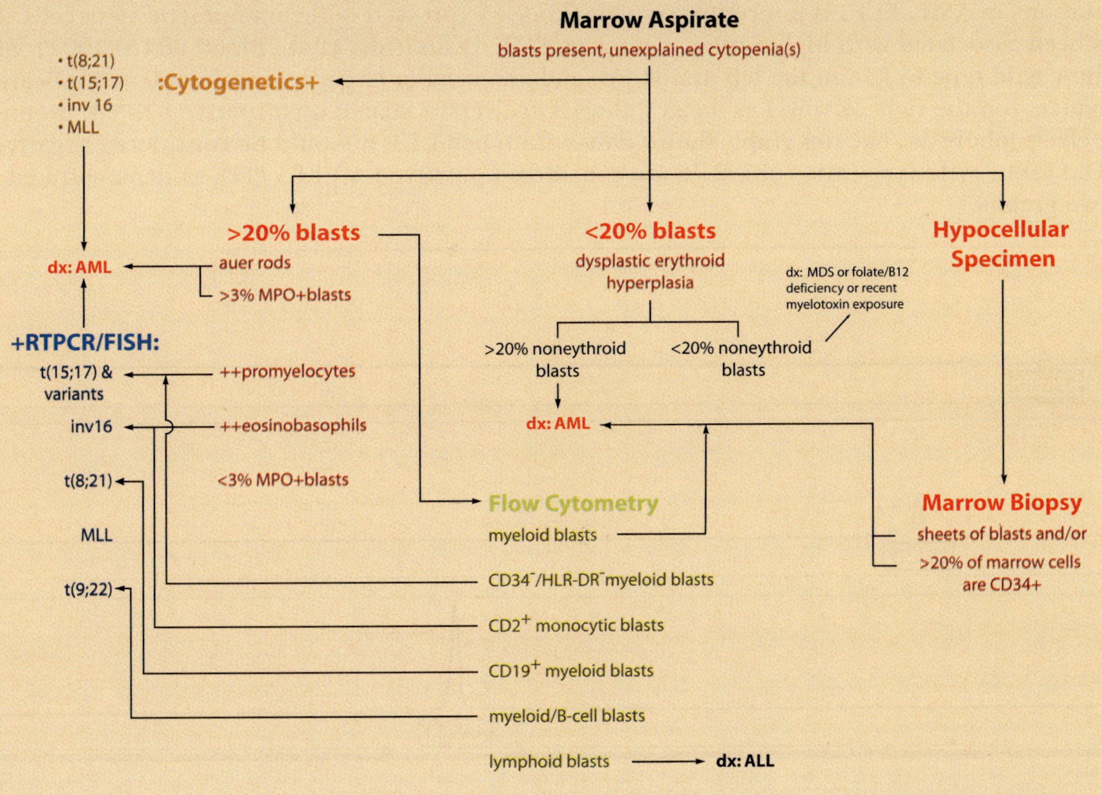

Table 2.4

Acute promyelocytic leukemia: chromosomal translocations and fusion products

Translocation	Frequency (%)	Molecular Fusion Product (X-RARα)	Function "X" Gene	Retinoid Sensitive	Chemotherapy Sensitive
(15;17) (q22,q21)	95	PML-RARα	Transcriptional	+	+
(11;17) (q23,q21)	<5	PLZF-RARα	Developmental/ differentiation control	−	−
(5;17) (q35,q21)	<1	NPM-RARα	Ribonucleoprotein maturation and transport	+	+
(11;17) (q13,q21)	<1	NuMA-RARα	Structural role in mitosis, apoptosis, and interphase nuclear matrix	±	±
(17;17) (q11,q21)	<1	STAT 5b-RARα	Signal transduction, transcriptional factor	−	?

+, sensitive; −, not sensitive; ±, may be sensitive; NPM, nucleophosmin; NuMA, nuclear mitotic apparatus; PLZF, promyelocytic leukemia zinc finger; PML, promyelocytic leukemia; RARα, retinoic acid receptor-α; STAT 5b, signal transducer and activator of transcription 5b; "X," RARα partner gene.
Reprinted with permission from *Wintrobe's Clinical Hematology*, 11th Edition, page 2196.

Diagram 2.4

FLT3 mutations in AML. FLT3 is a receptor tyrosine kinase expressed on hematopoietic stem cells. ITD FLT3 has been associated with higher relapse rates in AML. [Kottaridis et al., Blood 98 (6):2001]. These graphs show wild-type FLT3 (on the left at 364 bp) and abnormally larger internal tandem duplicated (ITD) FLT3 products (on the right, *arrows*) as mean fluorescence versus size of quantitative RT-PCR product from capillary electrophoresis. The top graph shows only wild-type FLT3; it would be considered negative for FLT3 ITD. ITD-to–wild-type ratios of >0.78 are considered positive for FLT3 ITD, as demonstrated in the bottom two graphs.

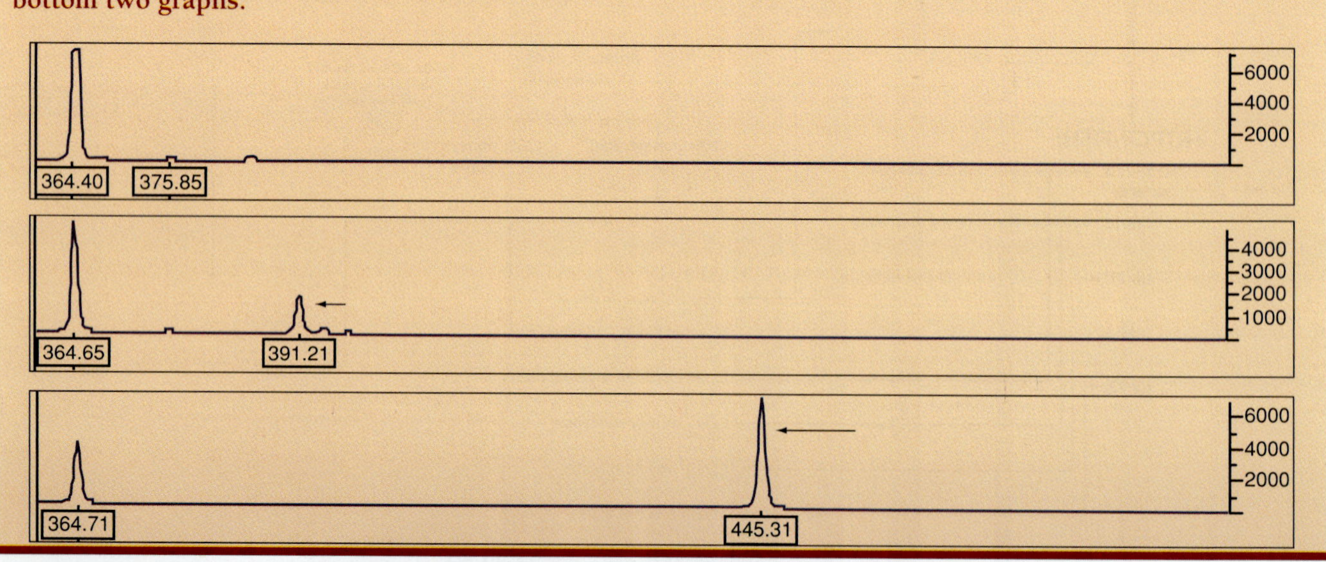

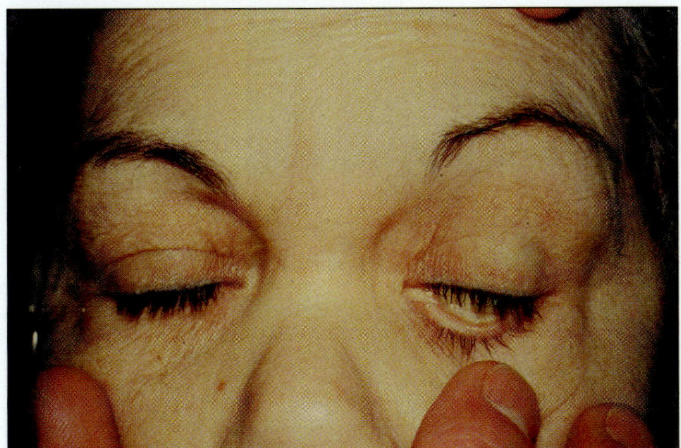

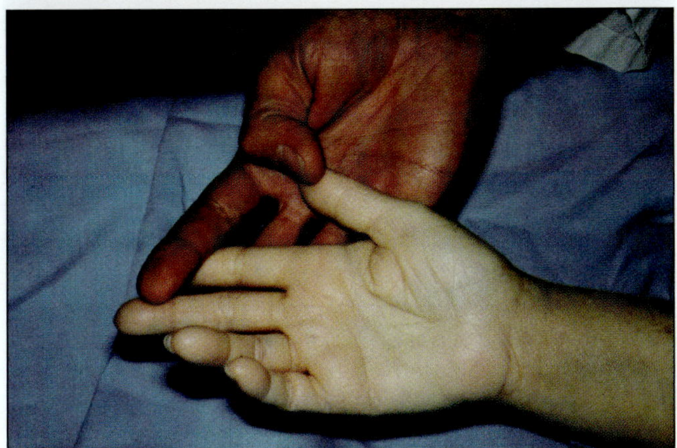

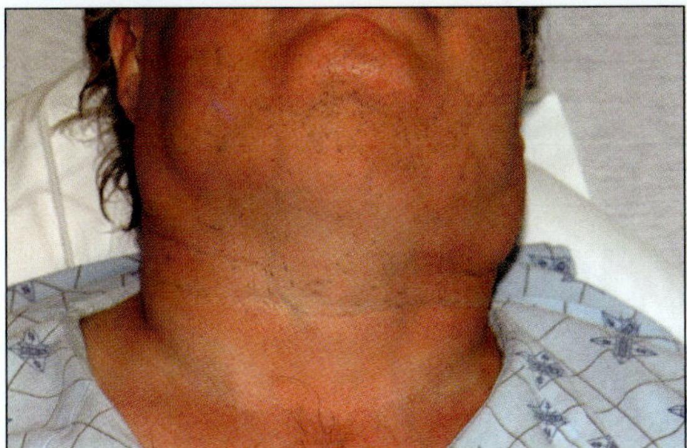

Figure 2.1   Clinical presentation of acute leukemia. Bone marrow replacement by leukemic blasts in acute leukemia can lead to decreased production of red blood cells (RBCs), platelets, and leukocytes resulting in anemia, thrombocytopenia, and leukopenia. The top two panels show conjunctiva and skin pallor in patients with severe anemia (Courtesy Dr. I. Quirt). The patient in the bottom panel presented with submandibular adenopathy from acute myelomonocytic leukemia.

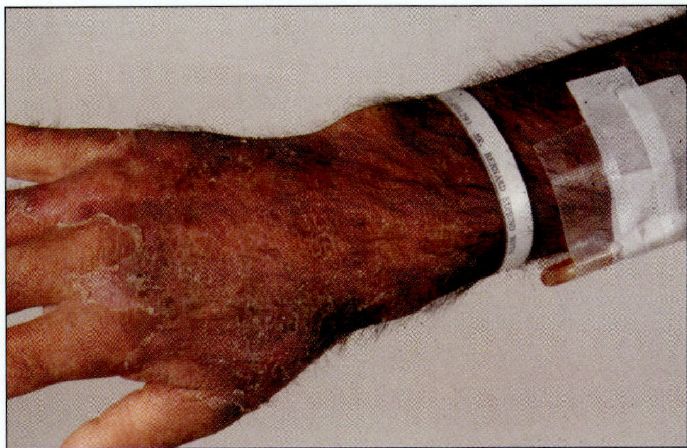

Figures 2.2 through 2.4   Sweet syndrome (acute febrile neutrophilic dermatosis) and AML. Sweet syndrome is most often idiopathic, but 10% to 20% of cases are associated with various malignancies, including AML, myelodysplastic syndrome, lymphoproliferative disorders, and multiple myeloma. The lesions are usually tender, swollen red papules or plaques that are most commonly distributed on the face, neck, and extremities. Compared with patients having idiopathic Sweet syndrome, those with malignancy more frequently have bullous and mucosal membrane lesions (Fig. 2.4). In addition to the skin findings, patients with Sweet syndrome usually also have fever and high erythrocyte sedimentation rates. (Courtesy of The Crookston Collection.)

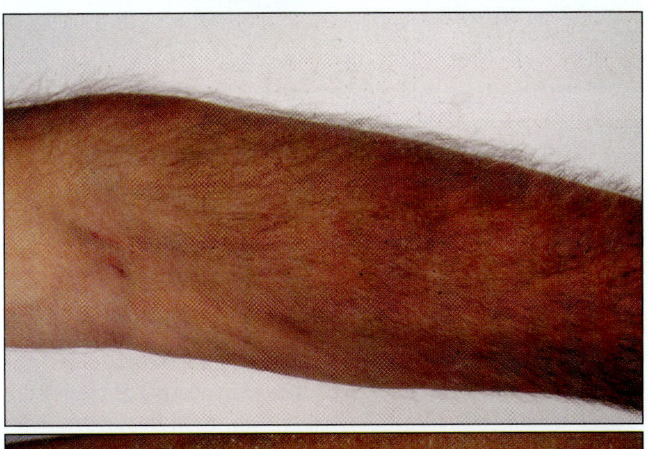

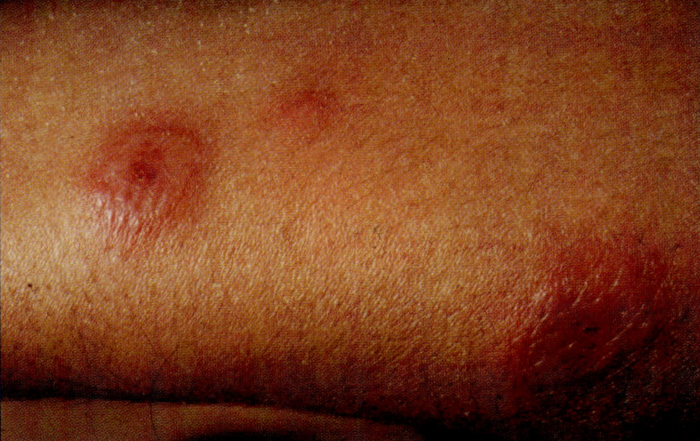

Figure 2.3

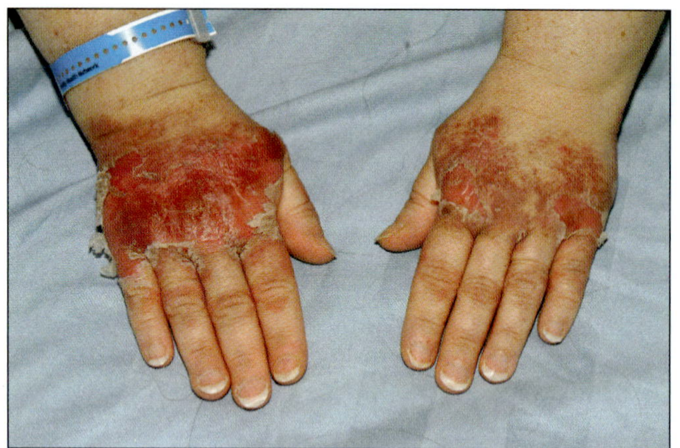

Figure 2.4

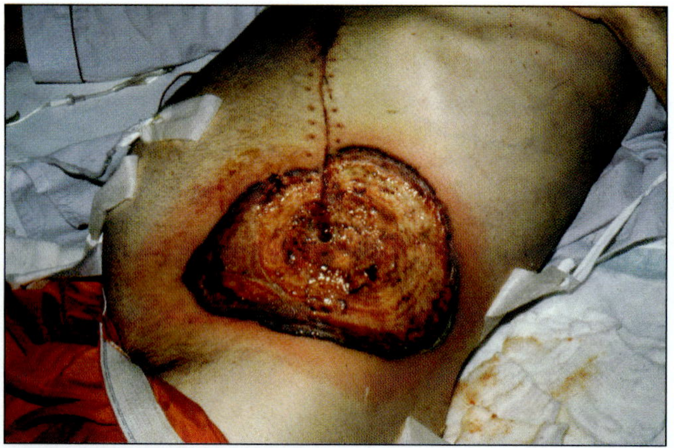

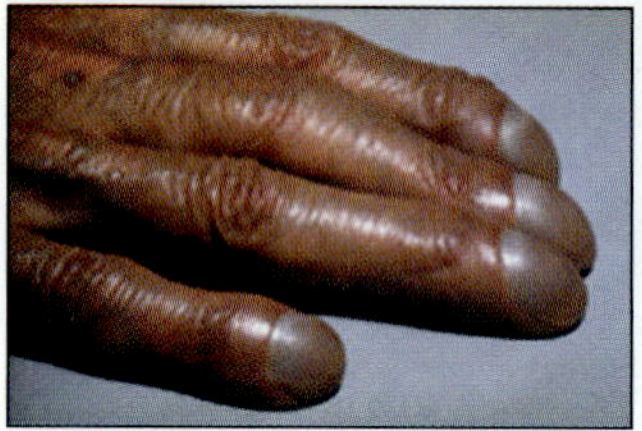

Figure 2.5 Conditions preceding AML. *Top panel:* Pyoderma gangrenosum. Approximately 10% of cases of pyoderma gangrenosum are associated with hematologic disorders, most commonly with AML, but also myeloproliferative syndromes and multiple myeloma. Pyoderma gangrenosum can precede the diagnosis of leukemia or be part of the initial presentation. The lesions are painful, coalescing papules or pustules that can evolve to large ulcers (Courtesy Dr. I. Quirt). *Bottom panel:* Clubbing of fingers can herald the onset of various malignancies including AML.

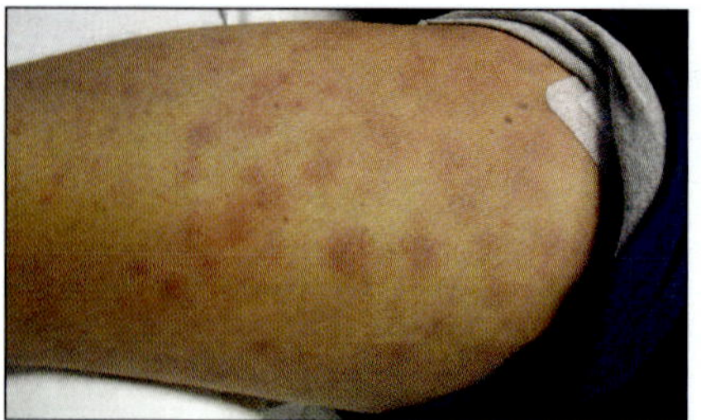

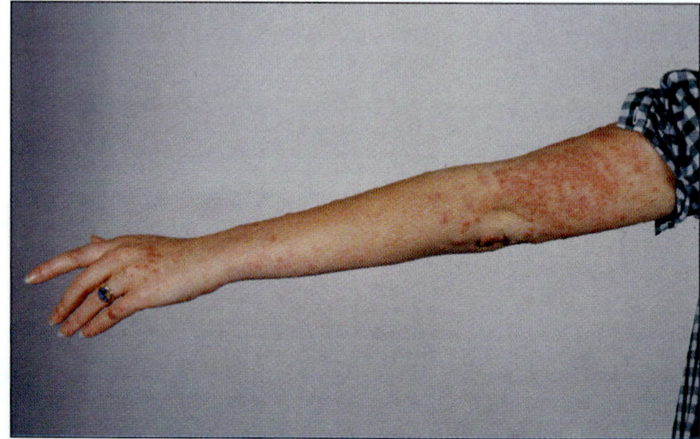

Figures 2.6 through 2.8 Leukemia cutis. Leukemia cutis most commonly occurs in monocytic forms of AML and represents skin infiltration by leukemic blast cells. It can also develop in any acute or chronic leukemia, including the leukemic phase of lymphomas and hairy cell leukemia. As shown in these figures from different cases of AML and leukemia cutis, this condition is highly variable in appearance and can include widespread papules, nodules, macules, palpable purpura, plaques, or ulcers. Pain, tenderness, and pruritus are uncommon. (Courtesy of The Crookston Collection.)

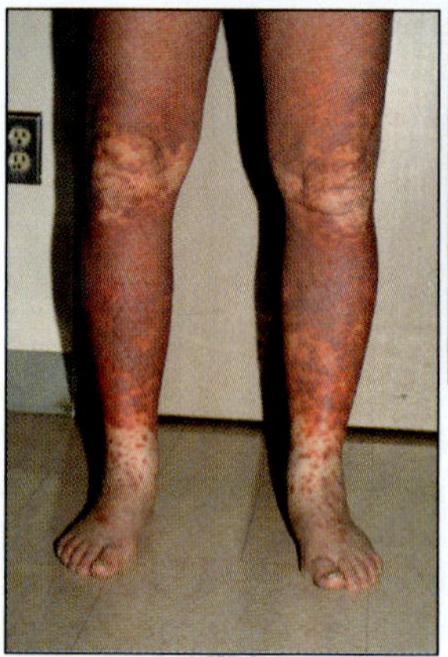

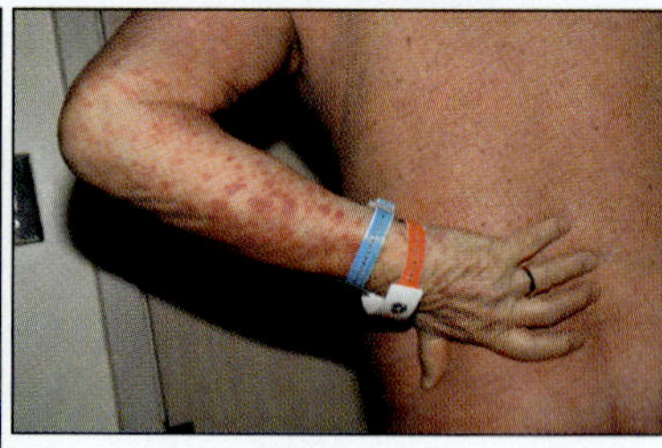

Figure 2.7

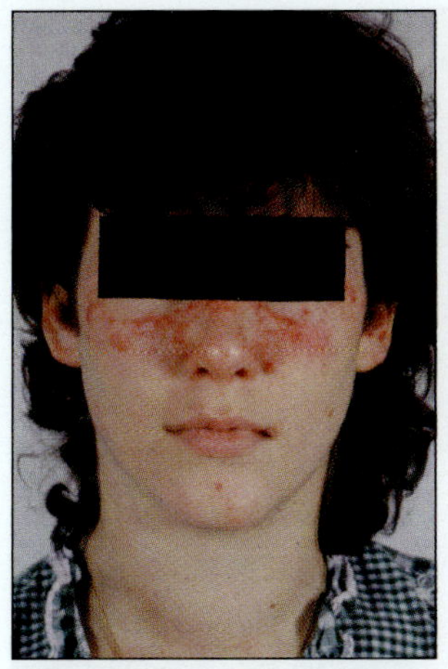
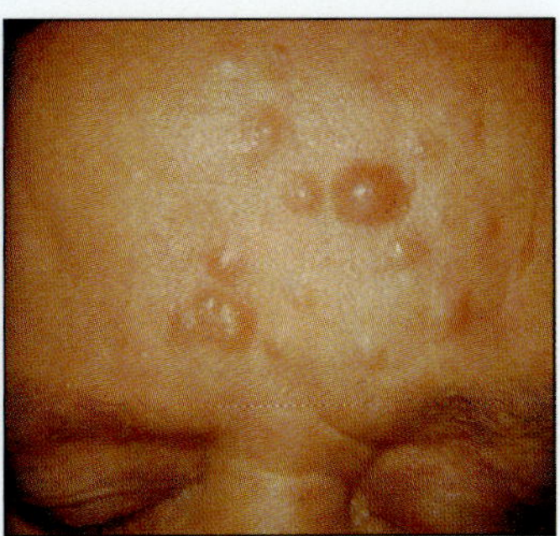

Figure 2.8

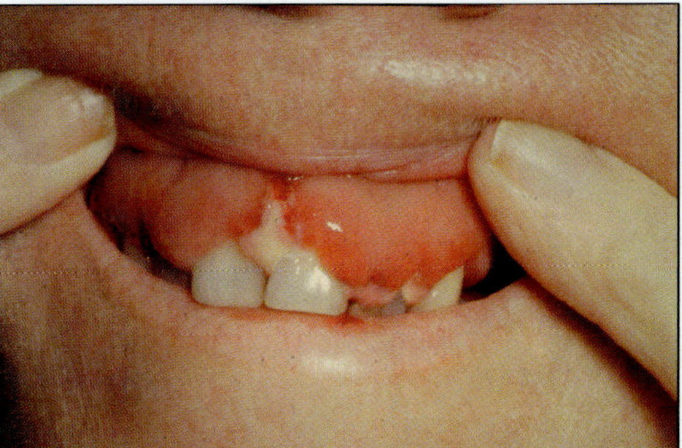
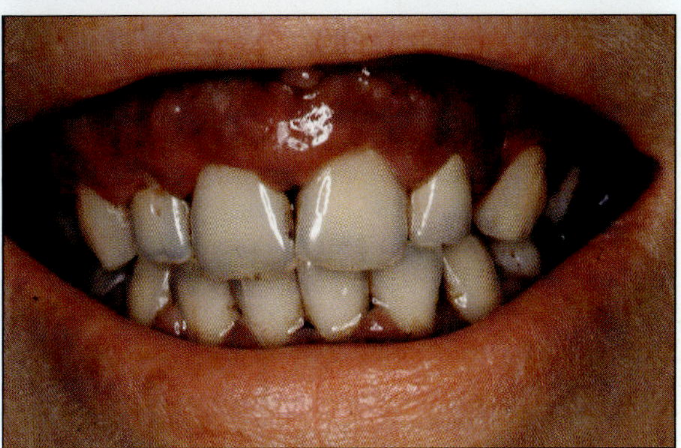
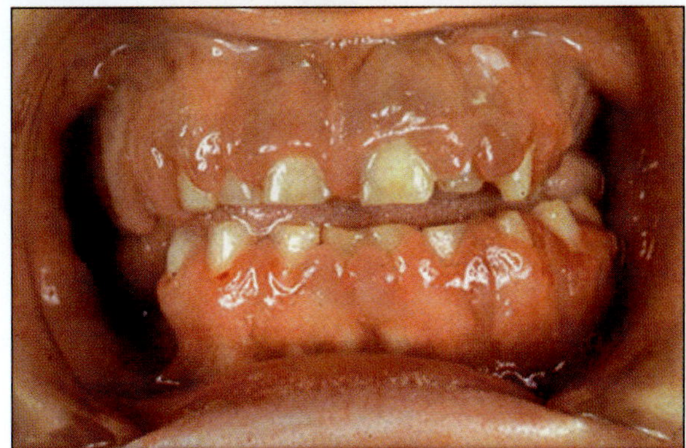
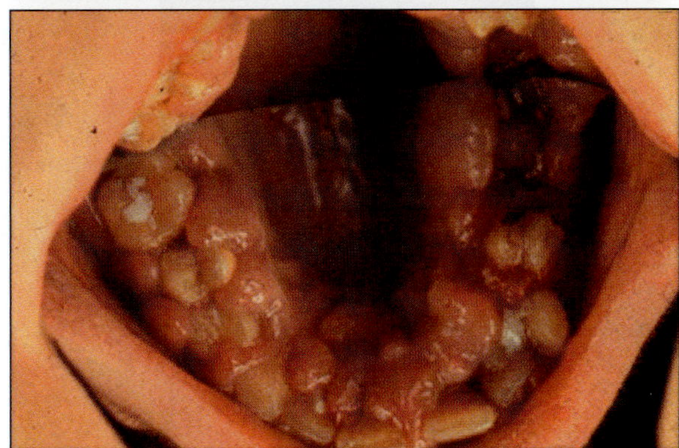

Figure 2.9 Extramedullary involvement by AML in the gums. Gingival hyperplasia, seen in these three cases of untreated AML at presentation, is most common in acute monocytic leukemias and usually resolves with effective leukemia chemotherapy. (Courtesy Drs. Galbraith and Quirt.)

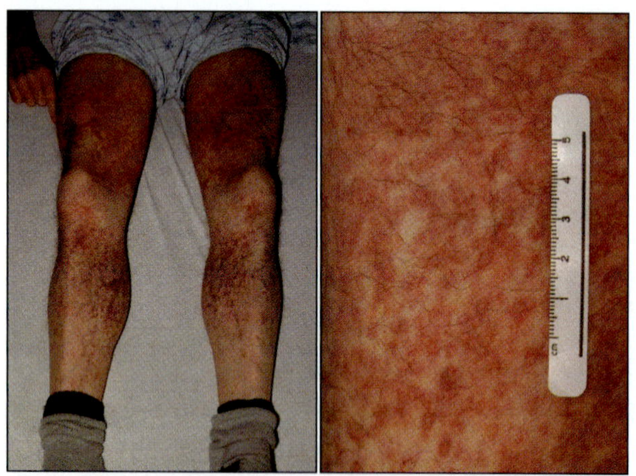

Figures 2.10 through 2.12   AML and thrombocytopenia. Purpura can be classified as petechiae, ecchymoses, or hematomas depending on the size, shape, and depth of blood extravasation. Petechiae are superficial, pinpoint (<3 mm), red or purple, nonblanching macules that mostly occur in dependent areas (Figs. 2.10 and 2.11). Ecchymoses (bruises) are larger, flat, extravasating lesions (Fig. 2.12). Hematomas are deep pockets of blood underneath the skin. (Courtesy Dr. D. Amato.)

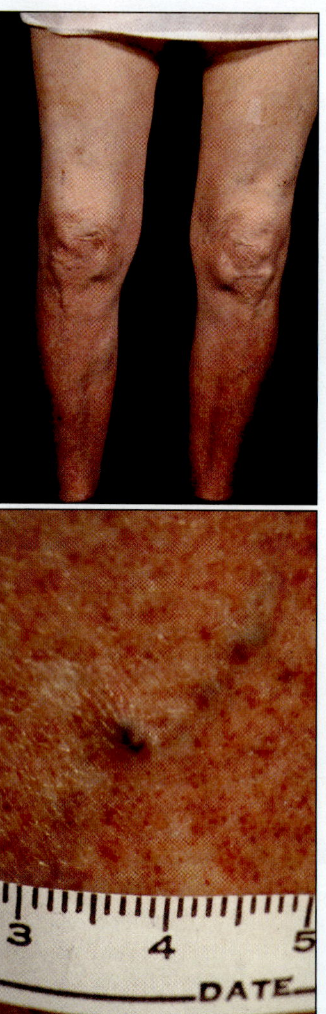

Figure 2.11

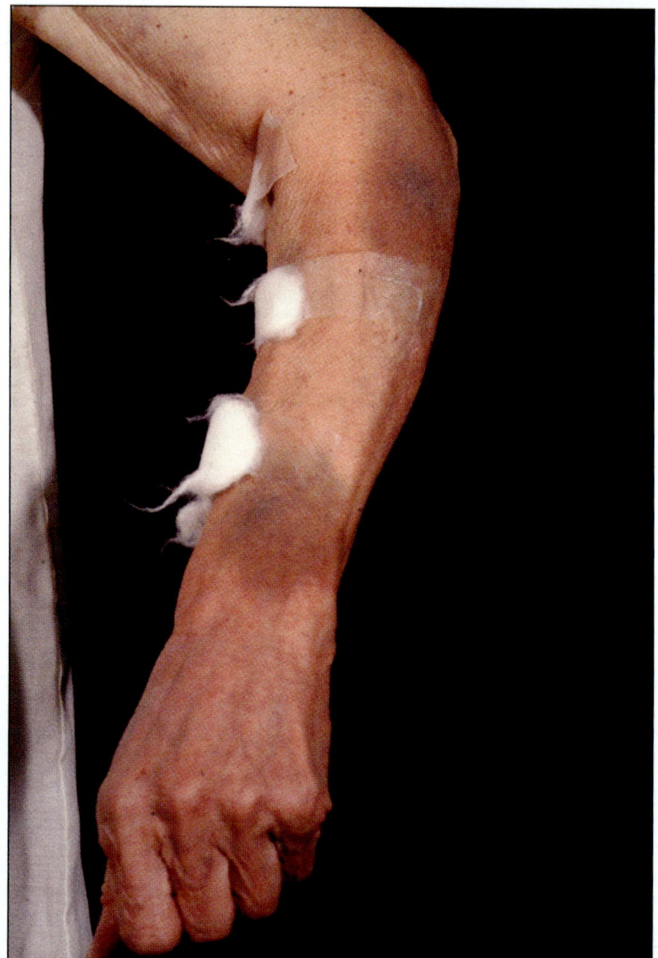

Figure 2.12

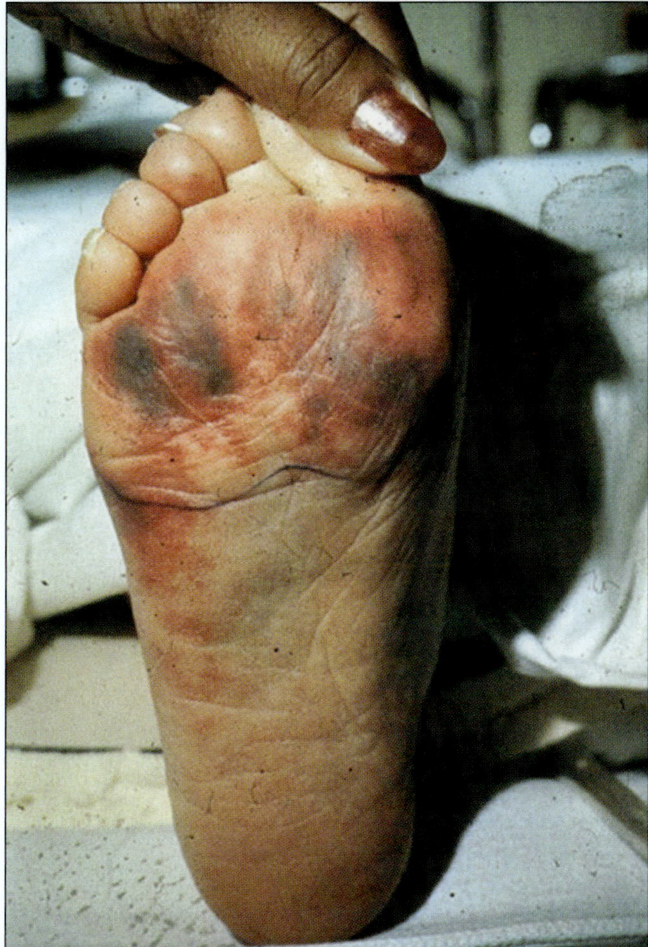

Figure 2.13 AML and disseminated intravascular coagulation (DIC). Extensive purpura is present on the soles of a patient with acute promyelocytic leukemia and DIC. (Courtesy Dr. I. Quirt.)

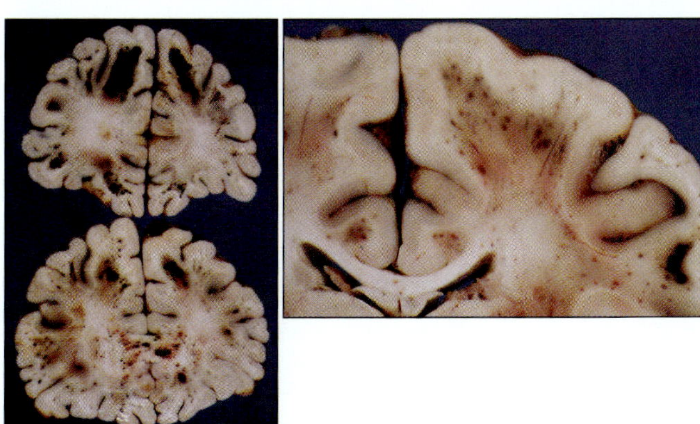

Figure 2.14 AML and DIC. This brain, from a case of AML complicated by DIC, demonstrates multiple tiny hemorrhages in white matter with some forming small hematomas. (Courtesy Dr. J. Bilbao.)

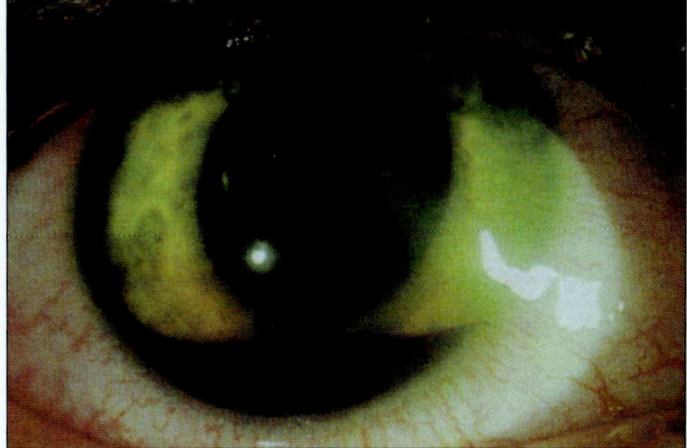

Figure 2.15 Hyphema. Thrombocytopenia has caused bleeding into the anterior chamber (hyphema).

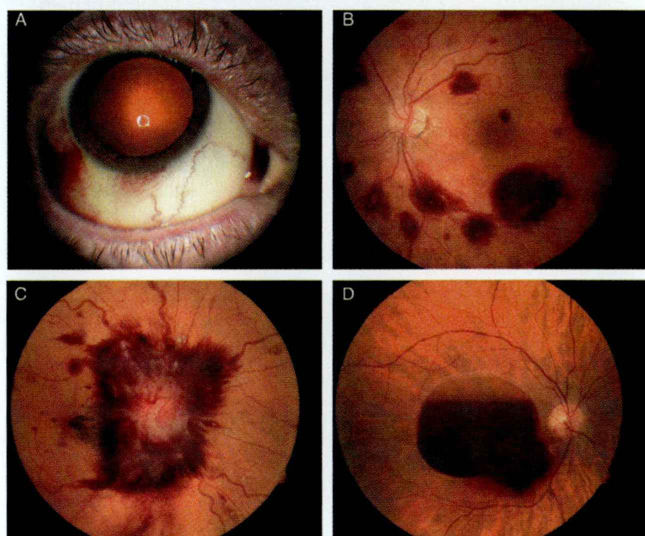

Figure 2.16 Ocular manifestations of AML and thrombocytopenia. **A.** Subconjunctival hemorrhage is present in the right eye. **B.** A fundus photograph shows intraretinal hemorrhages in the left eye. **C.** A fundus image demonstrates a hyperemic disc with peripapillary intraretinal hemorrhages and pseudo-Roth spots. **D.** Fundus of right eye has a subhyaloid hemorrhage with fluid level. (Courtesy Dr. F. Altomare.)

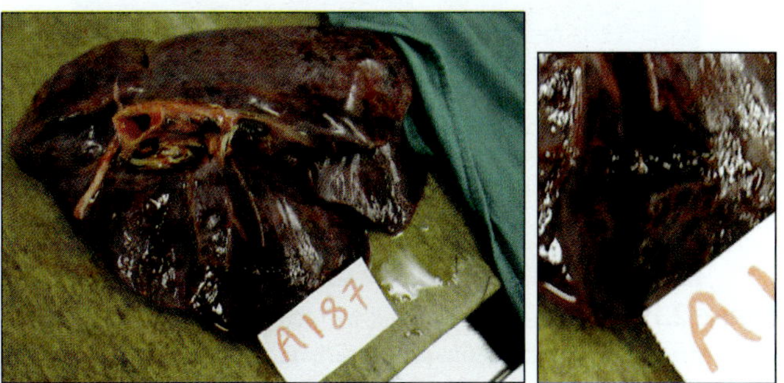

Figure 2.17 Pulmonary hemorrhage from AML-induced thrombocytopenia. An autopsy specimen from a case of diffuse pulmonary hemorrhage caused by thrombocytopenia secondary to AML shows a congested lung filled with blood.

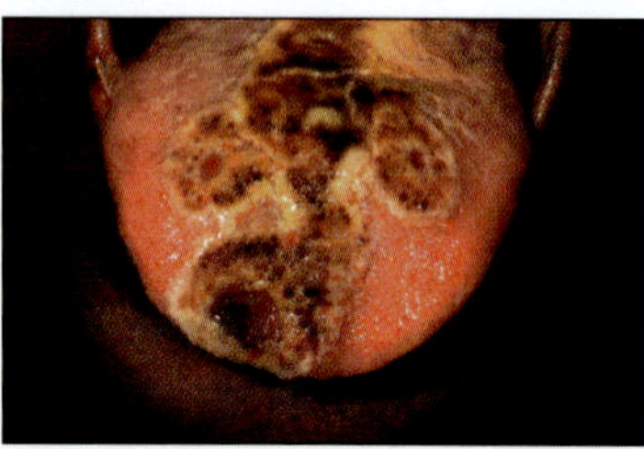

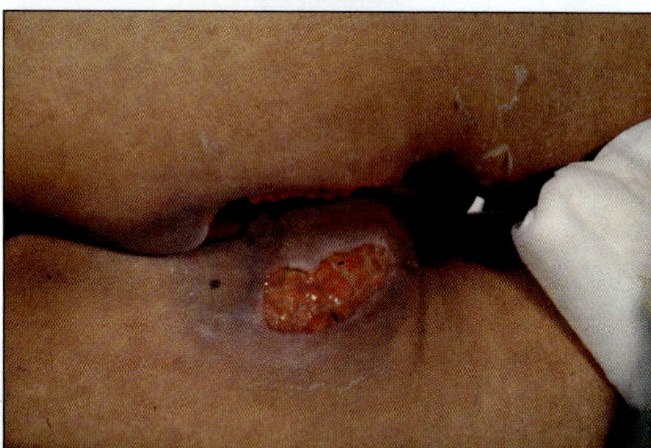

Figure 2.18   AML with neutropenia. Extensive fungal infection of tongue (*top panel*) and perirectal abscess (*bottom panel*) develop in cases of AML with neutropenia. (Courtesy Drs. A. Lutynski and I. Quirt.)

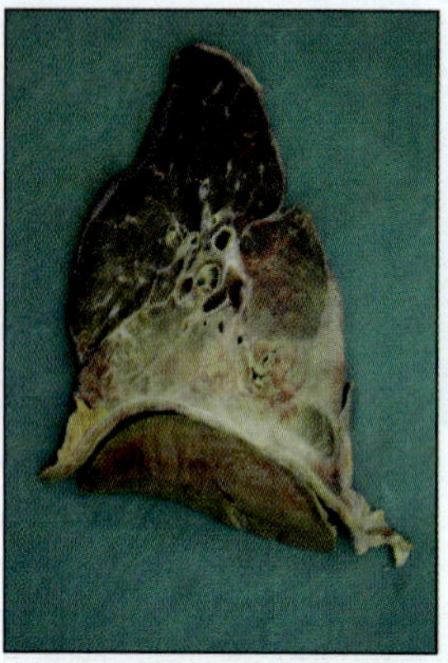

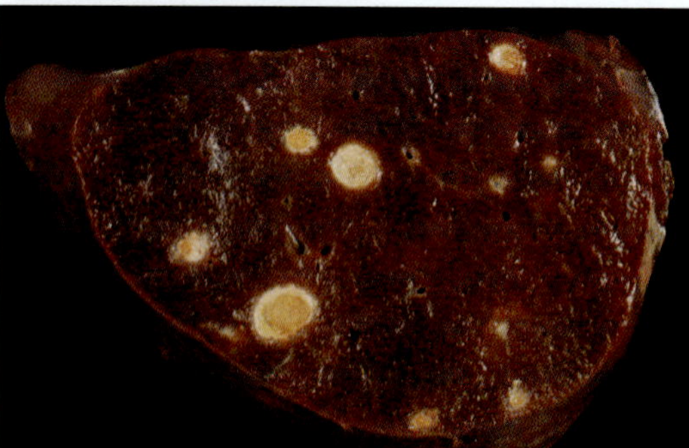

Figure 2.19   Autopsy lung (fixed in formalin) from a case AML presenting with neutropenia and extensive lobar pneumonia from aspergillosis (*top panel*). The liver from a different case of AML discloses multiple abscesses from aspergillosis. (Courtesy Dr. I. Wanless.)

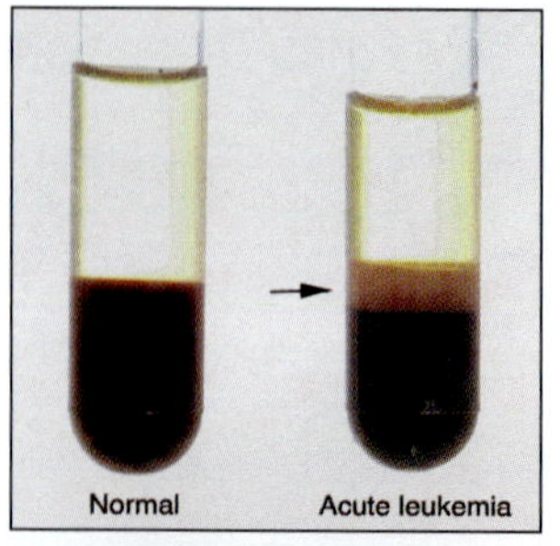

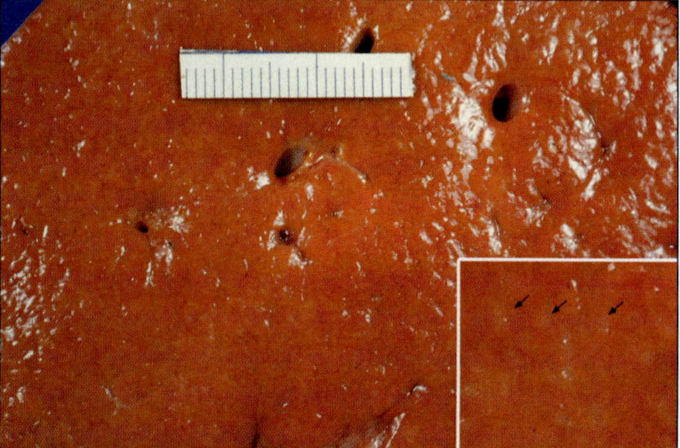

Figure 2.20   *Top panel:* Leukocytosis in acute leukemia. A tube of centrifuged whole blood from a patient with leukocytosis (WBC = 310K) due to acute leukemia is shown on the right, compared with normal (WBC = 5K) on the left. The prominent buffy coat consists entirely of leukemic blasts (*arrow*). *Bottom panel:* An autopsy liver specimen shows tiny nodules (*arrows*) of leukemic blasts filling the hepatic vasculature in a case of AML with a high blast count.

AML CLASSIFICATION, DEFINITION OF THE "BLAST"
Morphology: Wright-Giemsa stain

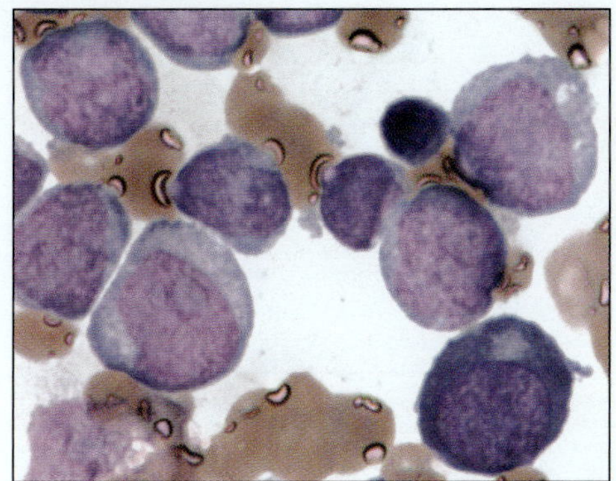

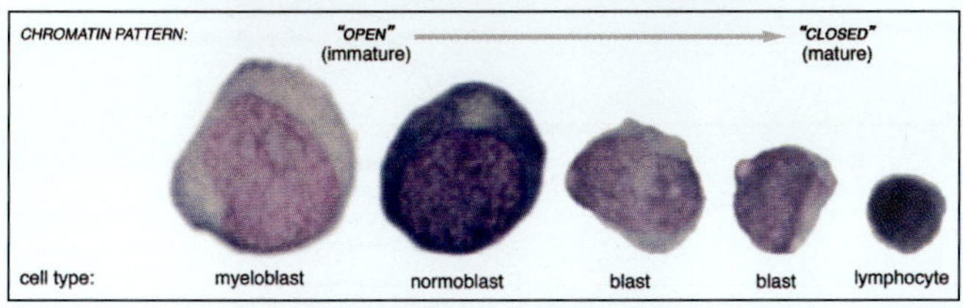

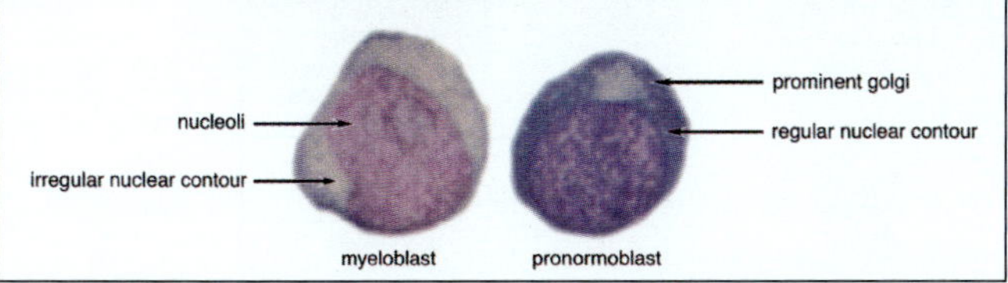

Figure 2.21 Blast morphology in AML. The upper panel shows a pleomorphic population of cells that are aligned in the middle panel according to size and chromatin patterns. The bottom panel illustrates the distinguishing features of the two blasts most commonly seen in aspirate smears, the mycloblast and erythoblast.

AML CLASSIFICATION, DEFINITION OF THE "BLAST"
Morphology: Wright-Giemsa stain

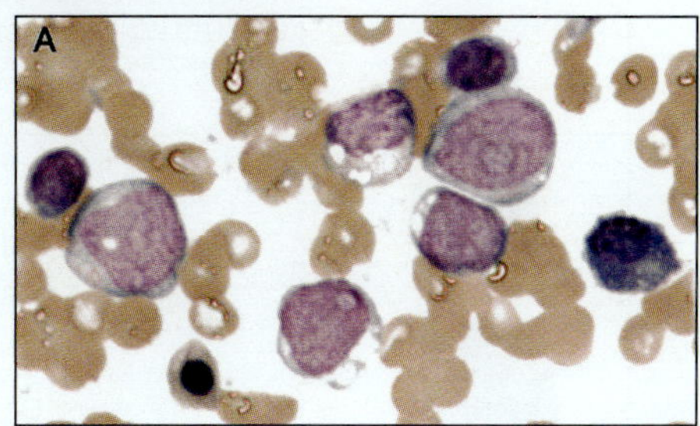

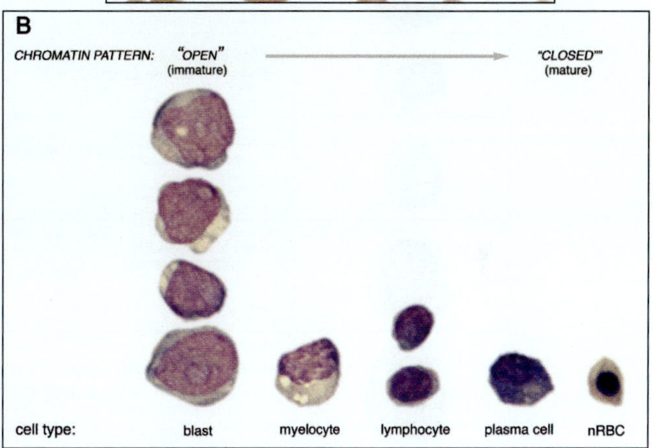

Figure 2.22 Chromatin patterns. **A.** An aspirate smear in AML shows diverse chromatin patterns in different marrow-cell populations. The blasts are characterized by "open" (uncondensed or lacy or immature) chromatin with prominent nucleoli. **B.** This schematic diagram categorizes cells from part **A.** with, from left to right, "open" (lacey or immature) to increasingly "closed" (condensed or mature) patterns of chromatin.

AML CLASSIFICATION, DEFINITION OF THE "BLAST"
Morphology: Myeloperoxidase (MPO) stain

AML, MINIMALLY DIFFERENTIATED (M0)   *AML, WITHOUT MATURATION (M1)*   *AML, WITH MATURATION (M2)*

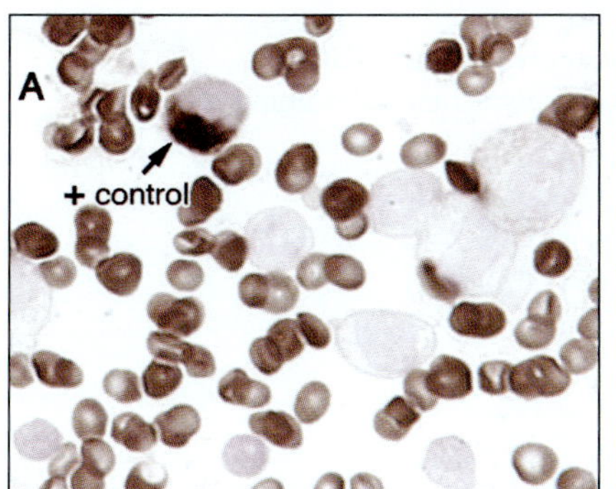

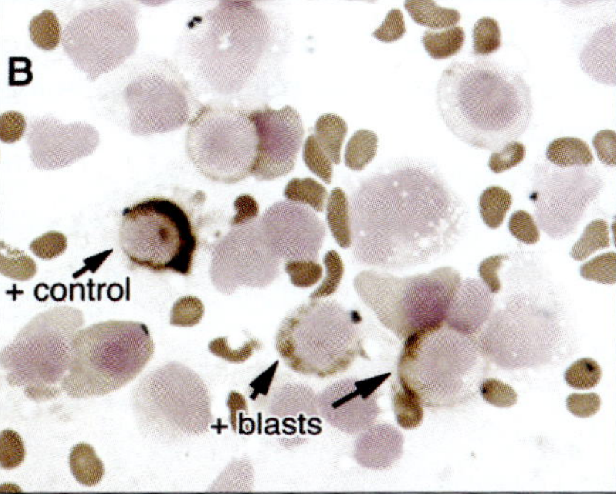

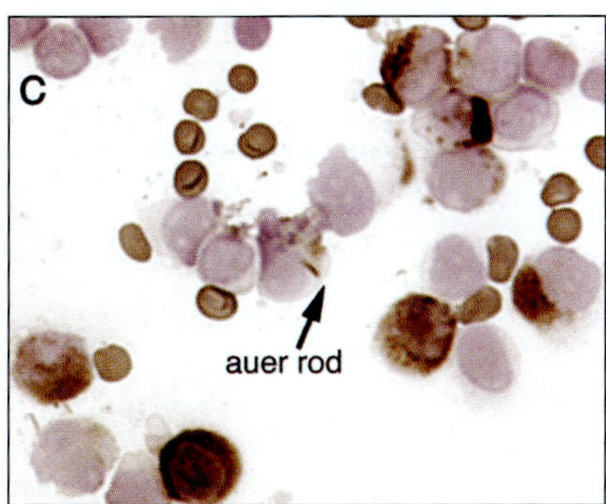

Figure 2.23 MPO staining in AML. **A.** AML, minimally differentiated. By definition this type of AML shows MPO staining in <3% of the total blast population. A mature granulocyte serves as positive control. **B.** MPO staining in AML, without maturation. Weak to moderate punctate staining is present in the cytoplasm of >3% of the blasts (a myelocyte serves as a positive control). **C.** MPO staining and AML with maturation. Strong cytoplasmic staining is present in blasts and abnormal maturing granulocytes. An Auer rod staining strongly with MPO is present.

MORPHOLOGY	CLASSIFICATION	NUCLEUS	NUCLEOLUS	CHROMATIN	CYTOPLASM
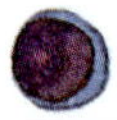	L1 ACUTE LYMPHOBLASTIC (principally pediatric)	Uniformly round, small	Single, indistinct	Slightly reticulated with perinucleolar clumping	Scant, blue
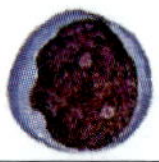	L2 LYMPHOBLASTIC (principally adult)	Irregular	Single to several, indistinct	Fine	Moderate, pale
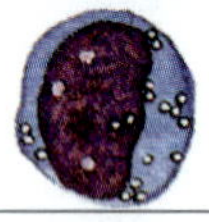	L3 BURKITT-TYPE	Round to oval	Two to five	Coarse with clear parachromatin	Moderate blue, prominently vacuolated
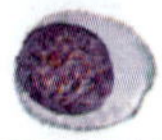	M0 MYELOBLASTIC (minimally differentiated)	Round to oval	Single to multiple, distinct	Fine to coarse	Scant, non-granulated
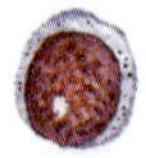	M1 MYELOBLASTIC (without maturation)	Round to oval	Single to multiple, distinct	Fine	Scant, variably granulated
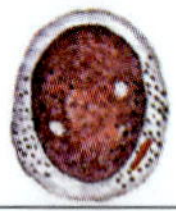	M2 MYELOBLASTIC (with maturation)	Round to oval	Single to multiple, distinct	Fine	Moderate azurophilic granules with or without Auer rods
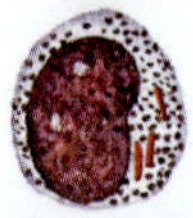	M3 MYELOCYTIC	Round to indented to lobed, "cottage-loaf"	Single to multiple, (granules may obscure)	Fine	Prominent azurophilic granules and/or multiple Auer rods
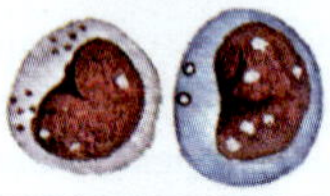	M4 MYELOMONOBLASTIC (biphasic M1 and M5)	Round to indented, folded	Single to multiple, distinct	Fine	Moderate, blue to gray, may be granulated
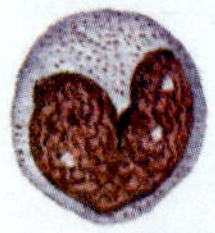	M5 MONOBLASTIC	Round to indented, folded	Single to multiple, distinct	Variable, lacy or ropy	Scant to moderate, gray-blue, dustlike lavender granules
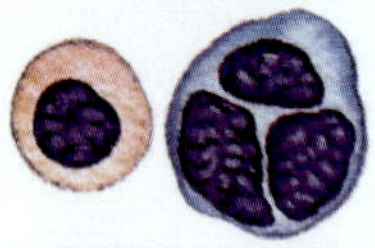	M6 ERYTHROBLASTIC	Single to bizarre multinucleated, multilobed	Single to multiple, distinct	Open "megaloblastoid"	Abundant, red to blue
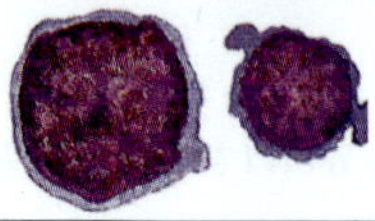	M7 MEGAKARYOBLASTIC	Round to oval	Single to multiple, distinct	Slightly to moderately reticulated	Scant to moderate, gray-blue, with blebbing

Figure 2.24 FAB classification of AML. Although largely replaced by the more popular WHO classification, the FAB classification is a scheme based solely on morphology and histochemical staining characteristics of leukemic blasts.

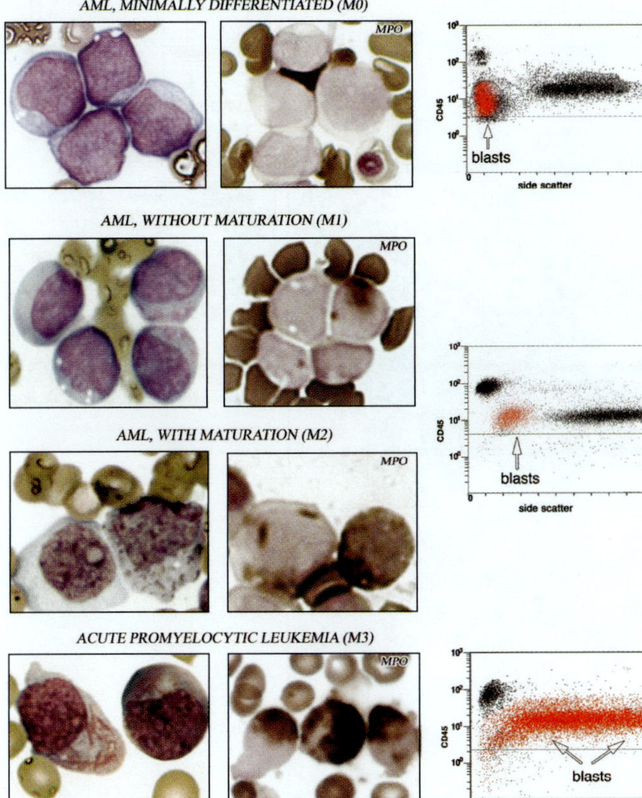

Figure 2.25 Patterns of cytoplasmic granulation in various types of AML. Cytoplasmic granulation as seen in standard Wright-Giemsa staining (*left column*), MPO histochemistry (*middle column*), and side scatter by flow cytometry (*right column*) correlates with the degree of blast differentiation in various types of AML. AML, minimally differentiated, is shown with the typical immature, agranular, MPO-negative blasts with low side scatter compared with the more mature cells of acute promyelocytic leukemia with the classic hypergranular cytoplasm (with multiple Auer rods here), strong MPO, staining, and the characteristic "comet-shaped" diffusely spread pattern characteristic of blasts with high side scatter.

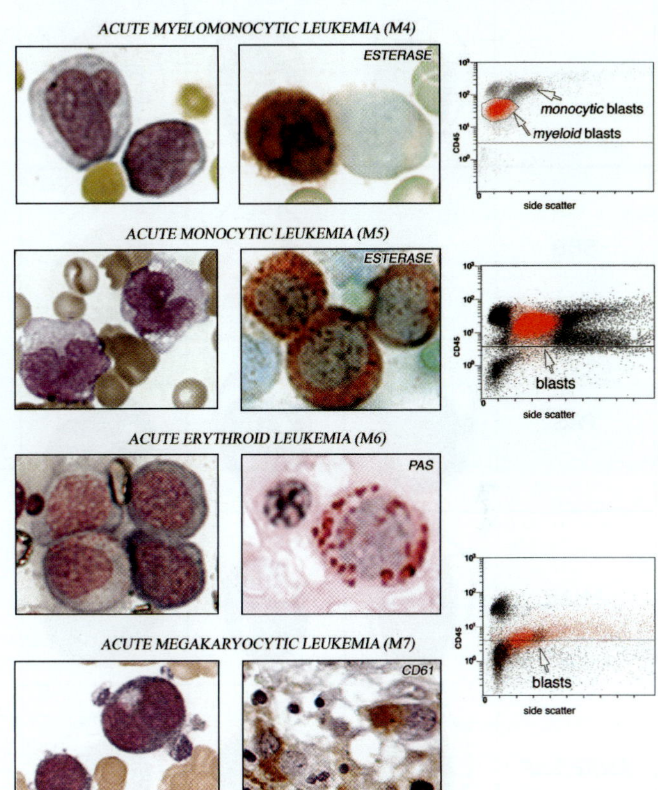

Figure 2.26 Morphology of cytoplasm in various types of AML. Cytoplasmic features are shown with standard Wright-Giemsa staining (*left column*), histochemistry (*middle column*), and CD45 versus side scatter by flow cytometry (*right column*) in various types of AML. Demonstrated here are: acute myelomonocytic leukemia with two distinct blast populations: acute monocytic leukemia with ample esterase+ cytoplasm, acute erythroid leukemia (pure erythroleukemia type shown here) with coarse PAS+ cytoplasmic granules, CD45 weak/negative blasts, and acute megakaryocytic leukemia with CD61+ blasts that are weakly CD45 positive. (Histograms courtesy J. Davidson and T. Anderson.)

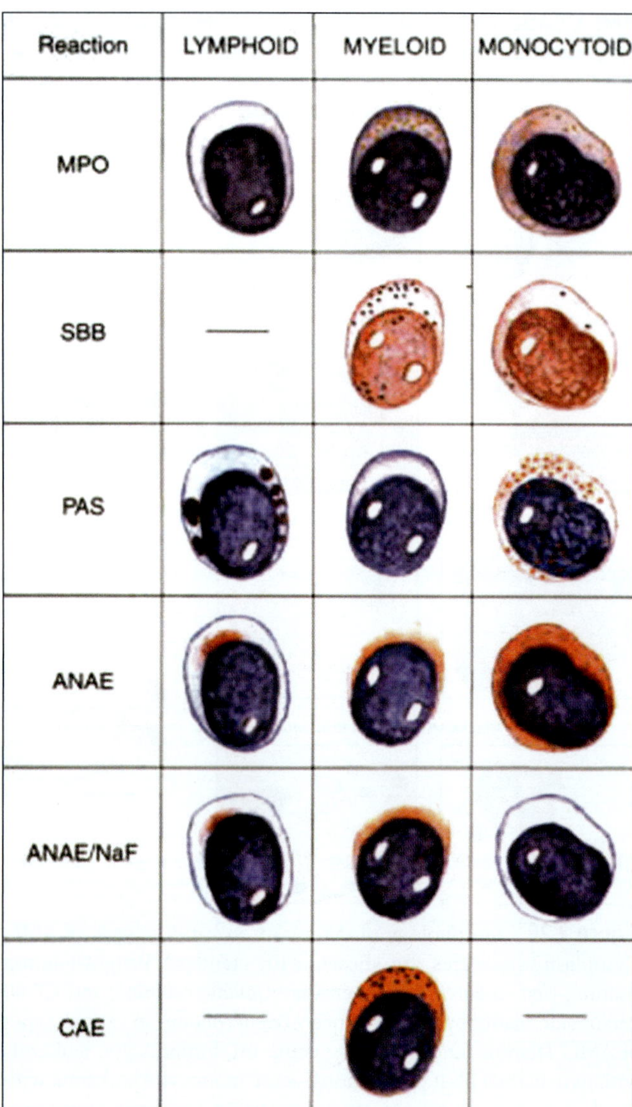

Figure 2.27 Morphology and histochemical staining characteristics of lymphoid, myeloid, and monocytoid leukemic blasts. MPO, myeloperoxidase; SBB, Sudan black B; PAS, periodic acid-Schiff; ANAE, alphanaphthyl acetate esterase; ANAE/NaF, ANAE with fluoride inhibition (butyrate substrates now more commonly in use); CAE, chloroacetate esterase.

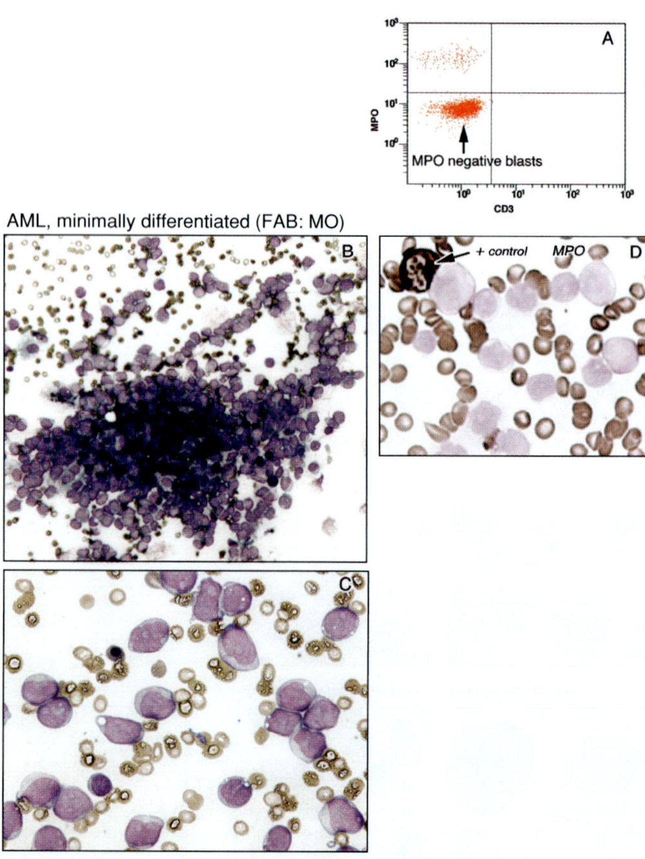

Figure 2.28 AML, minimally differentiated (FAB: M0). **A.** Flow cytometric scattergram shows blasts with low side scatter. **B.** Low-power magnification of aspirate smear demonstrates hypercellular marrow fragments consisting exclusively of monotonous sheets of primitive mononuclear cells. **C.** High-power view of aspirate smear discloses nucleolated undifferentiated blasts. **D.** Less than 3% of the blasts stain positively for MPO. A late myeloid precursor serves as a positive internal control (*arrow*).

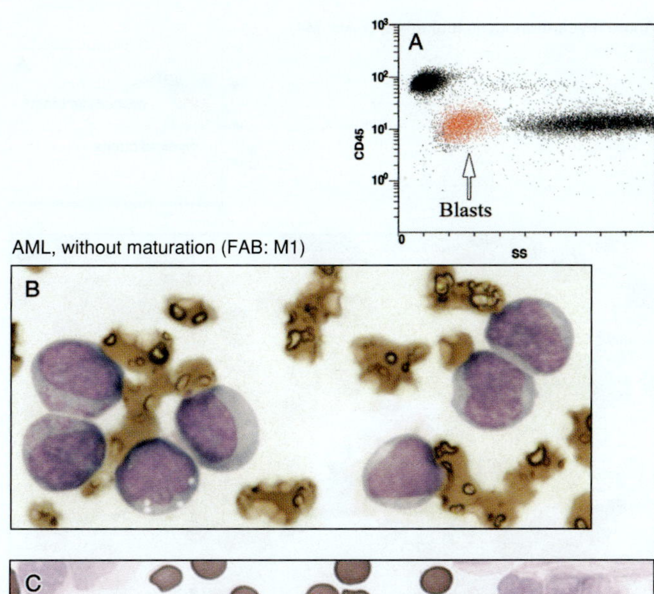

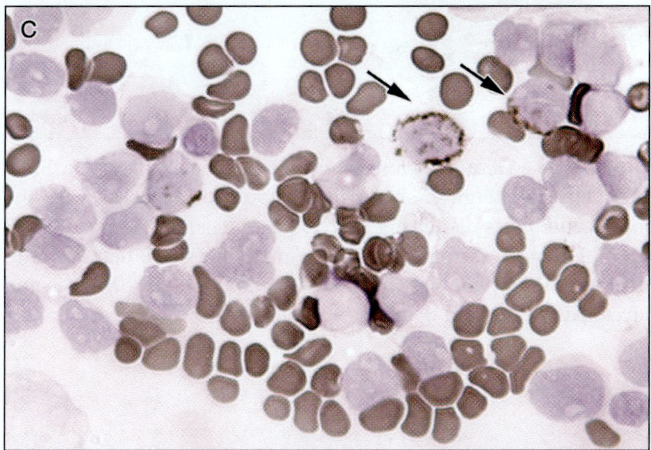

Figure 2.29 AML, without maturation (FAB: M1). **A.** Flow cytometry scattergram shows a discrete population of CD45+ blasts displaying weak side scatter signal consistent with low cytoplasmic granularity. **B.** An aspirate smear demonstrates immature myeloid precursors, some of which show the presence of numerous primary granules in the cytoplasm (so-called type III blasts). **C.** MPO stains of aspirate smear show a minor subpopulation of positive-staining blasts with punctate cytoplasmic staining (*arrows*).

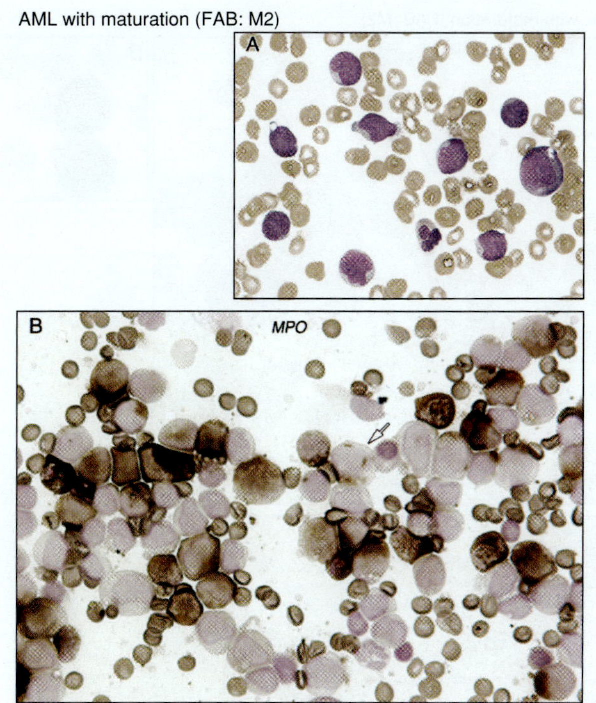

Figure 2.30 AML, with maturation (FAB: M2). **A.** Blood smear displays a spectrum of immature and mature myeloid precursors. **B.** MPO stains reveal strong granular cytoplasmic staining in many leukemic blasts. Two MPO positive Auer rods are present (*arrow*).

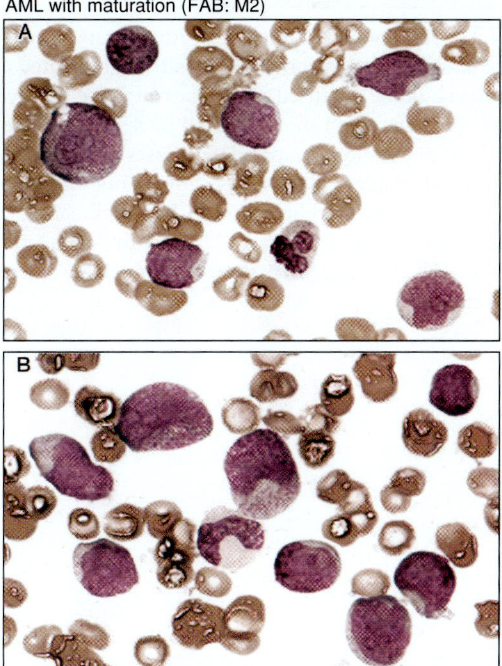

Figures 2.31 AML with maturation with t(8;21). Aspirates showing a spectrum of differentiated myeloid precursors ranging from blasts to mature segmented bands and neutrophils are shown in **A.** and **B.** With so many mature myeloid forms, AML with maturation can be confused with maturation arrest following marrow insults such as recent chemotherapy or recovery following bone marrow transplant.

AML with maturation (FAB: M2)

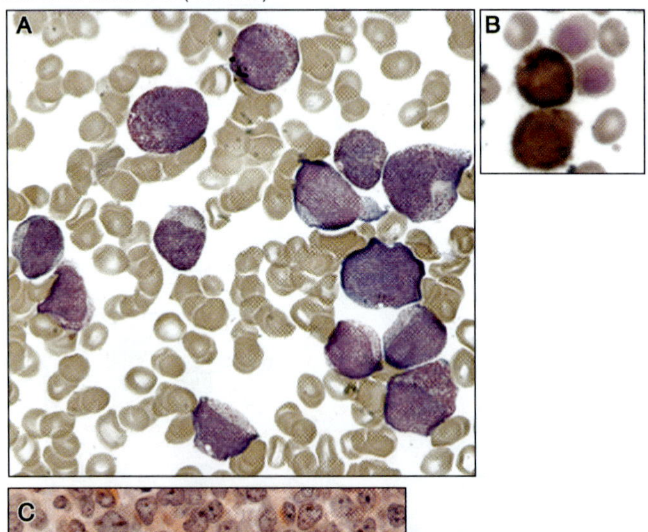

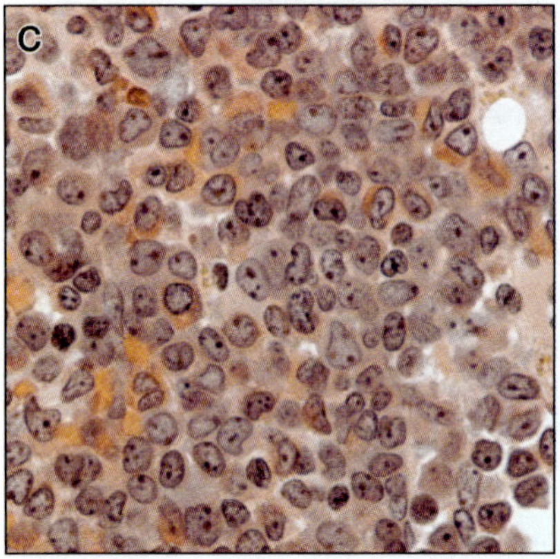

Acute myelomonocytic leukemia, (FAB: M4)

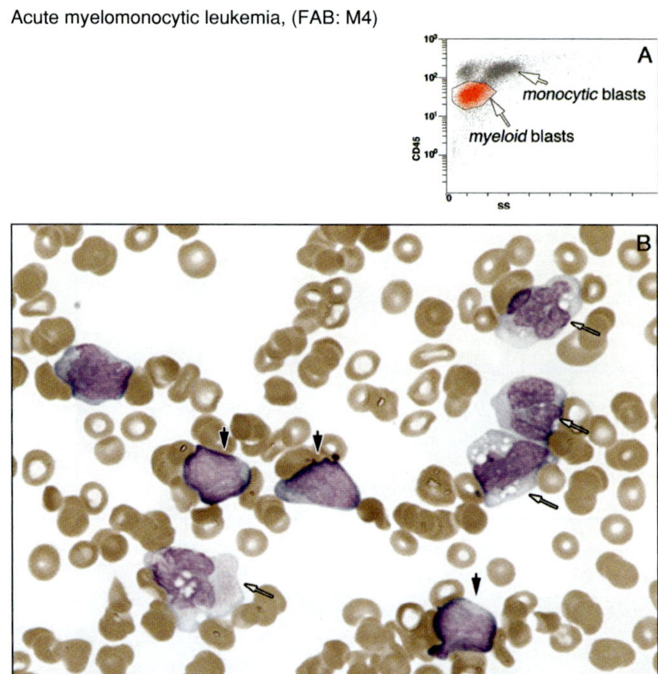

Figure 2.33   Acute myelomonocytic leukemia (AMML). **A.** Flow cytometric scattergram shows dual population of blasts with the monocytic blasts displaying more side scatter and stronger CD45 staining than do the myeloblasts. **B.** An aspirate smear demonstrates the same dimorphic blast population composed of monocytes and myeloblasts (*long* and *short arrows*, respectively).

Figure 2.32   AML with maturation. **A.** An aspirate smear shows a leukemic blast population composed mostly of granulated promyelocytes that could be confused with a case of acute promyelocytic leukemia. The latter often shows bilobed nuclei and a more homogeneous blast population compared with cases of AML with differentiation. **B.** Myeloperoxidase stains show strong diffuse staining that obscures nuclear morphology. **C.** A hypercellular clot section consists almost exclusively of large blasts with "open" chromatin pattern (vesicular nuclei), two to three small nucleoli, and indented nuclear contours.

Acute myelomonocytic leukemia, (FAB: M4)

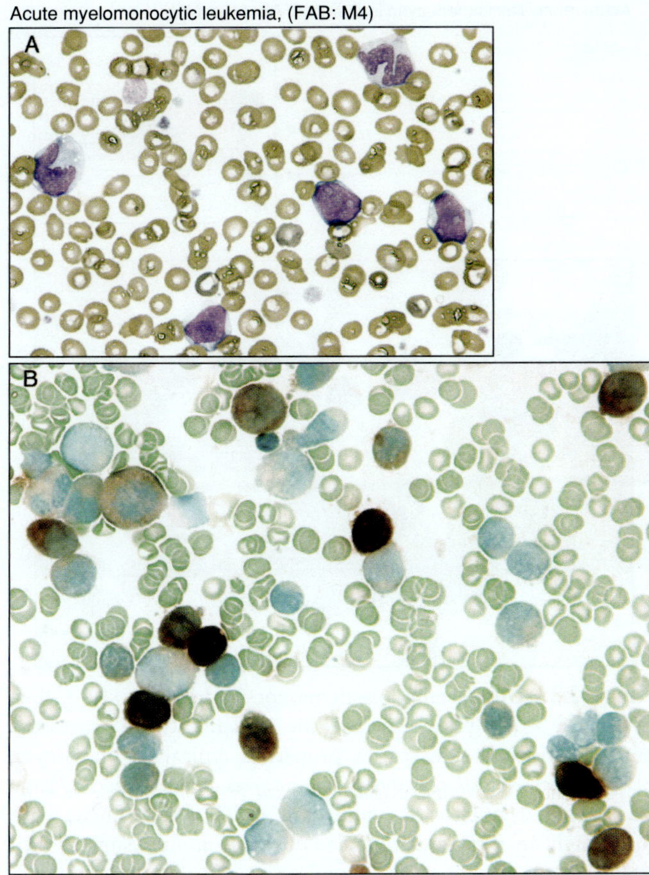

Acute myelomonocytic leukemia, (FAB: M4)

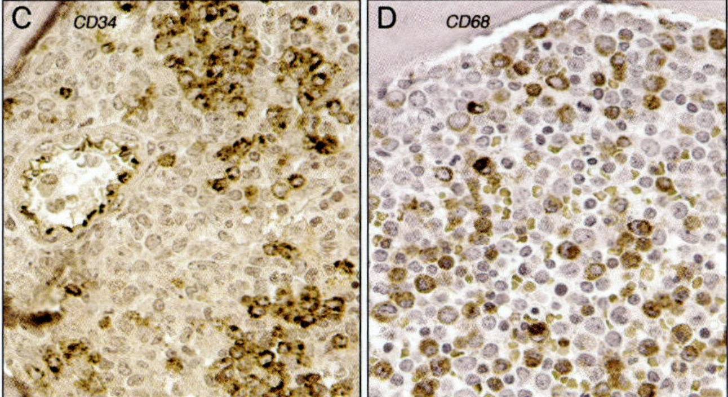

Acute myelomonocytic leukemia, (FAB: M4)

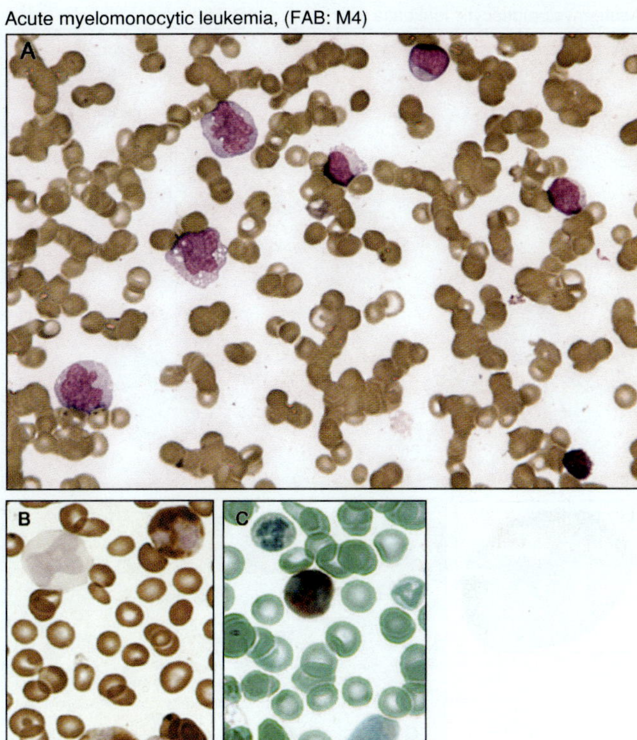

Figure 2.34   Acute myelomonocytic leukemia (AMML). **A.** A blood smear shows a distinctive dimorphic blast population consisting of immature nucleolated myeloblasts and mature monocytes. Fragments of cytoplasm also are present. **B.** An aspirate smear stained with butyrate esterase displays positive staining in only the larger-sized monocytic blast population. **C.** The bone marrow biopsy shows clusters of CD34⁺ myeloid blasts interspersed among negative-staining monocytic blasts. Note that the endothelial cells lining the vessel on the left side of the slide act as CD34 positive internal controls. **D.** Immunohistochemistry for monocytic marker CD68 shows positive staining in the monocytic blast subpopulation, corresponding to approximately 50% of all leukemia cells.

Figure 2.35   Acute myelomonocytic leukemia (AMML). **A.** A blood smear shows a dual population of small and large blasts; myeloblasts and monoblasts, respectively. On the left side are three mature monocytic blasts characterized by large size, low nuclear-to-cytoplasmic (N:C) ratios with somewhat condensed chromatin, absent nucleoli, irregularly folded nuclear contours, and vacuolated, finely granular, neutral-staining cytoplasm. The right upper corner of the slide contains three myeloblasts characterized by medium-size, higher N:C ratios, open chromatin, and scant cytoplasm. A small mature lymphocyte with closed chromatin is present in the right lower corner. **B.** Myeloperoxidase stains demonstrate strong granular cytoplasmic staining in a subpopulation of blasts. **C.** Butyrate esterase stains display strong positive staining in one blast. A neutrophil near the left upper corner serves as a built-in negative control.

Acute myelomonocytic leukemia with inv16, (FAB: M4)

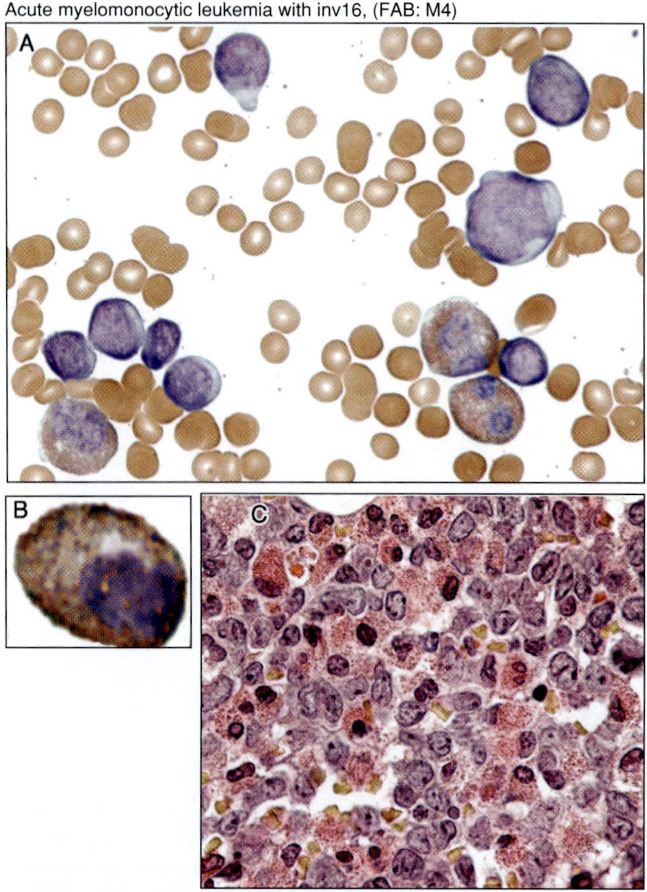

Figure 2.36   AMML with inv16 **A.** An aspirate with a dual population of small and large blasts with prominent eosinophilia. **B.** Some of the cells include the "eosinobasophils," which typically are associated with inv16. **C.** Biopsy shows hypercellular marrow with monocytic blasts and eosinophilia. Note the large monocytic blasts with folded nuclear contours.

Acute monoblastic/monocytic leukemia (FAB: M5a, M5b)

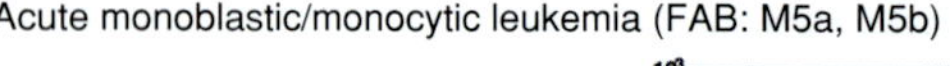

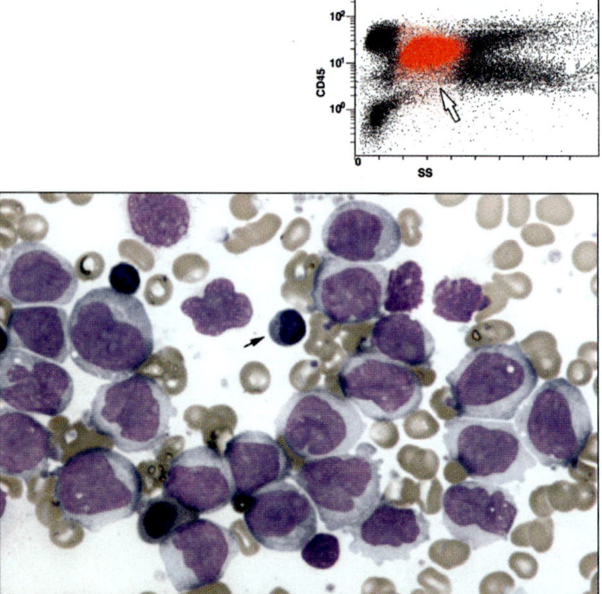

Figure 2.37   Acute monoblastic/monocytic leukemia. **A.** A flow cytometric scattergram illustrates the moderate CD45 expression and intermediate side scatter properties typical for monocytic blasts. **B.** An aspirate features promonocytes characterized by large size with low nuclear-to-cytoplasmic (N:C) ratios, nuclei with moderately open chromatin, folded nuclear contours (some kidney bean-shaped), absent nucleoli, and agranular, slightly basophilic-staining cytoplasm. For comparison, an arrow demonstrates a small mature lymphocyte with higher N:C ratio and closed chromatin. (Courtesy T. Anderson.)

Acute monoblastic leukemia (esterase negative).

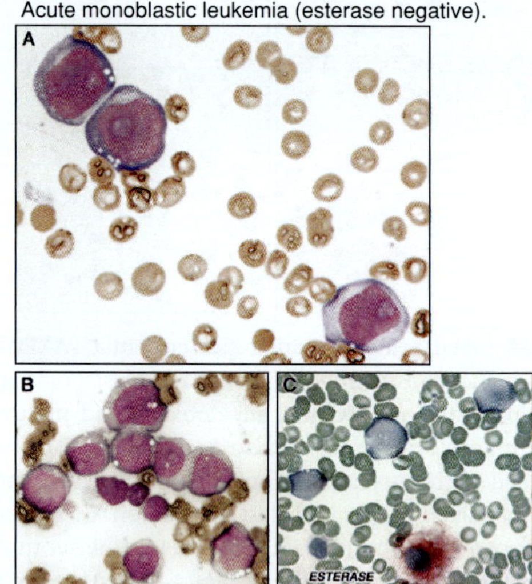

Figure 2.38   Acute monoblastic leukemia (esterase negative). **A.** This peripheral smear shows leukocytosis consisting of large undifferentiated blasts with low to moderate N:C ratios and basophilic staining cytoplasm. **B.** An aspirate smear shows clusters of these immature cells. By flow cytometric evaluation, these blasts displayed CD45 versus side scatter properties characteristic of monocytes and were CD11C^{+}/CD4^{+}. **C.** Butyrate esterase stains are negative in this particular case of acute monoblastic leukemia. A benign histiocyte located near the bottom of the slide serves as internal positive control.

Acute monoblastic leukemia, (FAB: M5): granular variant

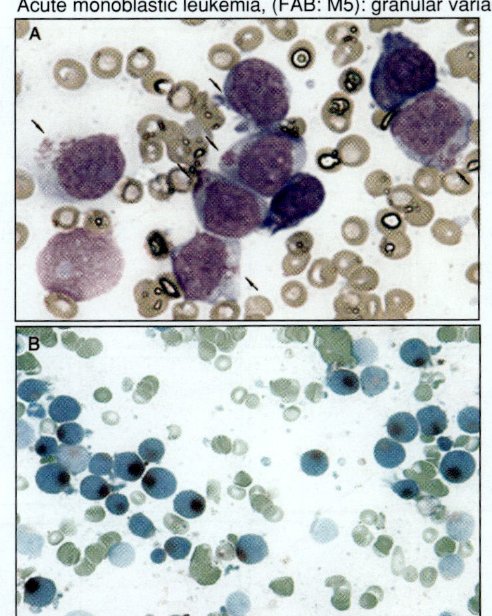

Figure 2.39 Acute monoblastic leukemia. **A.** An aspirate smear from acute monoblastic leukemia displays cytoplasmic granularity that is focally localized to the Golgi area (*arrows*). **B.** Butyrate esterase stains show localized positivity restricted to the perinuclear granules, confirming the monocytic origin for this case of acute monoblastic leukemia with heavily granulated blasts.

Acute monocytic leukemia, (FAB: M5): immunohistochemical findings on biopsy

Figure 2.40 Acute monoblastic leukemia with marrow fibrosis. **A.** and **B.** Bone marrow biopsy at low- and high-power, respectively: **A.** shows increased cellularity and architectural distortion such as swirling and lining up of individual marrow cells, (so-called Indian filing), suggesting the presence of significant bone marrow fibrosis, whereas **B.** demonstrates large, monotonous-appearing, wide-spaced, immature hematopoietic cells that replace the entire marrow cavity. **C** and **D.** In this case, CD68 stains only the benign reactive histiocytes interspersed among the negative-staining leukemic monoblasts. **E** and **F.** Immunohistochemistry for lysozyme stains with equal intensity in both the benign histiocytes and leukemic monoblasts.

Acute monocytic leukemia, (FAB: M5b)

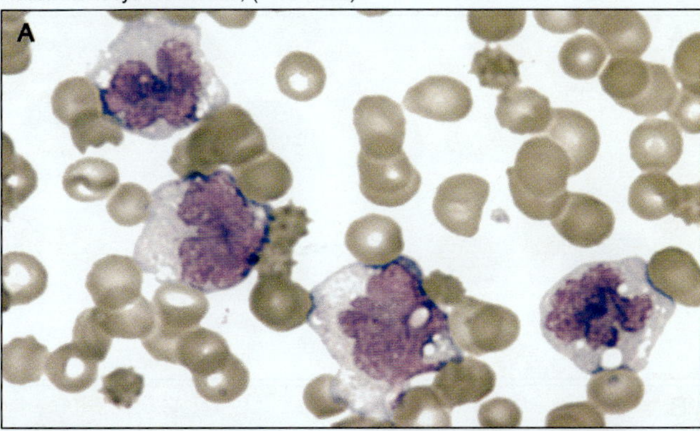

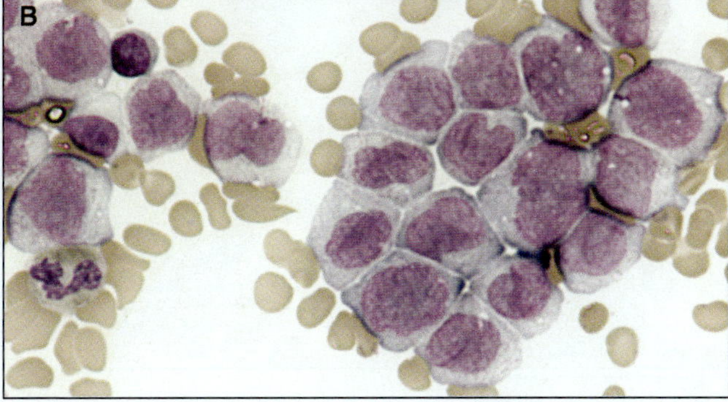

Figure 2.41 Acute monocytic leukemia. **A.** A high magnification view of a blood smear shows four large mature monocytes that have low N:C ratios, lobulated nuclei with moderately closed chromatin pattern and neutral staining, and finely granular, vacuolated cytoplasm. **B.** This aspirate smear shows clusters of monocytic blasts that have a more immature appearance than do the circulating blasts.

Acute monocytic leukemia, (FAB: M5a)

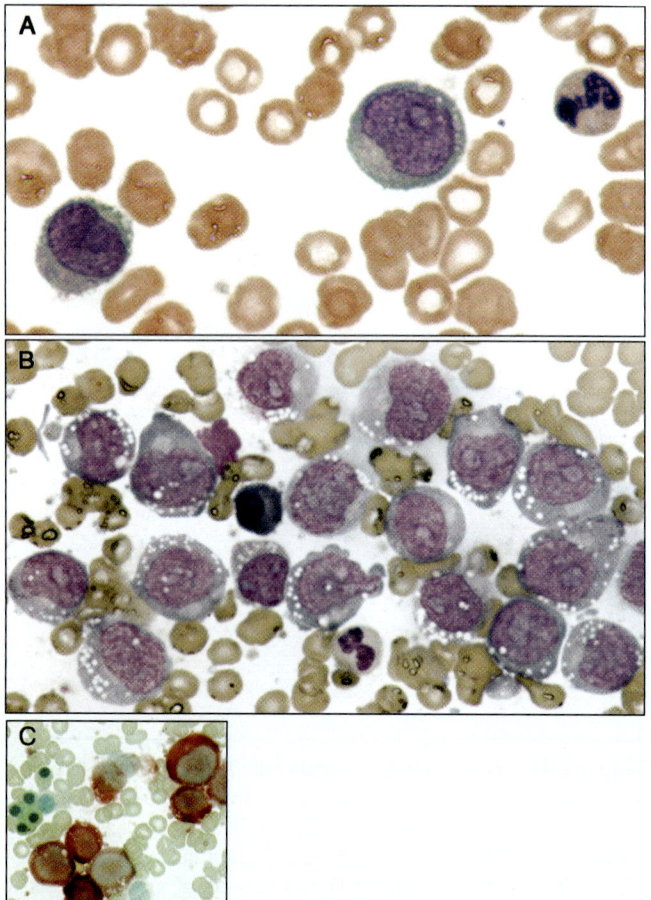

Acute monoblastic/monocytic leukemia: blast morphology

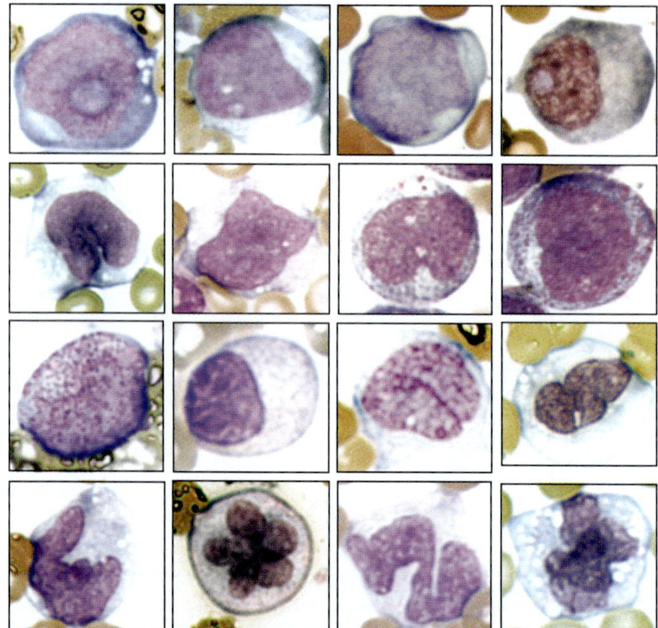

Figure 2.43   Blast morphology in acute monocytic leukemia. This mosaic, from 16 different cases of acute monoblastic and monocytic leukemias, illustrates the wide variation in blast morphology seen in this type of AML. Undifferentiated monoblasts with high N:C ratios, open chromatin, nucleoli, and basophilic staining cytoplasm are present in the upper panels, promonocytes in the middle panels and differentiated monocytic blasts with closed chromatin pattern and lobulated nuclei are shown in the lower panels.

Figure 2.42   **A.** Acute monoblastic leukemia. Nucleolated monoblasts are present in this peripheral blood smear. **B.** An aspirate smear shows monotonous sheets of monoblasts displaying open chromatin with multiple prominent nucleoli and vacuolated, basophilic-staining cytoplasm. These are somewhat reminiscent of the L3 blasts seen in Burkitt lymphoma. **C.** Strong, diffuse, cytoplasmic staining by butyrate esterase confirms the monocytic origin of these leukemic blasts. An erythroid cluster on the left side of the slide serves as a negative control.

Acute monoblastic leukemia (FAB: M5a)

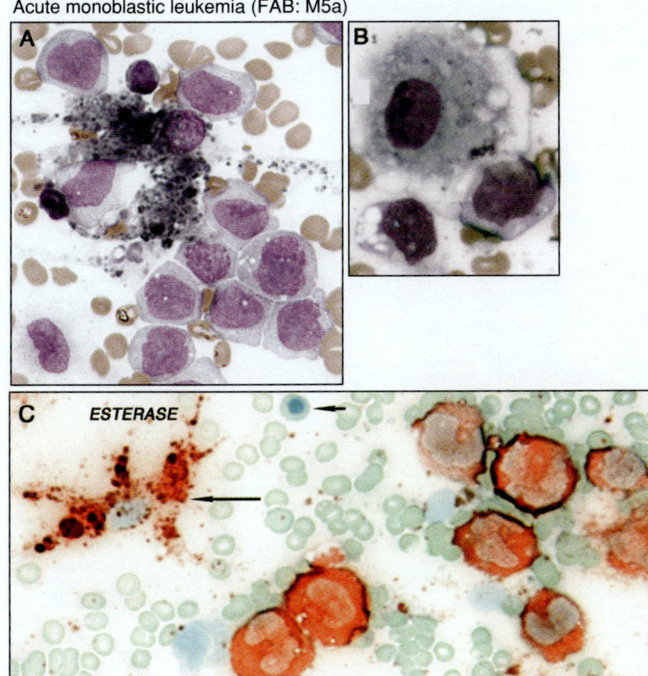

Figure 2.44   Acute monoblastic leukemia. **A.** Monoblasts surround a large, benign histiocyte with long tentacles of cytoplasmic projections packed with dark-staining pigment (likely iron) in this case of acute monoblastic leukemia. **B.** In this slide from the same case, the two lower cells are monocytic leukemic blasts and the larger cell in the upper area is a benign histiocyte. Histiocytes, usually "innocent" benign bystanders in marrow diseases, are characterized by oval-shaped nuclei, smooth nuclear contours, "bland" chromatin patterns and ample neutral-staining cytoplasm. Often, histiocytes are stuffed with iron pigment and/or digested cellular debris. **C.** Positive butyrate esterase staining is seen in: (1) the numerous leukemic monoblasts (*on the right*) and (2) a benign histiocyte (*long arrow*). An erythroid precursor serves as a negative control (*short arrow*).

Acute monoblastic leukemia (FAB: M5a)

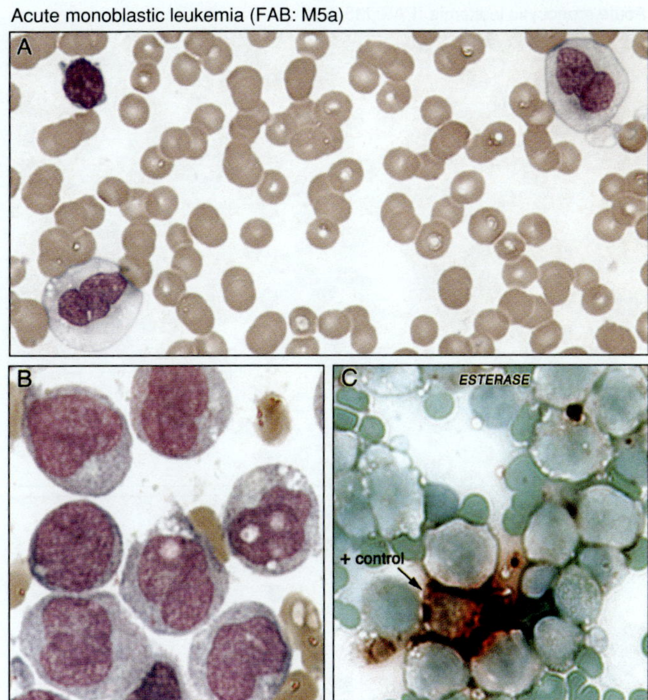

Figure 2.45   **A.** Acute monoblastic leukemia, esterase negative. A peripheral blood smear displays two circulating promonocytes and a small mature lymphocyte. The two promonocytes are characterized by large size, low N:C ratios, distinctly lobulated nuclear contours and ample "agranular" neutral-staining cytoplasm. **B.** A higher-power view of an aspirate smear shows monoblasts with bilobed nuclei reminiscent of the microgranular variant of acute promyelocytic leukemia. (Note the dissimilarity between the cytoplasmic granularity of the blasts in peripheral blood compared with the aspirate smear). **C.** Butyrate esterase histochemistry demonstrates negative staining in the promonocytes (a benign histiocyte serves as positive control).

Acute monocytic leukemia (FAB: M5b)

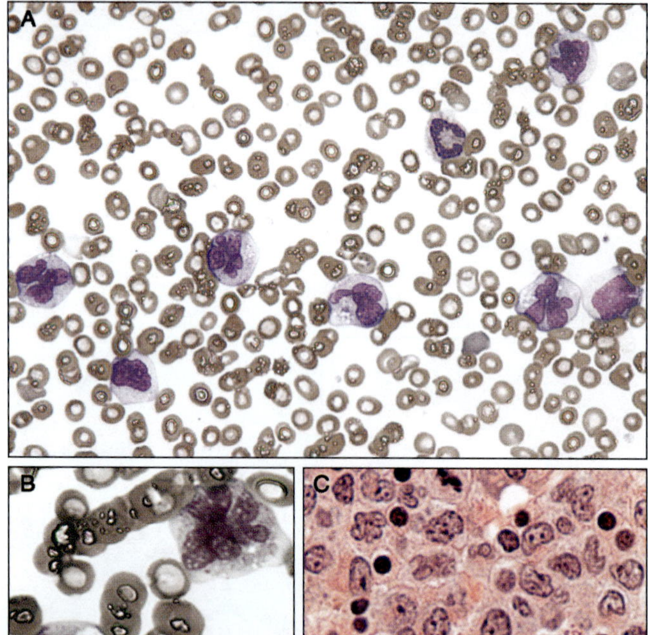

Chloromas (granulocytic sarcomas): CD45 negative acute monocytic leukemia

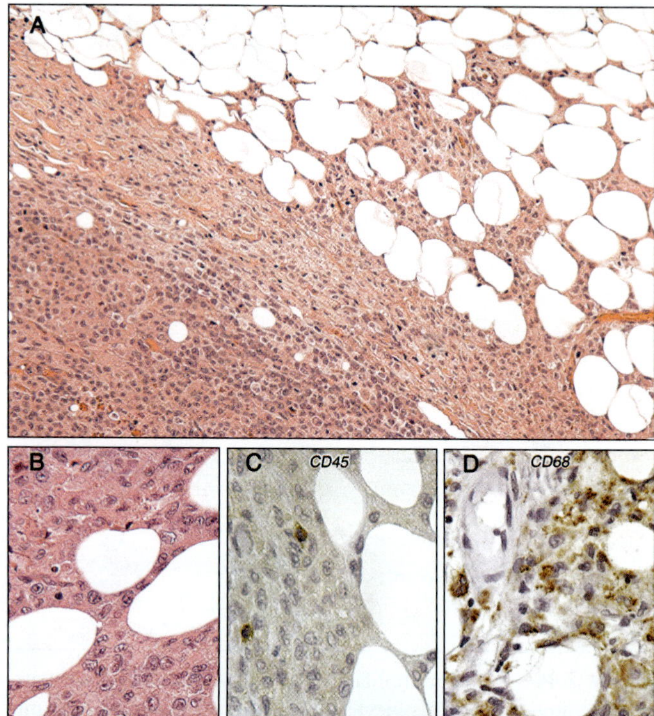

Figure 2.46 Acute monocytic leukemia. **A.** and **B.** Blood smears show peripheral monocytosis consisting of mature monocytes that have a closed chromatin pattern, lobulated nuclei, and abundant granular, vacuolated cytoplasm. **C.** A bone marrow biopsy demonstrates hypercellular marrow consisting almost exclusively of monocytoid precursors.

Figure 2.47 Chloroma. **A.** Low magnification of a chloroma (granulocytic sarcoma) arising in the chest wall of a patient suffering from acute monocytic leukemia. **B.** The malignant behavior of this lesion is shown by the invasive growth pattern consisting of finger-like projections of tumor reaching deep into the subcutaneous fat. **C.** Immunohistochemistry for CD45 shows negative staining in this tumor derived from leukemic monocytes. Two lymphocytes displaying strong CD45 staining are present on the left side of the slide and serve as positive controls. **D.** Anti-CD68 shows strong cytoplasmic staining in the monocytic leukemia cells.

Acute erythroid leukemias (FAB: M6a, M6b)

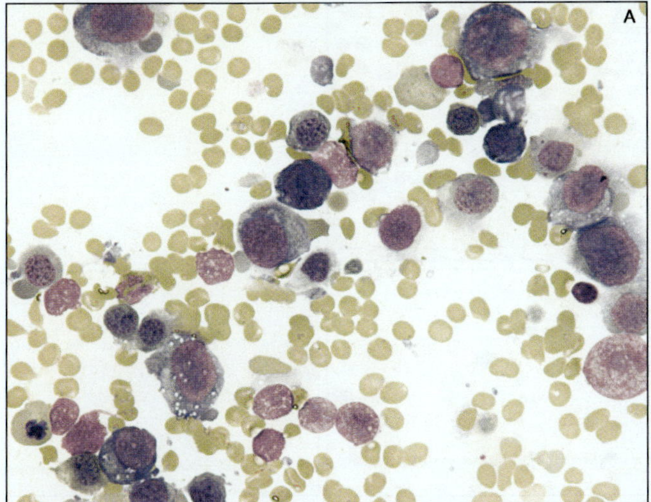

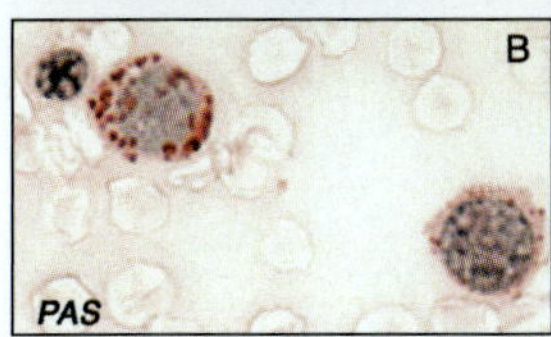

Figure 2.48 Acute erythroid leukemia, pure erythroid type. **A.** The aspirate smear consists entirely of a heterogeneous mixture of dysplastic erythroid blasts, many displaying cytoplasmic vacuolation. **B.** PAS stains show the characteristic coarse granular staining in immature leukemic erythroid precursors, compared with a negative staining mature erythroid precursor shown in the left upper corner.

Acute erythroid leukemia (erythroid/myeloid type): the "non-erythroid blast count"

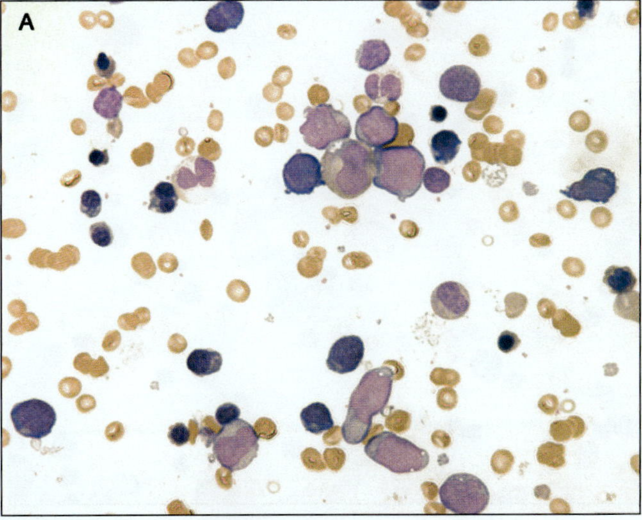

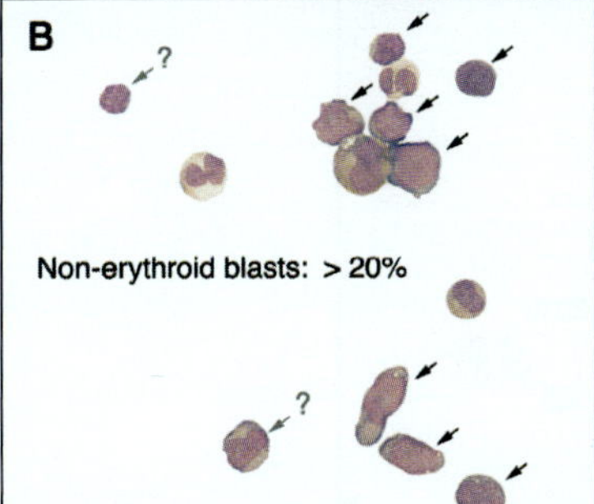

Figure 2.49 Acute erythroid leukemia, erythroid/myeloid type. **A.** An aspirate smear shows a mixture of dysplastic erythroid precursors and immature myeloid cells, including numerous blasts. **B.** In this panel, all the nonerythroid cells from the field above in **A.** are removed, clearly demonstrating a non-erythroid blast count exceeding 20% (blasts shown by *arrows*).

Acute erythroid leukemia (erythroid/myeloid type): the "non-erythroid" blast count

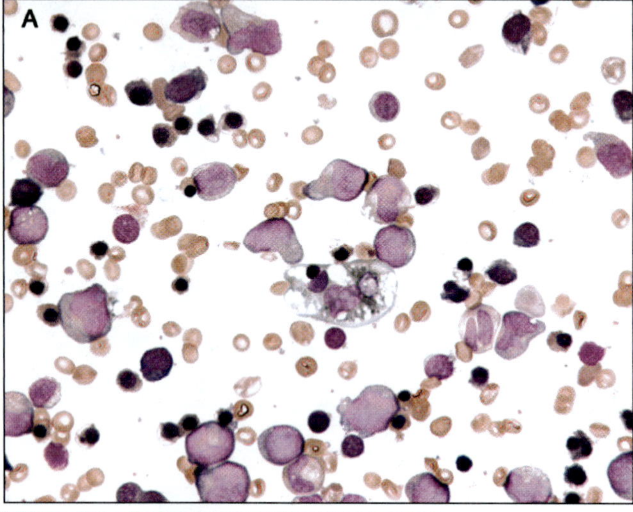

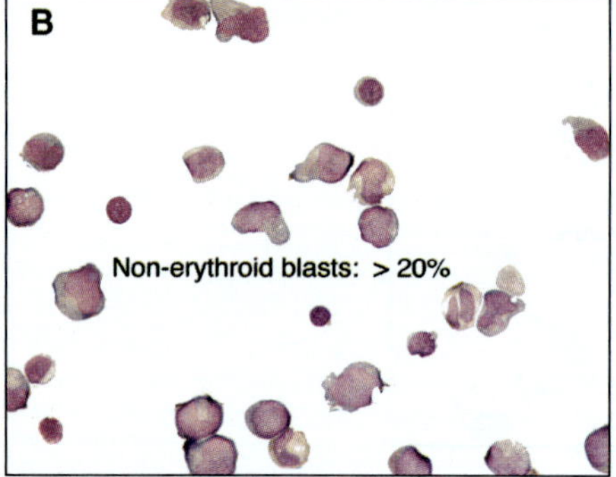

Figure 2.50 Acute erythroid leukemia, erythroid/myeloid type. **A.** An aspirate smear shows erythroid hyperplasia, increased numbers of blasts, and hemophagocytosis. In the center of the figure, a benign-appearing histiocyte engulfs cellular debris. Hemophagocytosis can occur in both benign and malignant bone marrow disorders, including acute erythroid leukemia. **B.** This figure excludes all the nonerythroid cells from the figure above in **A.** and clearly shows a non-erythroid blast count exceeding 20%.

Acute erythroid leukemia versus megaloblastic erythroid hyperplasia

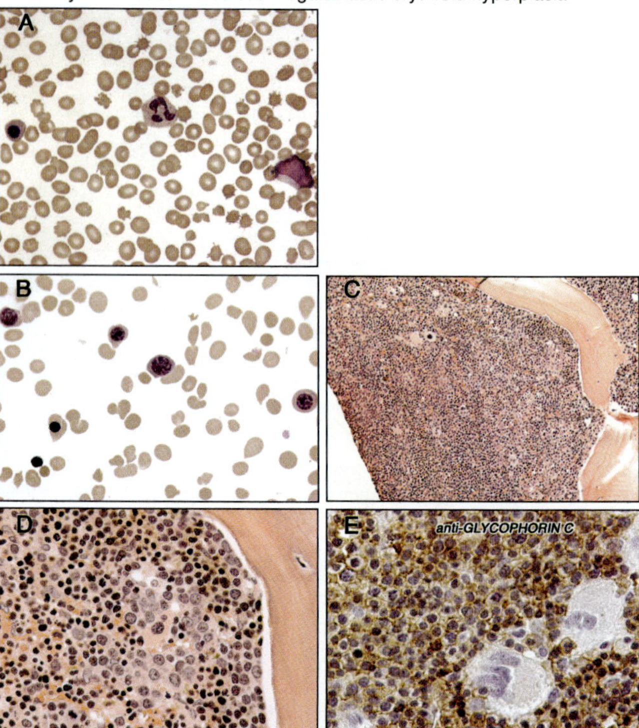

Figure 2.51 Acute erythroid leukemia, pure erythroid type. **A.** This blood smear shows a leukoerythroblastic picture with marked poikilocytosis. **B.** An aspirate smear reveals only scattered megaloblastic erythroid precursors. **C.** Biopsy at medium magnification shows a hypercellular marrow composed exclusively of a heterogeneous mononuclear cell population. **D.** Biopsy at high magnification shows replacement of the bone marrow cavity by a mixed erythroid population. **E.** Immunohistochemistry for the erythroid lineage marker glycophorin C demonstrates positive staining in the leukemic cells, and negative staining megakaryocytes serve as controls.

Acute erythroid leukemia versus dysplastic erythroid hyperplasia

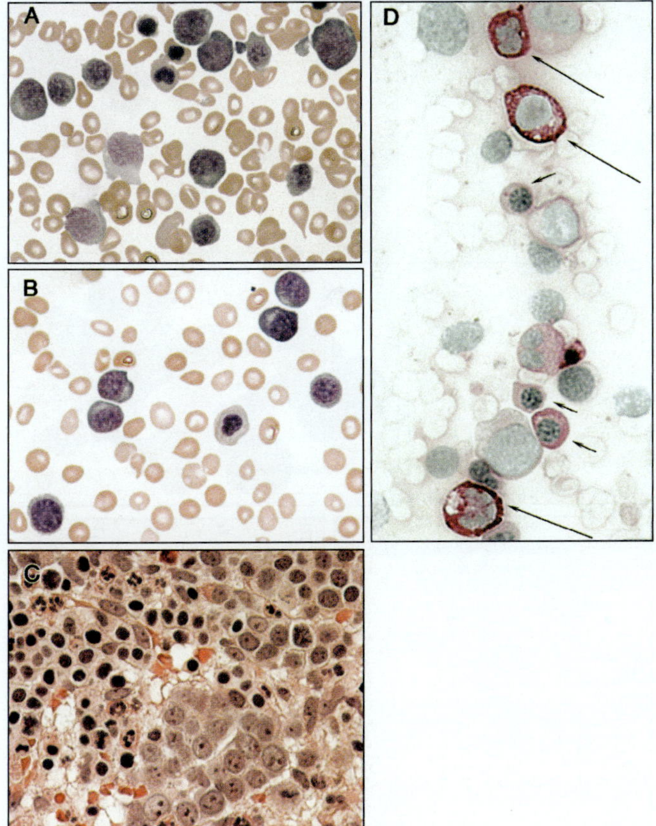

Acute erythroid leukemia (pure erythroleukemia type)

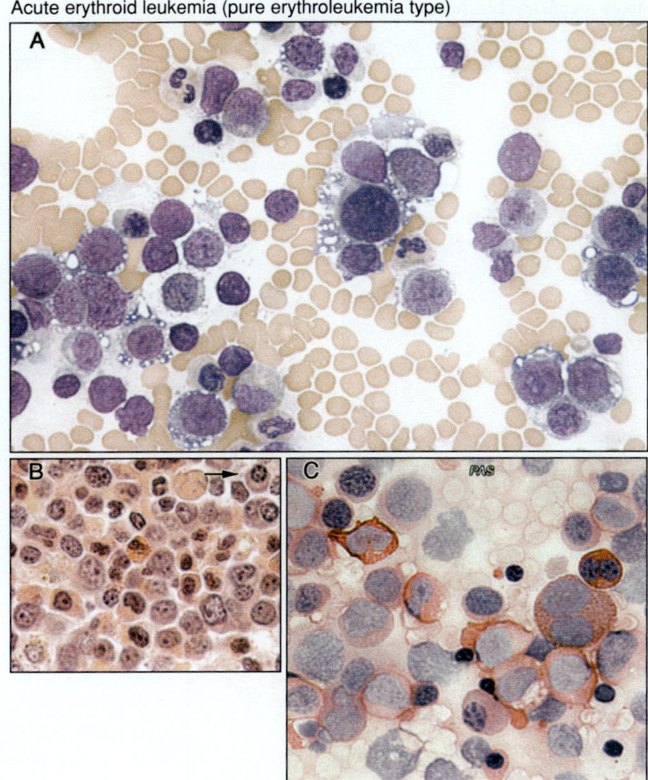

Figure 2.52   **A** and **B**. Acute erythroid leukemia versus dysplastic erythroid hyperplasia. Aspirate smears show increased numbers of erythroid blasts associated with dysplastic mature erythroid forms displaying irregular ("cookie cutter") nuclear contours. Teardrop RBCs related to the bone marrow fibrosis also are visible. **C**. A biopsy shows atypical erythroid hyperplasia with nests consisting exclusively of monotonous immature erythroid forms. **D**. A periodic acid-Schiff (PAS)–stained aspirate shows the typical coarse granular pattern of staining in immature erythroid precursors (*long arrows*) compared with the diffuse staining seen in the more mature forms (*short arrows*).

Figure 2.53   Acute erythroid leukemia (pure erythroid type). **A**. An aspirate smear shows erythroid hyperplasia and numerous dysplastic erythroid blasts with vacuolated cytoplasm. **B**. The biopsy demonstrates increased numbers of erythroid precursors, which, especially in biopsies, can be confused morphologically with plasma cells (a plasma cell is shown by an *arrow*). **C**. PAS stains of aspirate smear demonstrate granular and diffuse staining in immature and mature erythroid precursors, respectively.

Acute megakaryoblastic leukemia (FAB: M7)

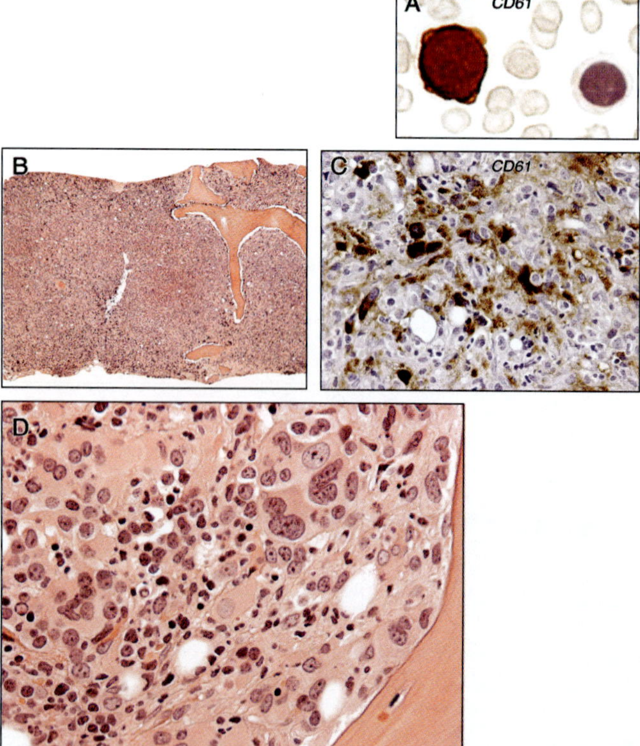

Acute megakaryoblastic leukemia (FAB: M7)

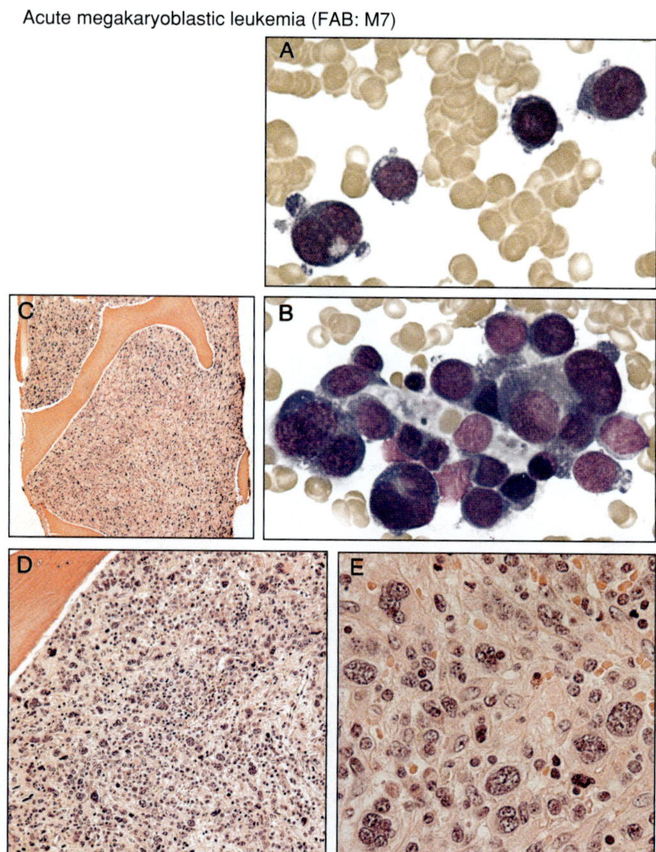

Figure 2.54   Acute megakaryoblastic leukemia. **A.** An aspirate shows a blast that is positive for the megakaryocytic marker CD61 (on the *left*) with a negative staining lymphocyte (on the *right*). **B–D.** A biopsy shows fibrotic, hypercellular marrow composed entirely of atypical megakaryocytes. In C, CD61 is only positive in the larger, more differentiated blasts. Fibrosis often precludes flow cytometry, and often the diagnosis of this disease rests solely on immunohistochemically stained biopsies.

Figure 2.55   Acute megakaryoblastic leukemia. **A.** An aspirate smear shows four blasts with multiple, broad-based cytoplasmic projections reminiscent of platelet production by megakaryocytes. **B.** Cohesive clustering of malignant cells appears in this aspirate smear. **C–E.** Bone marrow biopsies show marrow replaced by immature hematopoietic cells, some displaying megakaryocytic features.

Acute megakaryoblastic leukemia (FAB: M7)

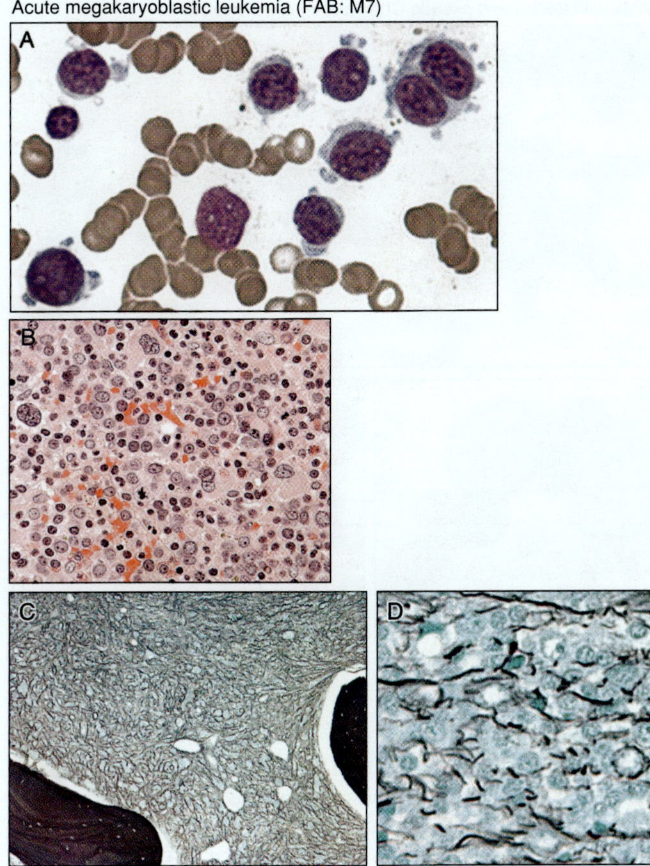

Figure 2.56 Acute megakaryoblastic leukemia. **A.** An aspirate smear shows blasts with cytoplasmic blebbing reminiscent of platelet production by megakaryocytes. **B.** A bone marrow biopsy demonstrates increased blasts, some of which display megakaryocytic differentiation. **C.** Reticulin stains of a biopsy at low magnification display a diffuse increase in the number of fibers throughout the bone marrow space. **D.** Higher magnification of the bone marrow biopsy stained for reticulin shows thickened fibers that encircle individual bone marrow cells.

AML with t(8;21)(q22;q22)

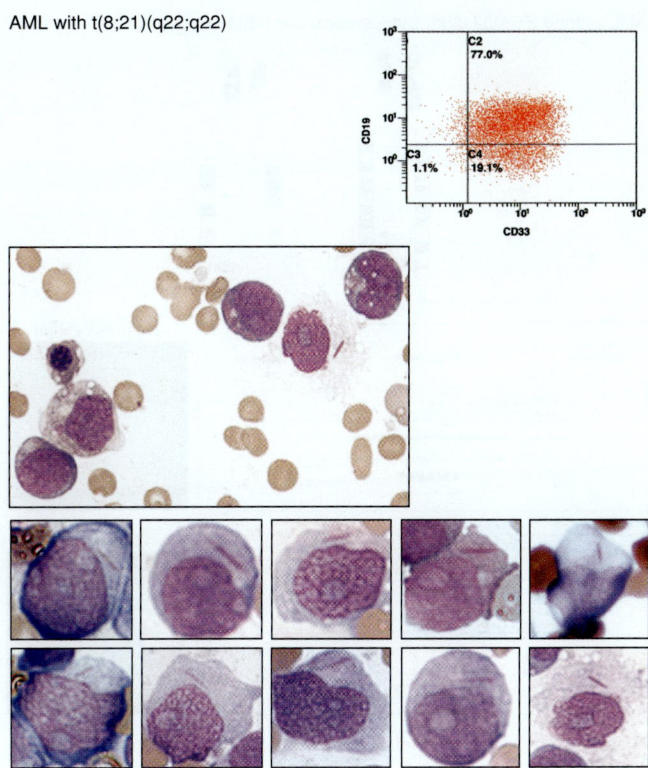

Figure 2.57 AML with t(8;21). **A.** Aberrant expression of the B-cell marker CD19 by myeloid blasts is commonly seen in AML with t(8;21) (detailed immunophenotype discussed in Fig. 6.7). **B.** An aspirate shows granulated blasts mixed with abnormal mature myeloid forms. A long slender, tapered Auer rod is present in the cytoplasm of a partially degenerated blast in the upper right area of the slide. **C.** Auer rod morphology is shown here from several cases of AML with t(8;21). The blasts in this type of AML often appear more differentiated and may contain long, tapering Auer rods.

AML with t(8;21)(q22;q22): Cytogenetics and FISH

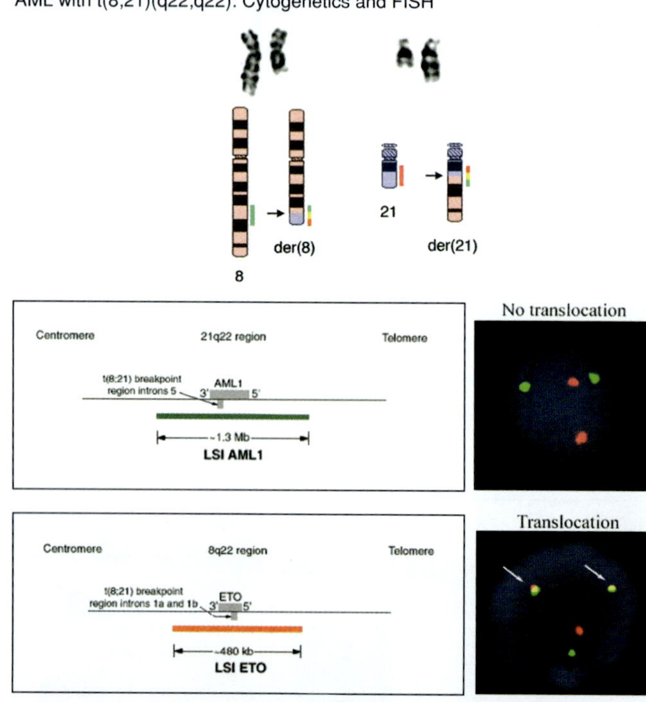

Figure 2.58 *Upper panel:* The t(8;21) (q22;q22) rearrangement. The ideograms of chromosomes 8, 21 and the respective derivative chromosomes are depicted below in color, and the corresponding G-banded chromosome pairs are shown above. The arrows indicate the breakpoints on the respective chromosomes. The green, red, and yellow colors indicate expected FISH signals using the LSI AML1 and LSI ETO probe as shown in lower panel. *Lower panel:* FISH of the AML1/ETO fusion gene. The AML1 gene at 8q22 (*green*) and the ETO gene at 21q22 (*red*) co-localize to generate yellow fusion signals (*arrows*), indicating a reciprocal translocation involving these loci.

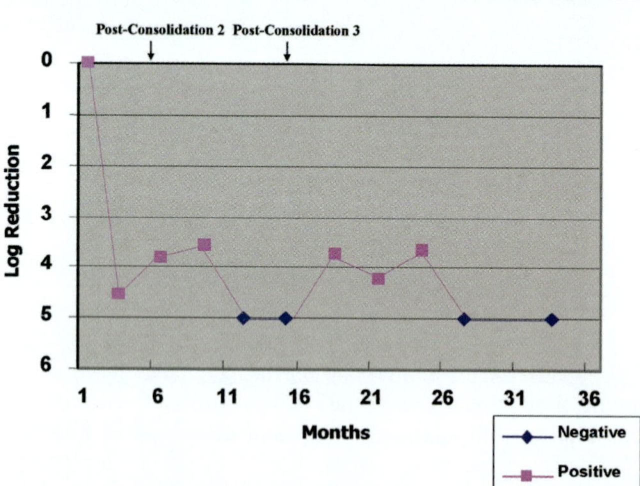

Figure 2.59 Minimal residual disease assessment in AML with t(8;21). Quantitative PCR for AML-ETO mRNA is shown here for a period of 3 years following diagnosis. (Courtesy Dr. S. Kamel-Reid.)

AML with t(8;21) and pseudo Chediak-Higashi inclusions

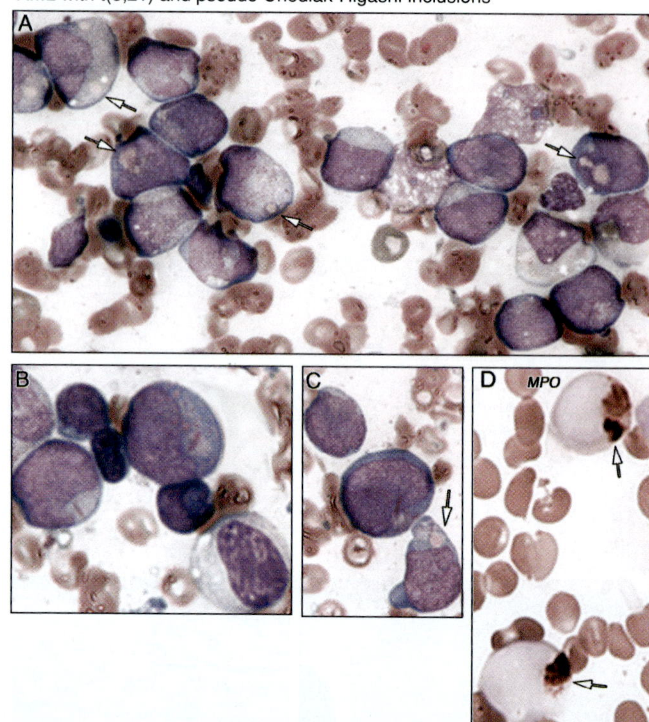

Figure 2.60 AML with t(8;21) and pseudo–Chediak-Higashi inclusions. **A.** An aspirate shows numerous granulated blasts and differentiated myeloid precursors. Many of the blasts contain unusual "blob-like" Auer rods or so-called pseudo–Chediak-Higashi inclusions (*arrows*). **B.** The t(8;21) leukemia cells include two blasts, each containing long thin Auer rods and, in the lower right corner, a myelocyte. **C.** Three blasts are shown here, one with a blob-like Auer rod. **D.** Myeloperoxidase stains show heavy block-like staining of the blob-like Auer rods (*arrows*) in this unusual case of AML with t(8;21). Pseudo–Chediak-Higashi inclusions also occur in other AML subtypes.

AML with t(15;17)(q22;q12) or acute promyelocytic leukemia (APL)

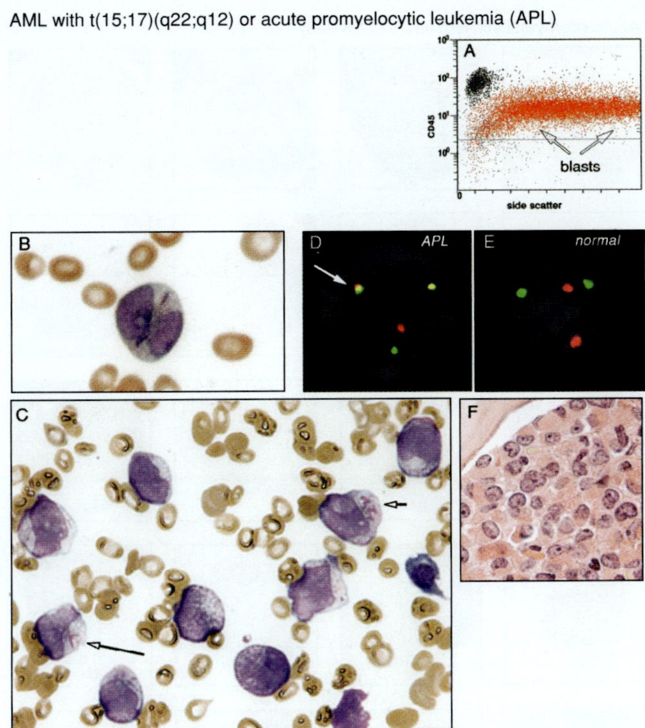

Figure 2.61 Acute promyelocytic leukemia. **A.** CD45 versus side scatter plot shows the classic comet-shaped pattern from granulated blasts. **B.** A blood smear displays pancytopenia, low platelets, and a rare abnormal bilobed promyelocyte. A single Auer rod appears in the two o'clock position of this APL cell. **C.** An aspirate shows numerous abnormal promyelocytes, many containing fused primary granules in the form of either classical Auer rods (*long arrow*) or other bizarre forms (*short arrow*). **D** and **E.** Fluorescent in situ hybridization (FISH) of the PML/RARA fusion gene. The PML gene at 15q22 (*red*) and RARA gene at 17q12~21 (*green*) co-localize to generate yellow signals, indicating a reciprocal translocation involving these loci. **F.** A biopsy demonstrates replacement of the marrow by uniformly spaced, large, immature cells with folded nuclei and ample cytoplasm.

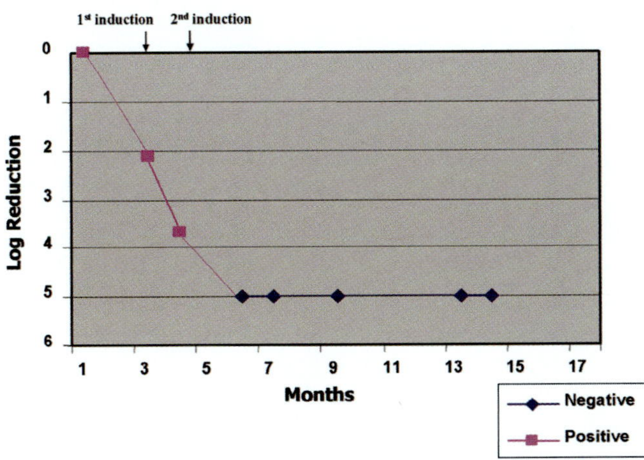

Figure 2.62 Minimal residual disease assessment in AML with t(15;17). Quantitative PCR for PML-RAR-α and mRNA is shown here for a period of 15 months following diagnosis. (Courtesy Dr. S. Kamel-Reid.)

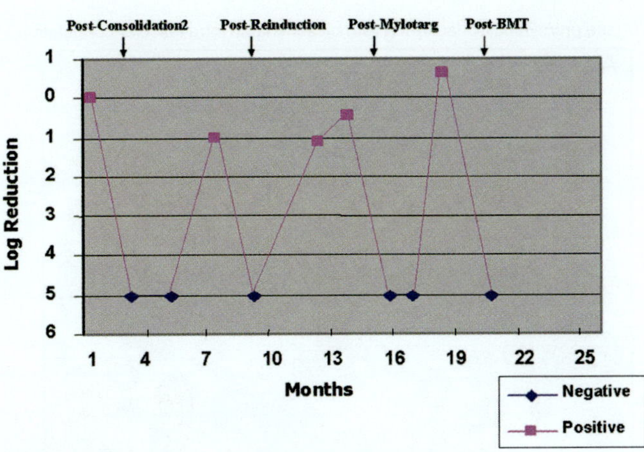

Figure 2.63 Minimal residual disease and response to treatment and in AML with t(15;17). Quantitative PCR for PML-RAR-α mRNA is shown here for a period of 21 months following diagnosis and shows cycles of treatment response and relapse that often occur in this disease. (Courtesy Dr. S. Kamel-Reid.)

Acute promyelocytic leukemia, microgranular variant

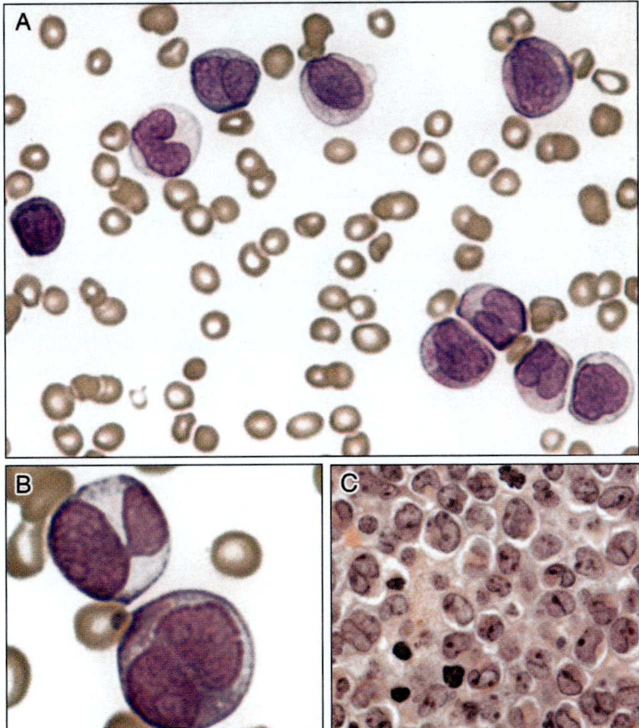

Figure 2.64 Acute promyelocytic leukemia, microgranular variant. **A.** A peripheral smear shows leukocytosis and severe thrombocytopenia with increased numbers of early myeloid cells displaying the characteristic bilobed nuclei of microgranular APL cells. **B.** Closer inspection of the APL cells demonstrates the characteristic bilobed or "pinched" nuclei and very fine, dust-like cytoplasmic granules. **C.** High-power view of a bone marrow biopsy reveals a hypercellular bone marrow with uniformly spaced, large immature hematopoietic cells with abundant eosinophilic-staining cytoplasm and bilobed (buttock-like) nuclei.

Acute promyelocytic leukemia with disseminated intravascular coagulation

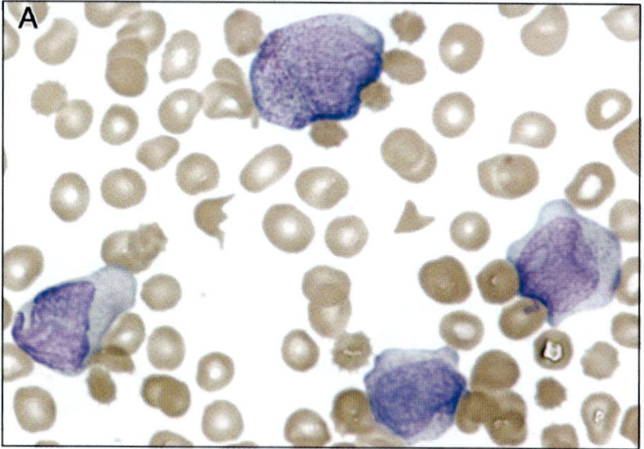

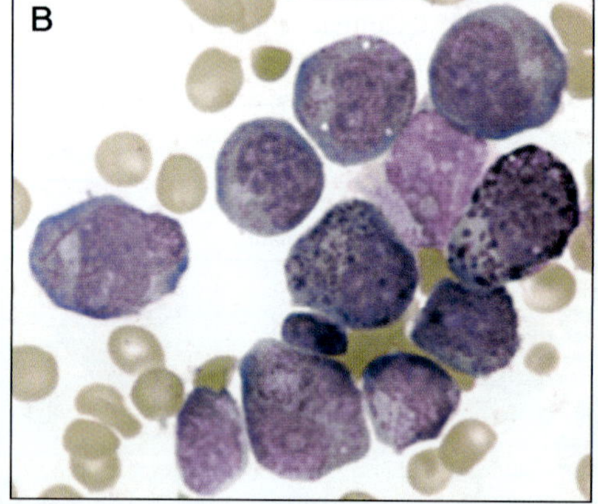

Acute promyelocytic leukemia, (FAB: M3)

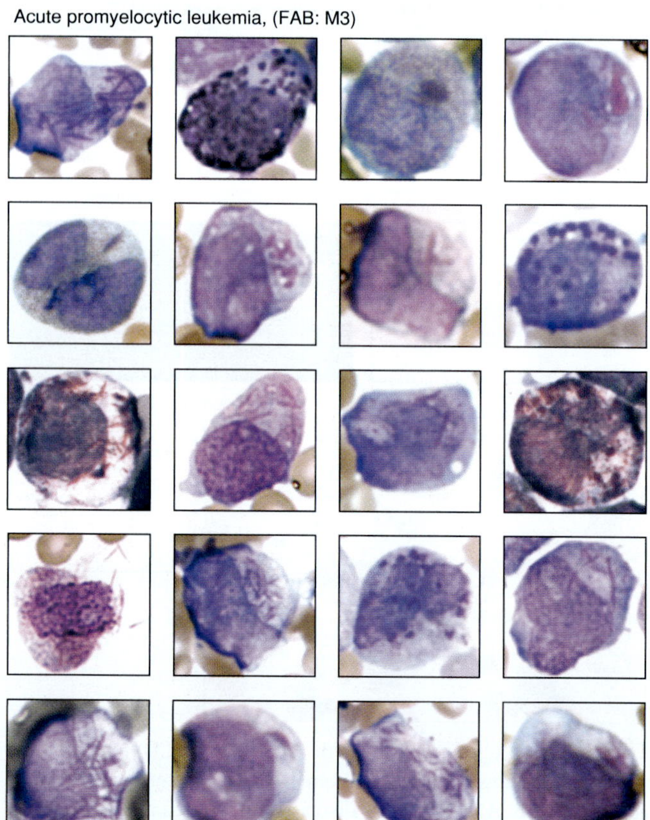

Figure 2.65 Acute promyelocytic leukemia with disseminated intravascular coagulation. **A.** A peripheral blood smear from a case of APL shows a leukocytosis with thrombocytopenia and schisto-cytes. **B.** Aspirate smears demonstrate increased numbers of abnormal promyelocytes with bizarre cytoplasmic granulation including typical Auer rods (shown on the *left*), large coarse granules (shown in the *right central area*), and fine, dust-like eosinophilic granules.

Figure 2.66 Auer-rod morphology in acute promyelocytic leukemia. This picture shows variations on the appearance of "faggot cells" in several different cases of APL.

Acute promyelocytic leukemia, microgranular variant

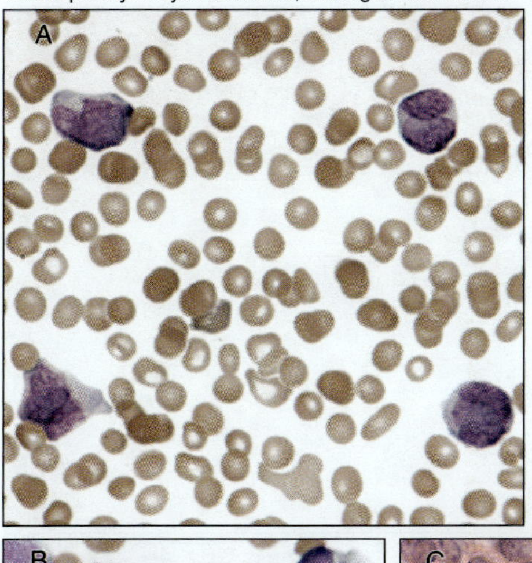

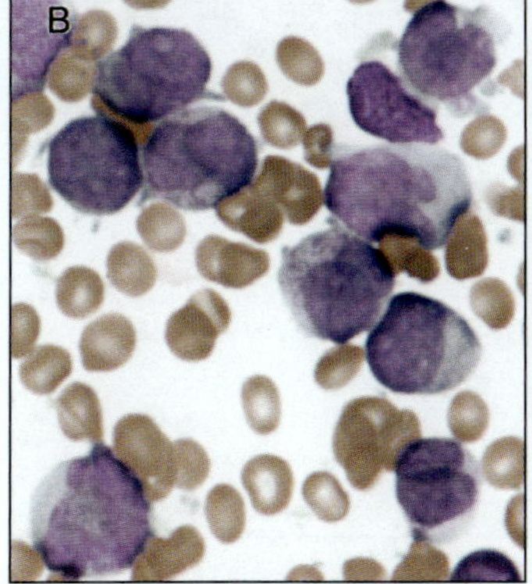

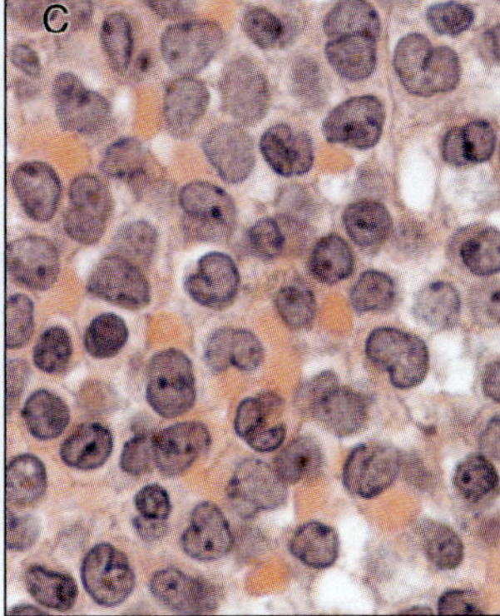

Figure 2.67   Acute promyelocytic leukemia, microgranular variant. **A.** A peripheral blood smear from a case of microgranular variant APL demonstrates leukocytosis and thrombocytopenia. The characteristic abnormal bilobed promyelocytes are present. **B.** Close examination of the abnormal promyelocytes in this case reveals fine, dust-like eosinophilic granules within the cytoplasm. Auer rods are difficult to find in many of these cases. **C.** A bone marrow biopsy shows replacement of bone marrow by monotonous sheets of uniformly spaced bilobed immature hematopoietic precursors.

Acute promyelocytic leukemia, microgranular variant

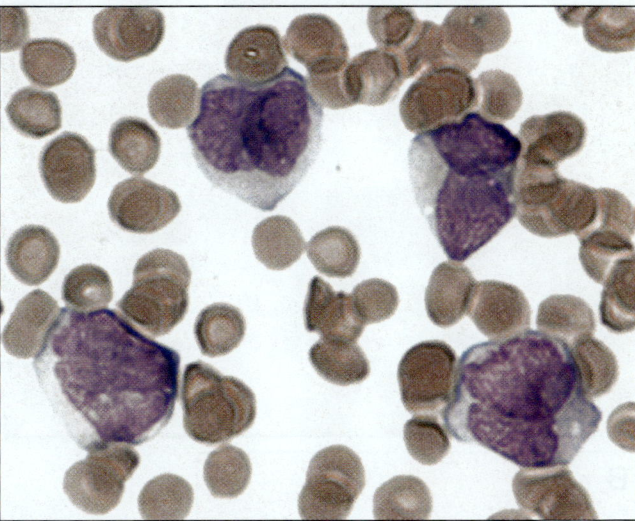

Figure 2.68   Acute promyelocytic leukemia, microgranular variant. A peripheral blood smear from a case of the microgranular variant of APL discloses leukocytosis and thrombocytopenia with increased numbers of abnormal seemingly agranular, bilobed promyelocytes.

Acute promyelocytic leukemia

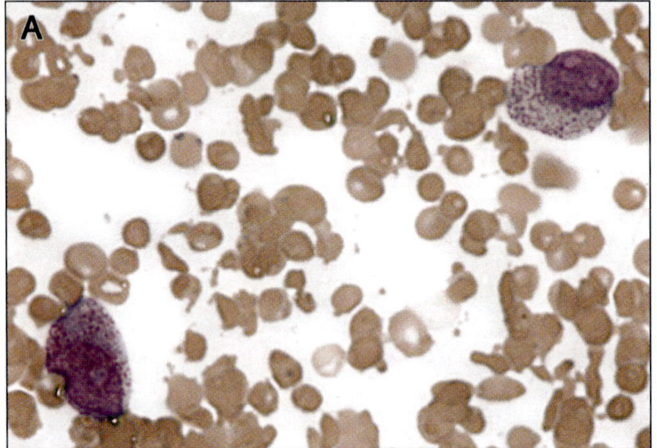

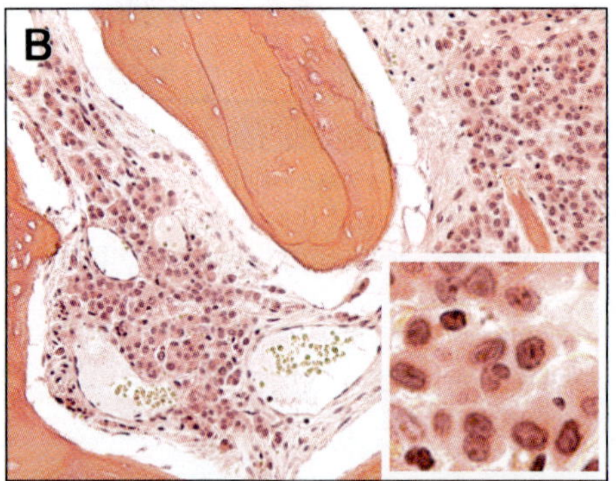

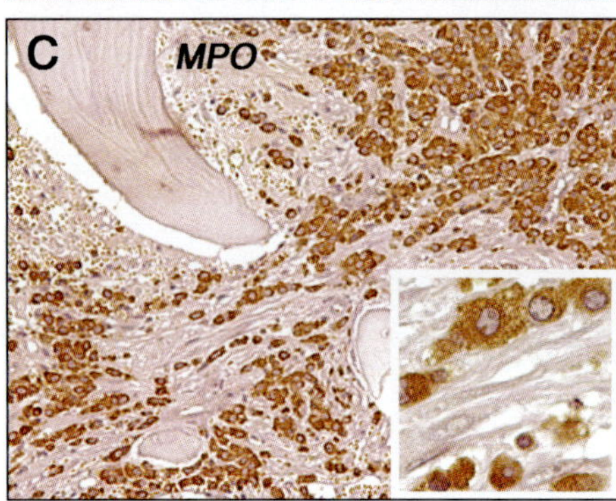

Figure 2.69 Acute promyelocytic leukemia with bone marrow fibrosis. **A.** This hypocellular aspirate smear demonstrates rare, abnormal, heavily granulated promyelocytes. **B.** A bone marrow biopsy shows architectural distortion suggesting significant marrow fibrosis and replacement by a monotonous immature hematopoietic cell population. Higher magnification of the biopsy (inset in *right lower corner*) discloses monotonous foci composed of uniformly spaced immature, bilobed hematopoietic precursors. **C.** A bone marrow biopsy reveals infiltration of bone marrow space by MPO-positive immature hematopoietic cells. Higher-power view of the bone marrow biopsy (inset in *right lower corner*) shows strong granular staining of APL cells with anti-MPO immunostaining.

Acute promyelocytic leukemia, microgranular variant

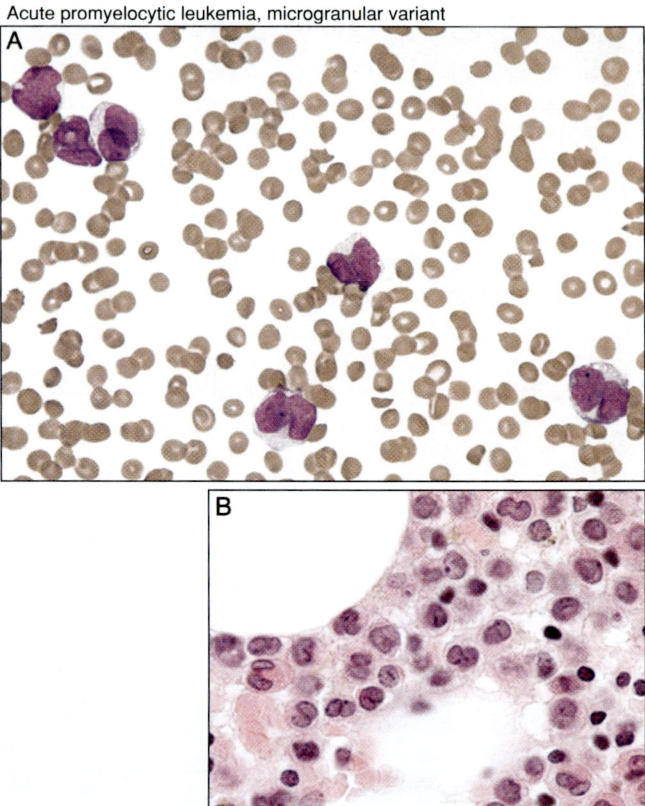

Figure 2.70 Acute promyelocytic leukemia, microgranular variant. **A.** This blood smear shows increased numbers of abnormal bilobed promyelocytes with hypogranular cytoplasm and thrombocytopenia. These large immature hematopoietic cells with folded nuclear contours can be confused with monocytic blasts. **B.** A bone marrow biopsy demonstrates a monotonous proliferation of uniformly spaced large cells with characteristic bilobed (buttock-like) nuclei and ample cytoplasm.

Acute promyelocytic leukemia versus maturation arrest

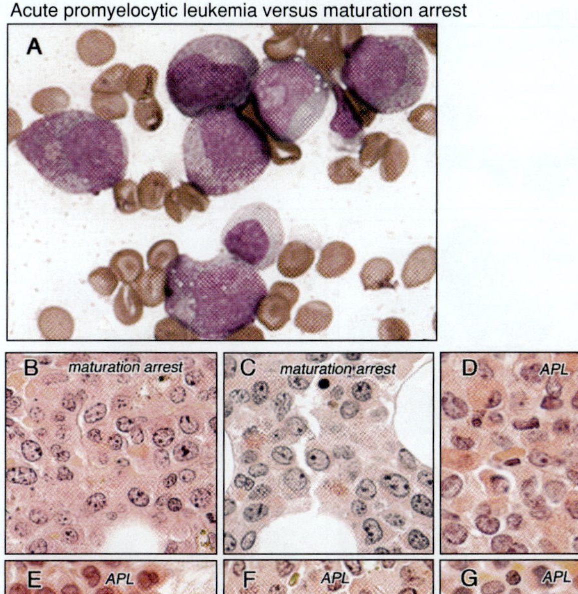

Figure 2.71 APL versus maturation arrest. **A.** An aspirate smear reveals scattered numbers of heavily granulated promyelocytes in a patient recovering from induction chemotherapy. This case of maturation arrest, without clinical-pathological correlation, could easily be mistaken for a case of APL. As demonstrated in this slide, cases of maturation arrest usually show moderate numbers of promyelocytes that are often, but not always, mixed with a spectrum of left-shifted myeloid forms. **B–F.** A collection of bone marrow biopsies from cases of maturation arrest (**B** and **C**) and APL (**D, E, F,** and **G**). Pleomorphism and lower marrow cellularity often are present in maturation arrest, whereas APL cases usually have more monotonous-appearing promyelocytes that may contain Auer rods and often, but not always, show the classical bilobed nuclei.

AML with inv16

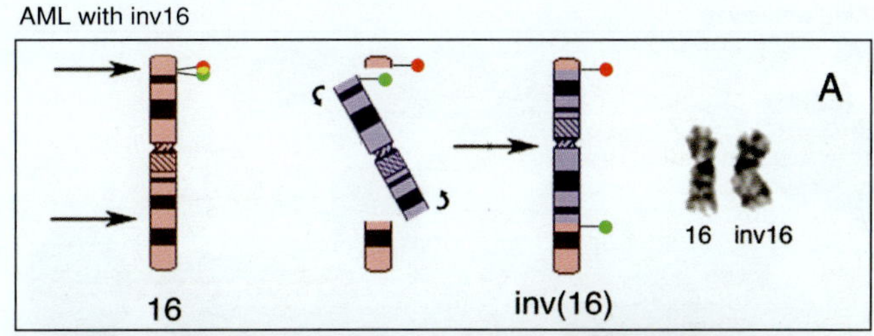

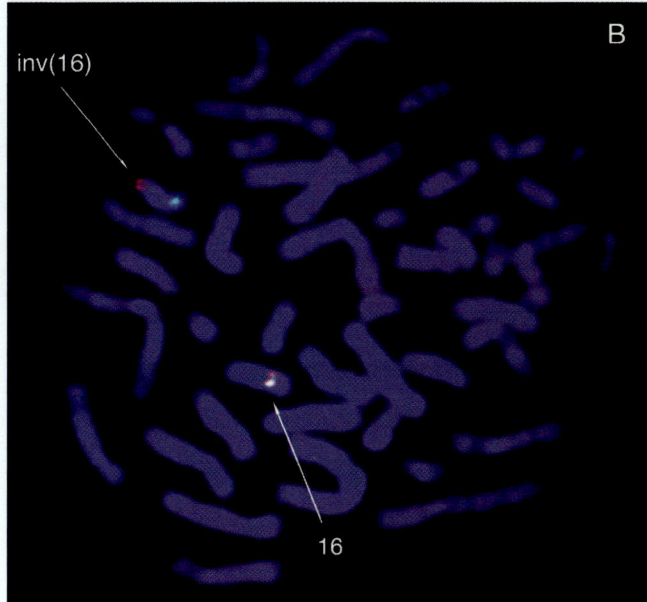

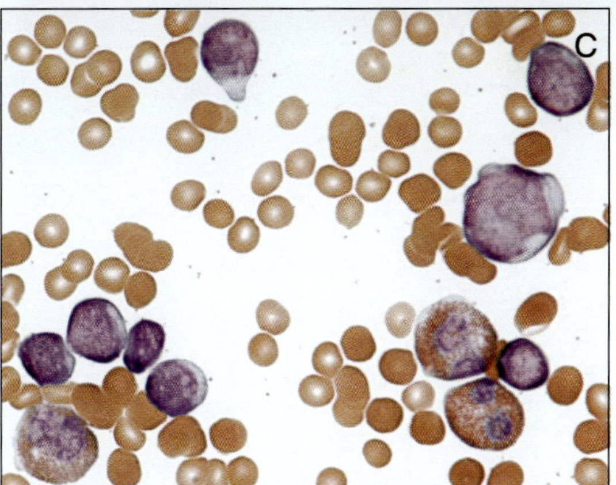

Figure 2.72 The inv(16)(p13.1q22) rearrangement. **A.** The ideograms of the normal and inverted chromosome 16s are to the left in color and the corresponding G-banded pair is to the right. The arrows on the normal chromosome 16 ideograms indicate the breakpoints on the short and long arms of chromosome 16. **B.** Metaphase FISH using a dual color CBFB (16q22) probe set. The CBFB gene is labeled with a red fluorochrome at the 5' end and with a green fluorochrome at the 3' end. When an inv(16)(p13.1q22) is present, the red and green signals split apart such that the red signal is now on the other arm. A yellow signal indicates the normal chromosome 16. **C.** Acute myelomonocytic leukemia with eosinophilia and inv16. An aspirate smear reveals a dimorphic blast population made up of large monocytoid and small myeloblast cells with eosinophilia.

AML with inv16

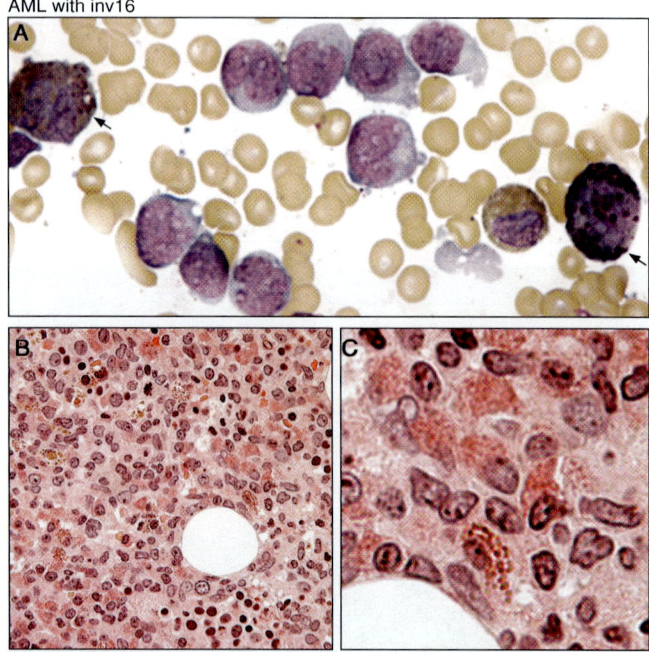

Figure 2.73   AML with inv16. **A.** This aspirate smear shows granular monocytoid blasts with dysplastic eosinophilic, basophilic precursors. **B.** A bone marrow biopsy displays a hypercellular marrow composed of sheets of uniformly spaced monocytoid blasts with eosinophilia. **C.** Higher-power view of the biopsy reveals uniformly spaced monocytoid blasts with characteristic folded nuclear contours associated with eosinophilia.

AML with inv16

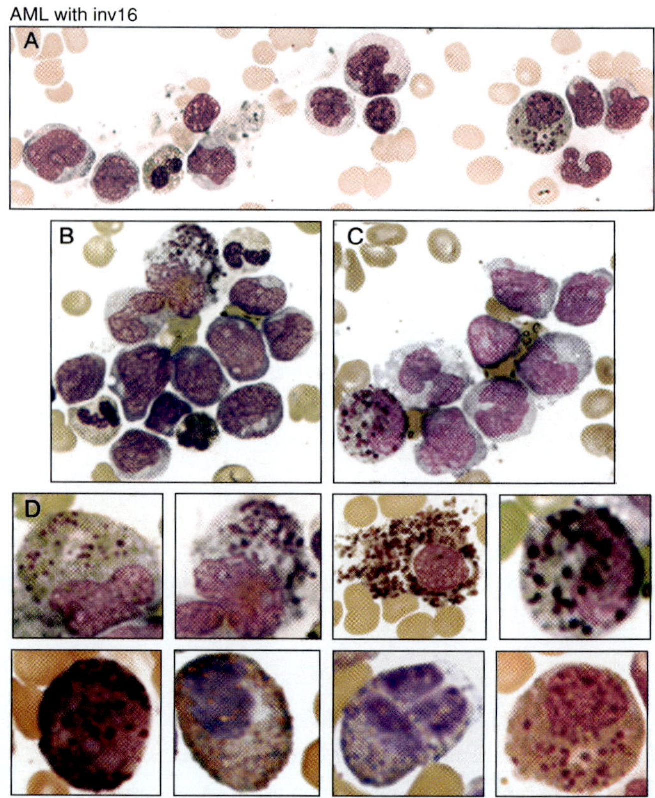

Figure 2.74   **A–C.** AML with inv16. Aspirate smears from three cases of AML with inv16 showing monocytic blasts mixed with dysplastic eosinophilic/basophilic precursors ("eosinobasophils"). The latter show the characteristic dual-staining cytoplasmic granules commonly seen in AML with inv16. **D.** Below are examples of the dysplastic eosinophilic, basophilic precursors seen in several different cases of AML with inv16.

Acute myelomonocytic leukemia with inv16

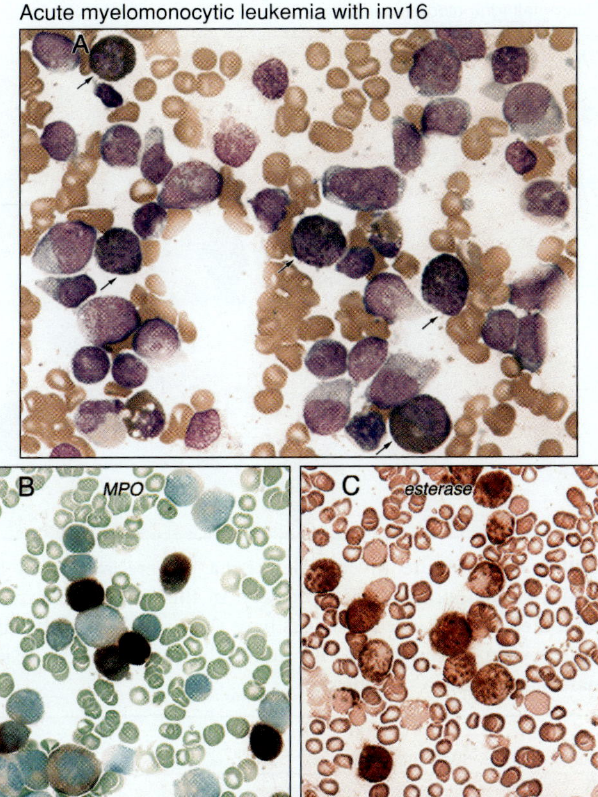

Figure 2.75 Acute myelomonocytic leukemia with inv16. **A.** A pleomorphic blast population composed of large cells with low nuclear:cytoplasmic (N:C) ratios, and smaller blasts with high N:C ratios is present in this aspirate smear. Dysplastic eosinophil precursors ("eosinobasophils") exhibiting the classical dual-staining cytoplasmic granules are prominent (*arrows*). **B.** Butyrate esterase stains show that approximately one-half of the blast population, particularly the larger blasts, display positive staining. **C.** Myeloperoxidase stains demonstrate strong "block-like" cytoplasmic staining in approximately one-half of the blast population, including the abnormal "eosinobasophils."

AML with 11q23 abnormalities

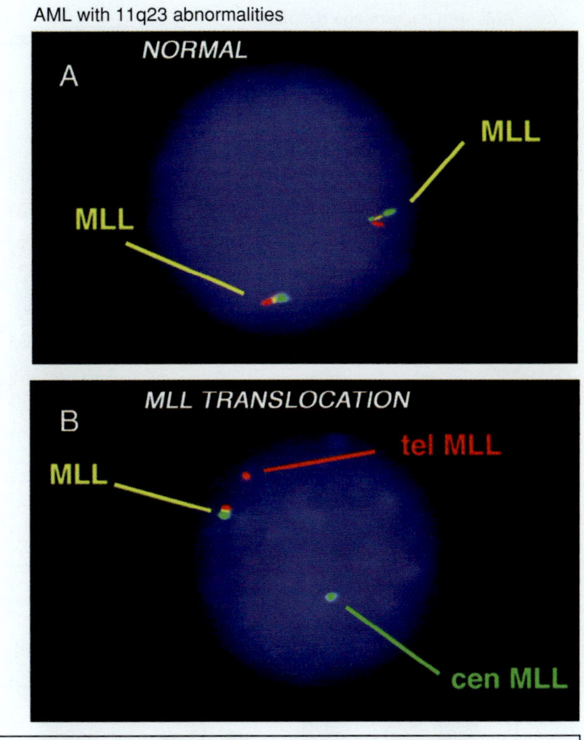

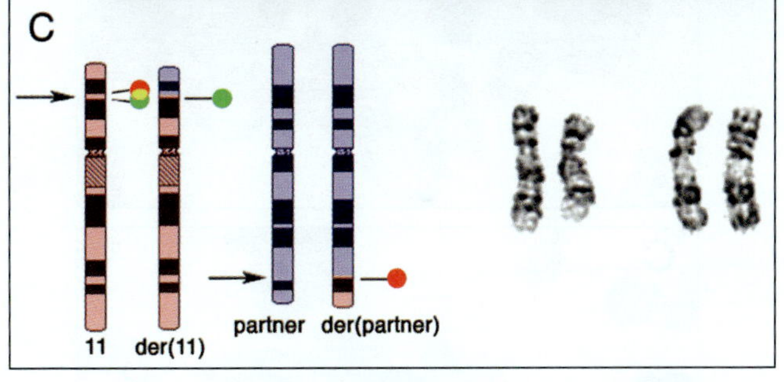

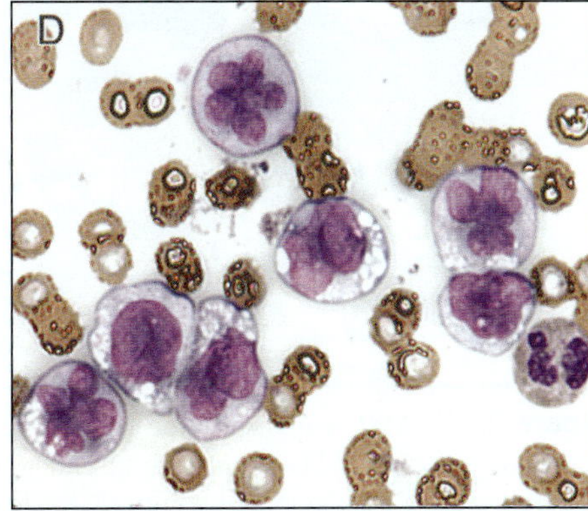

Figure 2.76 AML with 11q23 abnormalities. **A** and **B.** FISH of a MLL rearrangement. The MLL gene at 11q23 is labeled with a green fluorochrome at the telomeric (tel) end and with a red fluorochrome at the centromeric (cen) end. A yellow fusion signal indicates an intact MLL gene (**A**). Translocations involving the MLL (HRX) gene splits the red and green signals apart (**B**). **C.** The t(9;11)(p22;q23) rearrangement. The ideograms of chromosomes 9, 11 and the respective derivative chromosomes are to the left in color, and the corresponding G-banded chromosome pairs are to the right. The arrows indicate the breakpoints on the respective chromosomes. **D.** Acute monocytic leukemia with t(9;11). Well-differentiated monocytic blasts predominate in this aspirate smear.

AML with multilineage dysplasia

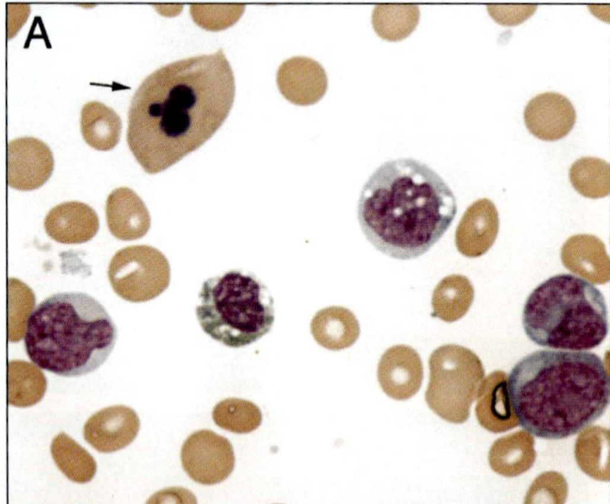

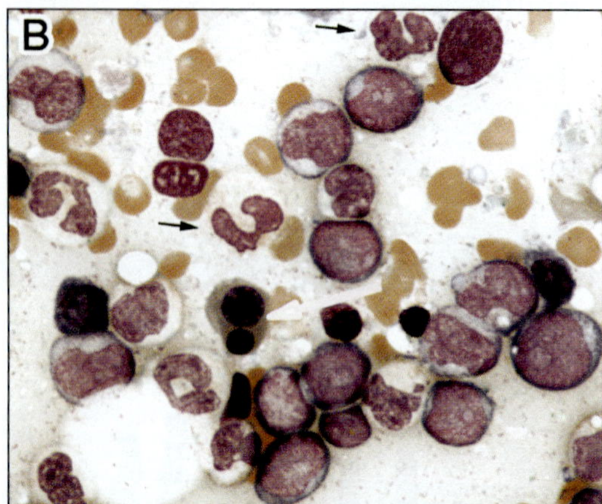

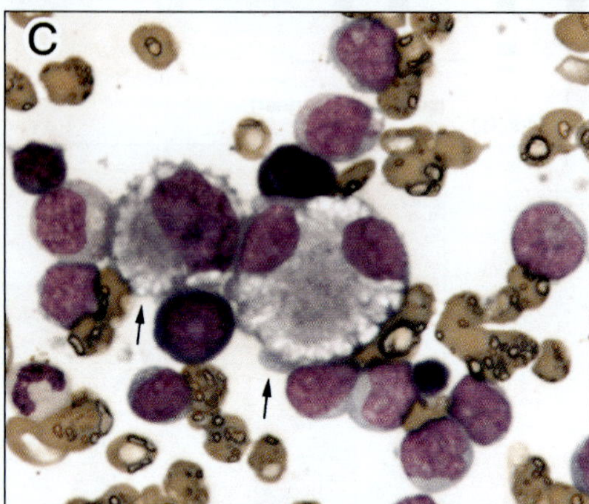

Figure 2.77   AML with multilineage dysplasia. **A.** An aspirate smear with increased blasts and a dysplastic mature erythroid precursor displays irregular ("cookie cutter") nuclear contours (*arrow*). **B.** This aspirate smear shows several giant hypogranular bands (*arrows*) and a dysplastic erythroid precursor with asymmetric binucleation is situated just below the centrally located hypogranular band. **C.** An aspirate smear reveals increased blasts and two dysplastic micromegakaryocytes (*arrows*).

Chloromas (granulocytic sarcomas)

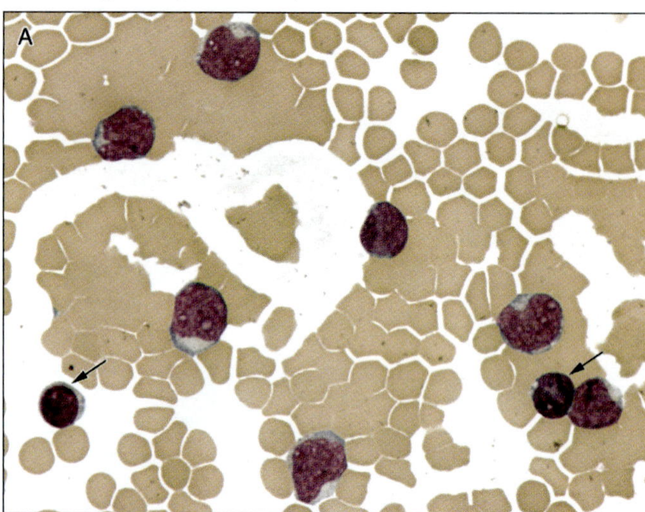

Figure 2.78   Acute myeloid leukemia in cerebral spinal fluid (CSF). Hematopoietic blasts are seen in this CSF specimen contaminated with blood. The blasts have the typical open chromatin pattern seen in immature cells, unlike the closed pattern of small mature lymphocytes (*arrows*).

Chloromas (granulocytic sarcomas)

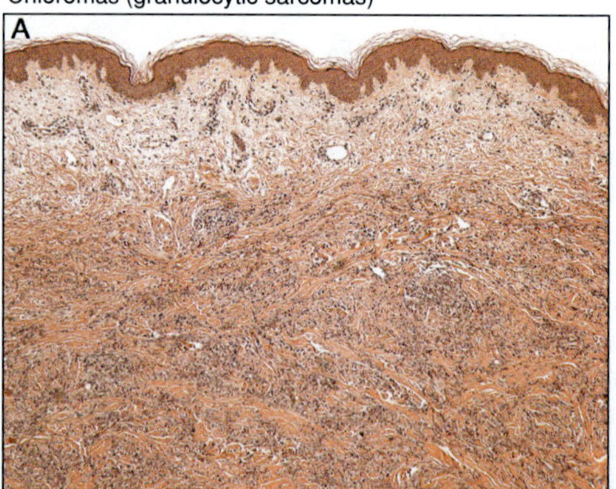

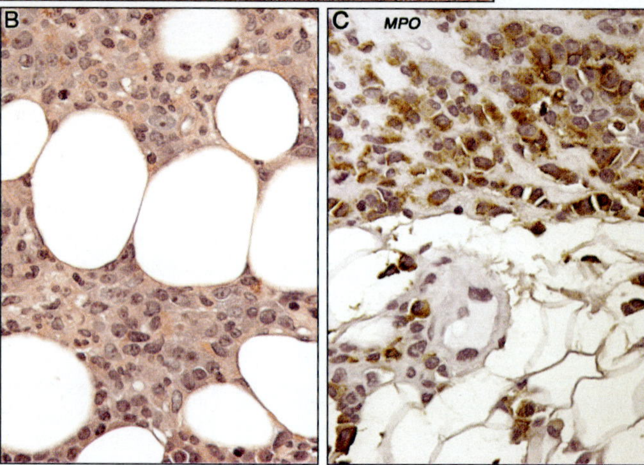

Figure 2.79   Leukemia cutis. **A.** Nests of large leukemic cells infiltrate the dermis in this skin biopsy from a patient with acute myeloid leukemia. **B.** Leukemic infiltration extends into the subcutaneous fat. **C.** Anti-MPO immunostains show positive-staining leukemia cells invading subcutaneous fat and a blood vessel.

Chloromas (granulocytic sarcomas)

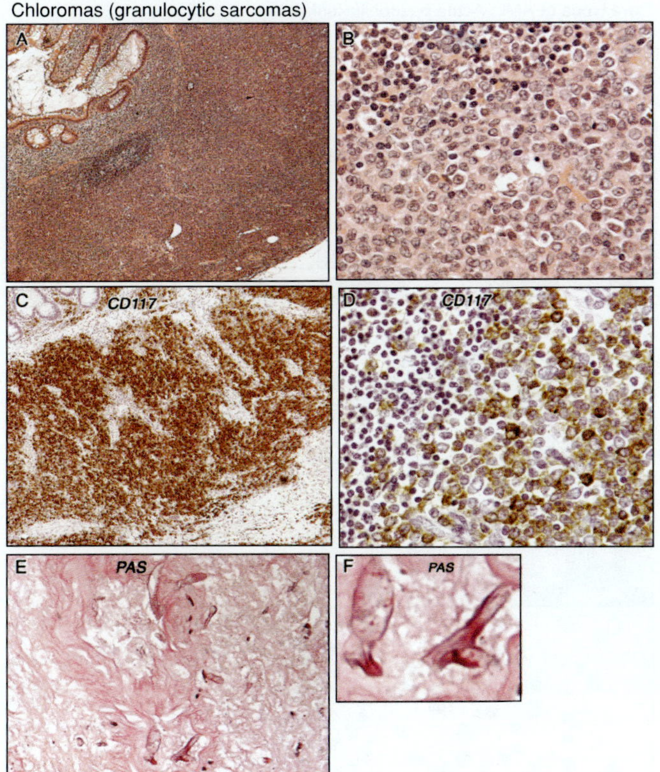

Figure 2.80   AML in appendix. AML presenting as acute appendicitis with neutropenia and systemic aspergillosis. **A.** This low-power view of the appendix shows transmural involvement by leukemic cells. **B.** Higher-power view of the appendix wall reveals infiltration by large leukemic cells with some residual small mature lymphocytes shown on the upper left side. **C** and **D.** Low- and high-power views, respectively, illustrating CD117$^+$ leukemic cells infiltrating the entire intestinal wall. In **D**, negative-staining residual lymphocytes are present in the upper left side of the slide. **E** and **F.** PAS stains show angioinvasive aspergillus.

Chloromas (granulocytic sarcomas)

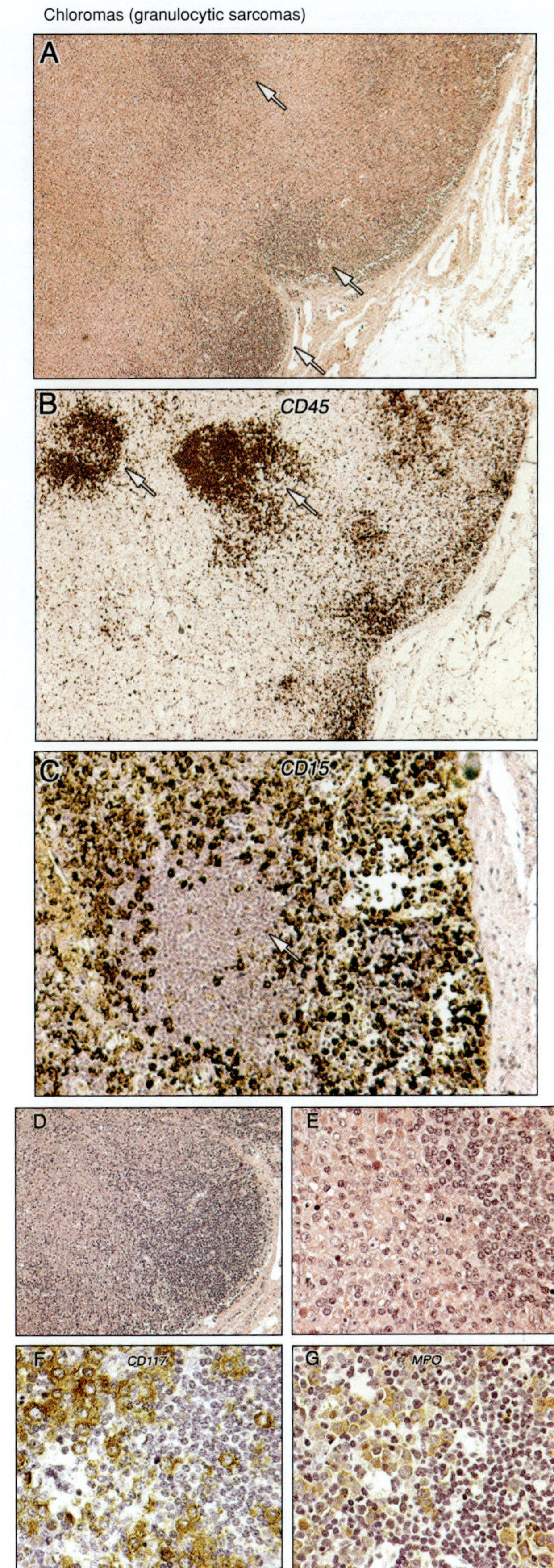

Figure 2.81   AML involving lymph node. **A.** Resected lymph node reveals almost total effacement by a diffuse proliferation of large pale-staining cells. Residual nodules of lymphocytes are present (*arrows*). **B.** CD45 immunostains show positive staining in residual lymphoid aggregates (*arrows*), with most of the metastatic leukemic cells showing a negative staining pattern. **C.** An immunostain for the myeloid marker CD15 shows positive-staining leukemic cells surrounding negative-staining nodule of residual lymphocytes (*arrow*). **D** and **E.** Low- and medium-magnification, respectively, of a surgically resected lymph node shows replacement of nodal tissue by pale-staining leukemic cells. Residual lymphocytes are present on the right side of both figures. **F.** An immunostain for CD117 demonstrates large positive-staining leukemic cells and negative-staining residual small lymphocytes. **G.** Anti-MPO stains show positive staining in the large leukemic cells, with negative-staining lymphocytes on the right.

Chloromas (granulocytic sarcomas)

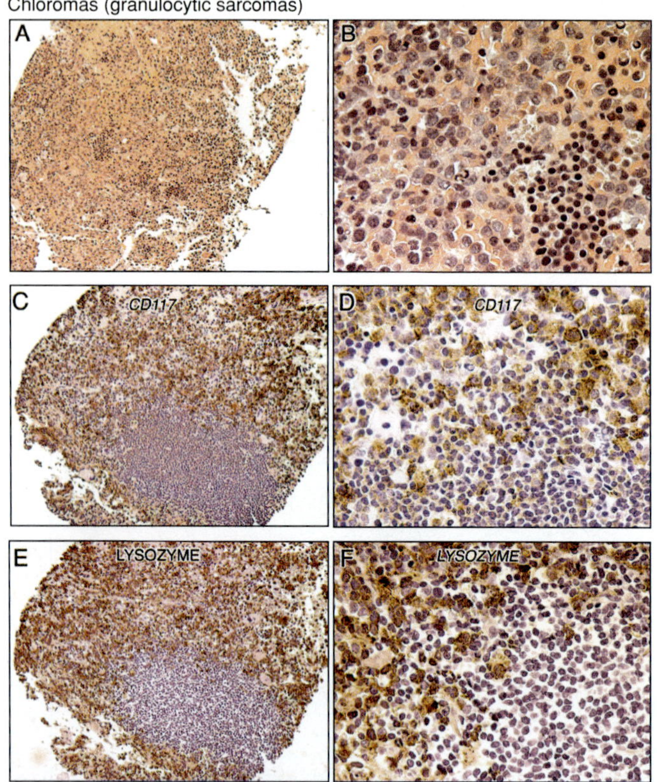

Figure 2.82 Acute monocytic leukemia involving lymph node. **A** and **B**. A fine-needle biopsy of a lymph node reveals effacement of architecture by sheets of large, uniformly spaced, monotonous, leukemic cells. Residual small, mature lymphocytes are present near the right lower corner of the slide. Immunostains for CD117 and lysozyme show positive leukemic cells surrounding negative-staining residual lymphocytes (**C,D** and **E, F**, respectively).

Rare types of AML: Acute basophilic leukemia

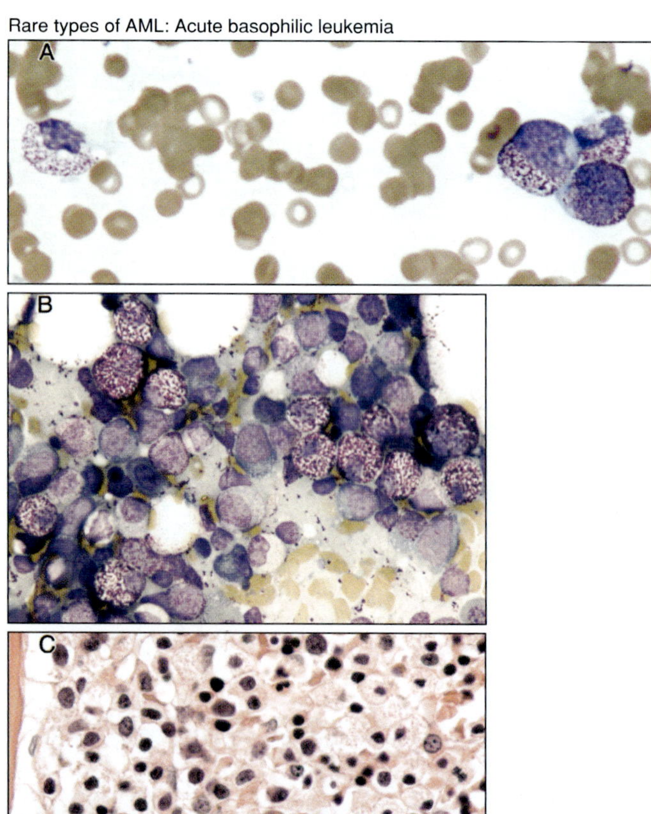

Figure 2.83 Acute basophilic leukemia. **A**. Blood smear shows circulating dysplastic basophilic precursors. **B**. An aspirate smear demonstrates cohesive clumps consisting exclusively of abnormal basophil precursors. **C**. A biopsy reveals a hypercellular bone marrow replaced by monotonous-appearing small cells with abundant "agranular" cytoplasm (representing basophils degranulated during tissue processing).

Rare types of AML: Hand mirror variant

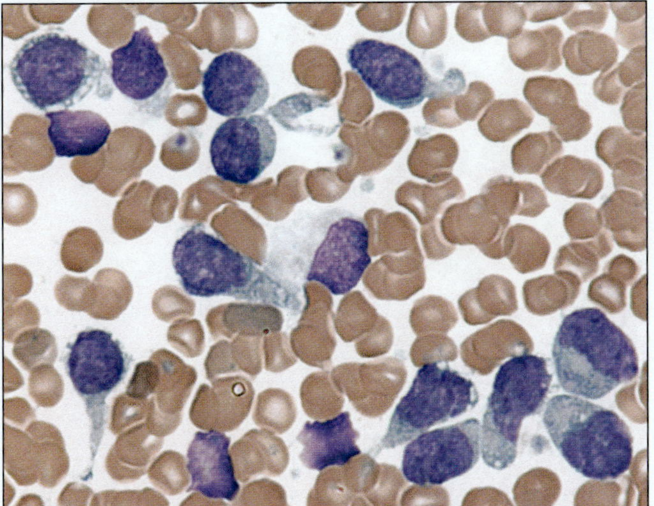

Figure 2.84   "Hand mirror variant" of acute leukemia. An aspirate smear from a case of AML shows unipolar cytoplasmic extensions that have the appearance of handles. This morphologic variant is not lineage-specific, occurs in various AML subtypes as well as in ALL, and is of uncertain prognostic significance.

Rare types of AML: AML with "thumbprinting"

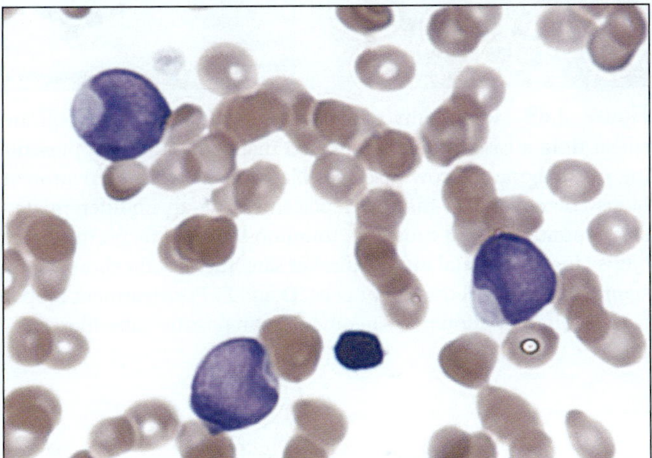

Figure 2.85   AML with cup-like nuclear indentation. In acute myeloid leukemia, this distinctive nuclear morphology, also referred to as "thumbprinting," has been associated with loss of HLA-DR expression and FLT3 internal tandem duplication. (Kussick et al, *Leukemia*, 2004;18(10):1591–1598.)

Rare types of AML: Acute monocytic leukemia with t(8;16)

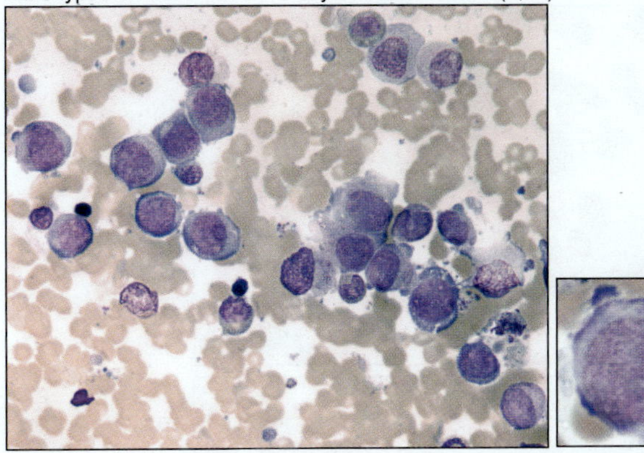

Figure 2.86   Acute monoblastic leukemia with t(8;16). An aspirate smear shows a pleomorphic population of immature monocytic precursors. Although this translocation has been associated with prominent hemophagocytosis, in this particular case only a rare blast was seen engulfing RBCs as shown on the right.

Acute leukemia mimics: small cell carcinoma

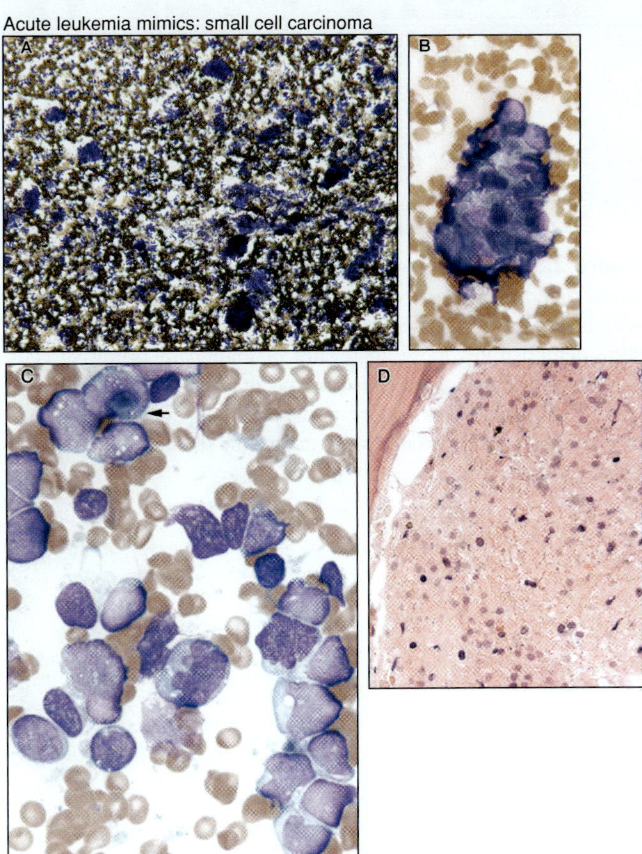

Figure 2.87   Small-cell carcinoma of lung. **A.** Low-power view of an aspirate shows tumor cell clumps. **B.** Medium-power view shows a cohesive nest of carcinoma cells with scalloped borders and nuclear molding is present in the aspirate. **C.** High power view of the aspirate shows very large pleomorphic malignant cells. An arrow delineates a paranuclear blue inclusion. **D.** Necrotic metastatic tumor composed of "ghost" cells appears in the biopsy specimen.

Acute leukemia mimics: Neuroblastoma

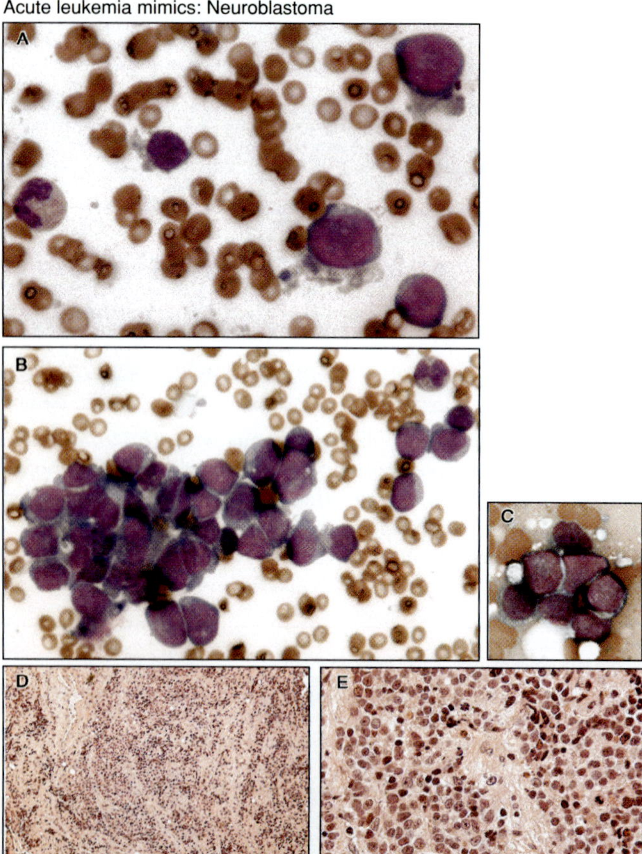

Acute leukemia mimics: rhabdomyosarcoma

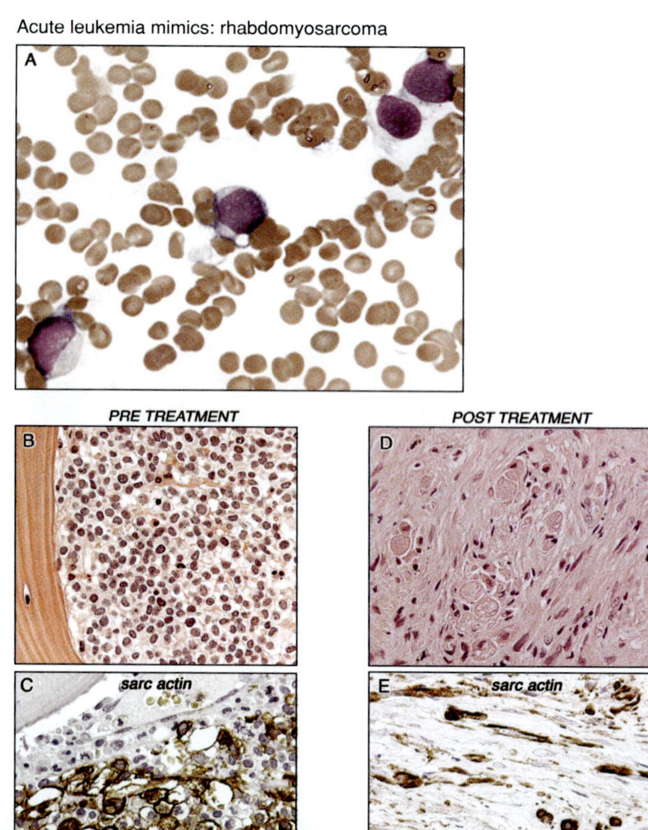

Figure 2.88 Neuroblastoma in bone marrow. **A.** An aspirate smear demonstrates an esthesioneuroblastoma in the bone marrow with blast-like cells possessing fine cytoplasmic projections. **B.** This slide demonstrates loose aggregates of malignant primitive cells. **C.** A clump of malignant cells displays nuclear molding. **D** and **E.** Low- and high-power views, respectively, of biopsy show bone marrow replacement by small, round, blue cells separated by fibrovascular bundles.

Figure 2.89 Rhabdomyosarcoma. **A.** A hypocellular aspirate smear from a case of undifferentiated rhabdomyosarcoma presenting in the bone marrow discloses blast-like cells. **B.** Pretreatment biopsy demonstrates marrow replacement by an undifferentiated small round blue-cell tumor. **C.** Immunostains on the pretreatment biopsy for the skeletal muscle marker sarcomeric actin show strong staining in many of the tumor cells. **D** and **E.** Posttreatment biopsy reveals differentiation into sarcomeric actin positive tube-like structures.

Acute leukemia mimics: Ewings sarcoma

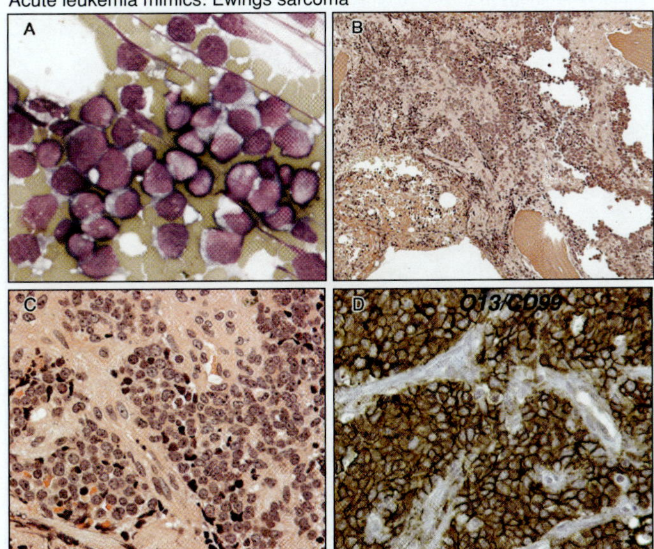

Figure 2.90   Ewing sarcoma of the bone marrow. **A.** A touch prep shows marrow replacement by undifferentiated, blast-like primitive cells. **B** and **C.** A biopsy displays infiltration of marrow by loose nests of malignant cells separated by fibrovascular bundles. **D.** Immuno-stains for O13 (CD99) reveal strong cytoplasmic staining.

Precursor B-cell lymphoblastic leukemia/lymphoma

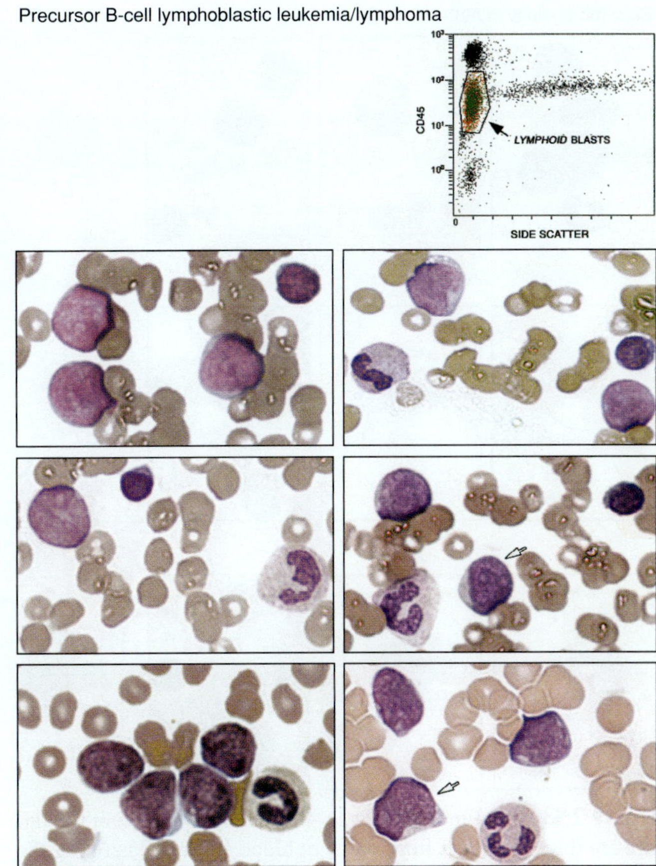

Figure 2.91   Precursor B-cell lymphoblastic leukemia/lymphoma (B-cell ALL). Lymphoid leukemic blasts with characteristic low CD45 expression and low side-scatter properties are shown by arrow in the upper right panel. Below are blood smears from six different case of B-cell ALL showing variations of morphology compared with small mature lymphocytes. Arrows delineate L2 blasts with lower N:C ratios and nucleoli.

Philadelphia chromosome positive acute leukemias

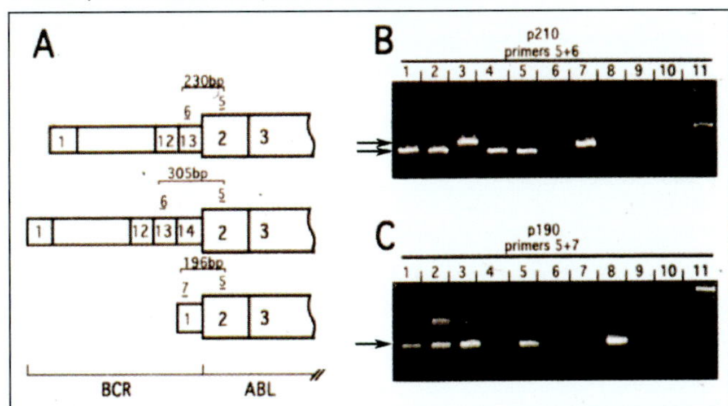

Figure 2.92   Philadelphia chromosome positive (Ph+) acute leukemia. Acute leukemia, in particular B-cell ALL, but also some AMLs, especially those coexpressing B-cell markers, harbors the t(9;22). This fact has important implications for initial treatment decisions, and RTPCR for BCR-ABL should be considered for all adult B-cell ALLs and those AMLs with B-cell marker expression profiles. RTPCR primers sets should include those that can detect the p190 BCR-ABL transcript (common in the Ph+ acute leukemia), as well as the p210 (common in CML) and p230 (found in rare Phi+ chronic neutrophilic leukemia). (Courtesy Dr. S. Kamel-Reid.)

Blast morphology in ALL

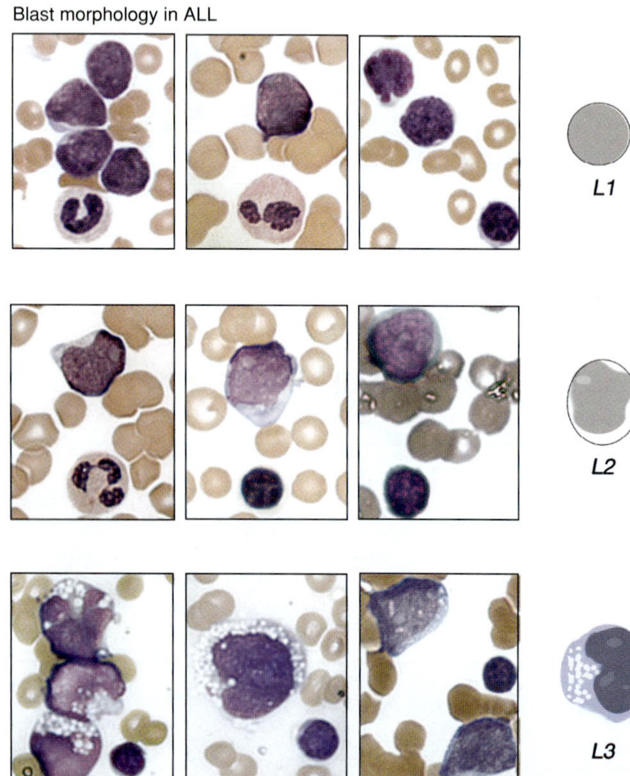

Figure 2.93 Blast morphology in ALL. On the left side of the figure are three examples from different blood smears illustrating the three morphologic variants of blasts: L1, L2, L3 seen in acute lymphoid leukemias. On the right side are the corresponding cartoons. The L1 blast is common and can be confused, especially in infants, with the normal small mature lymphocytes that are shown in many of the blood smears for comparison.

Blast morphology in acute leukemia

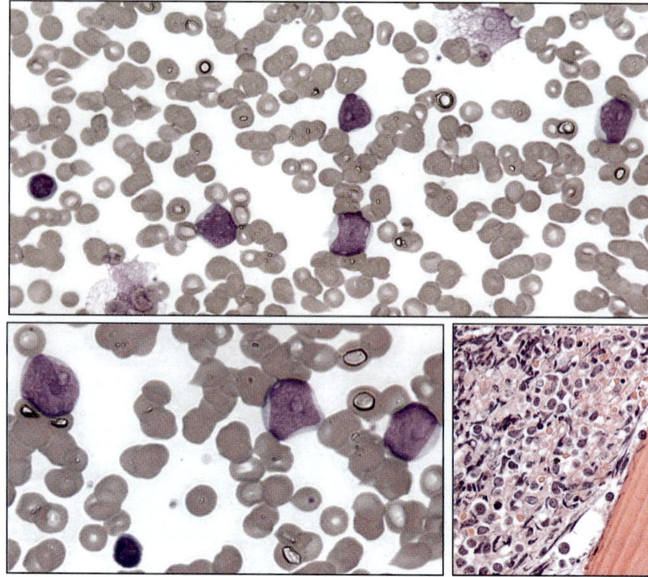

Figure 2.94 L2 ALL blasts. ALL blasts, in particular the L2 morphologic variants, can look very much like typical AML blasts (large cells with moderate N:C ratios and very prominent nucleoli). Morphology can be misleading when trying to determine lineage of blasts; immunohistochemistry and immunophenotyping are almost always necessary to distinguish ALL from AML.

ALL with fibrosis

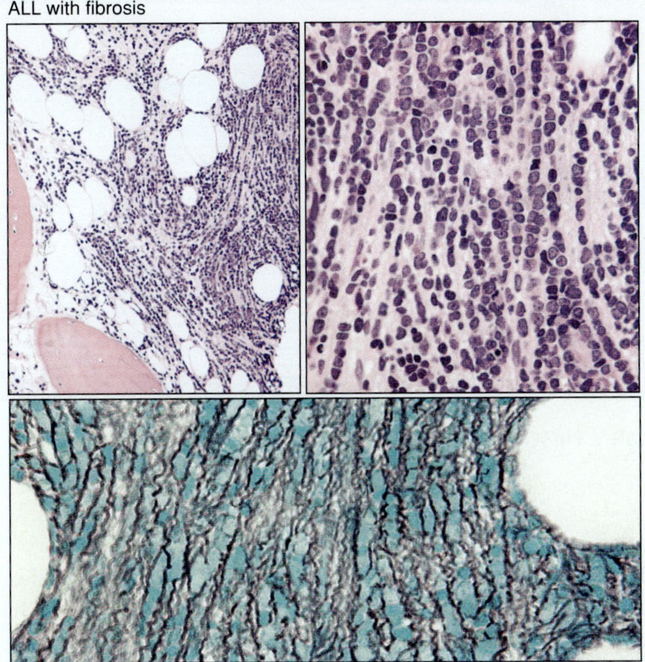

Figure 2.95 ALL with fibrosis. A case of B-cell ALL with architectural distortion on hematoxylin and eosin (H&E)-stained biopsy sections includes lining up of individual blasts (so-called Indian filing) and swirling patterns that suggest significant marrow fibrosis (*upper two panels*). The latter is confirmed with reticulin stains showing increased numbers of thickened fibers (*lower panel*). Marrow fibrosis often precludes flow cytometric evaluation of leukemic cells from dry aspirate smears. In these cases, efforts should be made either to disaggregate biopsy specimens for flow cytometry or, alternatively, to acquire biopsies for immunohistochemistry.

Precursor T-cell lymphoblastic leukemia

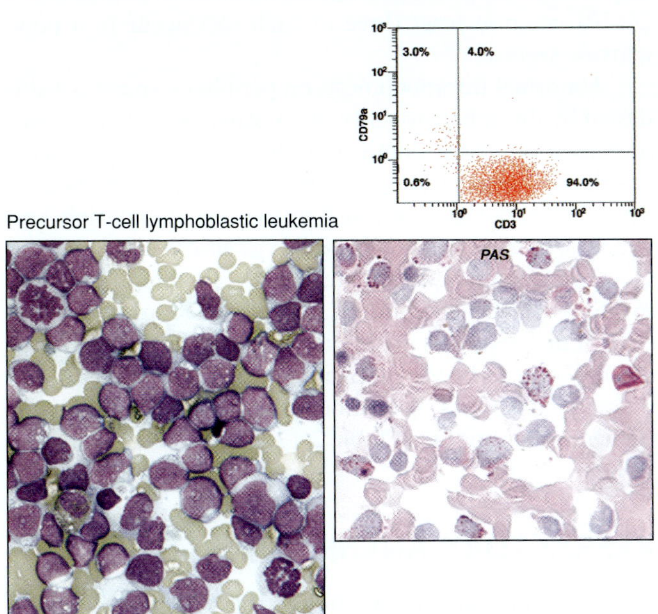

Figure 2.96 Precursor T-cell lymphoblastic leukemia/lymphoma (T-ALL). A scattergram shows blasts positive for cytoplasmic CD3 expression, a T-cell–specific marker that is usually positive in T-ALL (*upper panel*). Aspirate smears disclose sheets of L2 type blasts with high mitotic rate and strong block-like cytoplasmic PAS positivity (*left* and *right lower panels,* respectively).

Precursor T-cell lymphoblastic leukemia

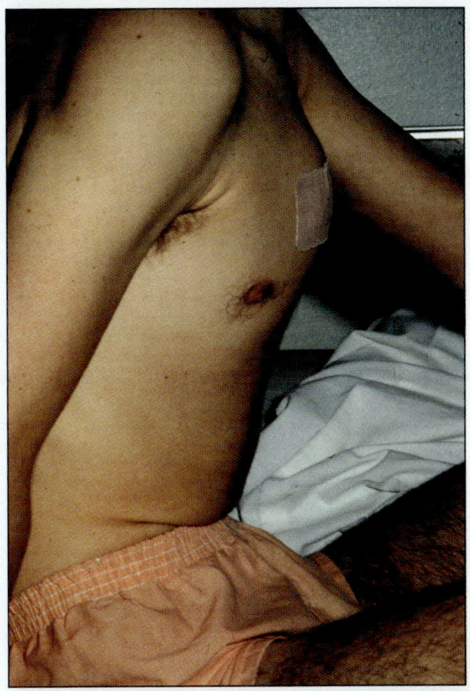

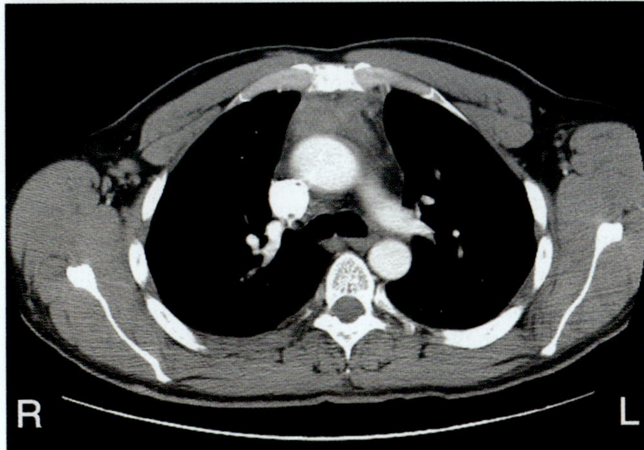

Figure 2.97 Precursor T-cell lymphoblastic leukemia/lymphoma (T-ALL). T-ALL often presents with a high blast count and a mass in the mediastinum or other tissues. This slide shows a young man with a mediastinal mass eroding through the sternum. An axial CT scan with intravenous contrast at the level of the upper thorax discloses an anterior mediastinal soft tissue mass consistent with leukemia/lymphoma. (Courtesy Dr. I. Quirt.)

Myelodysplastic Syndromes

Douglas C. Tkachuk, MD, FRCPC, Kathy Chun, PhD, FCCMG, and Jan V. Hirschmann, MD

The myelodysplastic syndromes (MDSs) are disorders caused by a clonal expansion of hematopoietic stem cells in which maturation is abnormal (dysplastic) and production ineffective, resulting in many cells being destroyed before they reach the systemic circulation. Anemia typically occurs, often accompanied by thrombocytopenia and/or neutropenia. Some cases develop from exposure to ionizing radiation or cytotoxic chemotherapy, usually with alkylating agents, and in these circumstances the bone marrow is characteristically hypocellular and partially fibrotic. More frequently, these diseases occur as a primary problem in older adults, with a median age of about 70 when diagnosed. In them, the bone marrow is usually hypercellular.

Blasts may be increased in the myelodysplastic syndromes, but they do not exceed 20% of the differential count of at least 200 leukocytes in the peripheral blood and 500 in the bone marrow. Dysplasia may involve one or more hematopoietic lines; to be significant it should affect at least 10% of that line's cells in the bone marrow, but evidence for dysplasia may also be present on the peripheral smear. In erythrocytes the smear may show macrocytosis, anisocytosis, basophilic stippling, and Pappenheimer bodies. Poikilocytosis is usual and includes target cells, acanthocytes, elliptocytes, stomatocytes, red-cell fragments, and teardrop cells. Bone marrow findings in the erythrocyte precursors comprise nuclear and cytoplasmic abnormalities. The former consist of budding, internuclear bridging, the presence of more than one nucleus per cell, karyorrhexis (fragmentation), abnormal chromatin (either fine or dense) and megaloblastic changes, in which the nucleus is enlarged and less mature than is the cytoplasm. Cytoplasmic abnormalities include vacuolization and ringed sideroblasts, which are erythroblasts that, on iron stain, contain ≥10 ferritin granules encircling at least one-third of the nucleus.

Evidence of abnormal granulopoiesis on peripheral smear includes neutropenia, hypersegmented neutrophils,

Döhle bodies, decreased or absent cytoplasmic granules, and the presence of immature cells, including blasts. The nuclei may have dense chromatin clumping, and many are hypolobulated, with a single lobe or two joined by a thin band of chromatin, resembling the congenital disorder, Pelger-Hüet anomaly. The presence of these pseudo-Pelger-Hüet cells on a blood smear strongly suggests an underlying myelodysplastic syndrome. Eosinophils and basophils may have diminished granules and decreased nuclear lobulation. These abnormalities also are apparent in the bone marrow, along with the small size of the granulocyte precursors, which may be present centrally rather than in their accustomed paratrabecular location, a finding labeled *atypical localization of immature precursors* (ALIP) when at least three of such foci occur in a bone marrow section.

Abnormal thrombopoiesis on peripheral smear is manifested by thrombocytopenia, giant platelets, and those with decreased or absent granules. In bone marrow specimens, dysplastic megakaryocytes are small (micromegakaryocytes), and possess abnormal nuclei that are multiple and widely separated or have decreased or absent lobulation.

Cytogenetic abnormalities are common in the myelodysplastic syndromes and all types are at varying risk for developing acute leukemia, which is almost always myelogenous. The World Health Organization (WHO) has defined eight types of myelodysplasia based primarily on bone marrow findings (Table 3.1).

REFRACTORY ANEMIA (RA)

This entity accounts for about 5% to 10% of cases of MDS, the median survival is about 5 years, and acute leukemia eventuates in approximately 5% of patients. Dysplasia occurs in the erythroid precursors alone, ranges from mild to pronounced, and consists of the findings described in the first section. On peripheral blood smear the red cells are normocytic or macrocytic. Nonspecific cytogenetic abnormalities occur in about 25% of cases.

REFRACTORY ANEMIA WITH RINGED SIDEROBLASTS (RARS)

This disorder is responsible for about 10% of cases of MDS, has a median survival of about 6 years, and has about a 1% chance of evolving into acute leukemia. Dysplasia occurs only in the erythroid line, and at least 15% of the red cell precursors are ringed sideroblasts. Cytogenetic abnormalities occur in <10% of cases.

REFRACTORY CYTOPENIA WITH MULTILINEAGE DYSPLASIA (RCMD)

This disorder accounts for about 25% of MDS, and the diagnosis requires cytopenias and dysplastic changes in at least two lines. When, in addition, ringed sideroblasts constitute >15% of the erythroid precursors, the diagnosis is the subtype *refractory cytopenia with multilineage dysplasia and ringed sideroblasts* (RCMD-RS), which accounts for about 15% of cases of MDS. The median survival for both is about 3 years, and the risk of leukemia is approximately 10%. Cytogenetic abnormalities occur in up to 50% of cases.

REFRACTORY ANEMIA WITH EXCESS BLASTS (RAEB)

In this MDS, the blasts are increased above normal, but not sufficiently to meet the criteria for leukemia, which is at least 20% of nucleated cells in the blood or bone marrow. Two subtypes exist: RAEB-1 has 5% to 9% blasts in the bone marrow and <5% in the blood; RAEB-2 has 10% to 19% blasts in the bone marrow and/or 5% to 19% blasts in the blood. Those with Auer rods are also considered RAEB-2. These two diseases account for approximately 40% of cases of MDS. About 25% of RAEB-1 and 33% of RAEB-2 develop acute leukemia, and their respective median survivals are 18 and 10 months. Approximately 33% to 50% of these patients have cytogenetic abnormalities.

MYELODYSPLASTIC SYNDROME, UNCLASSIFIABLE (MDS-U)

Patients are put in this category when they have dysplasia restricted to either the neutrophil or megakaryocytic lines. They fail to meet the criteria for the other MDSs. The number of patients who belong in this group, their median survival, and the risk of developing leukemia are uncertain.

MYELODYSPLASTIC SYNDROME ASSOCIATED WITH ISOLATED DEL(5Q) CHROMOSOME ABNORMALITY (5Q– SYNDROME)

Unlike the other MDSs, this entity is primarily defined not by hematologic findings but by a cytogenetic abnormality, a deletion between bands q31 and 33 on chromosome 5, with variability in the actual break points and the size of the deletion. Most patients are middle-aged to older women, whose major problem is refractory macrocytic anemia. Some patients have thrombocytosis. The bone marrow is usually hypercellular, dysplasia is present in the erythroid precursors, many megakaryocytes have hypolobulated nuclei, and blasts are <5%. Patients typically have a long survival, and progression to acute leukemia occurs in <25% of cases.

Table 3.1

World Health Organization classification of the myelodysplastic syndromes

Classification	Peripheral Blood	Bone Marrow
Refractory anemia	Anemia No or rare blasts	Erythroid dysplasia only <5% blasts <15% ringed sideroblasts
Refractory anemia with ringed sideroblasts	Anemia No blasts	>15% ringed sideroblasts Erythroid dysplasia only <5% blasts
Refractory cytopenia with multilineage dysplasia	Cytopenias (bicytopenia or pancytopenia) No or rare blasts No Auer rods $<1 \times 10^9$/L monocytes	Dysplasia in >10% of the cells of two or more myeloid lines <5% blasts in the marrow No Auer rods <15% ringed sideroblasts
Refractory cytopenia with multilineage dysplasia and ringed sideroblasts	Cytopenias (bicytopenia or pancytopenia) No or rare blasts No Auer rods $<1 \times 10^9$/L monocytes	Dysplasia in >10% of the cells of two or more myeloid lines <5% blasts in the marrow >15% ringed sideroblasts No Auer rods
Refractory anemia with excess blasts 1	Cytopenias <5% blasts No Auer rods $<1 \times 10^9$/L monocytes	Unilineage or multilineage dysplasia 5% to 9% blasts No Auer rods
Refractory anemia with excess blasts 2	Cytopenias 5% to 19% blasts Auer rods present $<1 \times 10^9$/L monocytes	Unilineage or multilineage dysplasia 10% to 19% blasts Auer rods present
Myelodysplastic syndrome, unclassified	Cytopenias No or rare blasts No Auer rods	Unilineage dysplasia: one myeloid cell line <5% blasts No Auer rods
5q– syndrome	Anemia Usually normal or increased platelet count <5% blasts	Normal to increased megakaryocytes with hypolobated nuclei <5% blasts Isolated del(5q) cytogenetic abnormality No Auer rods

Reprinted with permission from *Wintrobe's Clinical Hematology*, 11th Edition, page 2209.

Table 3.2

Morphologic abnormalities in myelodysplastic syndromes

Lineage	Peripheral Blood	Bone Marrow
Erythroid	Ovalomacrocytes	Megaloblastoid erythropoiesis
	Elliptocytes	Nuclear budding
	Acanthocytes	Ringed sideroblasts
	Stomatocytes	Internuclear bridging
	Teardrops	Karyorrhexis
	Nucleated erythrocytes	Nuclear fragments
	Basophilic stippling	Cytoplasmic vacuolization
	Howell-Jolly bodies	Multinucleation
Myeloid	Pseudo-Pelger-Huët anomaly	Defective granulation
	Auer rods	Maturation arrest at myelocyte stage
	Hypogranulation	Increase in monocytoid forms
	Nuclear sticks	Abnormal localization of immature precursors
	Hypersegmentation	
	Ring-shaped nuclei	
Megakaryocyte	Giant platelets	Micromegakaryocytes
	Hypogranular or agranular platelets	Hypogranulation
		Multiple small nuclei

Reprinted with permission from *Wintrobe's Clinical Hematology*, 11th Edition, page 2211.

Table 3.3

Predisposing factors and epidemiologic associations

Heritable predisposition
  Constitutional genetic disorders
    Down syndrome (trisomy 21)
    Trisomy 8 mosaicism
    Familial monosomy 7
  Neurofibromatosis 1
  Germ cell tumors (embryonal dysgenesis)
  Congenital neutropenia (Kostmann syndrome or Shwachman-Diamond syndrome)
  DNA repair deficiencies
    Fanconi anemia
    Ataxia telangiectasia
    Bloom syndrome
    Xeroderma pigmentosum
  Mutagen detoxification (GSTq1-null)

Acquired
  Senescence
  Mutagen exposure
    Genotoxic therapy
      Alkylators
      Topoisomerase II interactive agents
      β-Emitters (phosphorus-32)
      Autologous bone marrow transplantation
    Environmental or occupational exposure (e.g., benzene)
    Tobacco
  Aplastic anemia
  Paroxysmal nocturnal hemoglobinuria
  Polycythemia vera

Reprinted with permission from *Wintrobe's Clinical Hematology*, 11th Edition, page 2214.

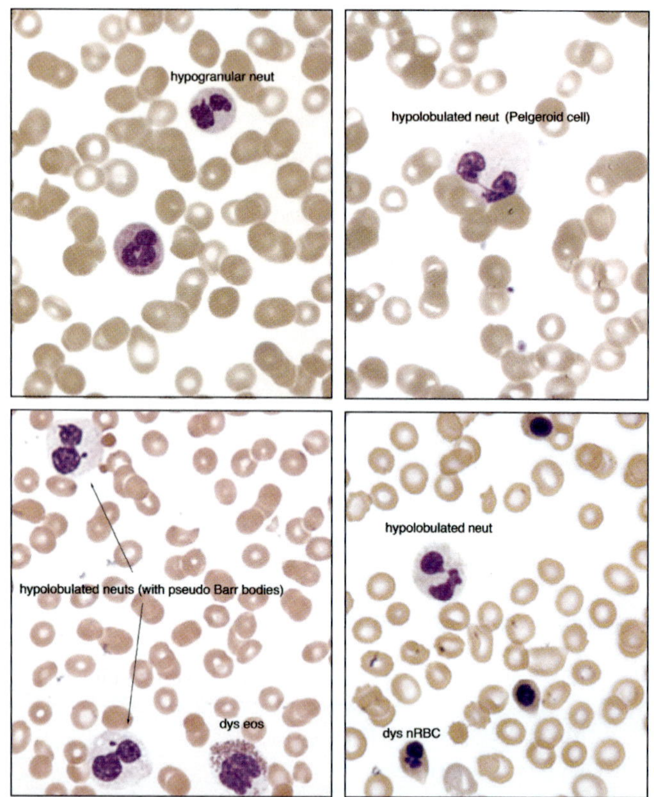

Figure 3.1 Myeloid dysplasia, blood smear. Dysplastic cytoplasmic and nuclear features in neutrophils from four cases of MDS are illustrated here.

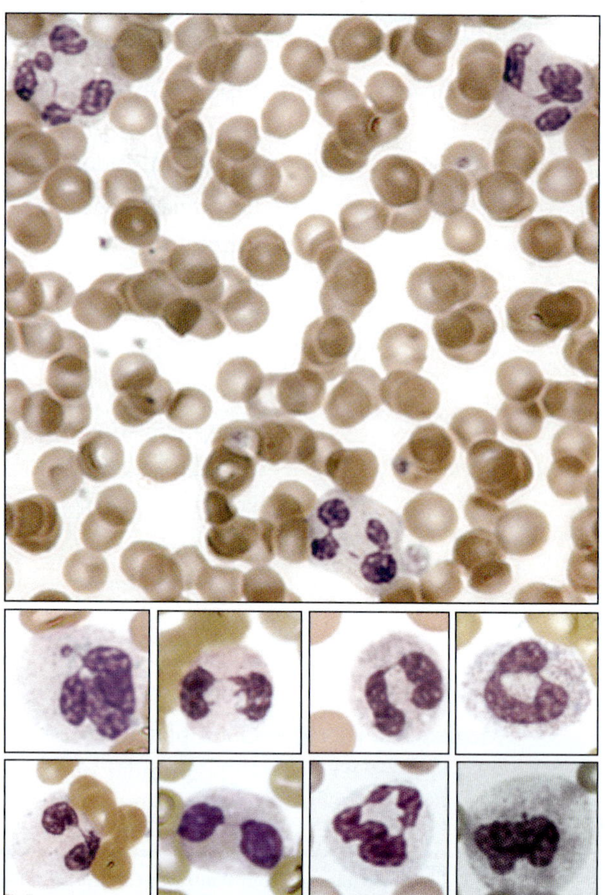

Figure 3.3 Dysplastic nuclear features in circulating neutrophils. Hypolobulation, "stringy" chromatin, and pseudo-Barr bodies are included in the spectrum of the abnormal nuclear features seen in MDS.

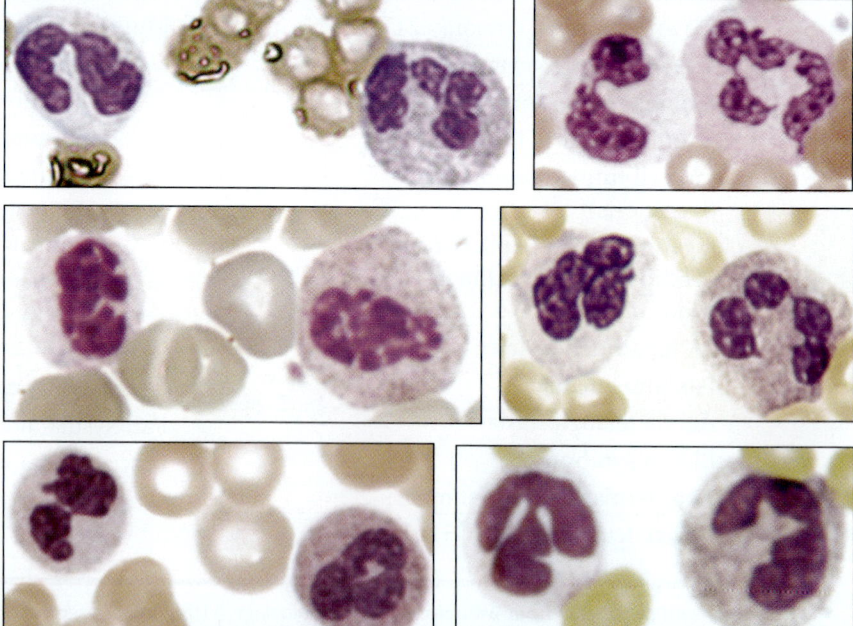

Figure 3.2 Dysplastic hypogranular neutrophils. Several examples of dysplastic, hypogranular neutrophils are shown here. In MDS, dysplastic features are seen usually only in a subpopulation of the affected lineage, whereas staining artifacts usually cause all granulocytes to appear hypogranular in the smear. In the blood smears displayed here, the dysplastic hypogranular neutrophils are all depicted on the left side of each panel.

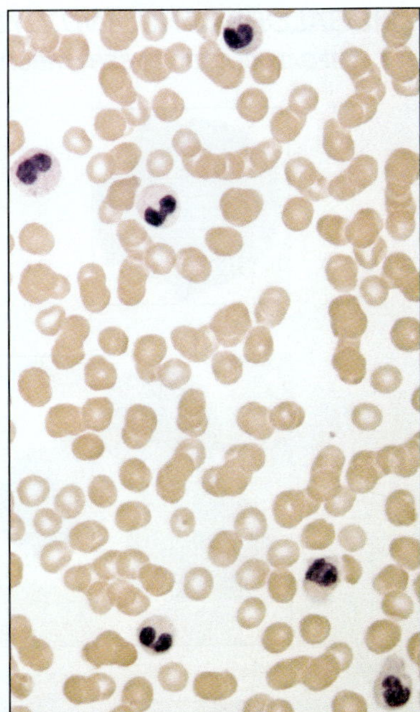

Figure 3.4 Inherited Pelger-Hüet anomaly. Low-power view of peripheral blood showing only hypolobulated neutrophils with very condensed chromatin from a case of inherited Pelger-Hüet anomaly. In myelodysplastic syndromes, hypolobulated neutrophils are usually seen as subpopulations mixed with normal appearing cells.

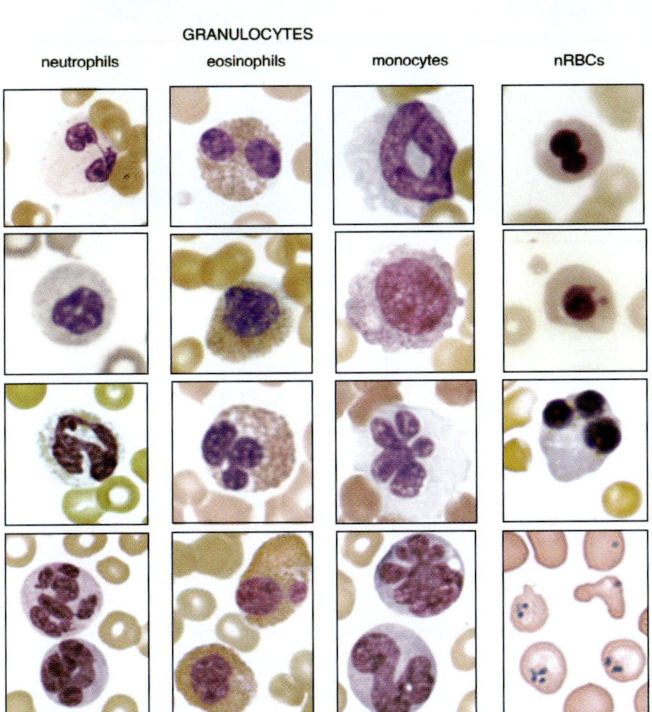

Figure 3.5 Dysplastic nuclear features in circulating cells. Composite image taken from several cases of myelodysplastic syndrome showing dysplastic nuclear features seen in circulating granulocytes and nucleated RBCs. The right lower figure shows numerous Pappenheimer bodies.

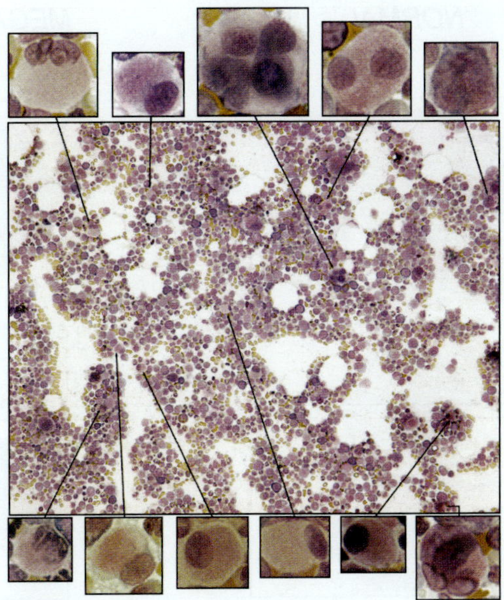

Figure 3.6 Dysplastic megakaryocytes. This low-power view of an aspirate smear from a case of MDS shows numerous dysplastic megakaryocytes that include micromegakaryocytes and forms displaying separate nuclear lobulations. Small dysplastic megakaryocytes (micromegakaryocytes) can be difficult to detect during low-power examination of aspirate smears.

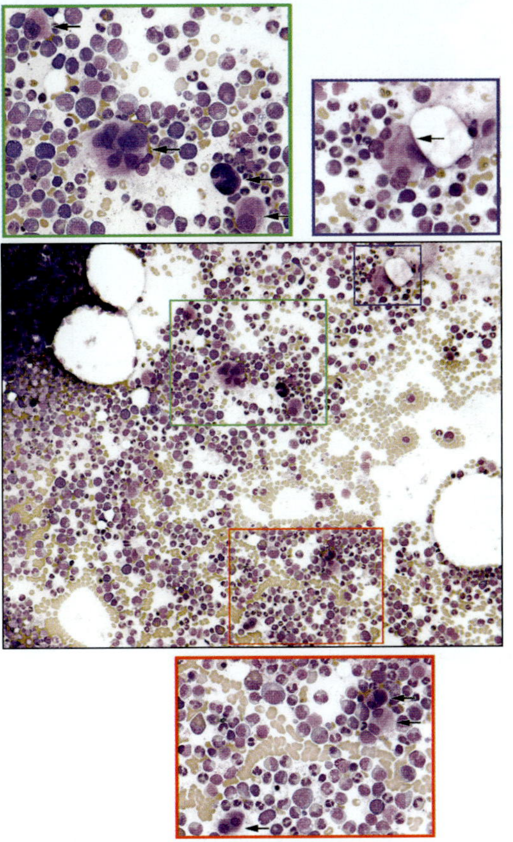

Figure 3.7 Dysplastic megakaryocytes. This low-power view of an aspirate smear from a case of RAEB-1 shows numerous dysplastic megakaryocytes displaying separate nuclear lobulations (*arrows*).

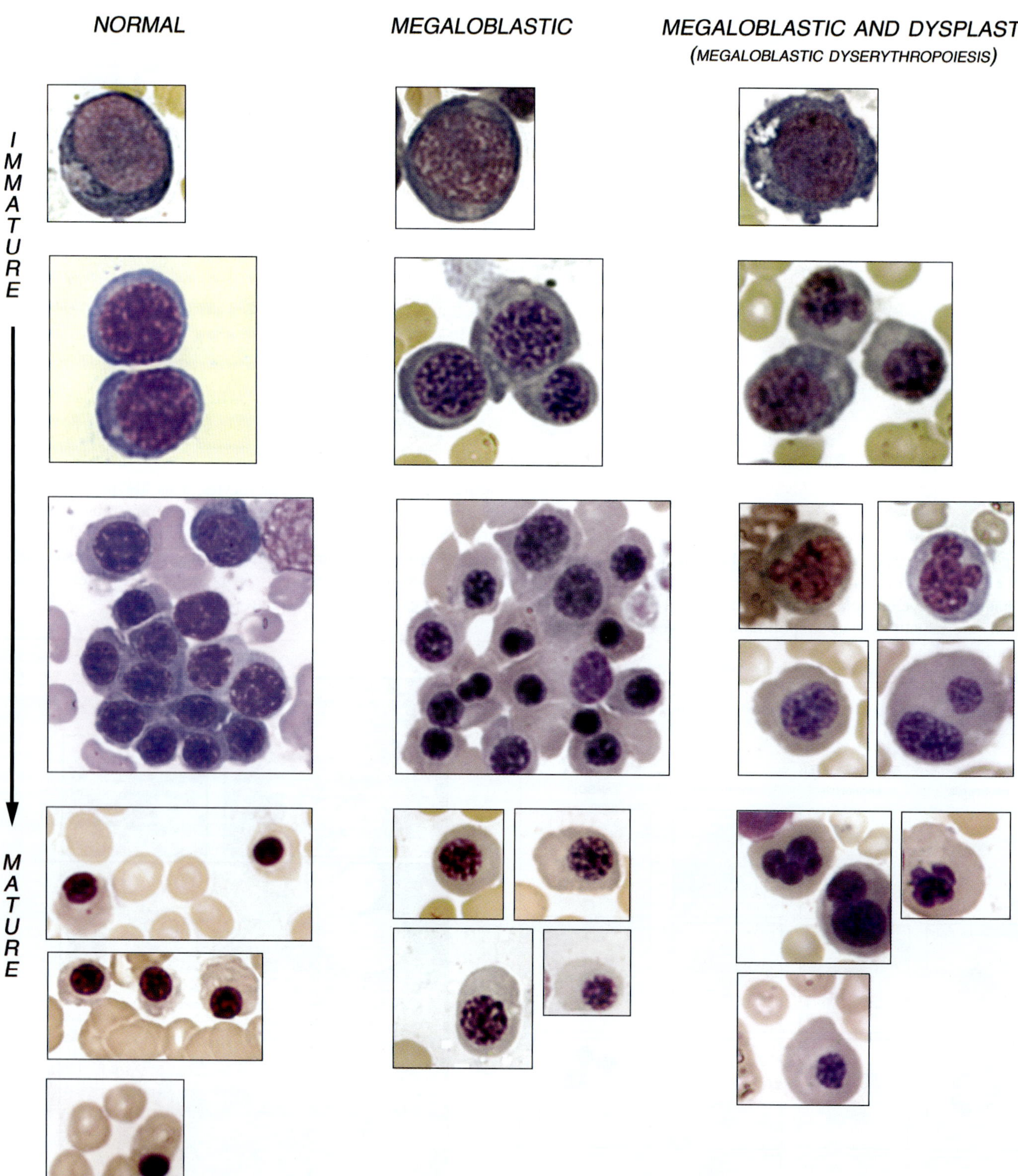

Figure 3.8   Normocytic, megaloblastic, and dysplastic features of the erythroid lineage. Composite figure showing several examples of normal (normocytic) versus megaloblastic and dysplastic erythroid precursors at different stages of maturation. Megaloblastic precursors are typically larger in size than normal precursors and exhibit asynchronous nuclear and cytoplasmic maturation. The latter features are best appreciated in more mature forms, where cytoplasmic maturation proceeds in the form of hemoglobin production while nuclear maturation is delayed. Dyserythropoiesis is manifested primarily by nuclear contour abnormalities such as budding, irregularity ("cookie cutter" appearance), and asymmetric multinucleation.

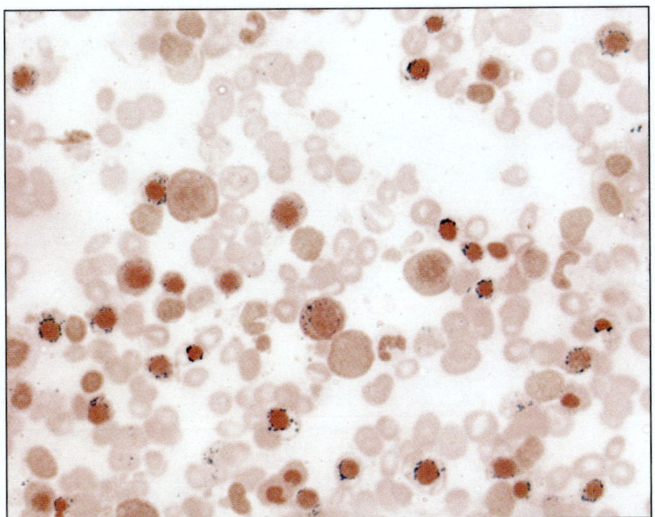

Figure 3.9 Dysplastic erythroids, iron stain. Low-power view of a Prussian blue–stained aspirate from a case of refractory anemia with ringed sideroblasts. More than 15% of the nucleated erythroid precursors display perinuclear necklaces of iron-laden mitochondria that encircle at least one-third of the circumference of the nucleus (ringed sideroblasts).

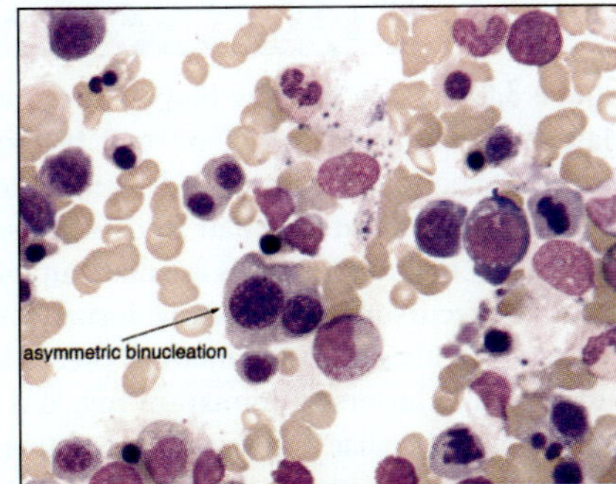

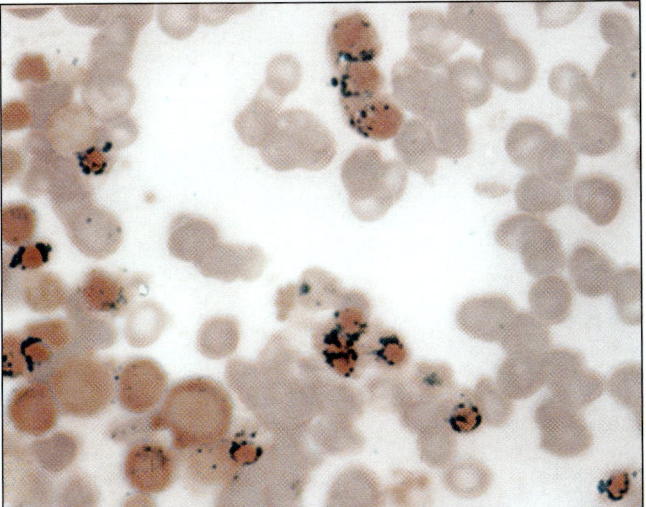

Figure 3.10 Dysplastic erythropoiesis. Hyperplastic megaloblastic dyserythropoiesis in an aspirate smear (*top panel*). The bottom panel is an iron-stained aspirate smear showing numerous ringed sideroblasts with perinuclear "necklaces" made of siderotic granules.

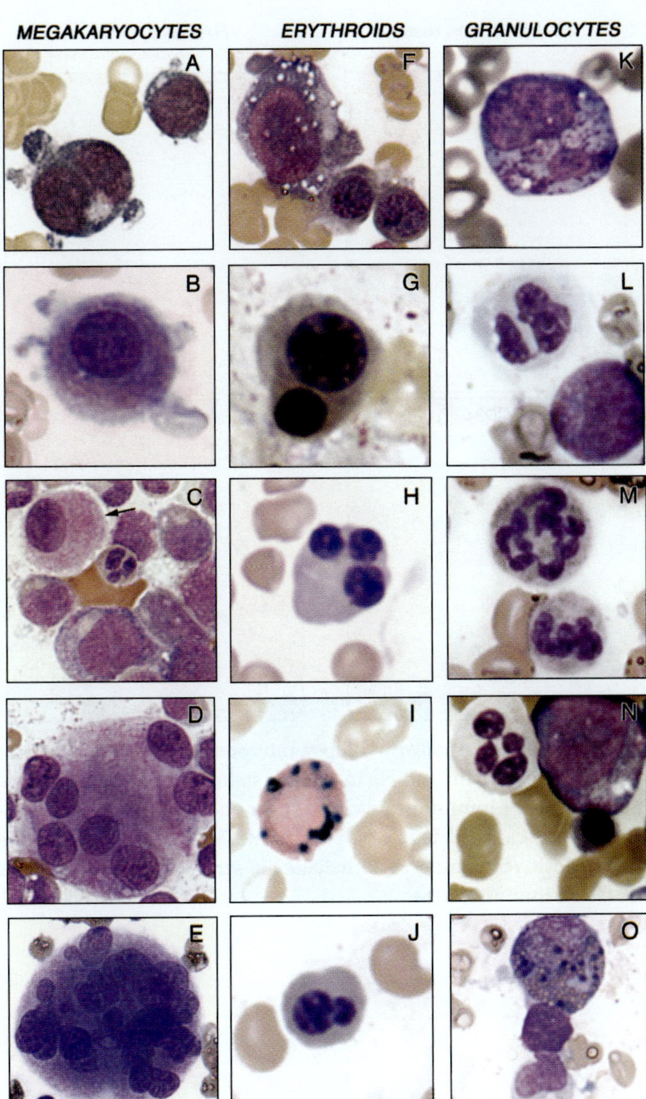

Figure 3.11 Dysplastic megakaryocytic (A–E), erythroid (F–J), and myeloid (K–O) precursors in aspirate smears. **A.** Bizarre megakaryoblasts. **B.** and **C.** Unilobular micromegakaryocytes. **D.** and **E.** Megakaryocytes with separate nuclear lobulations. **F.** Dysplastic vacuolated pronormoblast. **G.** Asymmetric binucleation in mature erythroid. **H.** Trinucleate mature erythroid. **I.** Ringed siderocyte (iron stain). **J.** Mature erythroid with "nuclear budding." **K.** Promyelocyte with dysplastic nucleus. **L.** Hyposegmented neutrophil. **M.** Hypersegmented neutrophil. **N.** Hypogranular neutrophil. **O.** Abnormal eosinobasophilic precursor.

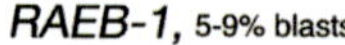
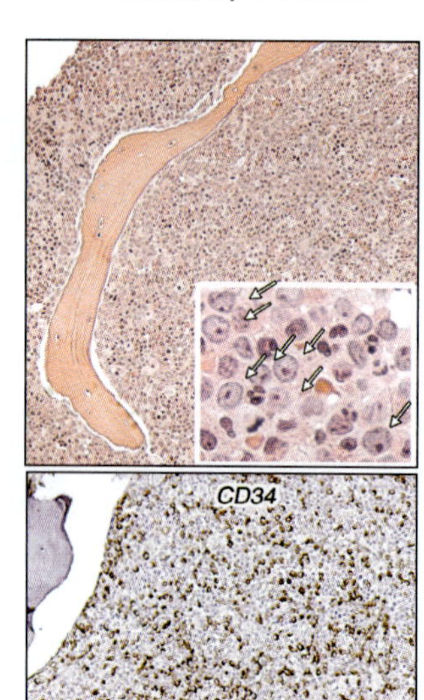

Figure 3.12   Bone marrow biopsy interpretation in MDS. Hypercellular hematoxylin and eosin (H&E)-stained bone marrow biopsies and CD34 immunostains are shown above and below, respectively, from cases of low- and high-grade MDS. Arrows delineate blasts. Positive-staining endothelial cells serve as built-in controls for CD34 immunostains.

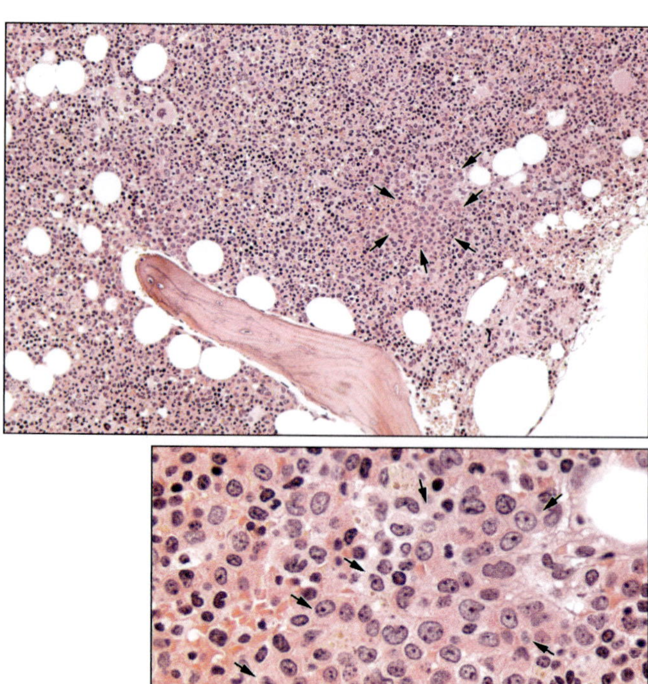

Figure 3.13   Bone marrow biopsy interpretation in MDS, ALIPS. Maturing granulopoiesis in normal biopsies usually appears as indiscrete, poorly circumscribed foci, centered primarily, but not exclusively, in paratrabecular and perivascular locations. These normal foci of granulopoiesis are made up of a mixture of maturing myeloid precursors with mature forms predominating. In MDS, abnormal localization of immature precursors (ALIPS) occurs, in which small clusters of immature myeloid forms are found away from bony trabeculae and vascular structures (*arrows*).

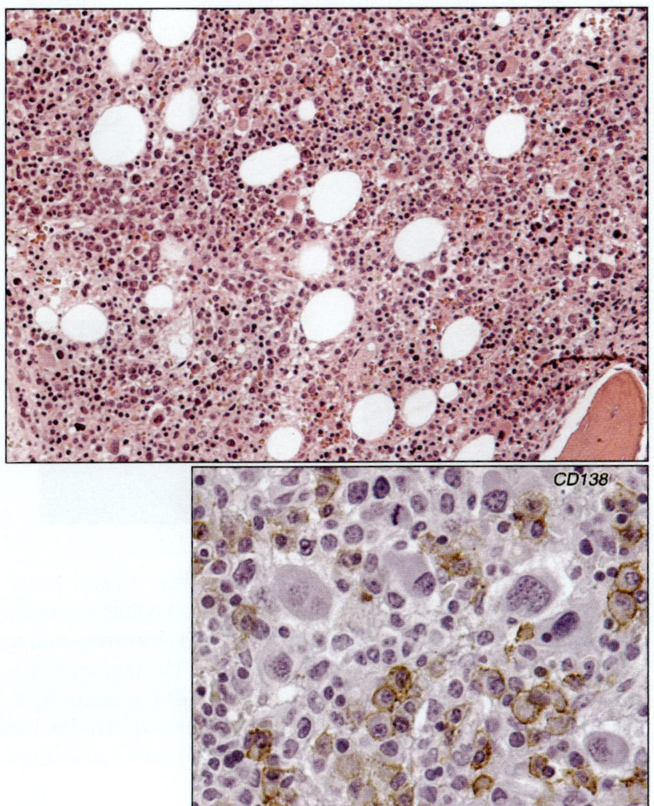

Figure 3.14 Bone marrow biopsy interpretation in MDS. Dysplastic small, unilobular megakaryocytes are readily seen in this case of secondary MDS occurring following unsuccessful treatment for myeloma. The upper panel shows numerous small dysplastic megakarocytes. CD138 immunostains show increased numbers of plasma cells admixed with numerous dysplastic megakaryocytes (*lower panel*).

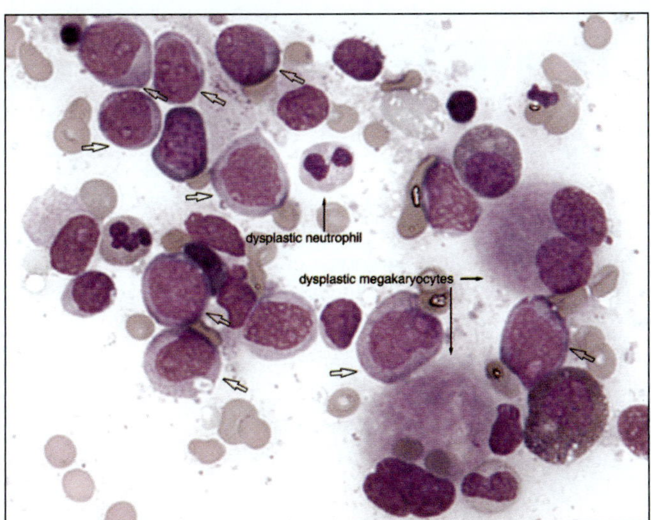

Figure 3.15 Refractory anemia with excess blasts, type 2 (RAEB-2). Aspirate smear from a case of RAEB-2 showing dysplastic small megakaryocytes (micromegakaryocytes), a dysplastic hypogranular/hypolobulated neutrophil, and increased numbers of blasts (*open arrows*).

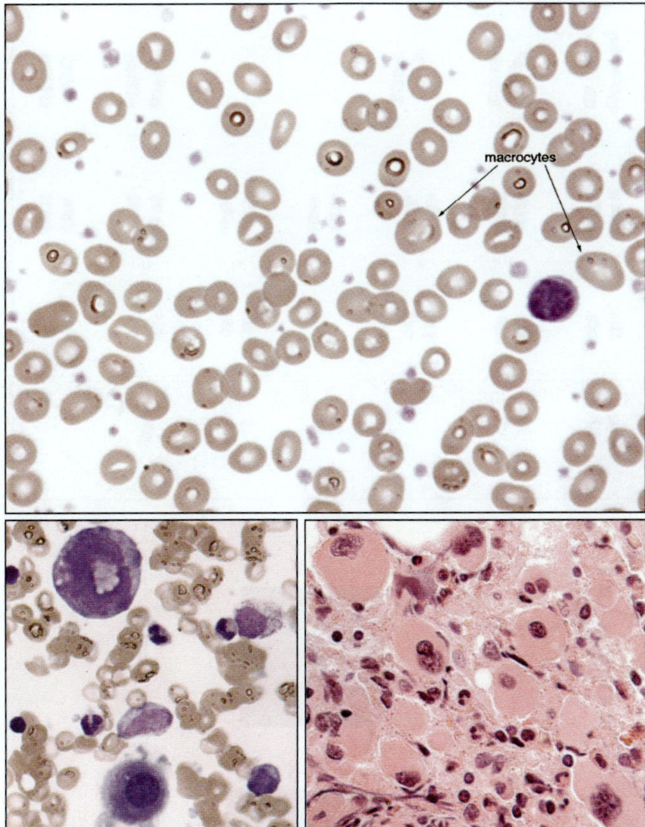

Figure 3.16 5q⁻ syndrome. The top panel is a blood smear showing macrocytic anemia and thrombocythemia. Macrocytic RBCs with cellular diameters that exceed the nucleus of a small mature lymphocyte are seen. Aspirate smear and biopsy in the left and right bottom panels, respectively, show increased numbers of the characteristic unilobular megakaryocytes. The isolated del(5q) cytogenetic abnormality is part of this syndrome or it may be found with or without other cytogenetic abnormalities in other MDS subtypes (see Fig. 3.18).

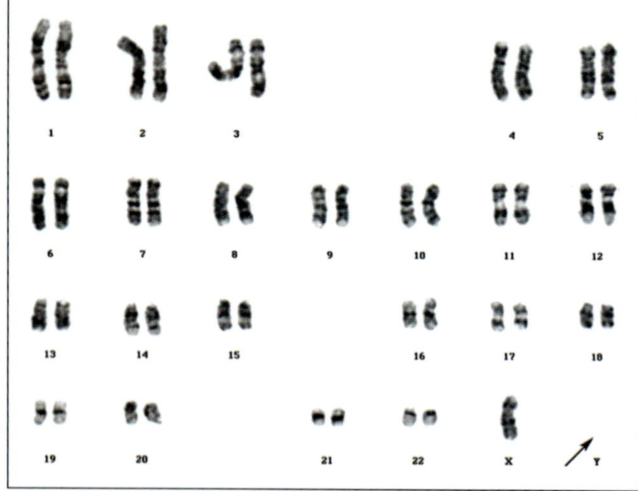

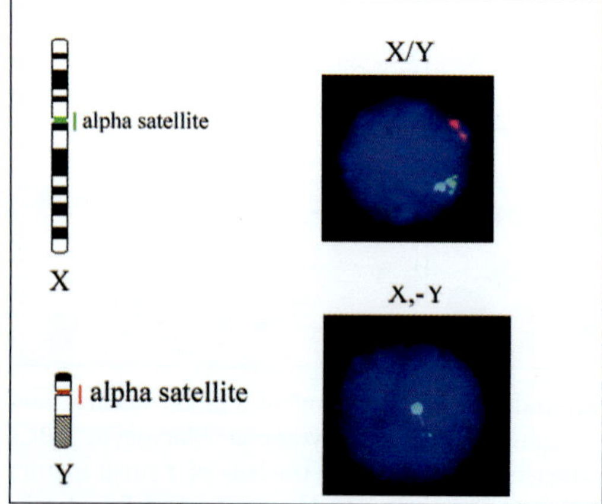

Figure 3.17 45,X,–Y. Karyotype with a missing Y chromosome (*upper panel*). Fluorescent in situ hybridization (FISH) of chromosome X/Y (*lower panel*). The α-satellite region on the X chromosome is labeled with a green fluor, whereas the α-satellite region on the Y chromosome is labeled with a red fluor. When the Y chromosome is missing, only the green signal is present.

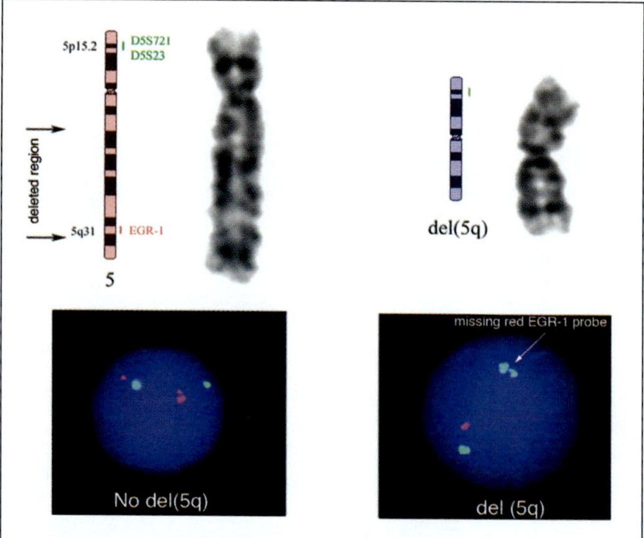

Figure 3.18 del(5q) cytogenetic abnormality. *Upper panel:* Ideograms of the normal chromosome 5 with breakpoints shown by arrows and the del(5q) are shown to the left. The corresponding G-banded chromosomes are shown to the right. The bottom panels show the corresponding FISH results. The EGR-I gene at 5q31, labeled with a red fluor, is usually deleted (*arrow*). The loci at 5p15.2, including D55721 and D5523, are labeled with a green fluor and serve as intrachromosomal controls.

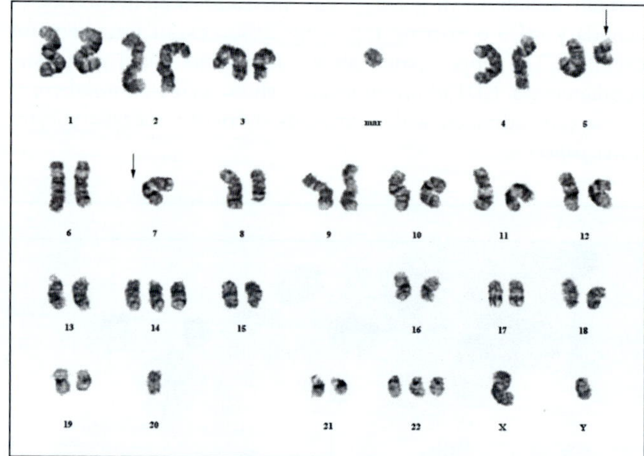

Figure 3.19 Complex karyotype of an MDS patient. This karyotype from a case of RAEB-2 includes, among other aberrations, a del(5q) and monosomy 7.

Chronic Myeloproliferative Syndromes

Tracy I. George, MD

Chronic myeloproliferative diseases (CMPDs) are clonal disorders of the hematopoietic stem cells in which marrows are usually hypercellular and acute leukemia may evolve, similar to myelodysplastic syndromes. CMPDs differ from myelodysplastic syndromes (MDSs), however, in that bone marrow dysplasia is absent, maturation is normal, and production of cells is effective, causing elevated blood levels of one or more cell lines (i.e., erythrocytosis, leukocytosis, and thrombocytosis). Patients also tend to have hepatosplenomegaly (an unusual finding in MDSs) because of sequestered blood cells, extramedullary hematopoiesis, or infiltration by neoplastic cells. These diseases differ from acute leukemias in the slower onset and more protracted course, measured in months to years for CMPDs, compared to weeks for untreated acute leukemias.

CMPDs usually occur in middle-aged adults. The clinical and hematologic features of the various CMPDs (Tables 4.3 and 4.4) overlap, and one type can transform into another. Some do not conform readily to current criteria, and these should be labeled as unclassifiable CMPDs. Moreover, myelofibrosis is a common element, probably caused by the release of various cytokines and growth factors from megakaryocytes and other marrow cells that cause fibroblasts to proliferate and produce collagen and fibronectin. In many cases, the disease evolves with stepwise increases in fibrosis, leading to end-stage myelofibrosis. In others, an increase in blasts may occur, progressing through an "accelerated" phase (10%–19% blasts in the bone marrow) to overt acute leukemia (≥20% blasts). The various CMPDs differ in the incidence of such transformations.

A point mutation in the gene regulating Janus kinase 2, a cytoplasmic protein-tyrosine kinase that is important in cell proliferation and survival, occurs in the majority of patients with polycythemia vera, and approximately one-half of patients with essential thrombocythemia, and with chronic idiopathic myelofibrosis. This mutation (JAK2^{V617F}) is rarely, if ever, present in chronic myelogenous leukemia or in the normal population, and it is uncommon in chronic myelomonocytic leukemia, hypereosinophilic syndrome, MDSs, and systemic mastocytosis. Nonspecific cytogenetic abnormalities are present in about 50% of patients with idiopathic myelofibrosis, 10% to 20% with polycythemia vera, and <5% with essential thrombocythemia.

CHRONIC MYELOGENOUS LEUKEMIA (CML)

The most common of the CMPDs, chronic myelogenous leukemia (CML), accounts for about 20% to 35% of all adult leukemias. It typically occurs at ages 40 to 60, with about 20% to 40% of patients asymptomatic, the diagnosis having been suggested by hepatosplenomegaly on physical examination or abnormal results—leukocytosis, anemia, or thrombocytosis—on routine hematologic testing. When symptoms occur (Table 4.3), they usually relate to splenomegaly (left upper quadrant discomfort or early satiety), problems from an increased white cell production (bone pain, mild fever, night sweats, weight loss), or anemia (dyspnea, fatigue, pallor).

The disease often goes through three stages: chronic phase (CML-CP), accelerated phase (CML-AP), and blast phase (CML-BP) (Table 4.4). In the chronic phase, the blood studies typically show mild anemia and leukocytosis that usually exceeds 25×10^9/L (median white count of about 170×10^9/L), primarily comprising neutrophils in various stages of maturation, especially increases in myelocytes and mature neutrophils (Table 4.5). Basophils are universally increased, and eosinophilia is common. The platelet count is normal or elevated, and may exceed $1,000 \times 10^9$/L, but resulting thrombosis is unusual. The serum lactate dehydrogenase (LDH) and uric acid are commonly increased, reflecting the underlying excessive cell proliferation. The bone marrow shows hypercellularity in the neutrophil line, blasts constitute <5% of the cells, and megakaryocytes are small and hypolobular. In about 50% of patients, the megakaryocytes are increased in number, and, especially in this group, but also in others, reticulin fibrosis may be apparent. Because of the excessive hematopoiesis, the number of cells that eventually die increases, and macrophages containing the lipids from the dead cells may be visible as sea-blue histiocytes or pseudo-Gaucher cells.

According to the World Health Organization (WHO), the accelerated phase is defined by fulfilling at least one of the following: (1) increasing white count and spleen size despite therapy; (2) persistent thrombocytopenia ($<100 \times 10^9$/L) or thrombocytosis ($>1,000 \times 10^9$/L) despite treatment; (3) blasts making up 10% to 19% of bone marrow or peripheral blood white cells; (4) peripheral blood basophilia of $\geq$20%; and (5) evidence of clonal evolution. Bone marrow findings suggestive of, but not definitive for, CML-AP are marked dysplasia of neutrophil precursors and the appearance of abundant aggregates of small, dysplastic megakaryocytes associated with marked reticulin or collagen fibrosis.

The blast phase is defined by one or more of these features: (1) blasts accounting for $\geq$20% of peripheral white cells or nucleated bone marrow cells; (2) blasts proliferating in extramedullary sites, such as the skin, lymph nodes, and spleen; and (3) large aggregates of blasts occuring in the bone marrow. The blasts are usually myeloid but, in about 20% to 30% of cases, they are lymphoid, usually precursor B lymphoblasts. Occasionally, both types are present simultaneously.

Cytogenetic abnormalities now define CML. About 95% of cases have a translocation—t(9;22)(q34;q11)—that results in the Philadelphia chromosome, which fuses the *BCR* gene from chromosome 22 with parts of the *ABL* gene on chromosome 9. The remaining cases of CML have other cytogenetic abnormalities that also result in the *BCR/ABL* fusion gene, which may be detected by Southern blot techniques, reverse transcriptase polymerase chain reaction, or fluorescent in situ hybridization (FISH) analysis.

POLYCYTHEMIA VERA (PV)

In PV, the clonal stem cell population produces excessive numbers of erythrocytes, usually accompanied by increased platelets and granulocytes as well. The average age is about 60 at diagnosis, which, in asymptomatic patients, may be suspected by finding plethora and splenomegaly on examination or abnormalities on a routine blood count. Symptoms typically arise from the erythrocytosis, which causes hyperviscosity and a tendency for venous and arterial thromboses, such as myocardial infarctions, strokes, and venous thromboses of the legs (Table 4.6). In some patients, concomitant platelet abnormalities abet this propensity to clot. Venous occlusion of the intraabdominal vessels, such as the portal, hepatic (Budd-Chiari syndrome), and mesenteric veins is especially suggestive of PV. Other features pre-

sumably related to the erythrocytosis include dizziness, tinnitus, headache, paresthesias, visual disturbances, and painful feet, sometimes associated with digital ischemia and ulcerations despite palpable pulses. A finding probably originating from platelet abnormalities is erythromelalgia—a combination of a burning sensation, erythema, and warmth in the hands and feet that is worsened by exercise, dependency of the extremity, and heat and that is reduced by elevation, cooling, and aspirin.

Hemostatic problems, such as epistaxis, gingival hemorrhage, and gastrointestinal bleeding are common and probably relate to abnormal platelet function and, in about one-third of patients, primarily those with marked thrombocytosis, to the development of acquired von Willebrand disease. The reduction in von Willebrand factor apparently occurs from absorption of large von Willebrand multimers onto platelets, resulting in their removal from the circulation and subsequent destruction.

Another symptom, present in about one-half of patients, is itching on exposure to water (aquagenic pruritus), probably caused in part by histamine release from basophils. Excessive cell production can lead to weight loss and sweating, presumably from hypermetabolism, and to hyperuricemia, which often leads to attacks of gout.

Findings on examination include hypertension and ruddy cyanosis, apparent on the nose, cheeks, lips, ears, neck, and digits. The eyes can appear bloodshot because of conjunctival plethora, and funduscopy may reveal distended, tortuous, and unusually violaceous vessels. Most patients have splenomegaly, and almost half have hepatomegaly.

The hematocrit is elevated, frequently to values above 60%. Leukocytosis (white cells >12,000/μL) occurs in most cases and typically involves immature granulocytes, basophils, and eosinophils as well as mature neutrophils. Thrombocytosis (platelets >400,000/μL) occurs in about one-half of patients and may exceed 1 million/μL. Because the excessive red cell production depletes the iron stores, the erythrocytes may be microcytic and hypochromic. Other findings sometimes seen on a peripheral blood smear include polychromatophilia, basophilic stippling, nucleated red cells, and markedly enlarged and misshapen platelets. On bone marrow evaluation, hyperplasia of the erythroid line is often accompanied by increased megakaryocytes and granulocyte precursors. Maturation is normal, but megakaryocytes may be large and hyperlobulated. Some patients, especially those with megakaryocytic hyperplasia, have substantial bone marrow fibrosis. Iron stores are nearly always absent.

The diagnosis of polycythemia vera rests on finding a genuine increase in red cells without another explanation, such as hypoxia, abnormal hemoglobins, or erythropoietin-secreting tumors. Elevation in the erythrocyte mass typically corresponds with hemoglobin levels of >16.5 g/dL (Hct about 49.5) in women and 18.5 g/dL (Hct about 55.5) in men. Sometimes, however, these values occur in the absence of an actual increase in circulating red cells.

Hematocrits above 60% in the absence of obvious volume depletion, however, almost always indicate a true increase in red cell mass. Findings that support polycythemia vera as the cause of an increased red cell mass include the presence of splenomegaly, thrombocytosis, leukocytosis, oxygen saturation ≥92% when the patient breathes room air, a low serum erythropoietin level, and characteristic bone marrow histology.

The hematologic findings of polycythemia may evolve into acute leukemia, myelodysplasia, or, most commonly, into a "spent" or post-polycythemic phase characterized by anemia and other cytopenias caused by ineffective erythropoiesis, marrow fibrosis, hypersplenism, and extramedullary production of cells with shortened life spans. The spent phase occurs in up to 50% of patients and, on average, appears about 10 years after the diagnosis. The blood smear shows leukoerythroblastosis (the presence of nucleated red cells and cells in the granulocyte series that are more immature than bands (i.e., metamyelocytes, myelocytes, etc.), poikilocytosis, and teardrop cells. The bone marrow demonstrates reticulin and, sometimes, collagen fibrosis, along with trilineage hypocellularity. Dysmorphic megakaryocytes may be present.

CHRONIC IDIOPATHIC MYELOFIBROSIS

Also called *agnogenic myeloid metaplasia* or *myelofibrosis with myeloid metaplasia*, this disorder consists of clonal proliferation of megakaryocytes and granulocytic precursors in the bone marrow, accompanied by reactive, marrow fibrosis thought to be secondary to local release of fibrogenic growth factors. Replacement of the marrow by fibrosis leads to extramedullary hematopoiesis, which is most common in the spleen and liver, but can also affect many other sites, such as the dura mater, lymph nodes, lung, and pleura. In these locations, it may cause symptoms ranging from organ enlargement, bleeding, fluid formation, or compression of adjacent normal structures. Chronic idiopathic myelofibrosis has a prefibrotic phase, which is commonly asymptomatic and is characterized by a hypercellular marrow and minimal fibrosis. Progression leads to extensive bone marrow fibrosis. Occurring in the elderly, idiopathic myelofibrosis portends a shortened life expectancy with an increased risk of developing acute leukemia.

About 30% to 40% of patients are asymptomatic at diagnosis, which may be suggested by splenomegaly or abnormal blood tests. Symptoms typically occur from anemia, hypermetabolism from high cell turnover, splenomegaly, or thrombocytopenia (Table 4.8). Hypermetabolism may cause weight loss, fever, sweats, or problems associated with hyperuricemia, including attacks of gout or renal stones. Anemia can lead to complaints of fatigue, dyspnea, weakness, and palpitations. Splenomegaly can produce left upper quadrant discomfort, a sensation of early satiety from compression of the stomach, or diarrhea from pressure on the bowels. On examination,

splenomegaly is nearly universal and often enormous, and hepatomegaly is present in about one-half of patients. Thrombocytopenia or altered platelet function may cause cutaneous hemorrhage, and, occasionally, extramedullary hematopoiesis in the skin produces erythematous or purplish nodules, papules, and plaques. Extramedullary hematopoiesis affecting the serosal surfaces can cause pleural or pericardial effusions and ascites, which can also originate from portal hypertension due to hepatic involvement or increased blood flow from an enlarged spleen. Esophageal varices produced by the portal hypertension can lead to gastrointestinal hemorrhage.

About one-third of patients are diagnosed during the *prefibrotic phase*, in which the characteristic findings are anemia, thrombocytosis, and mild leukocytosis. The blood smear may show occasional nucleated red cells, teardrop-shaped erythrocytes (dacrocytes), immature granulocytes, and large platelets. The bone marrow at this stage is hypercellular, with increased neutrophils and atypical megakaryocytes, characterized by large size, abnormal chromatin clumping, altered nuclear-to-cytoplasm (N:C) ratios, and abnormally lobulated nuclei, some of which may lack surrounding cytoplasm. Fibrosis is absent or minimal. The prominent hematologic findings of the *fibrotic phase* are anemia and a leukoerythroblastic blood smear (nucleated erythrocytes, immature granulocytes) with numerous dacrocytes. White cell and platelet counts vary widely, but a few myeloblasts are common, and platelet abnormalities include large size, bizarre shape, circulating megakaryocyte nuclei, and micromegakaryocytes. Bone marrow aspiration is usually unsuccessful, but the bone marrow biopsy demonstrates variable cellularity, with marked reticulin or collagen fibrosis and numerous atypical megakaryocytes in large aggregates. Osteosclerosis (new bone formation) may be visible. Various criteria for the diagnosis of chronic idiopathic myelofibrosis exist. They typically require the absence of *BCR/ABL* and the presence of diffuse marrow fibrosis, associated with a variable number of other features, including splenomegaly, atypical megakaryocyte hyperplasia, myeloid metaplasia, and the presence on a peripheral smear of teardrop erythrocytes, immature granulocytes, and nucleated red cells. Myelofibrosis may accompany a large number of neoplastic and non-neoplastic conditions (Table 4.9) which should be excluded before the diagnosis of chronic idiopathic myelofibrosis is made. Other common laboratory abnormalities include hyperuricemia, elevated serum lactic dehydrogenase (LDH), and abnormal liver tests. Some patients have cytogenetic abnormalities, most commonly deletions of chromosomes 20q and 13q. About 50% have an acquired mutation in the Janus kinase 2 (JAK2) gene.

ESSENTIAL THROMBOCYTHEMIA

In essential thrombocythemia, a clonal population of mature megakaryocytes in the bone marrow produces excessive numbers of platelets. The average age at diagnosis is about

50 to 60 years, and most cases are discovered by routine blood tests of asymptomatic patients. When symptoms occur, they usually are related to vessel thrombosis or abnormal vascular reactivity, such as dizziness, headaches, visual disturbances, transient ischemic attacks, digital ischemia, and paresthesias. One form of vascular abnormality is erythromelalgia, a combination of erythema, burning pain, and warmth of the hands and feet that is exacerbated by dependency, heat, or exercise and is relieved by elevation, cooling, and aspirin. It is typically asymmetric. Thromboses usually involve the arteries, but venous occlusion also can occur. Hemorrhage is less frequent, most commonly from the upper respiratory and gastrointestinal tracts. Sometimes bleeding occurs from acquired von Willebrand disease associated with marked thrombocytosis, in which the large von Willebrand multimers adhere to platelets and are removed from the circulation. Splenomegaly, usually moderate and nonprogressive, is present in about 50% of patients, hepatomegaly in approximately 20%.

The platelet count commonly exceeds $1,000 \times 10^9$/L, and the most prominent finding on blood smear is the large number of platelets, which vary considerably in size, ranging from small to giant (diameter larger than an erythrocyte). White cells are typically normal in number and appearance, as are the erythrocytes, unless hemorrhage has led to iron-deficiency anemia. The bone marrow discloses markedly increased numbers of large megakaryocytes, which commonly form loose aggregates and possess abundant cytoplasm with normal maturation, along with deeply lobulated nuclei. Minimal reticulin fibrosis may occur, but larger amounts or collagen fibrosis suggests another diagnosis. The serum LDH and uric acid can be elevated from the increase in cell turnover. About one-half of patients have an acquired mutation in the Janus kinase 2 (JAK2) gene.

Because many diseases, such as inflammatory states, malignancy, iron deficiency, and other myeloproliferative disorders, can produce thrombocytosis, and no definitive test exists, the diagnosis depends on the presence of certain features and the exclusion of others. Various criteria, including those by the WHO, have been proposed, but most have in common the requirements of: (1) sustained thrombocytosis (platelet count $>600,000/\mu$L; (2) characteristic bone marrow biopsy findings of increased large, mature megakaryocytes; (3) no evidence of malignancy, inflammatory state (including infections), or prior splenectomy that could explain the thrombocytosis; (4) the exclusion of chronic myelogenous leukemia as confirmed by absent Philadelphia chromosome and *BCR/ABL* fusion gene; (5) the exclusion of chronic idiopathic myelofibrosis by demonstrating absent or mild reticulin fibrosis and no collagen fibrosis in the bone marrow; (6) the absence of a myelodysplastic syndrome; and (7) no evidence of polycythemia vera or iron deficiency based on the presence of a normal hematocrit or red cell mass and stainable marrow iron or a normal mean corpuscular volume (MCV) or serum ferritin. If iron deficiency is present,

a trial of iron therapy will determine whether it alone is the underlying cause, in which case the thrombocytosis should abate, or whether occult polycythemia vera is present, in which case erythrocytosis will occur.

The life expectancy of patients with essential thrombocythemia is nearly normal, but a small percentage will develop acute myeloid leukemia, myelodysplasia, or myelofibrosis.

RARE CHRONIC MYELOPROLIFERATIVE DISEASES

Chronic neutrophilic leukemia is a very rare disorder in which marrow granulocytic hypercellularity results in persistent blood neutrophilia. Mature neutrophils and bands constitute most of the neutrophils, with few being less immature forms. The neutrophils may appear normal, but sometimes contain coarse granules. The bone marrow shows normal numbers of blasts or promyelocytes, but myelocytes and mature neutrophils are increased. Splenomegaly and hepatomegaly usually are present. The WHO criteria for diagnosis are: (1) blood leukocytosis $\geq 25 \times 10^9$/L, with mature neutrophils and bands constituting $>80\%$ of the white cells; (2) promyelocytes, myelocytes, and metamyelocytes making up $<10\%$ of white cells and myeloblasts $<1\%$; (3) hypercellular bone marrow biopsy with increased neutrophils, normal neutrophil maturation, and myeloblasts $<5\%$ of nucleated marrow cells; (4) no alternative explanation of neutrophilia, such as infection or tumor; (5) hepatosplenomegaly; (6) no Philadelphia chromosome or *BCR/ABL* fusion gene; and (7) no evidence of another myeloproliferative or myelodysplastic disorder. Patients often have a long life span, but the neutrophilia progresses, and anemia and thrombocytopenia can develop. A few transform into acute leukemia. About 20% of cases occur with an associated malignancy, most commonly multiple myeloma.

Chronic eosinophilic leukemia (CEL) and *hypereosinophilic syndrome* are disorders with persistent blood eosinophilia ($\geq 1,500/\mu$L) without another cause. In both, organ damage occurs from infiltration with eosinophils or from the toxic materials that they produce. The two differ in that, in CEL, the proliferation of eosinophils is clonal, but proof of that feature may be difficult to establish; if so, then the diagnosis of CEL is made if blasts are increased in blood or bone marrow. Both diseases are much more common in men than in women. Most patients with these disorders are symptomatic with constitutional complaints, such as pruritus, fever, and fatigue, or with problems related to a specifically affected area, such as cough, peripheral neuropathy, or rashes. Heart involvement includes a restrictive cardiomyopathy caused by endomyocardial fibrosis and scarring of the mitral or tricuspid valves, leading to valvular regurgitation. The blood smear shows markedly increased eosinophils, with mainly mature forms, but with variation in size, granulation, and nuclear segmentation. Basophilia, neutrophilia, or monocytosis may be present. The bone marrow demonstrates eosinophilic proliferation, usually with normal maturation and no significant dysplasia. Charcot-Leyden crystals are often plentiful. The WHO diagnosis of CEL requires: (1) persistent blood eosinophilia and increased bone marrow eosinophils; (2) <20% myeloblasts in the blood and bone marrow; (3) exclusion of other diseases that can cause eosinophilia, such as allergies, infections, lymphomas, and other myeloproliferative and myelodysplastic disorders; and (4) evidence of a clonal chromosomal abnormality or blast cells >2% in the peripheral blood or >5% in the marrow but <20% in both. Cytogenetic and/or molecular genetic testing (i.e., FISH) is recommended in all patients with CEL/HES, because a subset of patients has a fusion gene with tyrosine kinase activity, *FIP1L1-PDGFR-α*, caused by an interstitial deletion on chromosome 4q. HES patients with this tyrosine kinase have rapid and complete hematologic remissions to imatinib mesylate therapy, the tyrosine kinase inhibitor used to treat CML. HES patients with this fusion gene have marrows with increased fibrosis and increased serum tryptase levels. This fusion gene also appears related to a subset of patients with systemic mastocytosis and eosinophilia who also are responsive to imatinib mesylate. Patients with HES may subsequently develop a myeloid malignancy or acquire a clonal abnormality. Several clonal cytogenetic abnormalities are reported in CEL. The t(5;12) and other abnormalities involving 5q33 show features of chronic myelomonocytic leukemia with eosinophilia, with production of a fusion oncogene, *TEL-PDGFR-β* with constitutive activation of the kinase domain of *PDGFR-β*. Eosinophilia also is seen with myeloproliferative syndromes involving translocations with 8p11; these disorders show an association with non-Hodgkin lymphomas, including T-lymphoblastic lymphoma.

Chronic myeloproliferative disease, unclassifiable refers to disorders in which myeloproliferative disease is definitely present, based on clinical and laboratory findings, but the features fail to conform to the diagnostic entities delineated above. The disease may: (1) be early in its course and not yet fully developed into a clear diagnostic category; (2) be late in the course and end-stage findings, such as advanced myelofibrosis or osteosclerosis, have replaced earlier diagnostic features; or (3) possess characteristics of two or more myeloproliferative disorders. The patients do not have a Philadelphia chromosome or *BCR/ABL* fusion gene.

MYELODYSPLASTIC/ MYELOPROLIFERATIVE DISEASES

These clonal disorders have, at presentation, both myeloproliferative and myelodysplastic features. The bone marrow is hypercellular, and some cell lines have increased numbers in the peripheral blood, although they have dysplastic characteristics; other cell lines have ineffective proliferation with cytopenias. Organomegaly and marrow fibrosis may occur.

The presence of fibrosis alone in a case that is otherwise typical of myelodysplasia, however, is better classified as MDS with fibrosis. Similarly, patients with a long history of CMPD who develop dysplasia are not considered a mixed MDS/CMPD. The three main disorders of MDS/CMPD are chronic myelomonocytic leukemia, atypical chronic myeloid leukemia, and juvenile myelomonocytic leukemia.

Chronic Myelomonocytic Leukemia

The average age at diagnosis is about 65 to 75 years, and males predominate. With a short median survival of a few years, up to one-third of patients evolve into acute leukemia. The most common symptoms are weight loss, fever, fatigue, and night sweats. Hepatosplenomegaly is present in about 50% of cases. About one-half of patients have leukocytosis; the remaining have either normal or decreased white counts.

The WHO diagnostic criteria for chronic myelomonocytic leukemia are: (1) persistent monocytosis in the peripheral blood $>1 \times 10^9$; (2) no Philadelphia chromosome or *BCR/ABL* fusion gene; (3) <20% blasts (including myeloblasts, monoblasts, or promonocytes) in peripheral blood or bone marrow; and (4) dysplasia in one or more myeloid lines. The fourth criterion may be absent if bone marrow cells have an acquired clonal, cytogenetic abnormality or if unexplained monocytosis has been present for at least 3 months.

The circulating monocytes usually appear mature, but some can have abnormalities in granulation, nuclear lobulation, or nuclear chromatin. Dysplasia may be apparent in neutrophils, causing abnormalities in nuclear lobulation and cytoplasmic granulation. Large platelets sometimes are present. The bone marrow typically is hypercellular, with increased monocyte precursors and dysplasia in one or more myeloid lines.

Cytochemical stains, such as α-naphthyl acetate esterase or α-naphthyl butyrate esterase, can help identify the monocytes. The WHO classification recommends subcategorizing CMML into two types: (1) CMML-1, in which blasts are <5% in the blood and <10% in the marrow; and (2) CMML-2, in which any of the following occurs—blasts 5% to 19% in the blood, blasts 10% to 19% in the marrow, or Auer rods are present. When blood eosinophils are $>1.5 \times 10^9$/L, the disease should be called *CMML-1* or *CMML-2 with eosinophilia*. Nonspecific clonal cytogenetic abnormalities occur in 20% to 40% of patients, most commonly trisomy 8, monosomy 7/deletion 7q, and structural abnormalities of 12p and isochromosome 17q. Some patients with CMML with eosinophilia have t(5;12) involving the *PDGFR-β* gene partnering with the TEL gene.

Atypical Chronic Myeloid Leukemia (aCML)

Atypical CML, a disease primarily affecting elderly men, shares some features of usual CML including: splenomegaly, left-shifted leukocytosis sometimes $>100 \times 10^9$/L and anemia. Many granulocytes are dysplastic, with abnormalities in nuclear lobulation, cytoplasmic granulation, and condensation of nuclear chromatin. Dysplasia also may be present in erythrocytes and platelets. The bone marrow has granulocytic proliferation, with pronounced dysplasia, but <20% blasts. Dysplasia is common in erythrocyte precursors and megakaryocytes. In contrast to usual CML, the Philadelphia chromosome and the BCR/ABL fusion gene are absent. Nonspecific cytogenetic abnormalities are common, including trisomy 8, trisomy 13, deletions of 12p or 20q11 and isochromosome 17q. Rare cases have t(5;10), in which the fusion gene *PDGFR-β/H4* is expressed. Up to 40% of patients will progress to acute leukemia.

Juvenile Myelomonocytic Leukemia

Juvenile myelomonocytic leukemia (JMML) is a childhood MDS/CMPD that includes childhood leukemias previously classified as CMML, juvenile CML, and infantile monosomy 7 syndrome. Although rare, JMML is the most common MDS/CMPD of children, typically in boys, who develop the disease by age 4 years. Skin lesions often precede the diagnosis, and these children present with a leukocytosis that may be identical in appearance to CMML of adults. Organomegaly is common, and the children usually have elevations of fetal hemoglobin. The typical clinical findings of JMML include fever, skin rash, pallor, hepatosplenomegaly, and lymphadenopathy. JMML must be differentiated from infection, which can present with similar clinical and morphologic findings. Consensus criteria for the diagnosis of JMML require peripheral blood monocytosis greater than 1,000/μL, blasts and promonocytes less than 20% in blood and marrow to exclude acute leukemia, and

the absence of *BCR/ABL* ruling out childhood cases of CML. At least two or more of the following optional criteria must also be present: increased hemoglobin F for age, circulating immature granulocytes, white blood cell count greater than 10,000/μL, clonal chromosomal abnormality and growth factor hypersensitivity of myeloid progenitors *in vitro*.

Children with neurofibromatosis type 1 have a markedly increased risk of developing JMML. Abnormalities of the *NF1* gene lead to loss of neurofibromin, an activation protein for *RAS*, resulting in deregulation of normal *RAS* signaling pathways and subsequent hypersensitivity of JMML cells to granulocyte-macrophage colony–stimulating factor.

Other Myelodysplastic and Chronic Myeloproliferative Syndromes

Some patients have diseases that show features of MDS and CMPD, but do not fit well into any of the previously mentioned categories. Many of these cases show typical features of myelodysplasia and an atypical finding more suggestive of a myeloproliferative disorder, such as marked marrow fibrosis and/or organomegaly.

A provisional entity in the WHO classification is refractory anemia with ringed sideroblasts associated with marked thrombocytosis, in which the marrow contains >15% ringed sideroblasts with an accompanying atypical megakaryocyte proliferation, often resembling those seen in essential thrombocytopenia (ET). Another syndrome not described earlier is a mixed MDS/CMPD associated with isochromosome 17q occurring in adults, with a male predominance, characterized by hyposegmentation of neutrophils, monocytosis, and a high rate of transformation to acute myeloid leukemia.

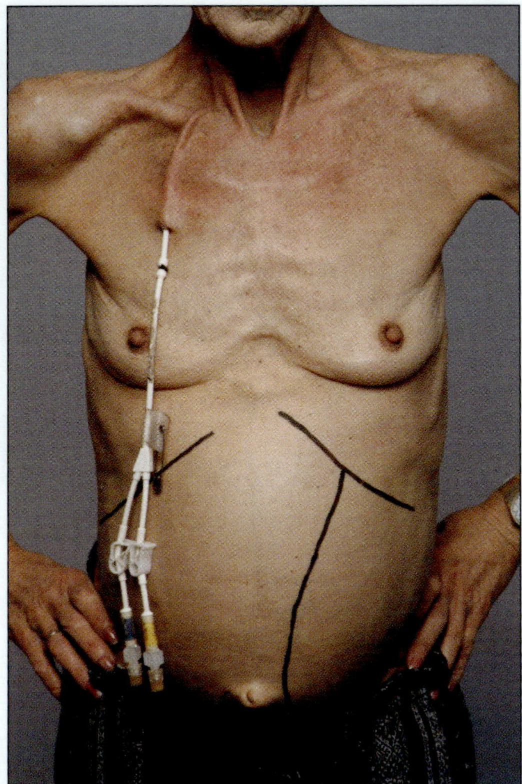

Figure 4.1   Cachexia and hepatosplenomegaly in chronic myelo-proliferative disorders. Massive hepatosplenomegaly in a woman with CML.

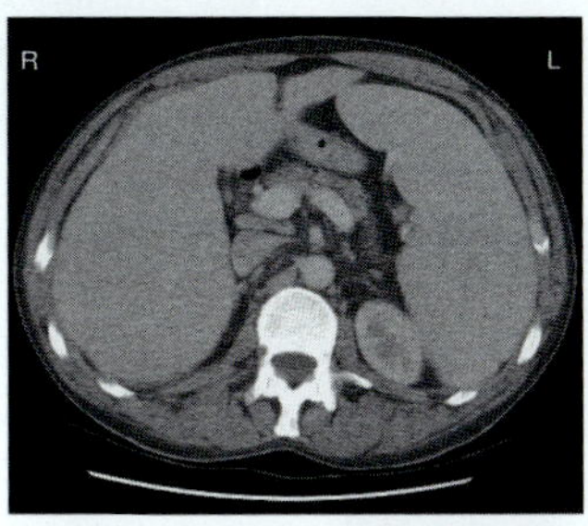

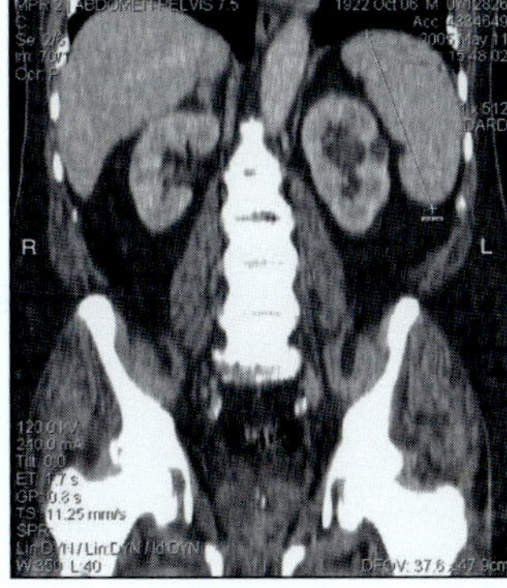

Figure 4.2   Hepatosplenomegaly and osteosclerosis in myeloproliferative disorders. *Upper panel:* Axial computed tomography (CT) scan of the upper abdomen showing homogenously enlarged spleen and liver in a patient with chronic idiopathic myelofibrosis. *Lower panel:* Coronal CT scan with bone windows in a patient with chronic idiopathic myelofibrosis showing a mildly enlarged spleen (normal is <14 cm). Increased density of the visualized bones is present.

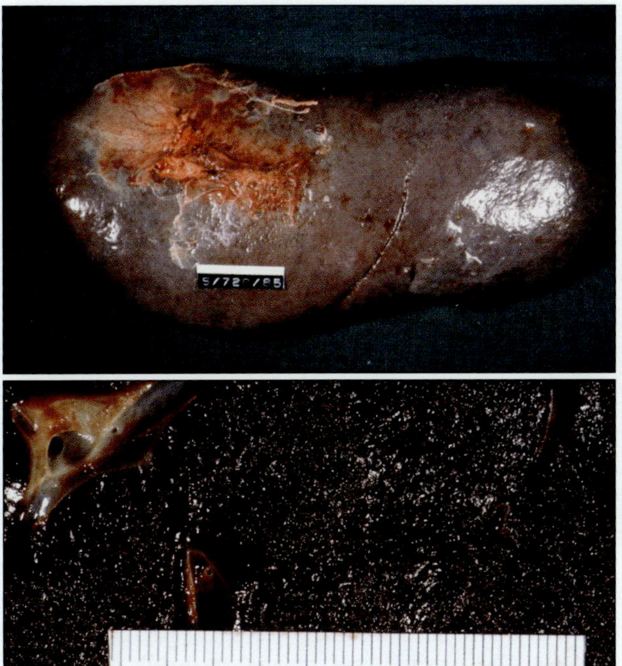

Figure 4.3   Splenomegaly in myeloproliferative disorders. Excised spleen from a case of CML showing a markedly enlarged spleen weighing >1,000 g and measuring approximately 30 cm in greatest dimension (label in *top figure* represents 5 cm). Bottom figure illustrates diffusely expanded red pulp made up of extramedullary hematopoiesis.

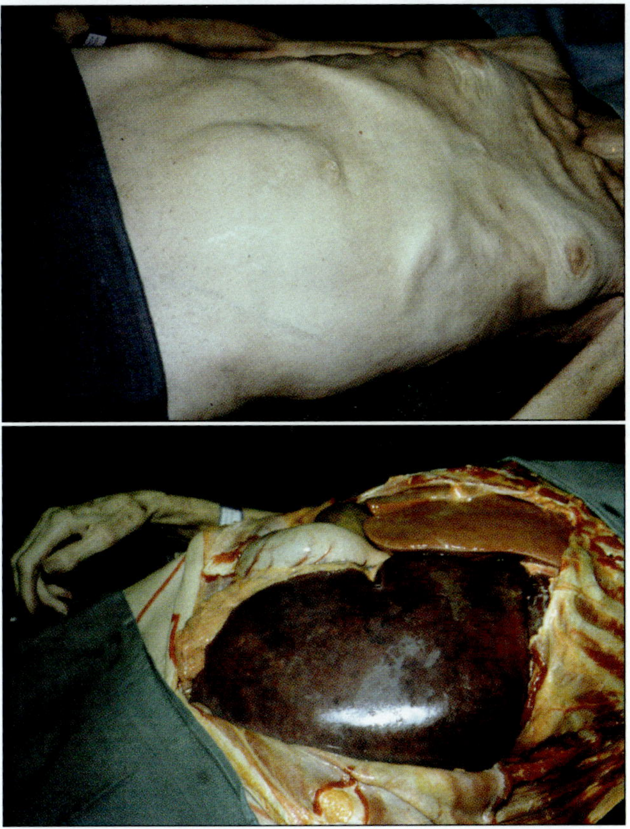

Figure 4.4   Cachexia and hepatosplenomegaly in chronic myelo-proliferative disorders. Autopsy showing an emaciated woman with CML and hepatosplenomegaly.

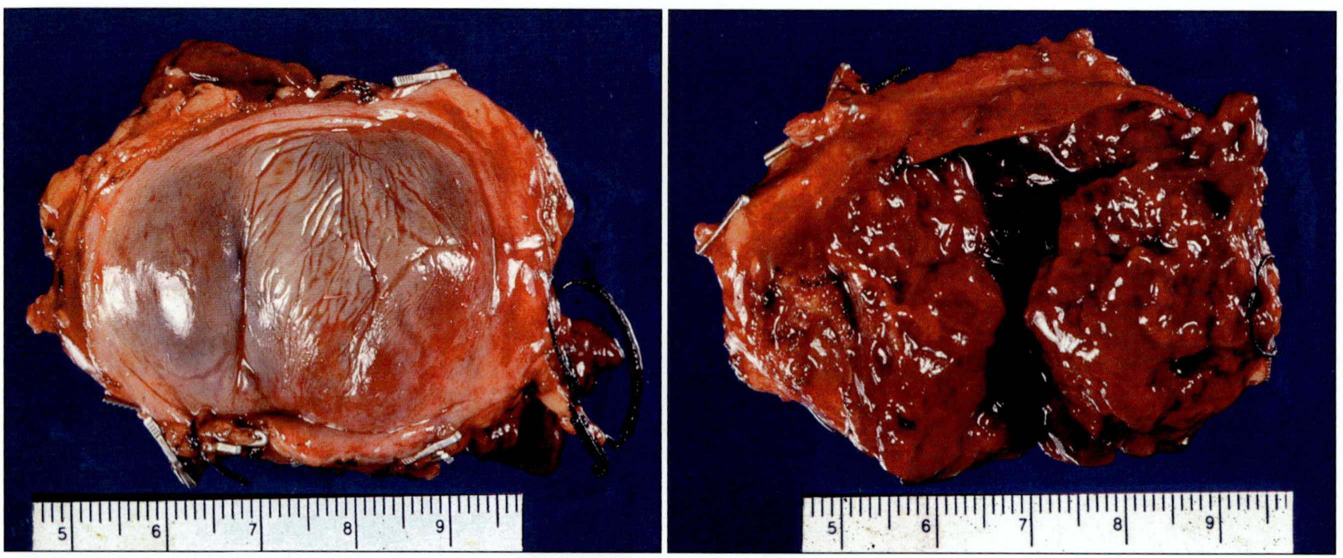

Figure 4.5 Extramedullary hematopoiesis in chronic myeloproliferative disorders. The liver and spleen are the most common site for extramedullary hematopoiesis; however, discrete tumor masses such as this retroperitoneal mass can occur virtually in any site. As shown on cut section in the right panel, these "tumors" are usually made up of bloody, friable tissue ("red currant jelly–like") pieces.

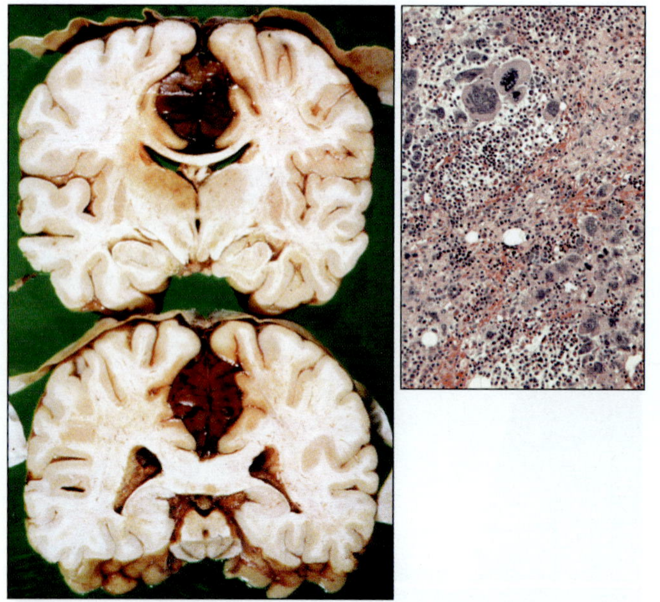

Figure 4.6 Extramedullary hematopoiesis in chronic myeloproliferative disorders. An unusual fatal case of intracranial extramedullary hematopoiesis situated between the two cerebral hemispheres involving the falx cerebri in a case of CML. The right panel is a photomicrograph showing trilineage hematopoiesis that includes numerous megakaryocytes.

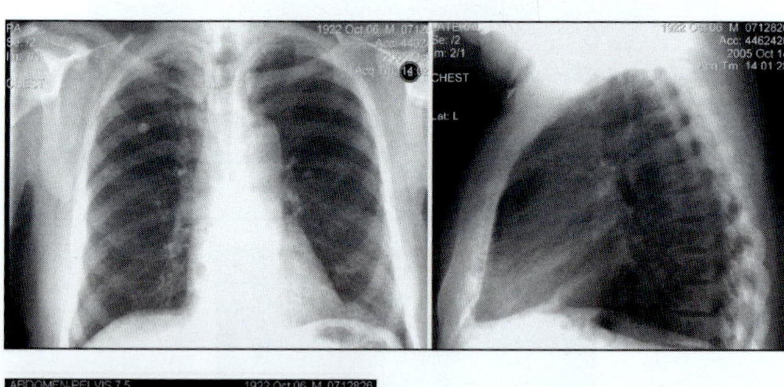

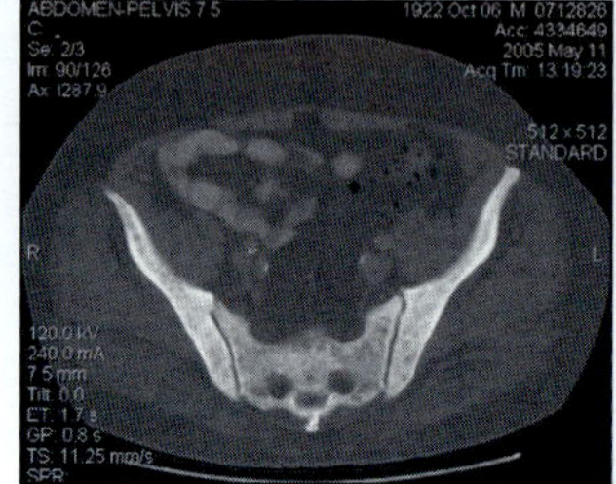

Figure 4.7 Osteosclerosis in chronic idiopathic myelofibrosis. Chest radiographs, PA and lateral views, showing diffuse increased density throughout bony skeleton in a patient with advanced chronic idiopathic myelofibrosis with osteosclerosis. Note prominent density of ribs.

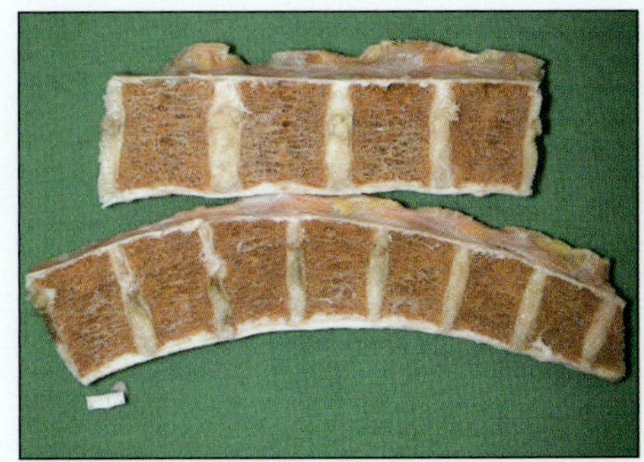
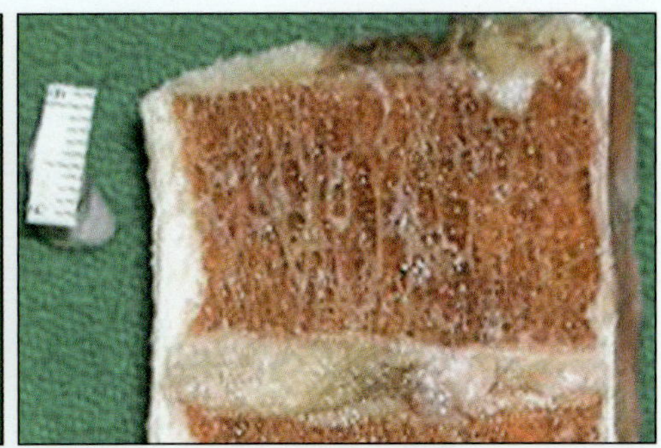
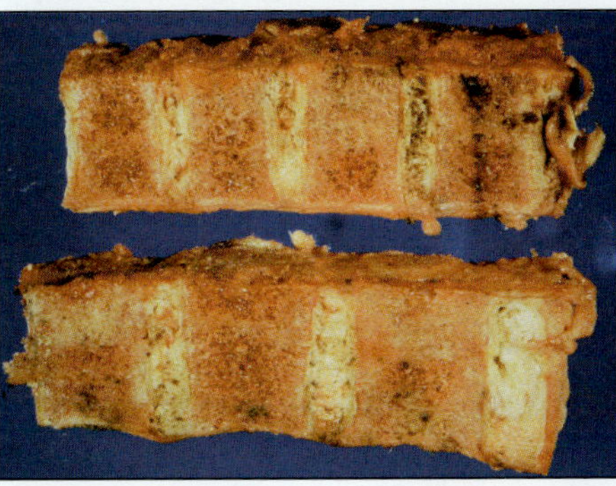
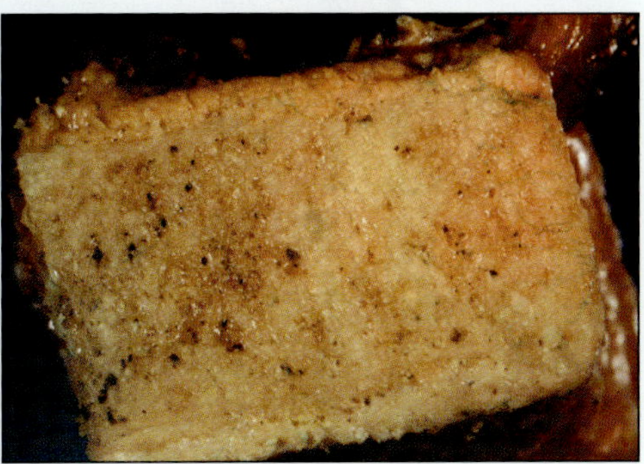

Figure 4.8 Osteosclerosis in chronic idiopathic myelofibrosis. Normal adult bone marrow is made up of cellular marrow and fat elements interspersed among thin bony trabeculae that appear, on gross examination, as red and white tissue, respectively (*upper panel*). In chronic idiopathic myelofibrosis, by contrast, cellular marrow is replaced by deposition of collagen and appears uniformly white (*lower panel*).

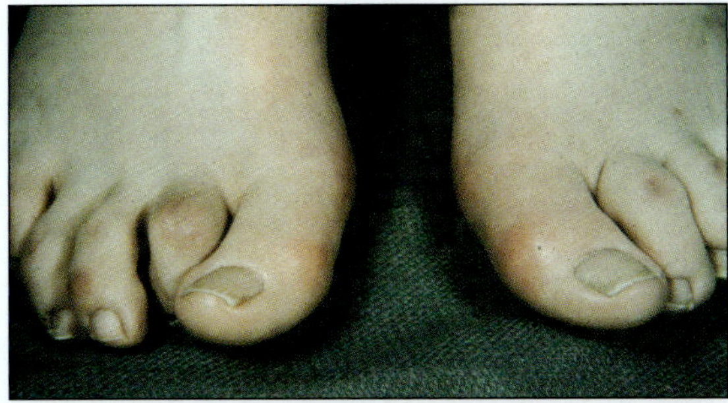
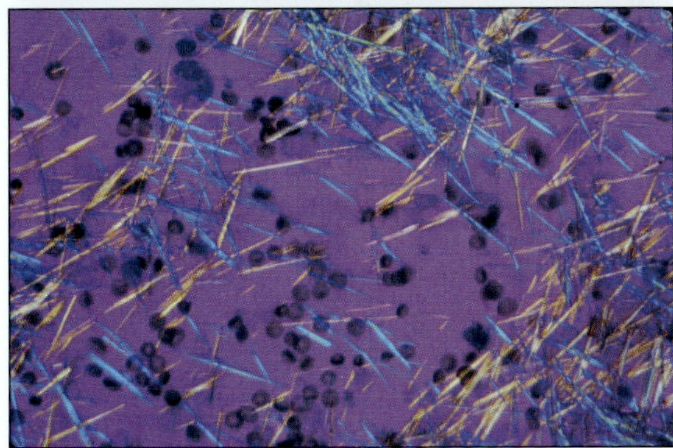

Figure 4.9 Hyperuricemia and gout in myeloproliferative disorders. Hyperuricemia caused by increased nucleic acid synthesis from high cell turnover in myeloproliferative disorders is not uncommon. The top panel shows red, swollen big toes (most marked on left toe) in a CML patient. The bottom panel displays joint fluid aspirated from a patient with gout. Needle-shaped sodium urate crystals are seen under polarized light with a red compensator. The crystals appear yellow (negatively birefringent) and blue in the opposite perpendicular direction of the main axis of the compensator.

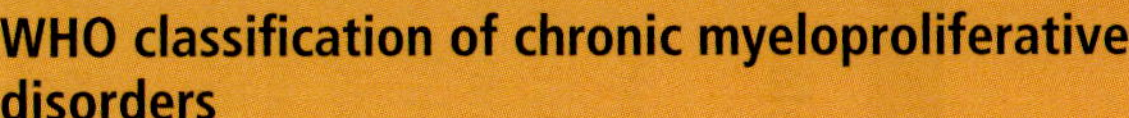

Table 4.1

WHO classification of chronic myeloproliferative disorders

Chronic myeloid leukemia
Polycythemia vera
Essential thrombocythemia
Chronic idiopathic myelofibrosis
Chronic neutrophilic leukemia
Chronic eosinophilic leukemia/hypereosinophilic
  syndrome

Table 4.2

Chronic myeloproliferative disorders: selected clinical, laboratory, morphologic, and cytogenetic/molecular genetic findings

Disease	Molecular Findings	Blood Smear	Bone Marrow	Fibrosis	Splenomegaly	Other
CML	*BCR/ABL*	Leukocytosis with immature granulocytes, basophilia	Marked myeloid hyperplasia with prominence of neutrophils and myelocytes	Variable	++	
PV	*JAK2* *PRV-1*	Normochromic or hypochromic anemia, may have thrombocytosis and mild basophilia	Panmyelosis +/− erythroid hyperplasia, atypical megakaryocytic hyperplasia	Increased in spent phase	++	Low erythropoietin
CIM	*JAK2*	Leukoerythroblastic with dacrocytes, giant and bizarre platelets	Panmyelosis with atypical megakaryocytic hyperplasia, pleomorphic and bizarre megakaryocytes	Increased in fibrotic phase	+++	
ET	*JAK2* *PRV-1*	Thrombocytosis, often with megakaryocytic nuclei	Atypical megakaryocytic hyperplasia with large/giant forms	Minimal	−/+	
CNL	*JAK2*	Leukocytosis > 25,000/μL with neutrophilia	Myeloid hyperplasia	Variable	++	~20% cases associated with underlying neoplasm
CEL/ HES	*PDGFR–* α and β	Eosinophilia > 1,500/μL for 6+ months	Marrow eosinophilia	Variable	+/−	Exclude other causes of eosinophilia

CEL/HES, chronic eosinophilic leukemia/ hypereosinophilic syndrome; CIM, chronic idiopathic myelofibrosis; CML, chronic myelogenous leukemia; CNL, chronic neutrophilic leukemia; ET, essential thrombocythemia; PV, polycythemia vera.

Dysregulated protein kinases appear to underlie the molecular basis of CMPD. CML is defined by evidence of the *BCR/ABL* fusion product, which results in overexpression of the *BCR/ABL* fusion protein encoding a dysregulated tyrosine kinase. Point mutations in *Janus kinase-2* (*JAK2*), a tyrosine kinase responsible for stimulating erythropoiesis, occur in the majority of patients with polycythemia vera and in approximately one-third to one-half of patients with chronic idiopathic myelofibrosis and essential thrombocythemia. A novel fusion tyrosine kinase involving *PDGFR-*α has been detected in a subset of patients with HES. *PRV-1* mRNA expression is increased in the blood of patients with PV and ET, but not in the other CMPDs.

Table 4.3

Symptoms and signs of chronic phase chronic myeloid leukemia (CML) at presentation

	Patients Experiencing Sign or Symptom (%)
Symptoms	
Fatigue	83
Weight loss	61
Abdominal fullness and anorexia	38
Easy bruising or bleeding	35
Abdominal pain	33
Fever	11
Signs	
Splenomegaly	95
Sternal tenderness	78
Lymphadenopathy	64
Hepatomegaly	48
Purpura	27
Retinal hemorrhage	21

Adapted with permission from *Wintrobe's Clinical Hematology*, 11th Edition, page 2237.

Table 4.4

Definitions of accelerated-phase (AP) or blastic-phase (BP) chronic myeloid leukemia

Symptoms of AP	Signs and Laboratory Features of AP
Fever	Increasing peripheral basophilia to >20%
Night sweats	Peripheral blood blasts >10%
Weight loss	—
Refractory splenomegaly	Marrow blasts >10%
Bone pain	Cytogenetic clonal evolution
	Difficult to control white blood cells with antiproliferative treatment
	Marrow reticulin or collagen fibrosis
	Thrombocytopenia (<100,000/µL) unrelated to treatment

Symptoms of BP	Signs and Laboratory Features of BP
Similar to AP Lymphadenopathy	Peripheral blood blasts >20%
	Marrow blasts >20%
	Clumps of blasts on marrow examination
	Extramedullary blastic chloroma

Adapted with permission from *Wintrobe's Clinical Hematology*, 11th Edition, page 2240.

Table 4.5

Morphologic abnormalities in blood smears of 50 untreated patients with chronic myeloid leukemia

Abnormality	Patients Exhibiting Abnormality (%)
Nucleated erythrocytes	98
Dyserythropoietic (binucleate)	12
Target cells	2
Giant platelets	2
Megakaryocytic nucleoli	24
Binucleate of lobular leukocyte nuclei	
Blasts	2
Promyelocytes	2
Myelocytes	6
Hypogranular leukocytes	
Myelocytes	8
Segmented neutrophils	2
Basophils	12
Eosinophils	4
Cells in mitosis	14
Giant metamyelocytes	24
Pelger-Hüet cells	4
Hypersegmented neutrophils	12
Leukocytes with mixed basophil-eosinophil granules	8

As shown in the following figures, a marked left-shifted leukocytosis with an accompanying basophilia is among the most important peripheral smear findings in CML. Numerous morphologic abnormalities, as described in this table also are observed. The white blood cell counts in CML may range from 20,000 to over 500,000/µL; the higher white blood cell count helps distinguish CML from reactive leukocytoses, atypical CML, and chronic myelomonocytic leukemia. Reprinted with permission from *Wintrobe's Clinical Hematology*, 11th Edition, page 2241.

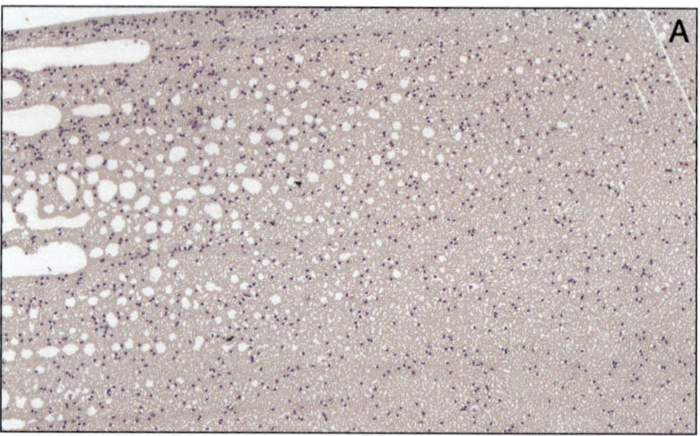

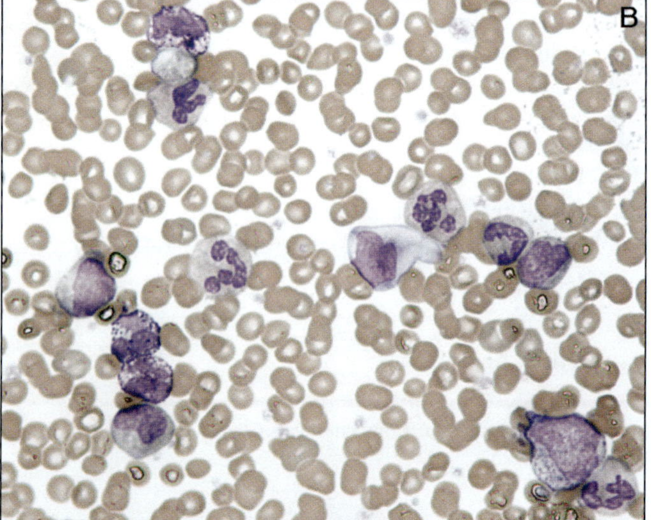

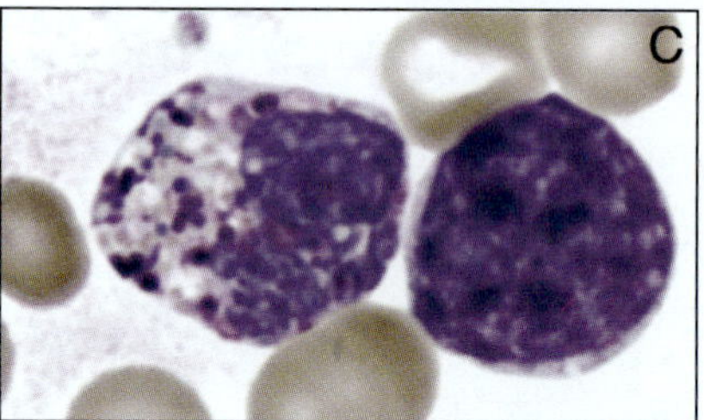

Figure 4.10 CML, chronic phase. **A** and **B**. Peripheral blood smear shows a marked leukocytosis with left-shift and basophilia. **C**. A high-power examination of a basophil at left contrasted with a lymphocyte is shown. To the left of the basophil, a purple haze of granule contents is present.

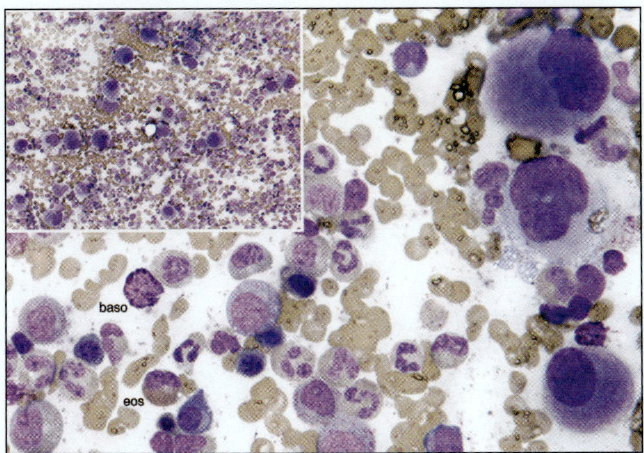

Figure 4.11   CML, chronic phase. The inset shows a low-magnification view of an aspirate smear with the numerous small, mononuclear megakaryocytes and hyperplastic, left-shifted granulocytes. The large image is a high-power view with small megakaryocytes and increased numbers of immature myeloid precursors that include eosinophils and basophils. The bone marrow aspirate in the chronic phase of CML usually contains fewer than 5% blasts, but they may range up to 9%.

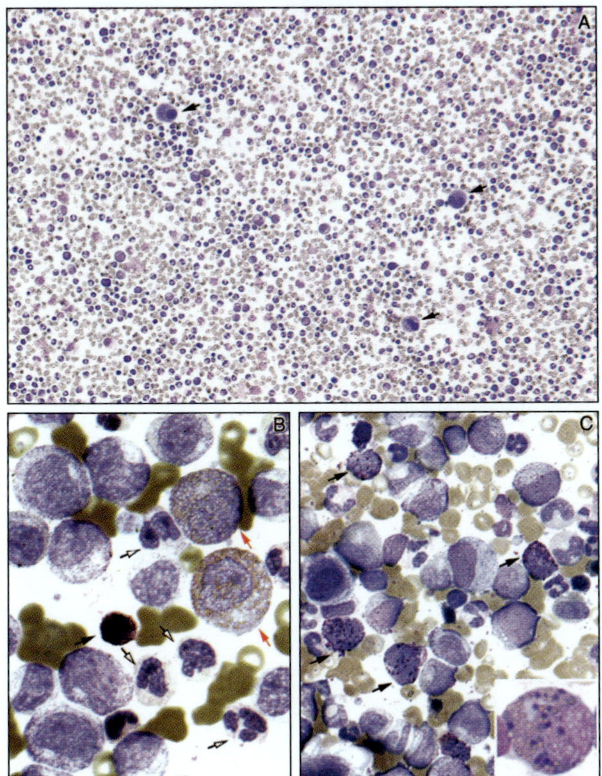

Figure 4.12   CML, chronic phase. **A.** Aspirate smear at low magnification showing the typical small megakaryocytes (*arrows*) and granulocytic hyperplasia seen in CML. **B** and **C.** Basophilia and eosinophilia are characteristic of CML. Basophils, both granulated (*closed black arrows*) and degranulated forms (*open black arrows*) along with eosinophil precursors (*red arrows*) are part of the myeloid hyperplasia in CML. Hybrid cells with mixed eosinophil-basophil granulation (eobasophils) also can be present (*arrows and inset in right lower corner*).

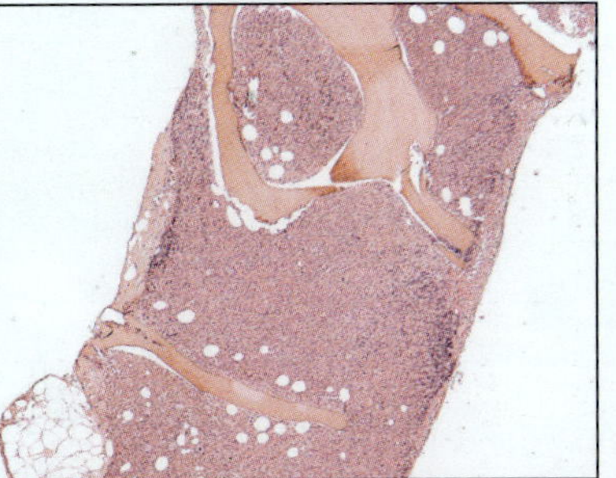

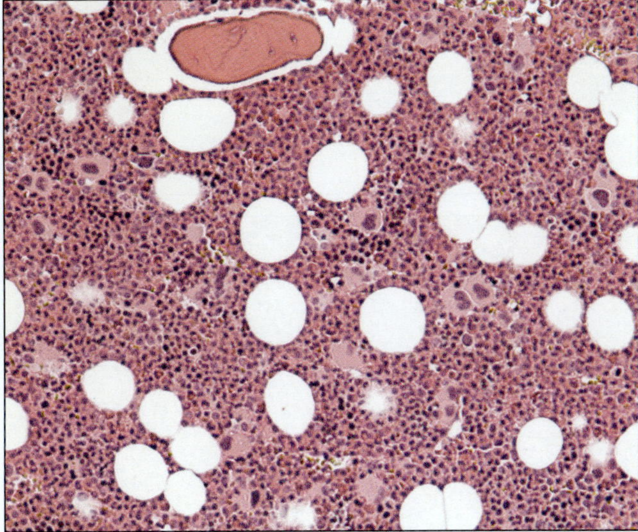

Figure 4.13   CML, chronic phase. A hypercellular marrow with granulocytic hyperplasia and the typical small megakaryocytes of CML.

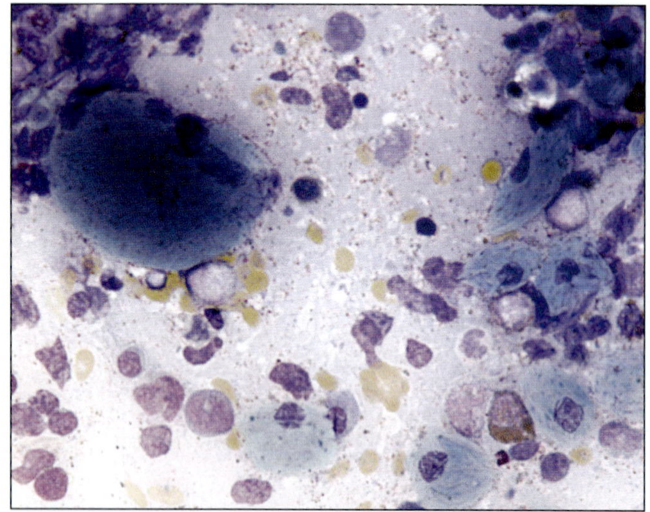

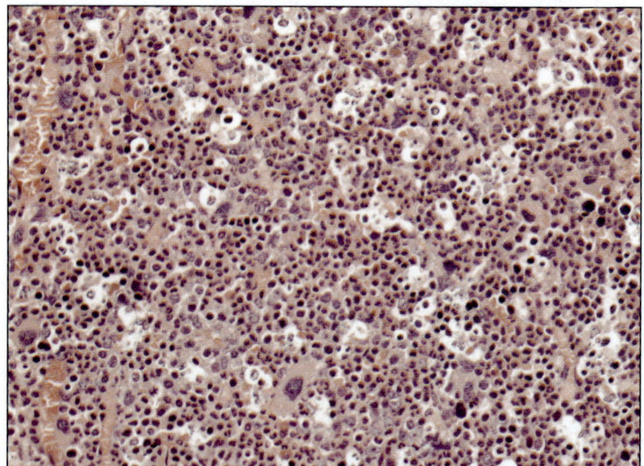

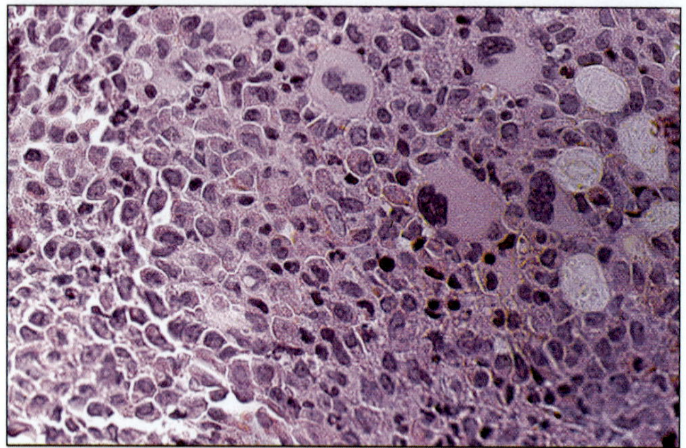

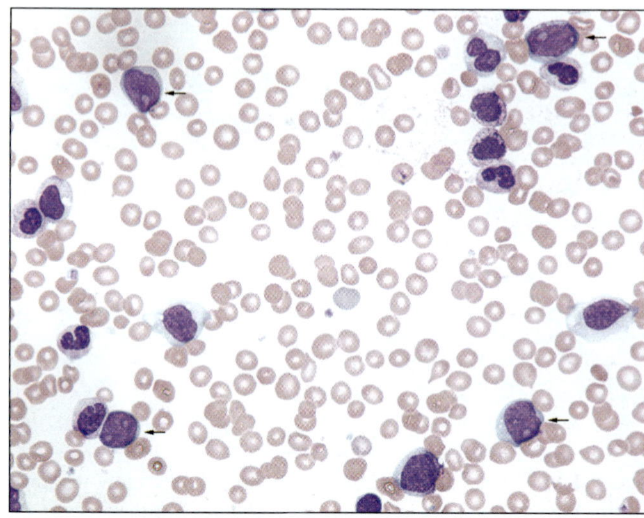

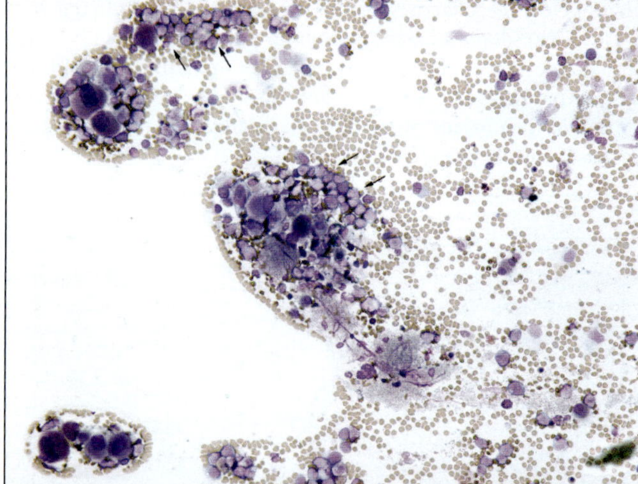

Figure 4.15   CML, blast crisis. Neutrophilia with left-shift and increased numbers of blasts (*arrows*) is illustrated in this blood smear (*top panel*). The bottom panel shows an aspirate smear with increased numbers of small megakaryocytes and clusters of cells made up almost entirely of blasts (*arrows*).

Figure 4.14   CML, chronic phase. Histiocytic response in CML. High cell turnover in rapidly growing neoplasms such as CML is often accompanied by increased phagocytic activity by reactive histiocytes. The top panel shows "sea blue" histiocytes in a CML aspirate smear. The middle panel reveals a "starry sky" pattern from scattered tingible-body macrophages. The bottom panel shows increased numbers of small megakaryocytes in the upper middle portion of panel, with five "pseudo-Gaucher" type histiocytes displayed on the right side.

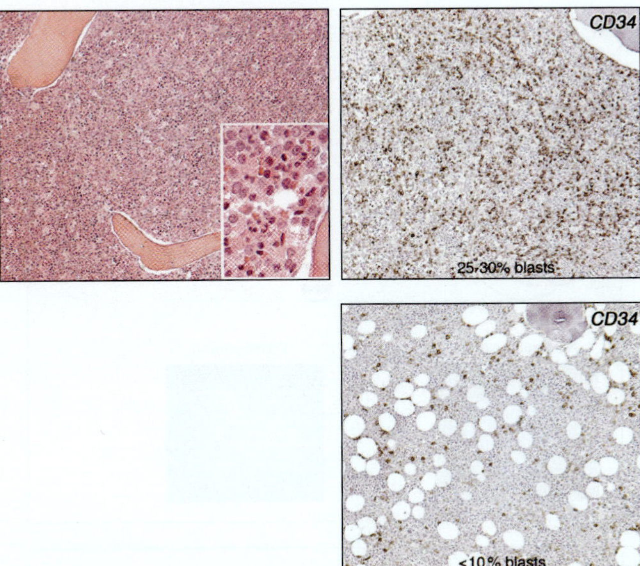

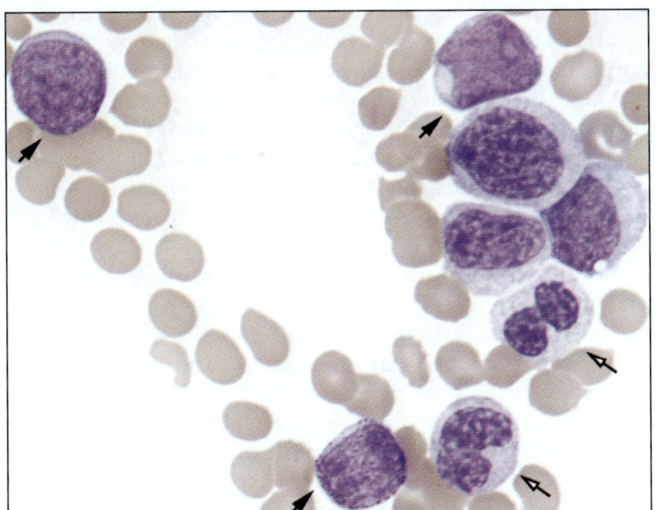

Figure 4.16 CML, blast crisis. *Upper two panels:* A hypercellular biopsy with increased numbers of blasts is shown on the left. By immunohistochemistry, approximately 25% to 30% of the bone marrow cells are CD34$^+$ blasts (*top right panel*). Blast phase or blast crisis in CML is defined by 20% or more blasts in the peripheral blood or bone marrow. Large numbers of blasts on the bone marrow biopsy, as shown here, also are sufficient for a diagnosis of blast phase. Similarly, the development of nonsplenic, extramedullary myeloid tumors is usually sufficient for blast phase according to WHO criteria. The bottom panel, from a case of CML in chronic phase, shows <10% CD34$^+$ marrow blasts.

Figure 4.17 CML, myeloid blast phase. A high-power field from an aspirate smear illustrating increased numbers of large blasts (*closed arrows*) with abundant granular cytoplasm, "open" chromatin pattern, and inconspicuous nucleoli. Dysplastic mature granulocytes accompany the leukemic blasts (*open arrows*).

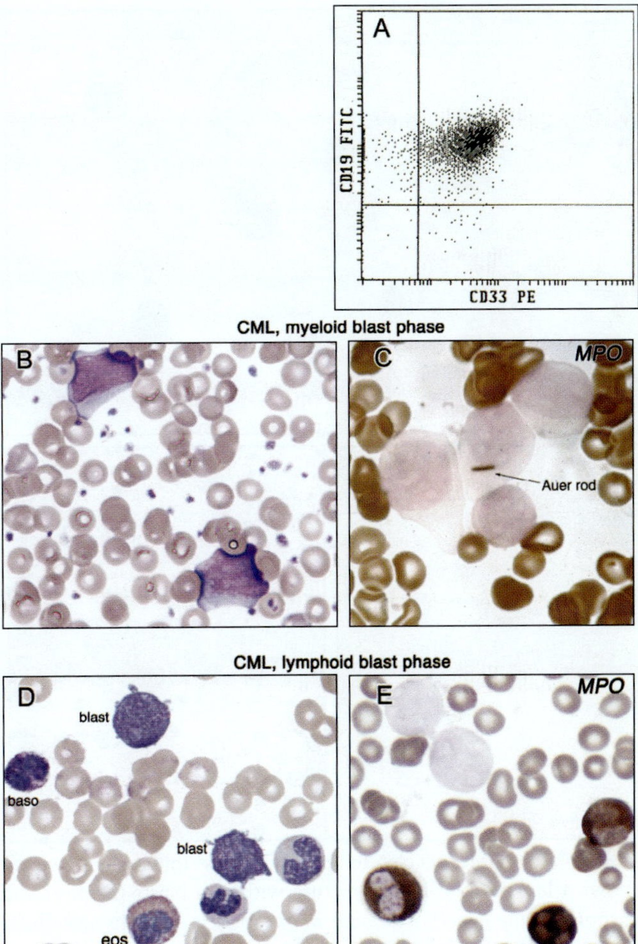

Figure 4.18 A–C. CML, myeloid blast phase. A. Flow cytometric scattergram displaying leukemic myeloid blasts coexpressing both myeloid (CD33) and B-cell (CD19) markers from a case of AML complicating CML. B and C. Blood smear showing blasts and increased platelets and myeloperoxidase (MPO) stains (C) highlight an Auer rod in one of the myeloid blasts.

D. and E. CML, lymphoid blast phase. Left-shifted neutrophilia, eosinophilia, basophilia, and increased blasts are shown in this blood smear from CML in lymphoid blast crisis (D). MPO stain demonstrates the lack of expression of MPO in the two lymphoid blasts in the upper left corner. E. The three darkly stained neutrophils near the bottom of the slide serve as an internal positive control. Lymphoid blast crisis has traditionally been defined as a blast cell proliferation that is TdT positive, but more detailed immunophenotyping shows expression of other precursor B-cell markers such as CD19 and CD10; weak coexpression of myeloid-associated antigens such as CD13 and CD33 also is common.

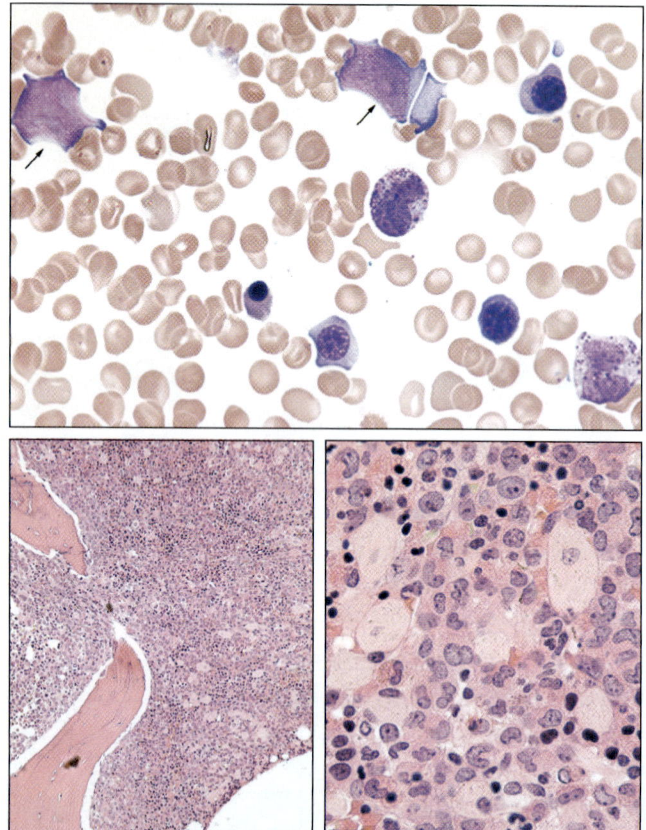

Figure 4.19 CML, accelerated phase. This peripheral blood smear shows a leukoerythroblastic picture with two blasts (*arrows*) and basophilia (*top panel*). The bottom two panels show hypercellular biopsies with granulocytic hyperplasia and scattered Gaucher-type histiocytes.

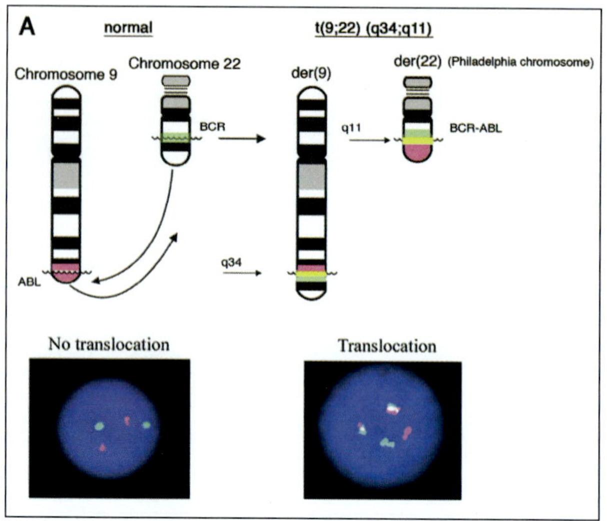

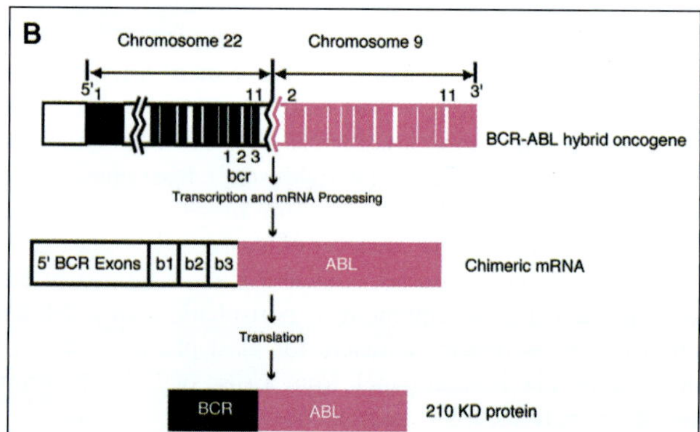

Figure 4.20 CML, chromosomal translocation results in formation of BCR-ABL fusion protein. **A.** FISH for *BCR/ABL*. CML is defined by the presence of the Philadelphia chromosome, the derivative chromosome 22 containing *BCR-ABL* that results from the reciprocal translocation of the *breakpoint cluster region gene (BCR)* from chromosome 22 with the *Abelson gene (ABL)* from chromosome 9, or molecular genetic evidence of the *BCR/ABL* fusion product. FISH analysis may be performed on interphase cells or metaphase spreads, blood or marrow. A probe directed at the *ABL* gene is labeled with a "red" fluorophore, whereas a probe directed at the *BCR* gene is labeled with a "green" fluorophore. After denaturation of DNA, both probes are added to the patient's cells and allowed to hybridize. Detection of two yellow signals resulting from the presence of the *BCR-ABL* fusion gene and reciprocal translocation indicates the presence of *BCR-ABL*, the t(9;22) (q34;q11.2) translocation. If two red and two green signals are detected, no translocation has occurred at *ABL* or *BCR*, and there is no evidence of CML. (Courtesy Cytogenetics Laboratory, Stanford Medical Center, Stanford, CA.) **B.** Chromosomal translocation between chromosomes 9 and 22, leads to juxtaposition of sequences from BCR and ABL (detected by cytogenetics or FISH) to form a chimeric 210-kiloDalton size mRNA (p210 transcript detected and measured by RTPCR) that is transcribed into the oncogenic fusion protein, BCR-ABL. In contrast to the t(9;22) of acute leukemias, which usually show the p190 *BCR/ABL* fusion protein, CML almost exclusively shows the p210 fusion product of this translocation. This reflects the breakpoint within the major breakpoint cluster region of the *BCR* gene, typically between exons b2 and b3, or, as shown here, between exons b3 and b4.

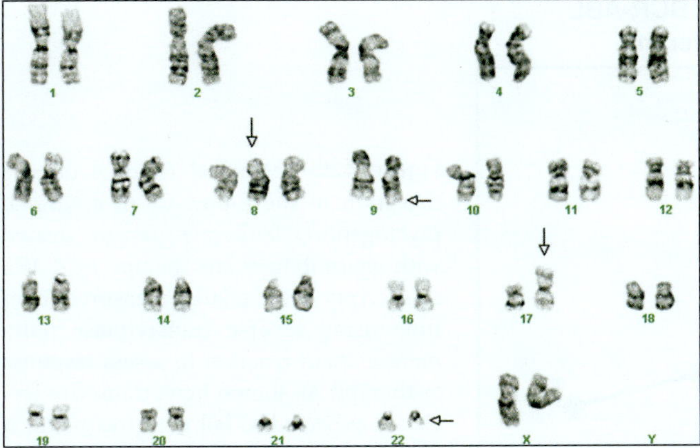

Figure 4.21   CML, karyotype. This karyotype from a patient with CML demonstrates clonal evolution, which may be present at the time of transformation to either the accelerated phase or the blast phase. Clonal evolution in this patient shows trisomy 8 and isochromosome 17q, in addition to the presence of the Philadelphia chromosome, t(9;22)(q34;q11). An extra Philadelphia chromosome also may be seen in clonal evolution in CML. (Courtesy Cytogenetics Laboratory, Stanford Medical Center, Stanford, CA.)

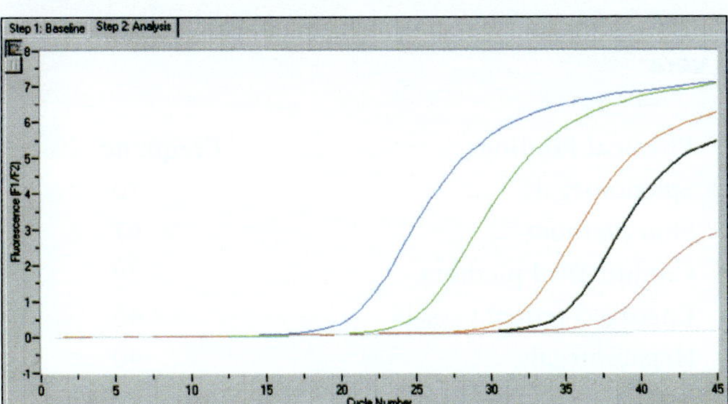

Figure 4.22   Quantitative reverse transcriptase-polymerase chain reaction (QRTPCR) for measuring *BCR/ABL* transcripts. Precise quantitation of transcript levels is done by real-time/reverse transcriptase PCR of peripheral blood or bone marrow samples, commonly utilizing a TaqMan-based assay. In the illustration, known standard transcripts are run in parallel with the patient sample. The Ct (threshold cycle) at which the amplified products are detectable depends on the number of transcripts present in the specimen and is calculated from the inflection points. The Ct of different transcript levels is used to plot a standard curve. The *BCR/ABL* transcript level of the patient sample is back-calculated from the standard curve. (Courtesy Molecular Pathology Laboratory, Stanford Medical Center, Stanford, CA.)

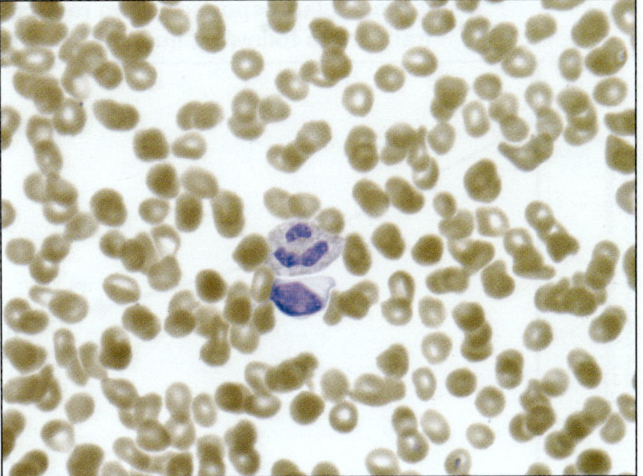

Figure 4.23   CML, peripheral blood smear after imatinib mesylate. Imatinib mesylate is a tyrosine kinase inhibitor that directly blocks the effects of the *BCR/ABL* fusion protein and has been used in all phases of CML. The peripheral blood responds first to imatinib mesylate therapy with a normalization of the white blood cell and platelet counts, a decrease in basophils, and normal-appearing platelets occurring after approximately 2 months of therapy. The hemoglobin levels tend to decrease slightly during therapy. A subset of patients may develop cytopenias, as did this patient.

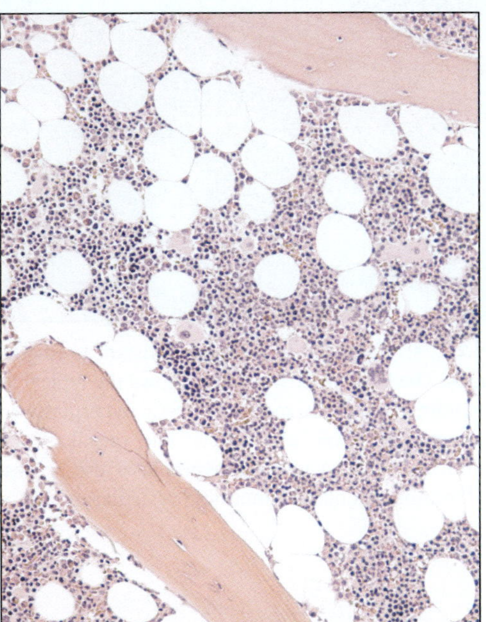

Figure 4.24   CML, biopsy after imatinib mesylate. After imatinib mesylate therapy, the bone marrow hypercellularity gradually decreases and, by 8 to 11 months, the marrow is normocellular or even hypocellular, with a normal or decreased myeloid-to-erythroid ratio. Bone marrow blasts and megakaryocytes decrease, and the number of hypolobated megakaryocytes diminishes, as does megakaryocyte clustering. Marrow fibrosis has even reversed in some patients. Here a bone marrow biopsy after approximately 1 year of imatinib mesylate therapy is normocellular with a slightly decreased myeloid-to-erythroid ratio.

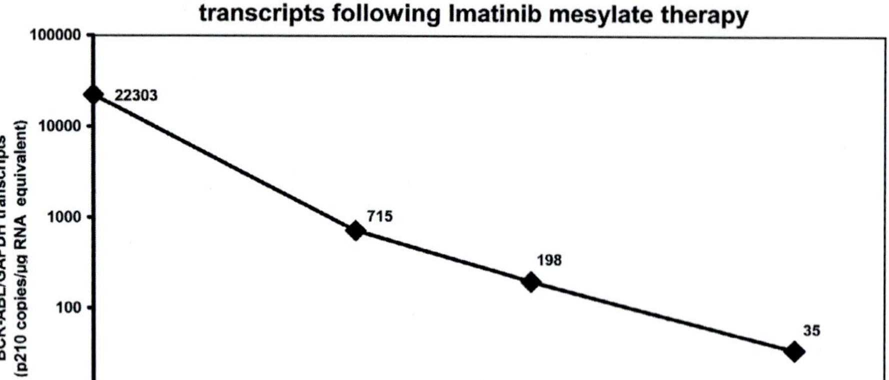

Figure 4.25 Minimal residual disease detection in the follow-up of a chronic myelogenous leukemia patient treated with imatinib mesylate therapy. *BCR/ABL* transcripts are serially measured over time using reverse transcriptase polymerase chain reaction to assess response to therapy. As shown here, transcript levels are expected to fall with treatment. A major molecular response occurs when the transcript levels decrease to greater than three log levels within 1 year, as seen in this patient. (Courtesy Molecular Pathology Laboratory, Stanford Medical Center, Stanford, CA.)

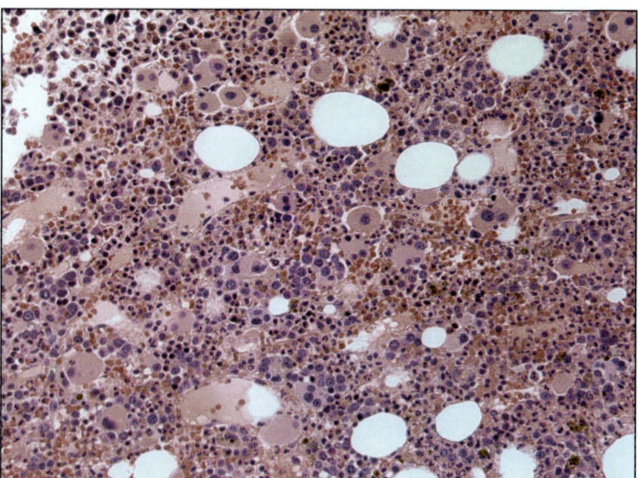

Figure 4.26 CML biopsy in a patient resistant to imatinib mesylate therapy. The bone marrow biopsy shows the typical features of CML, including an atypical megakaryocytic hyperplasia with dwarf forms possessing hypolobated nuclei and megakaryocytes with separate nuclear lobes. A myeloid hyperplasia also is present, with increased numbers of blasts containing vesicular nuclei.

Table 4.6

Physical findings and symptoms in polycythemia vera

Physical Findings	Frequency (%)
Splenomegaly	70
Skin plethora	67
Conjunctival plethora	59
Engorged retinal vessels	46
Hepatomegaly	40
Systolic blood pressure >140 mm Hg	72
Diastolic blood pressure >90 mm Hg	32
Symptoms	
Headache	48
Weakness	47
Pruritus	43
Dizziness	43
Diaphoresis	33
Visual disturbances	31
Weight loss	29
Paresthesias	29
Dyspnea	26
Joint symptoms	26
Epigastric discomfort	24

Data used with permission from Berlin NI. Diagnosis and classification of the polycythemias. *Semin Haematol* 1975;12:339–351.
Adapted with permission from *Wintrobe's Clinical Hematology*, 11th Edition, page 2260.

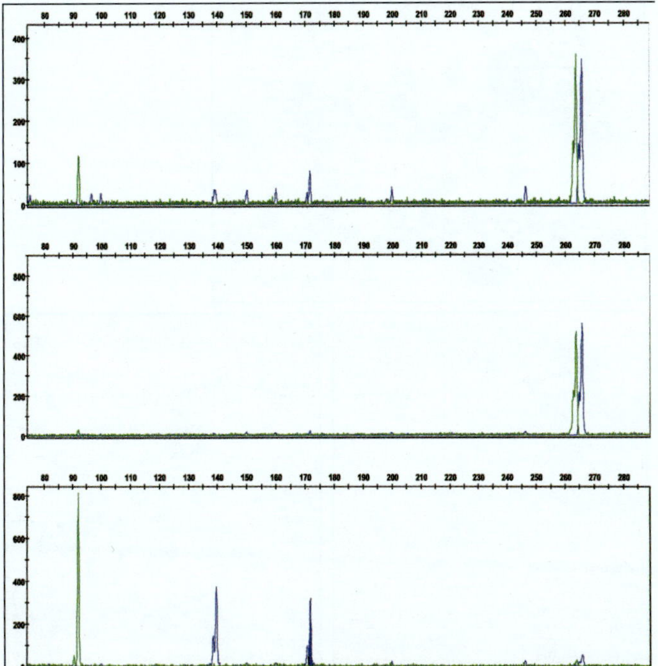

Figure 4.27 Detection of *JAK2* V617F mutation by PCR, digestion by restriction endonuclease and gel electrophoresis. JAK2 is a cytoplasmic protein kinase commonly mutated in myeloproliferative syndromes, particularily Polycythemia vera (PV). The *JAK2* mutation site is resistant to digestion by restriction endonuclease BsaXI. A 267-bp fragment that spans the mutation/restriction endonuclease (RE) site is amplified by PCR, digested with BsaXI, and separated by electrophoresis into different fragment sizes. In the case of a homozygous patient, RE digestion with BsaXI results in a 267-bp fragment that was resistant to digestion (*middle panel*). A wild-type patient shows RE digestion resulting in two products that are 140-bp and 97-bp in size. Incomplete digestion is indicated by the presence of a larger fragment of 170 bp. All three fragments are shown in the lower panel. The upper panel demonstrates a heterozygous state, where the mutant allele is resistant to digestion (267-bp peak) and the wild-type allele is digested by RE, resulting in smaller fragments similar to the lower panel. (Courtesy Molecular Pathology Laboratory, Stanford Medical Center, Stanford, CA.)

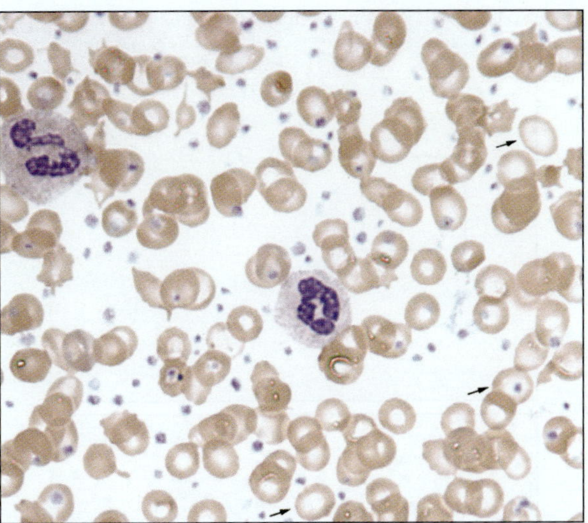

Figure 4.28 Polycythemia vera (PV). This blood smear demonstrates hypochromic microcytes (*arrows*), a feature of the iron deficiency commonly associated with PV. Absent stainable iron on marrow examination is typical. The red blood cell mass may be decreased in PV patients with concurrent iron deficiency; laboratory studies may need to be repeated following iron therapy. This 41-year-old man had splenomegaly with a white blood cell count of 29,000/μL, hemoglobin 19 g/dL, MCV 77 fl, and a platelet count of 804,000/μL. The proliferative or erythrocytotic phase typically has elevations of red blood cells, white blood cells, and platelets. White cells may be left-shifted and show a slight basophilia, but basophils are not typically as numerous as in CML. Platelet counts can exceed 600,000/μL, which may cause confusion with essential thrombocythemia.

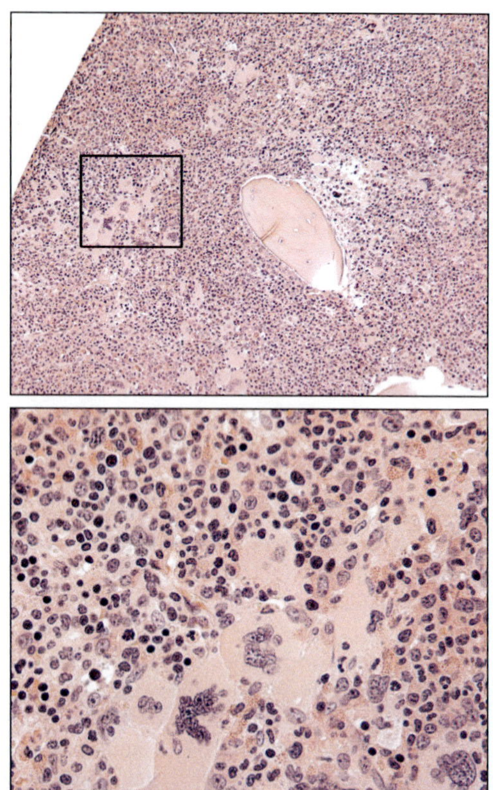

Figure 4.29 PV, proliferative phase. The bone marrow biopsy is hypercellular with trilineage hematopoiesis and loose clusters of pleomorphic megakaryocytes. Such atypical megakaryocytic hyperplasia of PV is not present in secondary polycythemias, and marrow fibrosis is typically minimal in this stage of the disease.

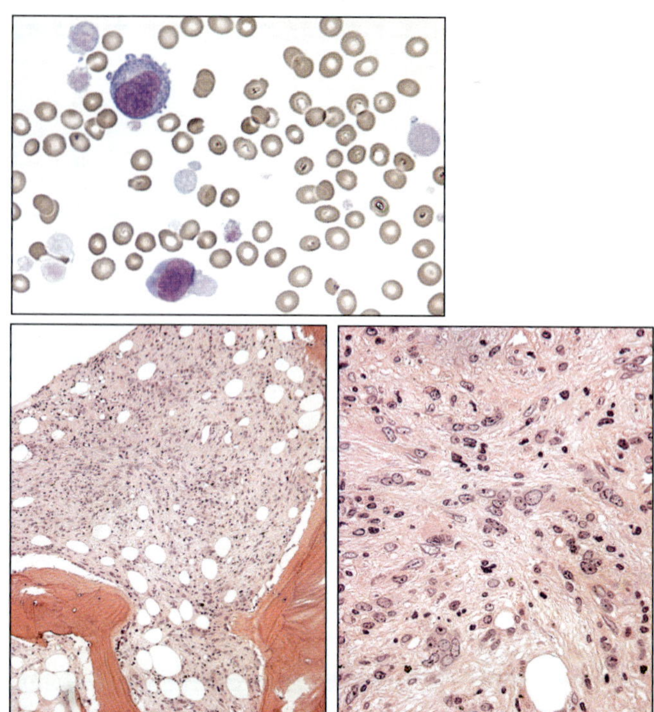

Figure 4.31 PV, transformation to AML. The *upper panel* is a blood smear from a patient with a long history of PV that shows increased blasts and numerous bizarre, giant platelets. Two large blasts dominate the field, with cytoplasmic blebbing reminiscent of platelet production by megakaryocytes. Positive expression of CD41 and CD61 confirmed megakaryocytic lineage of these blasts. Marrow replacement by a pleomorphic population of blasts associated with dense sclerosis is seen in the biopsy (*bottom panels*). Approximately 10% to 20% of PV patients will eventually transform to acute myeloid leukemia within 15 years of diagnosis.

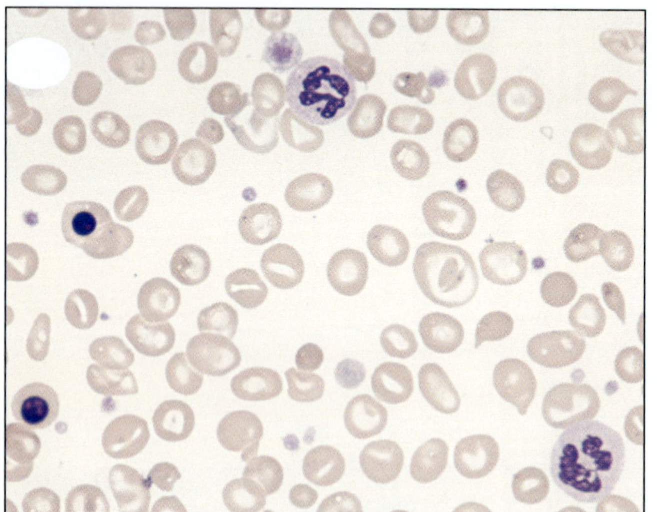

Figure 4.30 PV, post-polycythemic phase. The spent phase of PV is associated with marrow fibrosis and shows peripheral blood and bone marrow changes similar to or identical with changes seen in chronic idiopathic myelofibrosis, including a leukoerythroblastic smear with frequent dacrocytes and giant and bizarre platelets. This blood smear shows a leukoerythroblastic picture with dacrocytes and giant platelets. Differentiation between spent-phase PV and idiopathic myelofibrosis may not be possible without a history of PV. The spent phase will typically follow 10 to 15 years of the proliferative phase of the disease. Once in the post-polycythemic phase of the disease, median survival is a few years. Cases of myelodysplastic transformation are reported in the literature, which are favored to be therapy-related.

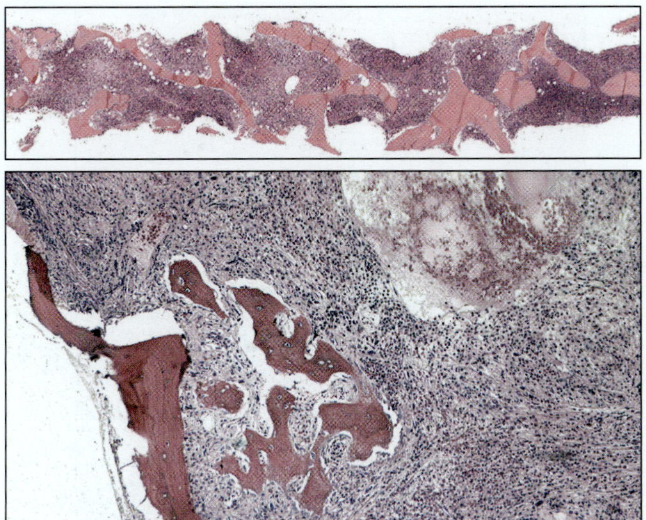

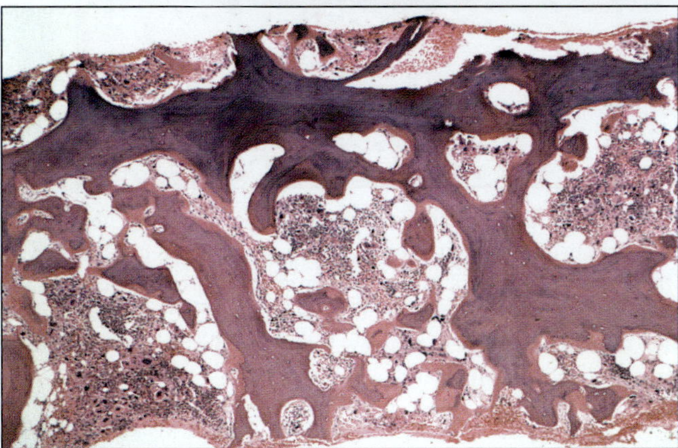

Figure 4.32 PV, post-polycythemic phase. The marked marrow fibrosis seen in this bone marrow biopsy from a patient with spent-phase PV manifests itself as a lining up of cells with a "streaming" quality on hematoxylin and eosin (H&E) stain. Reticulin and collagen stains can confirm the presence of fibrosis. Bone marrow aspirates at this stage of disease are typically "dry taps" yielding only blood. In this biopsy, a very large dilated sinus occupies the top right field (*middle panel*), while a focus of bony remodeling appears in the center of the field. Scattered foci of pleomorphic megakaryocytes in clusters were present on higher power.

Table 4.7

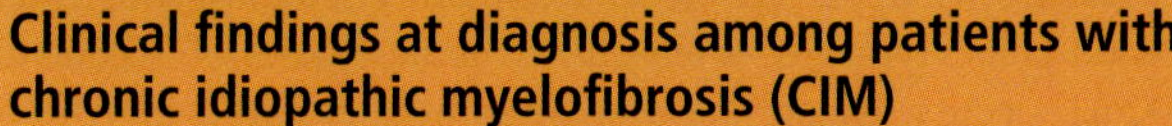

Causes of death in polycythemia vera patients

Cause of Death	PVSG (%)	GISP (%)
Thrombosis/ thromboembolism	31	29.7
Acute myeloid leukemia	19	14.6
Other malignancy	15	15.5
Hemorrhage	6	2.6
Myelofibrosis/ myeloid metaplasia	4	2.6
Other	25	35.0

GISP, Gruppo Italiano Studio Policitemia; PVSG, Polychthemia Vera Study Group.
Reprinted with permission from *Wintrobe's Clinical Hematology*, 11th Edition, page 2267.

Table 4.8

Clinical findings at diagnosis among patients with chronic idiopathic myelofibrosis (CIM)

Very common findings (>50% of cases)

Splenomegaly

Hepatomegaly

Fatigue

Anemia

Leukocytosis

Thrombocytosis

Common findings (10%–50% of cases)

Asymptomatic

Weight loss

Night sweats

Bleeding

Splenic pain

Leukocytopenia

Thrombocytosis

Thrombocytopenia

Uncommon findings (<10% of cases)

Peripheral edema

Portal hypertension

Lymphadenopathy

Jaundice

Gout

Adapted with permission from *Wintrobe's Clinical Hematology*, 11th Edition, page 2275.

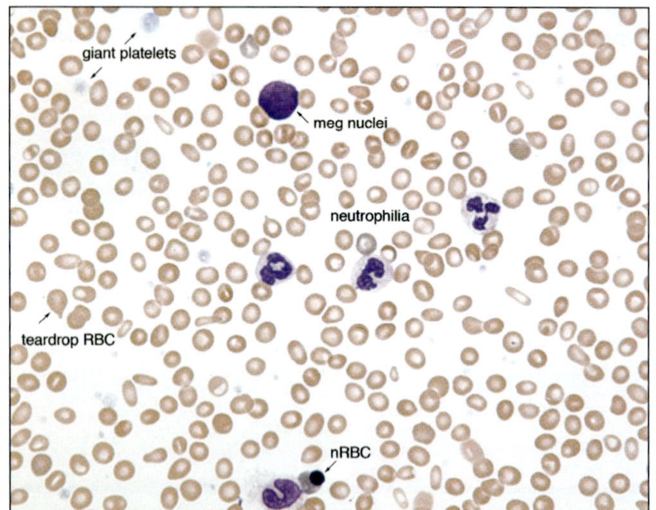

Figure 4.33   Chronic idiopathic myelofibrosis (CIM). This leuko-erythroblastic smear, displaying frequent dacrocytes and thrombocytosis with giant and bizarre platelets, is characteristic of the fibrotic phase of CIM, the phase of disease in which most patients are diagnosed. In this disease, the platelet count is variable, with giant and bizarre forms and sometimes bare megakaryocytes seen. The anemia typically is accompanied by a mild reticulocytosis, frequent teardrop-shaped red blood cells, and circulating nucleated red blood cells. Typically, a left-shifted leukocytosis of 15,000 to 30,000/μL occurs. Basophilia or eosinophilia is found in 10% to 30% of cases.

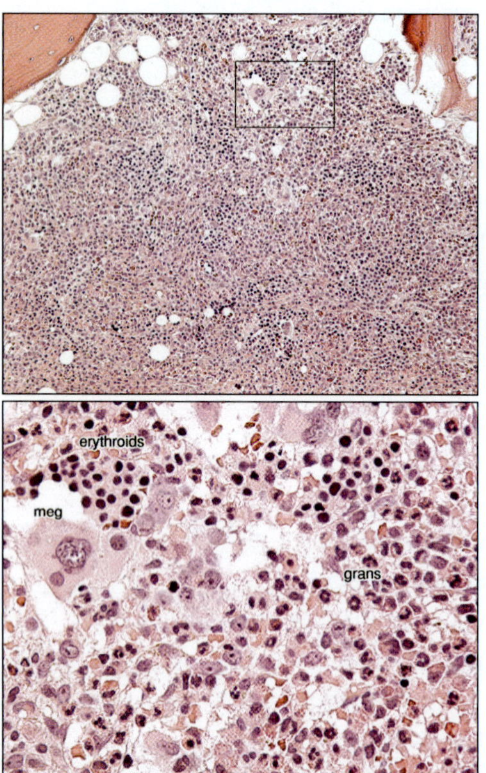

Figure 4.34   CIM, prefibrotic phase. The bone marrow biopsy may show trilineage hyperplasia as shown here, particularly early in the disease when marrow fibrosis is less prominent (the *prefibrotic* phase of CIM).

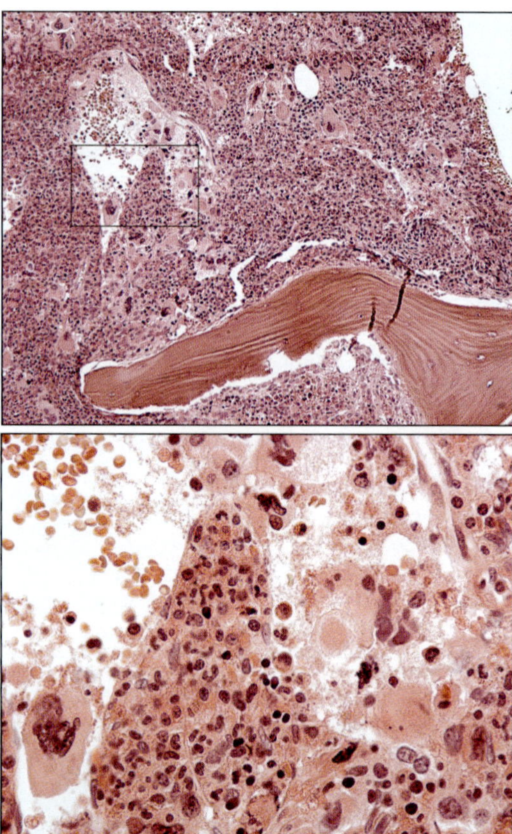

Figure 4.35   CIM, prefibrotic phase. Trilineage hyperplasia with dilated sinusoids and intrasinusoidal hematopoiesis is described in CIM and shown here. Distinguishing the prefibrotic phase of CIM from other CMPDs, especially essential thrombocythemia, can be quite difficult. Serial bone marrow biopsies will show an increase in fibrosis in patients with CIM.

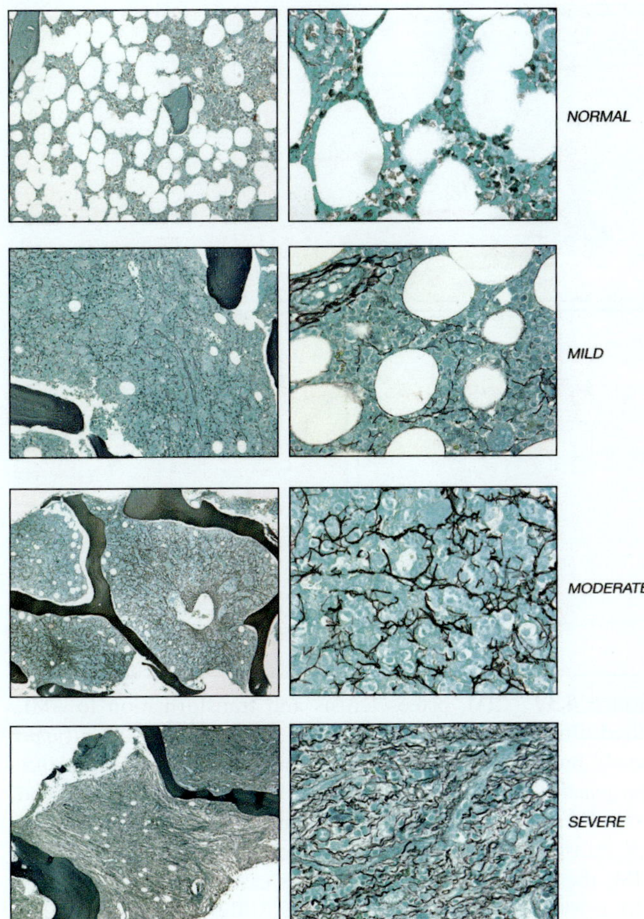

Figure 4.36   CIM, prefibrotic and fibrotic phases.

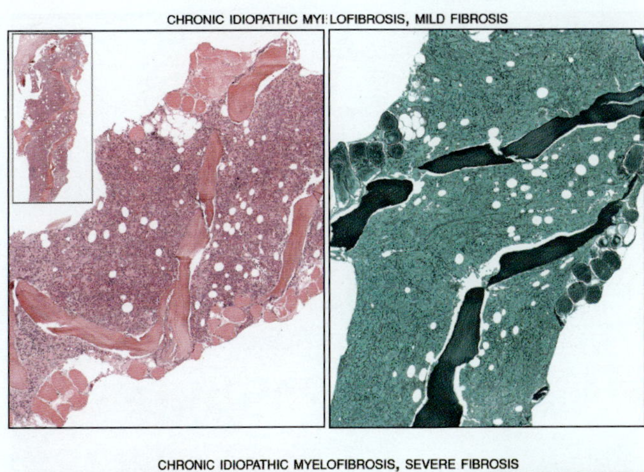

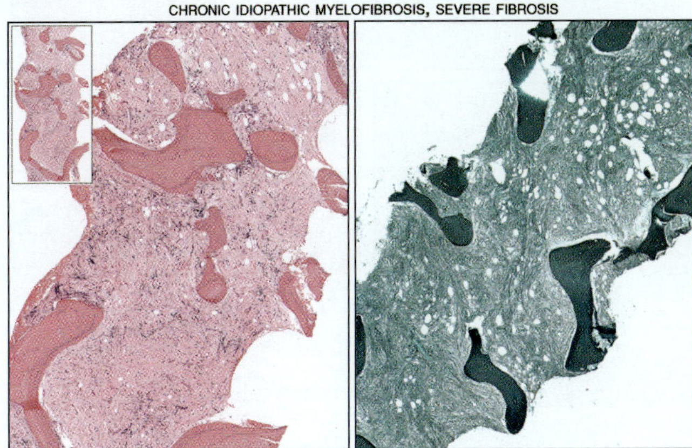

Figure 4.37   CIM, prefibrotic and fibrotic phases.

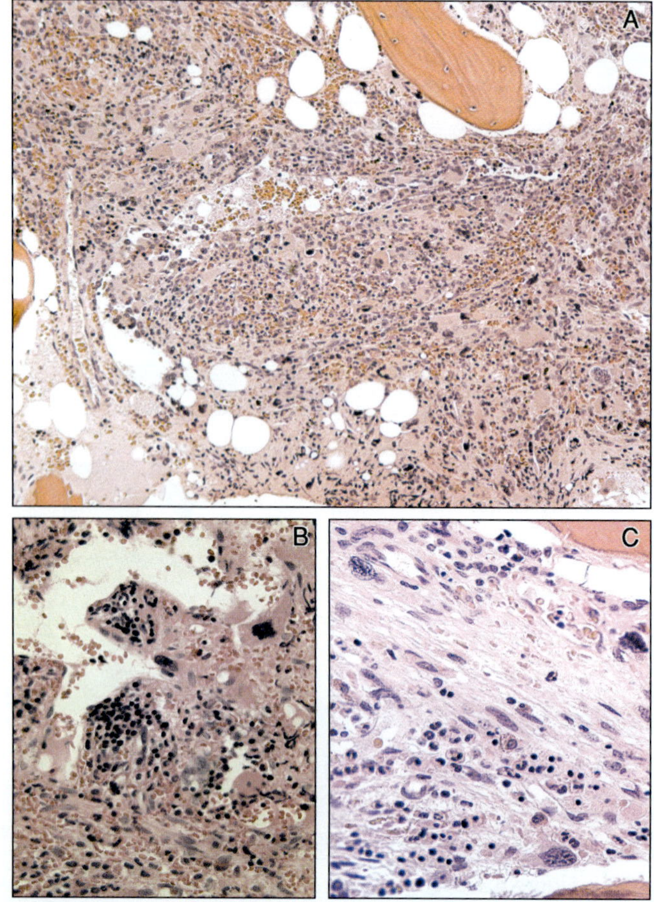

Figure 4.38   CIM, fibrotic phase. Bone marrow biopsies during the fibrotic phase of CIM show a replacement of marrow cellularity by fibrosis. Clonal studies demonstrate that the trilineage hematopoiesis is monoclonal in CIM patients and the fibrosis is reactive. Atypical megakaryocyte clustering is prominent, with collections of medium-sized to giant megakaryocytes, often adjacent to sinuses (as in **B**) and bony trabeculae. Features of architectural distortion, such as the lining up of individual marrow cells, is common. **C**. Megakaryocytes often contain hyperchromatic nuclei with coarse lobulations.

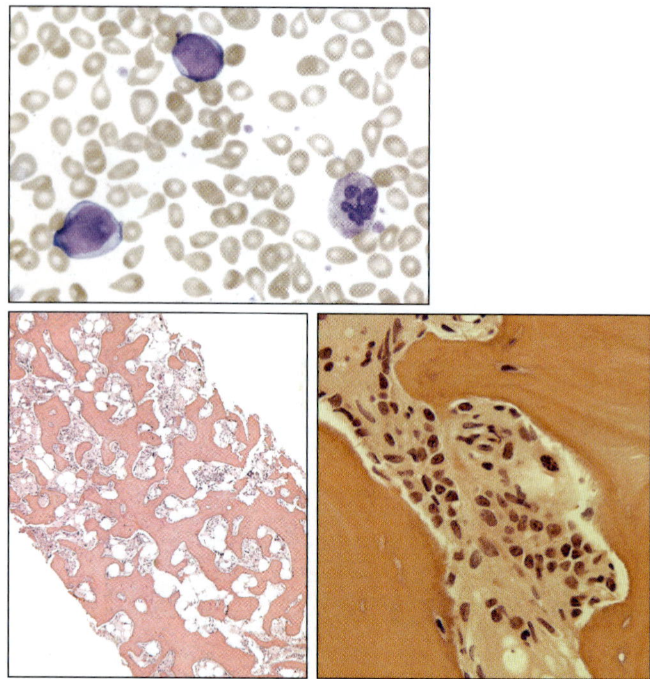

Figure 4.39   CIM, osteosclerosis and transformation to AML. Blood film shows blasts, neutrophilia, and teardrop RBCs (*upper panel*). Biopsies reveal sclerosis of bone trabeculae and blasts (*bottom panels*). Osteosclerosis occurs in late-stage CIM with broad, irregular trabeculae replacing the marrow space. Although stem cell transplant may reverse the marrow fibrosis in patients with CIM, the osteosclerosis remains. This case of longstanding CIM with osteosclerosis was complicated by AML.

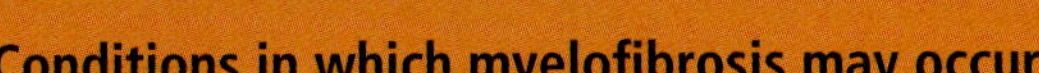

Table 4.9

Conditions in which myelofibrosis may occur

Neoplastic conditions

    Chronic myeloproliferative disorders

        Chronic idiopathic myelofibrosis

        Polycythemia vera

        Chronic myeloid leukemia

    Acute megakaryoblastic leukemia (M7)

    Myelodysplasia with fibrosis

    "Transitional" agnogenic myeloid metaplasia–myelodysplastic myeloproliferative syndrome

    Other acute myeloid leukemias

    Acute lymphoid leukemia

    Hairy-cell leukemia

    Myeloma

    Carcinoma

    Systemic mastocytosis

Non-neoplastic conditions

    Granulomatous disease

    Paget disease

    Hypoparathyroidism

    Hyperparathyroidism

    Osteoporosis

    Renal osteodystrophy

    Vitamin D deficiency

    Gray platelet syndrome

    Systemic lupus erythematosus

    Systemic sclerosis

Adapted with permission from *Wintrobe's Clinical Hematology*, 11th Edition, page 2274.

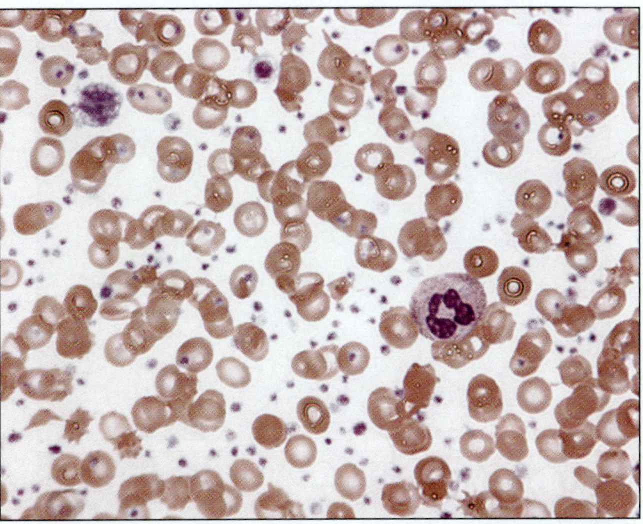

Figure 4.40 Essential thrombocythemia (ET). Peripheral blood findings in ET include a thrombocytosis with large and giant platelets and normal erythrocytes (as shown here). A mild leukocytosis, usually less than 30,000/μL, also may be present, as can circulating megakaryocyte nuclear fragments or even micromegakaryocytes.

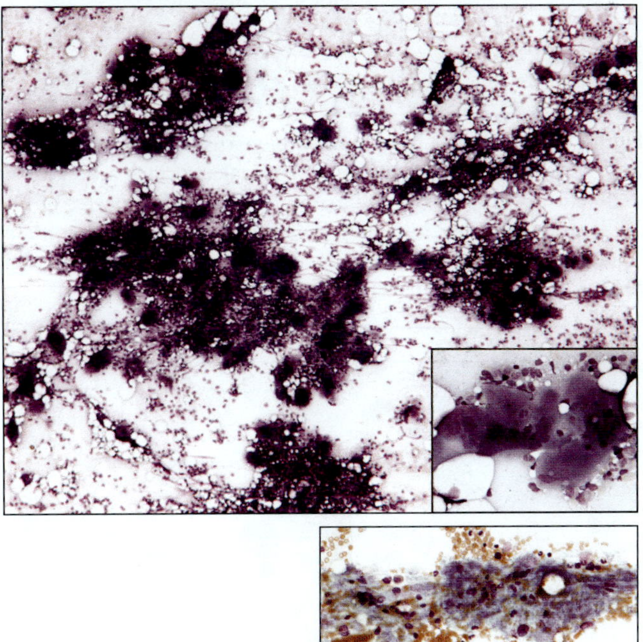

Figure 4.41 ET. Bone marrow aspirate at low power shows numerous large megakaryocytes with multilobulated nuclei and abundant cytoplasm (see *inset*). Clumps of platelets at low power, a common finding in ET, are shown in the lower panel.

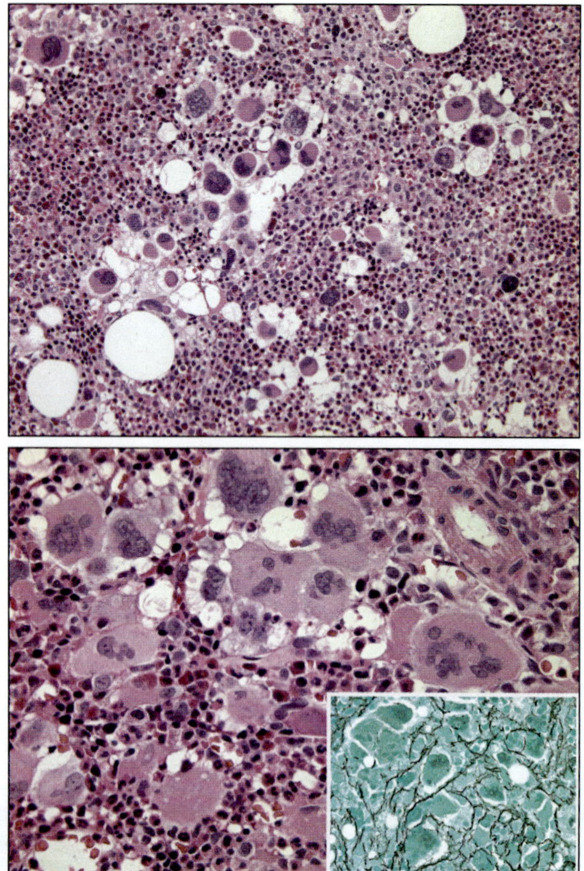

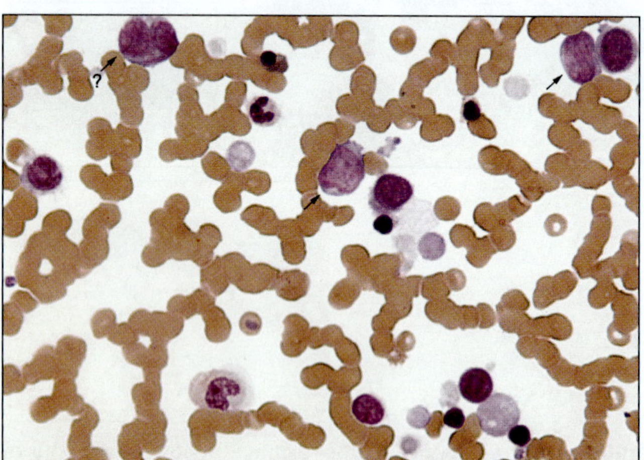

Figure 4.42 ET. The bone marrow biopsy is hypercellular with a marked increase in the numbers of megakaryocytes arranged in loose clusters throughout the marrow. The megakaryocytes of ET are larger than those in reactive conditions or CML and contain "cloud-like" nuclear lobations. A mild increase in thin reticulin fibers is present (*lower panel inset*).

Figure 4.43 ET transformation to acute myeloid leukemia. Two blasts (*arrows*) are shown in a background of marked thrombocytosis. Transformation to acute leukemia occurs in less than 5% of ET patients, although a therapy-related myelodysplastic syndrome and acute myeloid leukemia may occur in patients treated with hydroxyurea.

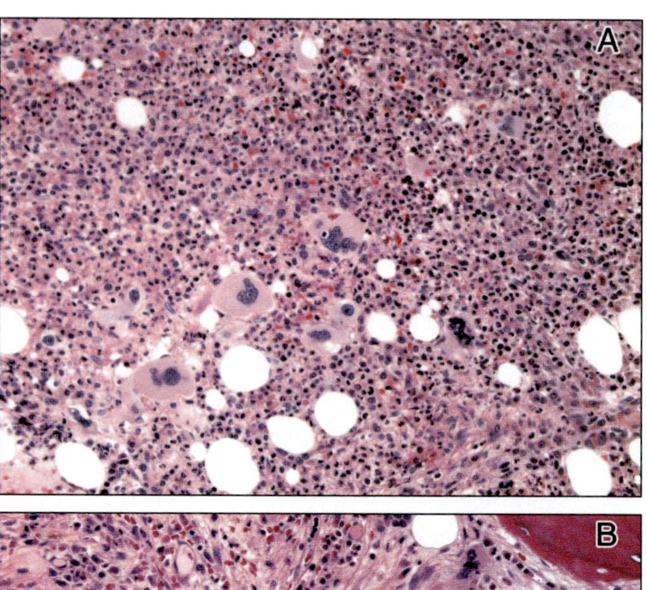

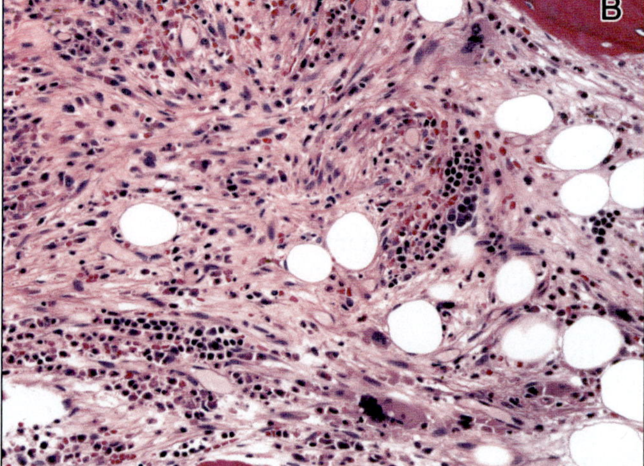

Figure 4.44 Morphologic overlap among myeloproliferative syndromes. This patient was originally diagnosed as ET (**A**), but subsequent bone marrow biopsy showed marked fibrosis and atypical hyperchromatic megakaryocytes characteristic of the fibrotic phase of CIM (**B**). Considerable morphologic overlap occurs between ET and the prefibrotic form of CIM. Sequential bone marrow biopsy specimens may allow for classification in difficult cases. Reticulin fibrosis is minimal in bone marrow biopsies of ET patients.

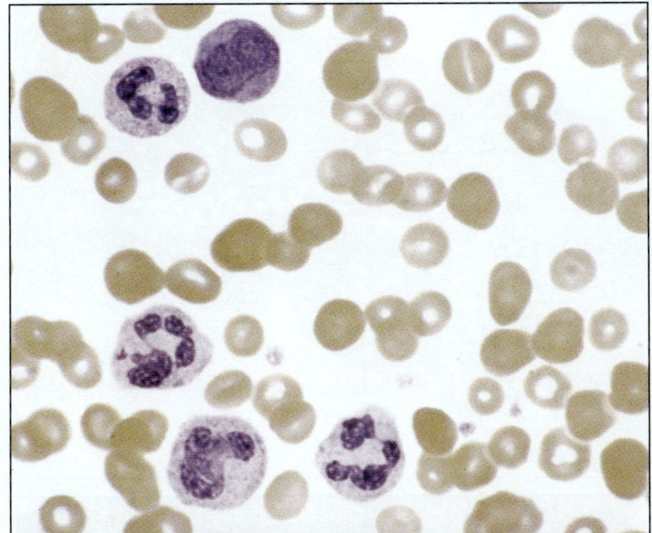

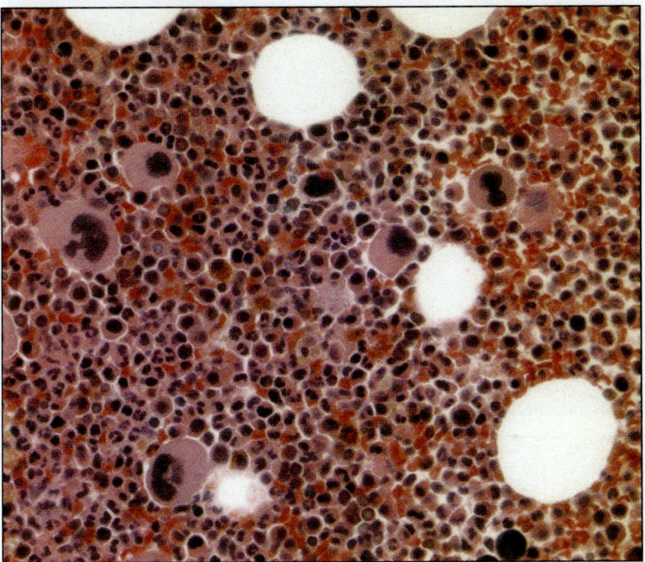

Figure 4.45 Chronic neutrophilic leukemia (CNL). Peripheral blood findings of CNL include a neutrophilia, usually with <5% immature granulocytes. Neutrophils may display toxic granulation or appear unremarkable. A bone marrow biopsy discloses a myeloid hyperplasia with no increase in blasts (*bottom panel*).

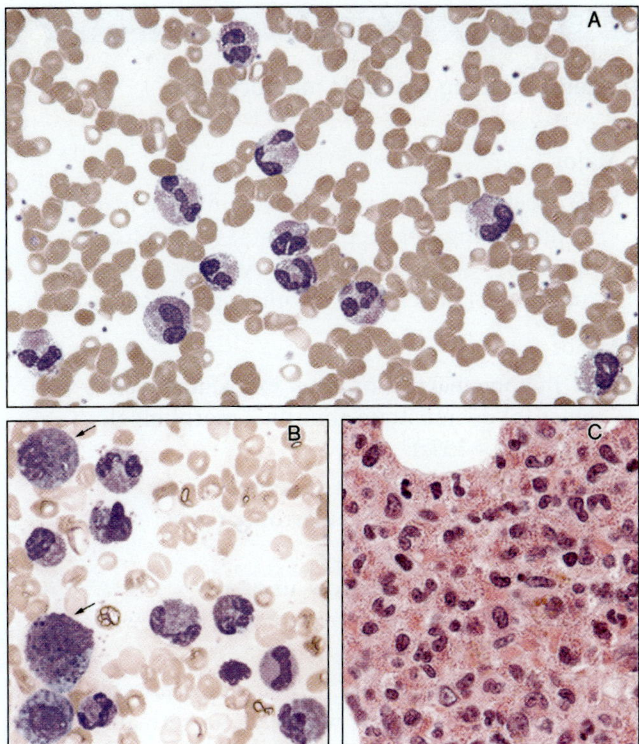

Figure 4.46 Chronic eosinophilic leukemia (CEL) and hypereosinophilic leukemia (HES). **A.** Peripheral blood smear shows chronic eosinophilic leukemia with normal or slightly atypical-appearing eosinophils. **B.** Aspirate smear reveals increased eosinophils and "eosinobasophils" (*arrows*). **C.** The biopsy shows sheets of eosinophils replacing marrow cavity. This case, as often seen in hypereosinophilic syndromes, was difficult to classify because no evidence existed for parasitic, allergic, or other known causes of eosinophilia and marrow cytogenetics were negative. CEL is usually distinguished from HES by the presence of increased blood (>2%) or marrow (5%–19%) blasts, or the presence of a clonal cytogenetic abnormality.

Table 4.10

Criteria defining systemic mastocytosis

Major

Multifocal dense infiltrates of MCs in bone marrow or other extracutaneous organ(s) (>15 MCs in aggregate) and confirmed by tryptase immunohistochemistry or other special stains

Minor

MCs in bone marrow or other extracutaneous organ(s) demonstrate abnormal morphologic features (>25%)

Detection of Kit mutation at codon 816 in peripheral blood, bone marrow, or other extracutaneous organs

MCs in blood, bone marrow, or other extracutaneous organs coexpress CD117 with CD2 or CD25

Serum total tryptase >20 ng/mL (not applicable in patients with systemic mastocytosis with an associated clonal hematologic nonmast cell lineage disease)

MCs, mast cells.
Note: The diagnosis of systemic mastocytosis is established if at least one major and one minor or at least three minor criteria are fulfilled. Reprinted with permission from *Wintrobe's Clinical Hematology*, 11th Edition, page 2288.

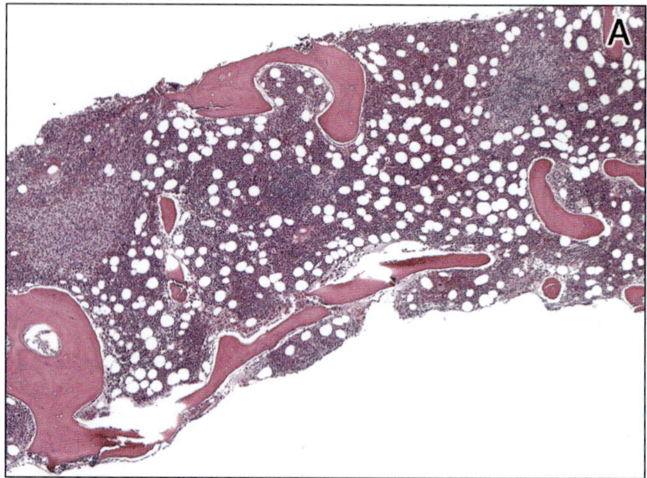

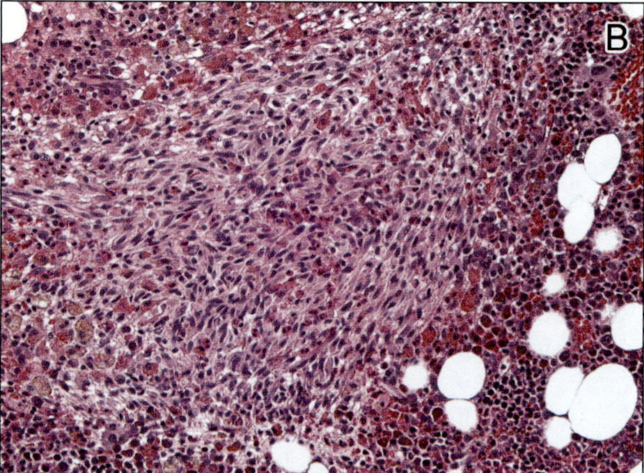

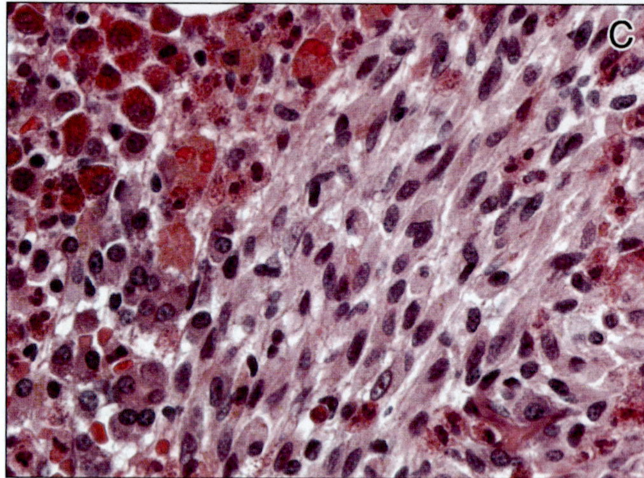

Figure 4.47 Systemic mastocytosis with eosinophilia and t(5;12). **A.** This low-power view of bone marrow biopsy shows a hypercellular marrow studded with pale and darkly staining nodules. **B.** On closer examination, the pale-staining nodule consists of mast cells admixed with numerous eosinophils. **C.** Most mast cells are spindled in appearance with abundant pink cytoplasm and elongated oval nuclei. Granules are not readily apparent in this preparation. A rim of eosinophils and scattered plasma cells encircle the nodule.

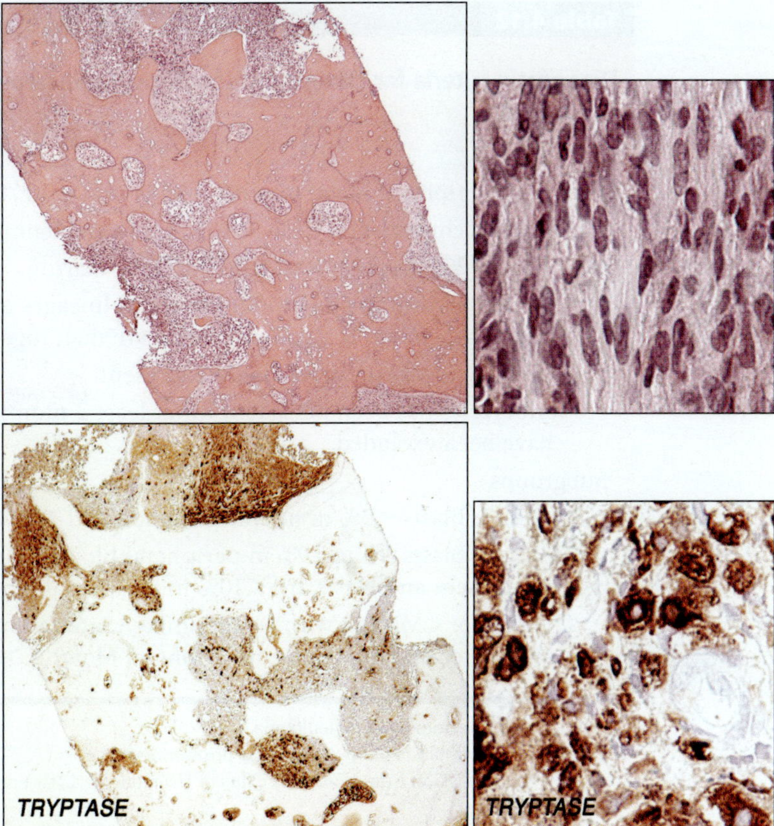

Figure 4.48 Systemic mastocytosis with osteosclerosis. *Top panel:* Low- and high-power views, left and right panels, respectively, of a biopsy displaying markedly thickened bony trabeculae with marrow replacement by proliferation of spindle-shaped cells. Low- and high-magnification reveal marrow replacement by tryptase-positive mast cells.

Table 4.11

Differential diagnosis of chronic myelogenous leukemia, atypical chronic myelogenous leukemia, and chronic myelomonocytic leukemia

Feature	CML	Atypical CML	CMML
BCR/ABL	+	−	−
WBC	+++	++	+
Basophils*	≥2%	<2%	<2%
Monocytes*	<3%	3%–10%	<2%
Immature granulocytes*	>20%	10%–20%	≤10%
Peripheral blasts*	<2%	>2%	<2%
Granulocyte dysplasia	−	++	+
Marrow erythroid hyperplasia	−	−	+

Chronic myelogenous leukemia, chronic phase, CML; chronic myelomonocytic leukemia, CMML; white blood cell count, WBC.

*Refers to peripheral blood. Of the three disorders, only CML is distinguished by the presence of the Philadelphia chromosome or *BCR/ABL*. CML usually has higher white blood cell counts than does either CMML or atypical CML, with WBC counts of greater than 200,000/µL on occasion. A prominent basophilia is more characteristic of CML, although a mild basophilia may occur in either atypical CML or CMML. A marked monocytosis, however, is more typical of CMML than either of the other diseases. The dramatic left-shift in granulocytes in overall numbers is higher in CML and much more modest in CMML, but increased numbers of circulating blasts may occur in atypical CML compared with either CML or CMML. Granulocytic dysplasia is most prominent in atypical CML and is conspicuous by its absence in CML; granulocyte dysplasia may be present or absent in CMML. Last, a marrow erythroid hyperplasia occurs more often in CMML than in *de novo* CML or atypical CML.

Table adapted with permission from George TI, Arber DA. Pathology of the myeloproliferative diseases. *Hematol Oncol Clin N Am* 2003;17:1101–1127.

Table 4.12

Diagnostic criteria for chronic myelomonocytic leukemia according to the World Health Organization

Persistent peripheral blood monocytosis is $>1 \times 10^9$/L.

Philadelphia chromosome or BCR/ABL rearrangement is absent.

Blasts[a] are $<20\%$ in peripheral blood or bone marrow.

Dysplasia is present in one or more myeloid lineages or, in the absence of dysplasia, CMML can be diagnosed if all other criteria are met, together with either of the following:

A clonal cytogenetic abnormality is present.

Monocytosis has been persistent for at least 3 months, and all other causes of monocytosis have been excluded.

Subgroups

CMML-1: Blasts $<5\%$ in peripheral blood and $<10\%$ in bone marrow.

CMML-2: Blasts 5% to 19% in peripheral blood, 10% to 19% in bone marrow, or Auer rods are present and blasts are $<20\%$ in peripheral blood or bone marrow.

CMML-1 or CMML-2 with eosinophilia: Criteria for CMML-1 and CMML-2 are present, and the eosinophil count in peripheral blood is $>1.5 \times 10^9$/L.

CMML, chronic myelomonocytic leukemia.
[a]Blasts include myeloblasts, monoblasts, and promonocytes.
Adapted with permission from *Wintrobe's Clinical Hematology*, 11th Edition, page 2209.

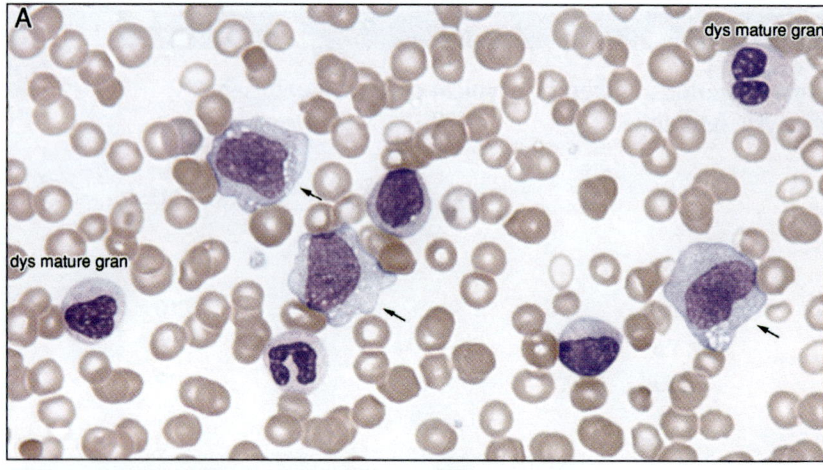

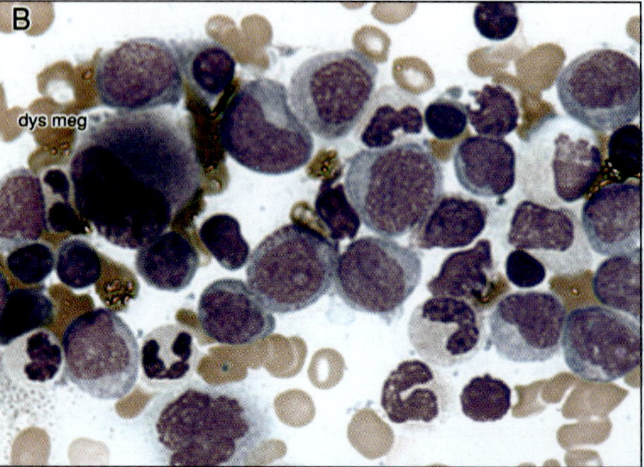

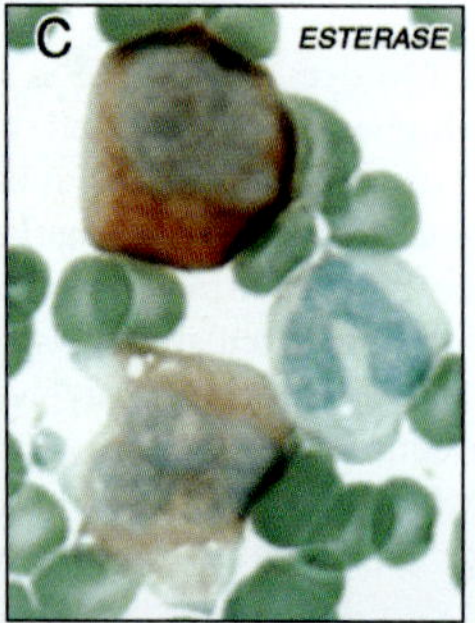

Figure 4.49 CMML-2, blood smear and aspirate smears. **A.** This blood smear shows monocytosis (*arrows*) and dysplastic neutrophils. **B.** Aspirate smear reveals increased numbers of nucleolated monoblasts and promonocytes, a dysplastic micromegakaryocyte, and dysplastic hypogranular myeloids. In C, a butyrate stain confirms the monocytic origin of the large mononuclear cells. The diagnosis of CMML requires more than 1,000/μL monocytes in the peripheral blood. The monocytes may be abnormal in appearance, and bizarre nuclei and promonocytes, with more immature nuclear chromatin, also may be present. Monoblasts are usually rare to absent. Cytopenias and often dysplastic changes, such as the hypogranular and hypolobated neutrophils shown here, also may be present and seen in blood smears.

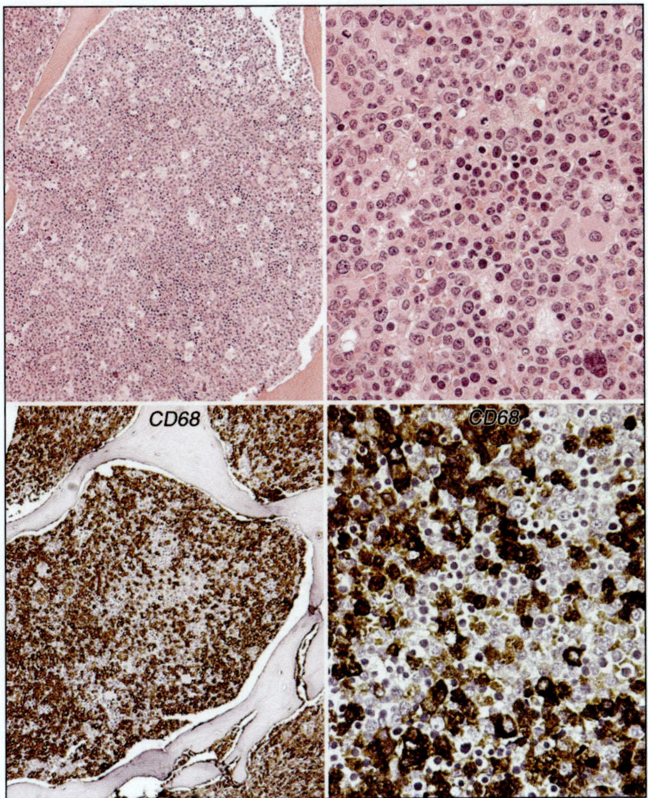

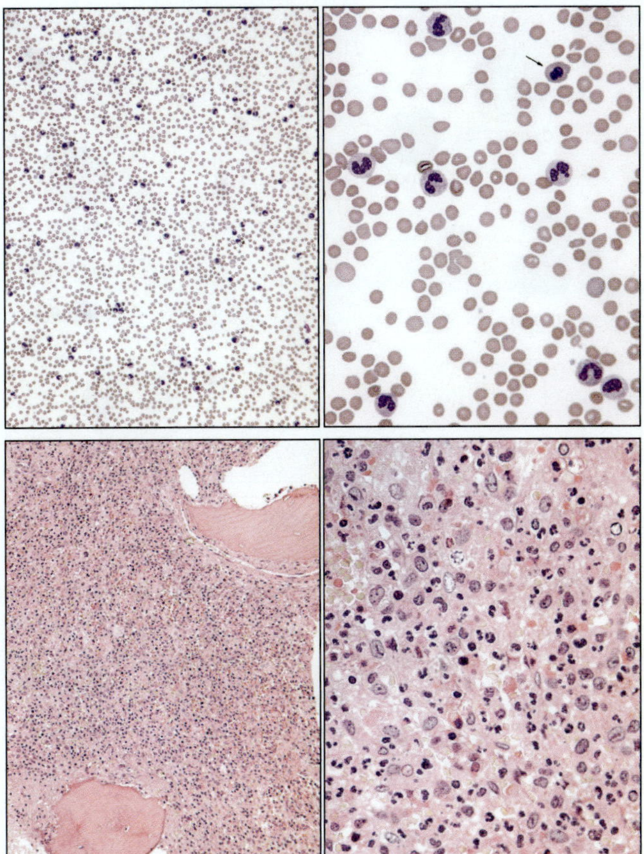

Figure 4.50   CMML-2, marrow biopsy. Low- and medium-power views, left and right panels, respectively, of a biopsy from the same case as shown in Figure 4.49 showing a hypercellular marrow infiltrated by sheets of CD68$^+$ monoblasts and promyelocytes. Increased blasts correlate with a poor prognosis and, when blasts and promonocytes exceed 20%, these patients are classified as AML. When blasts and promonocytes are <5% in the blood and <10% in the marrow, these cases are designated CMML-1. When peripheral blood blasts and promonocytes are 5% to 19%, or marrow blasts and promonocytes number 10% to 19%, these cases are diagnosed as CMML-2. When granulocytic hyperplasia is prominent, it may be difficult to distinguish the abnormal monocyte population from myelocytes, especially in the presence of dysplasia. Erythroid precursors and megakaryocytes may show prominent dysplastic features, but often these cell types are unremarkable in appearance.

Figure 4.51   Atypical CML. *Top panels:* Peripheral blood smear from a patient with atypical CML showed a leukocytosis with anemia and marked thrombocytopenia. Granulocytes are left-shifted, with dysplastic hypolobulated nuclei and a dysplastic nRBC is present (*arrow*). Blasts, promyelocytes, and myelocytes typically constitute 10% to 20% of cells in the blood, whereas monocytes are usually <10% and basophils <2% of cells. *Bottom panels:* Biopsy at low- and high-magnification (left and right, respectively) showing atypical granulocytic hyperplasia without sheets of blasts.

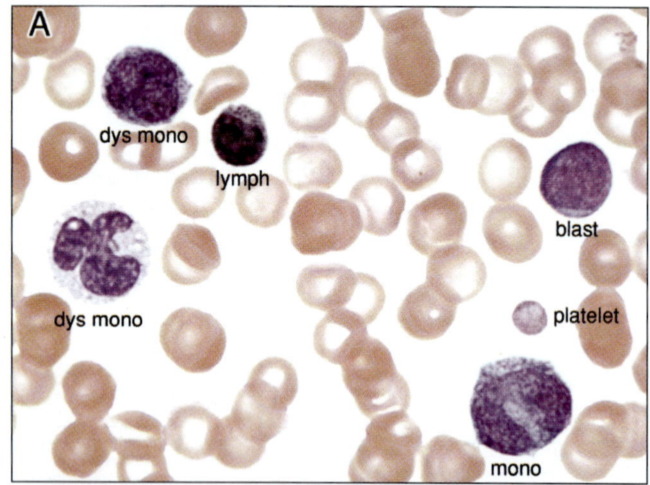

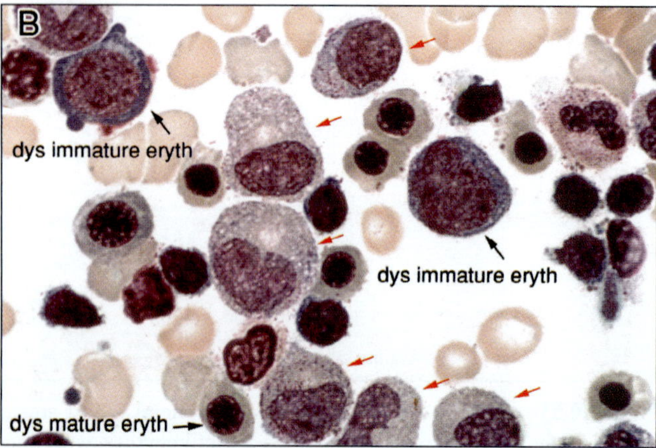

Figure 4.52 A–B Juvenile myelomonocytic leukemia (JMML). A. This peripheral blood smear from a child with JMML shows dysplastic monocytosis, left-shifted leukocytosis with a small blast, and thrombocytopenia. A lone sparsely granulated platelet is present. B. The aspirate discloses left-shifted granulocytes with dysplasia and a relative erythroid hyperplasia. (Fig. 4.52A courtesy Irma T. Pereira, MT(ASCP)SH.)

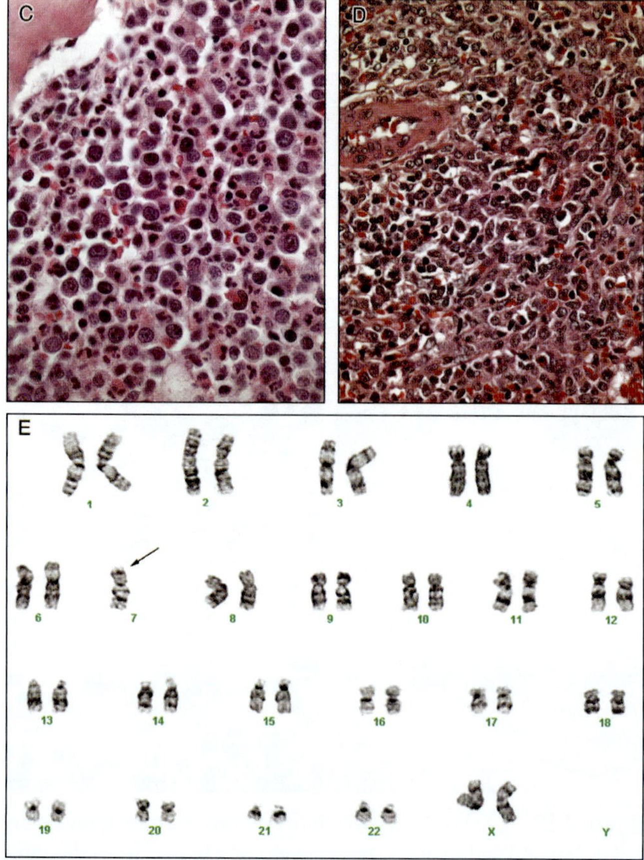

Figure 4.52 C–E C. The bone marrow biopsy is hypercellular, with a myeloid hyperplasia that includes increased numbers of immature myeloid precursors. D. The spleen is infiltrated by immature mononuclear cells with abundant cytoplasm, irregular nuclear contours, and delicate open chromatin resembling monocytes and immature myeloid precursors. E. Cytogenetic studies show monosomy 7. Infantile monosomy 7 syndrome is clinically similar to JMML and probably represents a subgroup of JMML patients. Cytogenetic abnormalities other than monosomy 7 are not specific for JMML. (Fig. 4.52E courtesy Cytogenetics Laboratory, Stanford Medical Center, Stanford, CA.)

Lymphoproliferative Disorders

Jan V. Hirschmann, MD, Denis J. Bailey, MD, FRCPC, and Douglas C. Tkachuk, MD, FRCPC

Among lymphoid tumors, the World Health Organization (WHO) classification has three major divisions: (1) B-cell neoplasms, (2) T- and NK-cell neoplasms, and (3) Hodgkin lymphoma. These categories include both lymphomas, traditionally identified as proliferative lymphoid tissue masses, and leukemias, indicating widespread bone marrow involvement, usually associated with circulating tumor cells. The distinction is arbitrary, and some "lymphomas" have extensive marrow involvement and circulating neoplastic cells initially, or they evolve into "leukemias" with progressive disease.

The classification of these disorders attempts to identify the tumors' putative cells of origin and their apparent maturity. The B and T/NK categories are divided into two types: precursor neoplasms, in which the cells are in the earliest stages of differentiation, and the peripheral neoplasms, which consist of cells in the later stages of maturation. Sometimes the cell of origin is apparent on morphologic criteria, but many are identified via immunophenotyping that identifies characteristic antigens on the cell surface. About 80% to 85% of lymphoid neoplasms are of B-cell origin; nearly all the rest derive from T cells. Tumors arising from NK cells are rare.

The entire B-cell line originates from precursor B lymphoblasts in the bone marrow that differentiate into naïve B cells that have surface immunoglobulin. The lymphoblasts are the putative cells of origin of precursor-B acute lymphoblastic leukemia and lymphoma. The naïve marrow B cells are the source of small lymphocytic lymphoma and chronic lymphocytic leukemia. The naïve B cells leave the marrow to circulate in the blood and travel to the cortex of lymph nodes, where they occupy primary follicles (those without germinal centers) and secondary follicles (those with germinal centers) in the mantle zone, which surrounds the germinal centers. These cells are the source of mantle cell lymphoma. When naïve B cells encounter antigen, they transform into blasts and travel to the center of primary follicles, forming the germinal center,

where the cells are called *centroblasts*. These large cells, whose vesicular nuclei contain nucleoli, are thought to be the source of most large B-cell lymphomas and Burkitt lymphoma. The centroblasts mature to centrocytes, which are medium-sized, cleaved cells with inconspicuous nucleoli from which follicular lymphomas are thought to arise. The centrocytes mature into: (1) antibody secreting plasma cells, from which plasma cell myeloma and Waldenström macroglobulinemia originate, and (2) memory B cells, which are found in the areas around follicles (marginal zone) and are the putative origin of marginal-zone lymphomas of the spleen, lymph nodes, and mucosa-associated tissue (MALT).

The earliest T cells reside in the thymus, and these are considered the source of precursor T-cell lymphoblastic leukemia/lymphoma. The circulating mature T cells are the source of peripheral (i.e., outside the thymus) T-cell neoplasms. The mature T-cell lymphomas account for about 12% of non-Hodgkin lymphomas. The most common subtypes are peripheral T-cell lymphoma and anaplastic large-cell lymphoma, which together constitute about half of all cases.

Mature B-Cell Neoplasms

The clonal proliferation of cells in mature B-cell neoplasms ranges in differentiation from naïve B cells—resting lymphoid cells that have surface immunoglobulin but have not yet encountered antigens—to mature plasma cells, which produce immunoglobulins in response to previous antigen exposure. The classification of these disorders, which account for >80% of lymphoid neoplasms, generally depends on morphologic characteristics, immunophenotyping of the cells, and anatomic involvement (i.e., whether the process is primarily disseminated [often leukemic], extranodal, or nodal). The disseminated disorders, which are usually indolent, typically involve the bone marrow and commonly affect the blood, lymph nodes, and spleen. This group includes chronic lymphocytic leukemia,

Waldenström macroglobulinemia, hairy cell leukemia, splenic marginal-zone lymphoma, and plasma cell leukemia. The primary mature B-cell extranodal neoplasm is marginal zone B-cell lymphoma of MALT. Common primary nodal mature B-cell lymphomas are follicular-center lymphoma and mantle cell lymphoma. Diffuse large B-cell lymphoma, the most common lymphoma worldwide, and Burkitt lymphoma may be nodal, extranodal, or disseminated. Most patients have no predisposing factors, but some have severe immunocompromise from infection with human immunodeficiency virus (HIV), primary immunodeficiencies, and immunosuppressive medications.

Chronic Lymphocytic Leukemia (CLL)

Chronic lymphocytic leukemia is a clinically heterogeneous disease consisting of monoclonal small B-cell lymphocytes expressing CD19, CD5, and CD23. The excessive number of cells occurs because of both increased proliferation and accumulation of cells with an increased lifespan. Most patients are asymptomatic at the time of diagnosis, their median age is about 65, and the male:female ratio is approximately 2:1. When symptoms occur, they commonly include weakness and fatigue, related to anemia from bone marrow replacement or immune-related hemolysis caused by a warm-reactive polyclonal IgG, which occurs in about 10% to 25% of patients during the course of disease. Other complaints may include fever, weight loss, and bleeding. The physical examination is often unremarkable, but common findings are hepatosplenomegaly and enlarged, nontender, firm, mobile lymph nodes in the cervical, axillary, and inguinal areas.

The diagnostic criteria for CLL are: (1) an absolute lymphocytosis $\geq 5 \times 10^9$/L; (2) $\geq 30\%$ lymphocytosis in a normocellular or hypercellular bone marrow; and (3) monoclonal B cells with low levels of surface immunoglobulins and CD5 positivity. The blood smear shows an increased number of mature small lymphocytes with little cytoplasm and dense, clumped chromatin. Nucleoli are not usually visible, and many cells, being more fragile than normal lymphocytes, disrupt during the preparation of the smear, producing "smudge cells," in which the cytoplasm is lost and the nucleus spread out. Some cells may be prolymphocytes, which are larger than mature lymphocytes, possess nucleoli, and have more cytoplasm. In a variant, *CLL with increased prolymphocytes*, a clinically more aggressive disease than CLL, prolymphocytes represent 10% to 55% of the lymphocytes. (When prolymphocytes are >55%, the diagnosis is B-cell prolymphocytic leukemia.) Bone marrow lymphocytes may assume one or more patterns: nodular—tightly packed aggregates of cells; interstitial—lymphocytes intermixed with other hematopoietic cells; or diffuse—extensive lymphocytic infiltration throughout the marrow. Rare hematologic findings include immune thrombocytopenia and pure red cell aplasia.

Several factors influence prognosis, but one especially important feature is whether somatic mutations exist in the specific immunoglobulin heavy-chain region (IgV_H) genes of the malignant lymphocytes. DNA sequences in which these genes in the B cells differ from those in the germ line by $\geq 2\%$ are considered "mutated," and CLL with this feature, which constitutes about 50% to 60% of cases, is much more indolent than that with unmutated genes. The presence of many cells that are CD38$^+$ or express ζ-chain-associated protein 70 (ZAP-70) also correlates with more aggressive disease.

Nonhematologic complications of CLL include infections related to hypogammaglobulinemia, decreased cell-mediated immunity, or neutropenia caused by CLL or its treatment. Paraneoplastic pemphigus, a blistering disorder of the skin and mucous membranes, rarely occurs. About 5% of patients with CLL develop Richter syndrome: The disease transforms into a non-Hodgkin lymphoma, usually diffuse large B-cell type. Characteristic features include fever, weight loss, rapid increase in lymph node size, and elevated serum lactic dehydrogenase (LDH).

B-Cell Prolymphocytic Leukemia

This rare disorder predominantly affects older adults (median age, 70), with a male:female ratio of 1.6:1. Most patients have marked splenomegaly without enlarged peripheral lymph nodes. By definition, prolymphocytes constitute >55% of the circulating lymphoid cells, but in most cases they exceed 90%. About half of patients have anemia and thrombocytopenia. The prolymphocytes are twice the size of small lymphocytes and possess a small amount of pale blue cytoplasm and round nuclei, which contain moderately condensed chromatin and a conspicuous central nucleolus. The bone marrow shows diffuse infiltration with these abnormal cells.

Waldenström Macroglobulinemia (Lymphoplasmacytic Lymphoma)

This clonal disorder is characterized by the production of monoclonal IgM in association with bone marrow infiltration by small lymphocytes showing plasmacytoid or plasma cell differentiation. The median age is about 65, and males slightly outnumber females. Some patients are asymptomatic, but most have problems related to: (1) tissue infiltration by the malignant cells; (2) circulating IgM; (3) IgM tissue deposition; (4) auto-antibody formation; (5) amyloid; and (6) constitutional symptoms of fever, weight loss, and night sweats. About one-third of patients have enlargement of lymph nodes, liver, or spleen from tumor infiltration. Uncommon sites of involvement include lungs (masses, nodules, pleural effusion) and skin (papules or nodules), although virtually any organ can be affected.

Circulating IgM, which usually exceeds 30 g/L, forms aggregates and binds water, sometimes resulting in hyperviscosity, which has several clinical manifestations. The level of IgM does not necessarily correlate well with clinical manifestations. Ophthalmologic features include visual blurring and decreased acuity, associated with retinal hemorrhages, exudates, and dilated, tortuous veins with segment of widening ("sausage links" or "boxcars"). The increase in plasma volume can cause congestive heart failure. The impaired blood transit through the microvasculature can cause neurologic symptoms of dizziness, headache, deafness, confusion, nystagmus, vertigo, and ataxia. The combination of damage to vessel walls from the diminished blood flow and the interaction of monoclonal IgM with clotting factors and platelets can lead to bleeding, such as epistaxis, oral mucosal hemorrhage, and cutaneous ecchymoses. The IgM can precipitate on cooling, creating a type I cryoglobulinemia in up to 20% of patients, but <5% have symptoms related to it, such as cutaneous vasculitis, Raynaud phenomenon, or cold urticaria.

Deposition of IgM in the kidneys can lead to proteinuria and renal insufficiency. Firm, flesh-colored papules and nodules can form from IgM in the dermis, and occasional patients can develop gastrointestinal problems of diarrhea, malabsorption, and bleeding from monoclonal protein present in the intestinal wall. Monoclonal light chains can form amyloid, which is clinically evident in about 2% of patients with Waldenström macroglobulinemia. The organs most commonly affected include the heart, peripheral nerves, kidney, liver, and lungs. The monoclonal IgM also can behave as an autoantibody, and up to 20% of patients have a peripheral neuropathy from antibodies against glycoproteins in the nerves. It is usually a distal, symmetrical, chronic demyelinating process. The macroglobulins also may interact with red cell antigens at temperatures <37°C, causing a chronic hemolytic anemia called *cold-agglutinin disease*.

A normocytic, normochromic anemia is common and can arise from bone marrow infiltration, hemolysis, dilution by increased plasma volume, and hemorrhage. On peripheral blood smear, rouleaux formation is common, and sometimes red-cell agglutination leads to clumping of erythrocytes. Increased numbers of small lymphocytes, some resembling plasma cells ("plasmacytoid lymphocytes") with abundant basophilic cytoplasm, are common. Plasma cells also may be visible.

The bone marrow shows lymphoid aggregates, a diffuse interstitial infiltrate, or a mixed nodular-diffuse pattern of the small lymphocytes, plasmacytoid lymphocytes, and plasma cells.

Hairy Cell Leukemia

The median age of patients with this disease is approximately 55 years, and the male:female ratio is about 4:1. In most patients, the neoplastic B-lymphoid cells affect primarily the bone marrow and spleen, causing splenomegaly and decreased circulating cells, including monocytes and neutrophils, in most patients. About 50% have pancytopenia at the time of diagnosis. The disease, which accounts for about 2% of adult leukemias, predisposes to bacterial infections because of neutropenia, but also causes diminished cell-mediated immunity. The result is an increased

susceptibility to non-tuberculous mycobacteria, fungi, *Listeria monocytogenes, Toxoplasma gondii, Pneumocystis pneumonia*, and various viruses. Hairy cell leukemia is also the most common cause of paraneoplastic vasculitis, whose features are fever, nodular skin lesions, palpable purpura, and arthritis. Some patients have other rheumatologic disorders, including systemic sclerosis, polymyositis, and polyarteritis nodosa. Nearly all patients with this disease have palpable splenomegaly, often to gargantuan size, and about 40% have hepatomegaly.

In addition to reduction in one or more cell lines, peripheral smears in about 85% of cases reveal the hairy cells—small- to medium-sized lymphoid cells that possess a round, kidney-shaped, oval or bilobed, and commonly eccentric, nucleus with ground-glass chromatin, but absent or inconspicuous nucleoli, and abundant, pale-blue cytoplasm with numerous irregular, thin projections resembling hairs. Because of associated reticulin fibrosis, aspirating a bone marrow specimen may be difficult or impossible but, if successful, usually discloses conspicuous hairy cells. Bone marrow biopsies are usually hypercellular and demonstrate patchy, diffuse, or interstitial infiltration with mononuclear cells possessing abundant cytoplasm and prominent cell borders, creating a "fried-egg" appearance. The reticulin fibrosis produces a net-like pattern affecting areas of hairy cell infiltration. Hairy cells have acid phosphatase activity that is resistant to tartrate and, in >95% of cases, a tartrate-resistant acid phosphatase stain (TRAP) is positive. In the rare variant form of hairy cell leukemia, however, the TRAP stain is usually negative, the white count is elevated, neutropenia and monocytopenia are absent, and the hairy cells have prominent nucleoli, similar to the cells of prolymphocytic leukemia.

Multiple Myeloma (Plasma Cell Myeloma)

Multiple myeloma is a clonal proliferation of plasma cells that occurs in older adults (median age at diagnosis is about 70 years), and it has a greater incidence in blacks than in whites. Exposure to ionizing radiation is a predisposing condition. The clinical features relate to: (1) marrow or other organ infiltration by plasma cells; (2) the production of a monoclonal protein in blood or urine, which occurs in 99% of patients; or (3) immune deficiency from inadequate immunoglobulin production from the normal plasma cells. Bone marrow infiltration by the plasma cells can cause several lytic bone lesions, from which the term multiple myeloma (tumor of the bone marrow) arises. These are often painful. Because the plasma cells produce substances that both resorb bone and impair its formation, diffuse osteopenia can develop, which can be painful when pathologic fractures occur, especially in the vertebrae and ribs. Sometimes, extramedullary aggregates of plasma cells— plasmacytomas—develop, especially in the skin, lymph nodes, liver, and spleen. Anemia is present in about 70% of patients with multiple myeloma, in part from impaired erythropoiesis caused by bone marrow replacement with plasma cells. Another consequence of bony involvement is hypercalcemia, which can lead to lethargy, confusion, polyuria, constipation, nausea, and vomiting. The polyuria can lead to renal insufficiency.

Reduced kidney function also arises from the effects of monoclonal protein, which is IgG in about 60% of cases of multiple myeloma, IgA in 20%, and light chains alone (κ in about two-thirds, λ in about one-third) in 20%. About 80% of patients of excrete light chains (Bence-Jones protein) in the urine, and their precipitation in the tubules can cause renal insufficiency. It also may occur when circulating light chains are deposited in the glomeruli. In about 35% of patients with multiple myeloma, excess light chains form AL amyloid, causing proteinuria most commonly, but sometimes renal insufficiency. Amyloidosis also may cause the carpal tunnel syndrome and, less frequently, cardiomyopathy, macroglossia, or periorbital ecchymoses. Some monoclonal proteins injure the peripheral nerves, producing a symmetrical, sensorimotor, demyelinating polyneuropathy, especially in the context of POEMS syndrome, an acronym for a disorder that includes in various combinations polyneuropathy, organomegaly, endocrinopathies, M (monoclonal) protein, and skin changes. The organomegaly is enlargement of the spleen and liver; the endocrinopathies may be diabetes, thyroid disease, gonadal, or adrenal disorders; and the skin changes typically include diffuse hyperpigmentation, hypertrichosis, and cutaneous thickening. Fewer than 10% of patients with multiple myeloma, usually IgA type, develop hyperviscosity, characterized by bleeding, mental changes, visual blurring and decreased acuity, and congestive heart failure.

Decrease immunoglobulin production increases the risk of bacterial infections, especially from encapsulated organisms, such as *Streptococcus pneumoniae* and *Haemophilus influenzae*. Infections from gram-negative bacilli are also common, typically a complication of neutropenia from therapy or progressive disease.

The diagnosis of multiple myeloma depends on a concurrence of features, and several different diagnostic criteria have been proposed. Perhaps the most common scheme requires fulfilling one major and one minor criterion or three minor criteria. The major criteria are: (1) marrow plasmacytosis >30%; (2) plasmacytoma on biopsy; and (3) M-component (monoclonal protein) in the serum of IgG >3.5 g/dL or IgA >2 g/dL or in the urine >1 g/24h of Bence-Jones protein. Minor criteria are: (1) marrow plasmacytosis of 10% to 30%; (2) M component, but less than the values of the major criteria; (3) lytic bone lesions; and (4) immunoglobulins <50% of normal: IgG <600 mg/dL, IgA <100 mg/dL, IgM <50 mg/dL.

The peripheral blood smear may appear more basophilic than normal because of the presence of the acidic paraproteins, which also cause the red cells to adhere, resulting in rouleaux, stacks of erythrocytes, in areas where they would normally be separated. The red cells are usually normochromic and normocytic. Sometimes, leukoerythro-

blastosis, the presence of nucleated red cells and immature white cells, is apparent, indicating disruption of the bone marrow from the infiltrating plasma cells. Occasional plasma cells may be visible. When plasma cells are >2,000/mm^3 (2 × 10^9/L) or constitute >20% of the circulating white cells, the term *plasma cell leukemia* is used. It can occur as the presentation of multiple myeloma or as a complication of a previously diagnosed case.

On bone marrow aspiration, the plasma cells may appear normal or may demonstrate altered maturation, such as a normal cytoplasm with a diffuse nuclear chromatin pattern, nucleoli, lobulated or multilobed nuclei, mitoses, and a high nuclear:cytoplasm (N:C) ratio. Immunoglobulins can appear in the cytoplasm as multiple small vacuoles (creating Mott cells), as large homogeneous spheres (Russell bodies), or as crystalline rods. The cytoplasmic margins may be eosinophilic, producing "flame cells." Inclusions present in the nucleus are called *Dutcher bodies*. On bone marrow biopsy, the pattern of plasma cells may be: (1) interstitial—intermixed with normal hematopoietic cells; (2) nodular—discrete aggregates of plasma cells; or (3) packed—with plasma cells occurring in sheets, replacing the normal fat and hematopoietic cells and obliterating the normal marrow architecture. As in aspirates, Russell bodies, Mott cells, crystals, and Dutcher bodies may be visible.

Splenic Marginal-Zone Lymphoma

This rare disorder, previously called *splenic lymphoma with villous lymphocytes*, is a B-cell neoplasm in which small lymphocytes replace the white pulp germinal centers of the spleen. The mantle zone of B lymphocytes that ordinarily surrounds the germinal center, and with it constitute the follicle, may be intact or effaced, and the marginal zone beyond that layer contains larger cells, including blasts. Most patients are >50 years old, and it affects both genders equally. The major clinical feature is splenomegaly. Some patients have immune thrombocytopenia or hemolytic anemia, but enlarged peripheral lymph nodes are uncommon, and extranodal disease is rare. About one-third of patients have a monoclonal gammopathy. Most patients have marrow involvement, but the peripheral blood usually shows only modestly increased numbers of pleomorphic small lymphocytes. Some are "villous" lymphocytes, which have a round or oval nucleus with moderately condensed chromatin, sometimes a small nucleolus, and basophilic cytoplasm, with short, thin projections, characteristically at one pole of the cell. Small numbers of plasmacytoid lymphocytes and plasma cells also may be present. In the bone marrow, the same combination of cells are present in a diffuse or nodular pattern.

Extranodal Marginal Zone B-Cell Lymphoma of Mucosa-Associated Lymphoid Tissue (MALT Lymphoma)

This neoplasm, usually an adult disease with a median age of about 60 years, constitutes about 8% of non-Hodgkin lymphomas. It often occurs in disorders associated with chronic lymphocytic inflammation, such as Sjögren disease, Hashimoto thyroiditis, and gastritis caused by *Helicobacter pylori*. The gastrointestinal tract is the most common site of disease, especially the stomach, and this neoplasm constitutes about 50% of all primary gastric lymphomas. Other common sites are the lungs, salivary glands, eye, skin, and thyroid. Bone marrow involvement is uncommon, and lymph nodes are variably affected, depending in part on the site of extranodal disease. In the involved tissue, the lymphoma cells are heterogeneous in appearance and include small lymphocytes, monocytoid B cells, sometimes plasma cells, and cells primarily residing in the marginal zone outside the lymphoid follicles. These cells look like centrocytes in being small to medium in size and having irregular nuclei with dispersed chromatin, inconspicuous nucleoli, and generous, pale cytoplasm. Large cells resembling centroblasts are usually present, but not predominant. When they involve the epithelium, marginal-zone cells typically accumulate in aggregates and distort or destroy it. In lymph nodes, the lymphoma cells occupy the marginal zone.

Follicular Lymphoma

Follicular lymphoma constitutes about 40% of non-Hodgkin lymphoma in the United States, affecting primarily adults, with a median age of about 60 years and equal gender distribution. Most patients have widespread disease at diagnosis, with diffuse lymph node enlargement, bone marrow involvement in about 40% of patients, and circulating neoplastic cells in about 10%. In 25% to 35% of cases the disease transforms into a large B-cell lymphoma, usually diffuse.

The lymphoma is called "follicular" because the neoplastic cells are those normally present in the germinal centers of lymphoid follicles—centrocytes and centroblasts—and because in affected tissue the cells maintain at least partially the follicular pattern of discrete aggregates rather than diffuse involvement. The predominant cells, the centrocytes, are small to medium in size, have scant pale cytoplasm, inconspicuous nucleoli, and nuclei that are twisted, elongated, or cleaved. The centroblasts are large, have noncleaved, round to oval nuclei with nucleoli, and possess sparse, basophilic cytoplasm. The proportion of centroblasts determines the grade of lymphoma based on microscopic examination of 10 neoplastic follicles at 40× high-power magnification: Grade 1 has 0 to 5 centroblasts/high-power field (hpf); Grade 2 has 6 to 15 centroblasts/hpf; Grade 3a has >15 centroblasts/hpf with centrocytes also present; Grade 3b has >15 centroblasts/hpf without centrocytes. In peripheral blood smears, the neoplastic cells are commonly smaller than normal lymphocytes, have very sparse cytoplasm, and possess cleft nuclei. In patients with bone marrow involvement, the process is typically focal and paratrabecular in location and, as in lymph nodes, the predominant cells are the centrocytes, which are small lymphocytes with cleaved

nuclei. Larger cells—either large centrocytes, with irregular or cleft nuclei, or centroblasts, with round or oval, noncleaved nuclei and prominent nucleoli—also are present.

Mantle Cell Lymphoma

This lymphoma, which constitutes about 5% to 10% of non-Hodgkin lymphoma, occurs primarily in adults, with a median age at diagnosis of about 60 years and a male predominance of at least 2:1. The disease is usually widespread, affecting lymph nodes, liver, spleen, and bone marrow. Some patients have gastrointestinal disease, with numerous lymphomatous polyps anywhere in the alimentary tract. The neoplastic cell closely resembles centrocytes, appearing as small- to medium-sized lymphocytes with sparse cytoplasm and irregular or cleaved nuclei containing moderately dispersed chromatin and inconspicuous nucleoli. In some cases, the cells tend to surround the germinal centers of lymph nodes in the mantle zone. The cell of origin is thought to be naïve B cells normally present in the mantle zone. Some cytologic variants occur, including a blastoid type in which cells resemble lymphoblasts with dispersed chromatin. Bone marrow involvement in mantle cell lymphoma includes interstitial, focal, paratrabecular, and diffuse patterns. The cells are small lymphocytes with irregular and cleaved nuclei, resembling centrocytes. Centroblasts are not present.

Diffuse Large B-Cell Lymphoma

This disorder accounts for about 40% of non-Hodgkin lymphomas. It occurs at all ages, but the median age at diagnosis is about 60 years. Patients typically have a rapidly enlarging mass at the sites of disease, which include lymph nodes, stomach, ileocecal region of the intestinal tract, and a wide variety of other extranodal areas. Bone marrow involvement, however, is rare. The histologic pattern is diffuse replacement of the normal tissue with large neoplastic cells of various morphologies that are at least twice the size of normal lymphocytes. The most common is the *centroblastic* type, in which the cells have oval to round vesicular nuclei with two to four nucleoli and sparse basophilic cytoplasm. In the *immunoblastic* variant, >90% of cells have a single, central nucleolus in the nuclei and abundant basophilic cytoplasm. In the *T-cell/histiocytic-rich* type, most cells are normal T cells and histiocytes, with <10% being large neoplastic B cells. The anaplastic variant has very large cells with bizarre, pleomorphic nuclei.

Mediastinal Large B-Cell Lymphoma

This is a subtype of diffuse large B-cell lymphoma in which the proposed cell of origin is a B cell normally present in the medulla of the thymus. It especially occurs in adolescents and young adults: The median age at diagnosis is in the third decade. Most patients are female. The clinical scenario is a rapidly enlarging anterior mediastinal mass, often producing the superior vena cava syndrome and airway obstruction. Extranodal involvement is uncommon initially, but disease can spread to various sites, including brain, skin, liver, kidneys, and adrenals. The neoplastic cells resemble those of other large B-cell lymphomas, with varying sizes and nuclear shapes, but usually with abundant basophilic cytoplasm.

Burkitt Lymphoma

This rapidly growing neoplasm commonly involves extranodal areas and occurs in three different settings. *Endemic Burkitt lymphoma* affects young children in equatorial Africa and Papua, New Guinea, typically causing masses in the jaw and other facial bones. Other common sites of involvement are the distal ileum, cecum, omentum, ovaries, kidneys, and breasts. Evidence of Epstein-Barr viral infection is present in all patients, and co-infection with malaria may predispose to the development of lymphoma. *Sporadic Burkitt lymphoma* occurs worldwide, affecting predominantly children and young adults, with a male:female ratio of about 3:1. In the United States, this neoplasm causes about 30% of childhood non-Hodgkin lymphoma. The commonest presentation is with abdominal tumors involving the ileocecal area and peritoneum, but ovaries, kidneys, and breasts often are affected. Evidence of Epstein-Barr virus in tumor cells is <30%. *Immunodeficiency-associated Burkitt lymphoma* occurs primarily in people infected with the human immunodeficiency virus (HIV), but it can occur in other immunosuppressed patients, such as organ transplant recipients. The presentation is similar to that of patients with the sporadic form, but nodal, bone marrow, and meningeal involvement is more common. Epstein-Barr virus is found in 25% to 40% of the neoplasms.

The relatively uniform, medium-sized neoplastic cells diffusely infiltrate the affected areas and show numerous mitotic figures and spontaneous cell death (apoptosis). They have round nuclei with clumped chromatin and multiple, central nucleoli. The basophilic cytoplasm usually contains lipid vacuoles. The benign histiocytes ingesting the dead cells have a clear cytoplasm, and their presence in the dark background of the abundant lymphoma cells gives the appearance of a "starry sky." Two variants are *Burkitt lymphoma with plasmacytoid differentiation* and *atypical Burkitt/Burkitt-like lymphoma*. Both have more pleomorphic nuclear sizes and shapes. In the former, some tumor cells contain a single nucleolus and a monotypic immunoglobulin in eccentric basophilic cytoplasm. In the latter, the nucleoli are more prominent and fewer in number than they are in typical Burkitt lymphoma.

MATURE T-CELL AND NK-CELL NEOPLASMS

The classification of these neoplasms depends on combining histologic, immunophenotypic, genetic, and especially, clinical features because morphologic and immunophenotypic abnormalities may be diverse in a specific disorder and yet similar among different diseases. As a group, these disorders have specific geographic foci (especially Asia), have infrequent lymph node involvement, demonstrate cell death (apoptosis) and necrosis, are accompanied by an increased incidence of the hemophagocytic syndrome, and often are associated with viral infections, especially with the Epstein-Barr virus.

T-Cell Prolymphocytic Leukemia

This disorder accounts for about 2% of adult small lymphocytic leukemias and is primarily a disease of people >50 years old, with most patients having impressive splenomegaly. Generalized lymph node enlargement and hepatomegaly are common. Skin nodules or diffuse papular rashes occur in about 25% of cases, pleural effusions or ascites in about the same number. The major laboratory finding is a very high white count, exceeding 200×10^9/L in about two-thirds of patients. Anemia and thrombocytopenia are also common. The diagnosis is established on peripheral blood films, where most cells are prolymphocytes, with a well-defined central nucleolus and a deeply basophilic cytoplasm that often demonstrates blebs or protrusions. These cells are larger than normal small lymphocytes, but in 20% of cases of T-cell prolymphocytic leukemia (the small-cell variant), the cells are small, with more condensed nuclear chromatin and no apparent nucleolus, which, however, is apparent on electron microscopy.

Bone marrow aspirates show the same cells that are present on blood smears. Bone marrow biopsies show heavy infiltration that can be interstitial, nodular, diffuse, or mixed. The number of reticulin fibers is increased.

T-Cell Large Granular Lymphocytic Leukemia

The median age of patients with this disorder is about 60 years, and many have clinical and serologic evidence of rheumatoid arthritis. About 40% are asymptomatic at the time of diagnosis. The most prominent clinical feature is splenomegaly, present in about 50%; lymph node enlargement is rare. The white cell count is elevated because of an increased number of large granular lymphocytes, which usually appear normal and have round or oval, eccentric nuclei with condensed chromatin and abundant basophilic cytoplasm containing small or large purplish granules. To fulfill diagnostic criteria these cells should exceed 2×10^9/L for at least 6 months without an alternative explanation. Severe neutropenia, sometimes associated with bacterial infections, is present in about 50% of patients, and a few have pure red cell aplasia. Bone marrow involvement is variable and often minimal, the typical pattern being interstitial or diffuse, but rarely nodular. Patients with neutropenia usually have normal immature granulocytes but decreased neutrophils (maturation arrest), and patients with thrombocytopenia characteristically demonstrate adequate or increased megakaryocytes. Anemia may be accompanied by red cell aplasia or hypoplasia.

Aggressive NK-Cell Leukemia

This disorder typically occurs in adolescents or young adults and is more common in Asians than in whites. The clinical features are usually fever and hepatosplenomegaly, associated with anemia, thrombocytopenia, and neutropenia. The peripheral blood film shows the leukemic cells, which may be sparse or numerous, as slightly bigger than normal large granular lymphocytes, some with irregular, hyperchromatic nuclei and coarser or more open chromatin. In the abundant pale or light-blue cytoplasm are fine or coarse azurophilic granules. The bone marrow demonstrates minimal to pronounced infiltration with neoplastic cells, sometimes accompanied by erythrophagocytic histiocytes (hemophagocytosis). Evidence of Epstein-Barr virus infection detected by *in situ* hybridization is present in most cases.

Adult T-Cell Leukemia/Lymphoma

This disorder, caused by infection with the retrovirus human T-cell leukemia virus type 1, is endemic in Japan, the Caribbean, and parts of central Africa. Most patients have acquired the infection at an early age through breast milk or exposure to blood, and the lifetime cumulative risk of later developing leukemia or lymphoma, which occurs at a median age of about 55 years, is approximately 2%. The typical clinical features include generalized lymph node enlargement, hypercalcemia, hepatosplenomegaly, and skin lesions, which can be nodules, papules, or a diffuse scaly rash. Four clinical patterns occur. Most common is the *acute variant*, which includes constitutional symptoms, diffuse lymph node enlargement, skin rash, hepatosplenomegaly, hypercalcemia with or without lytic bone lesions, high numbers of circulating leukemic cells, and an elevated serum lactic dehydrogenase (LDH). Some patients have opportunistic infections from decreased cell-mediated immunity. The *lymphomatous variant* consists of generalized lymph node enlargement without circulating leukemic cells. Hypercalcemia and elevated LDH may be present. The *chronic variant* has prominent skin lesions, mostly an exfoliative process, but no hypercalcemia. The white count is elevated, with >10% being leukemic cells. Serum LDH is slightly increased. The *smoldering variant* has a normal white cell count with <3% neoplastic cells, normal serum calcium and LDH, and no enlargement of lymph nodes, spleen, or liver. Pulmonary involvement and skin rashes may be present.

On peripheral smear the leukemic cells are markedly pleomorphic. The chromatin is coarsely clumped, nucleoli are present, and the nuclei often have numerous lobes that resemble flowers or clover. The cytoplasm is deeply basophilic. A small number of cells may resemble blasts, with dispersed nuclear chromatin. The bone marrow pattern may be patchy, interstitial, or diffuse. Cell size varies from small to large but, in most cases, the nuclei are pleomorphic in shape, lobulation, and chromatin appearance. Nucleoli are usually prominent. In the chronic and smoldering variants, small cells with minimal cellular abnormalities may be present. Osteoclasts and bone marrow resorption commonly are increased, sometimes even when neoplastic cells are not apparent.

In some patients with early or smoldering disease the lymph nodes resemble Hodgkin lymphoma in having diffuse paracortical infiltrates of small- to medium-sized lymphocytes and interspersed Reed-Sternberg–like cells (large cells with multiple nuclei containing prominent nucleoli) and giant cells with convoluted or lobulated nuclei. These cells, which express CD30 and CD15, are EBV-positive B lymphocytes, thought to proliferate in this disease because of the immunodeficiency that the T-cell neoplasm causes.

Extranodal NK-/T-Cell Lymphoma, Nasal Type

This disorder, virtually always associated with Epstein-Barr virus when it involves the nose, is more common in males than females and is more frequent in Asia and Latin America than elsewhere. It may develop in immunocompromised patients, including organ transplant recipients. The disease typically occurs in adults and originates as a mass or diffuse neoplastic infiltration causing nasal obstruction, pain, or bleeding. The process can extend to neighboring structures, causing swelling or destruction of the affected tissues. From these areas, it can disseminate to distant sites, such as the gastrointestinal tract, cervical lymph nodes, and the skin, where nodules and ulcers may form. When the disease originates outside the nasal cavity, systemic symptoms can occur, and multiple sites, such as skin and alimentary tract, often are involved.

The lymphoma cells commonly are intermingled with numerous benign cells, such as small lymphocytes, histiocytes, eosinophils, and plasma cells, making the disease often appear inflammatory rather than neoplastic. The process is destructive, typically causing ulceration and necrosis. It tends to occur around vessels, which it destroys. The cells are diverse in size and appearance. They may have irregular and elongated nuclei, often undergoing mitosis, with granular chromatin. The cytoplasm is commonly pale.

The peripheral blood film rarely discloses neoplastic cells, which have azurophilic cytoplasmic granules. Similarly, the bone marrow rarely is involved with neoplastic cells.

Hepatosplenic T-Cell Lymphoma

This rare disorder typically occurs in adolescents and young adults, affecting males much more frequently than females. Some patients have had previous solid organ transplants. The main clinical feature is marked hepatosplenomegaly, usually accompanied by thrombocytopenia. Lymph nodes usually are not enlarged. Anemia, sometimes from hemolysis, and leukocytosis also may occur. The peripheral blood film rarely shows neoplastic cells, but they usually are present on the bone marrow aspirate as medium-sized lymphocytes with dispersed chromatin and mildly basophilic cytoplasm. The marrow biopsy shows interstitial or intrasinusoidal infiltration with medium- to large-sized lymphoid cells with a rim of pale cytoplasm.

Mycosis Fungoides and Sézary Syndrome

This disorder occurs most commonly in adults, with a male:female ratio of about 2:1. It is a T-cell cutaneous lymphoma that begins as flat areas of scaling and erythema that may be asymptomatic or pruritic. At varying intervals, but typically after several years, it may progress to cause dusky red to violaceous plaques—sharply demarcated lesions that are elevated above the surrounding normal skin. Sometimes, lymph nodes are enlarged, but biopsies commonly show a reactive pattern, rather than neoplastic infiltrates. If the disease continues to advance, the next stage is the formation of cutaneous tumors. Only then does the lymphoma tend to spread to extracutaneous sites, typically, lymph nodes, spleen, liver, and lungs.

Confident pathologic diagnosis of mycosis fungoides can be very difficult, especially in the early stages, and numerous skin biopsies, sometimes taken over intervals of months to years, may be necessary before the characteristic findings are clearly present. The diagnostic abnormality consists of dermal and epidermal infiltration of small- to medium-sized T cells with irregular nuclei whose convolutions resemble the brain (cerebriform nuclei). In the dermis, infiltrates typically are present at the epidermal border and consist of small lymphocytes, eosinophils, and the neoplastic cells. Single or small numbers of the neoplastic cells may be present in the epidermis, but sometimes many aggregate there to form *Pautrier's abscesses*. Enlarged lymph nodes commonly represent *dermatopathic lymphadenopathy*, which consists of numerous histiocytes expanding the paracortical areas. A few cerebriform lymphocytes may be present, but not in clusters. This Grade I disease is considered to be uninvolved by neoplasm. Early involvement with mycosis fungoides (Grade II) shows focal disruption of lymph node architecture by aggregates of atypical cerebriform lymphocytes. Grade III lymph nodes have complete replacement of the lymph node by diffuse infiltrates of atypical cerebriform cells. One variant of mycosis fungoides is *pagetoid reticulosis*, in which a chronic solitary plaque is present, and the neoplastic cells are located only in the epidermis. Another is follicular mucinosis, in which the lymphoma cells are present only in hair follicles, where they cause mucinous degeneration. Clinically, the lesions are indurated papules or plaques, which in hairy areas can cause alopecia.

Sézary syndrome may be another variant of mycosis fungoides or, at least, closely resembles it. It occurs in adults and is defined by erythroderma (cutaneous redness and scaling involving nearly all the skin surface), generalized lymph node enlargement, and the presence of circulating neoplastic cells. Pruritus is typically present, and the disease may cause alopecia. As in mycosis fungoides, the skin shows dermal and epidermal infiltration with cerebriform lymphocytes. Lymph nodes show Grade II or III involvement. The peripheral blood film has numerous small or large neoplastic cells with cerebriform nuclei containing condensed chromatin. The N:C ratio is large. Because these cells may appear in small numbers in both benign skin diseases and early stages of mycosis fungoides, most criteria require that their level exceed 1,000/mm^3. Because mycosis fungoides can cause erythroderma, some experts distinguish it from Sézary syndrome according to this hematologic criterion.

Peripheral T-Cell Lymphoma, Unspecified

This category includes about 50% of the peripheral T-cell lymphomas in Western countries. Most cases occur in adults, and the disease usually presents with nodal involvement, but disseminated disease is common, often with circulating neoplastic cells and affected extranodal sites, especially the skin. Constitutional symptoms, such as weight loss, fever, and fatigue, are frequent.

These lymphomas cause diffuse infiltration of lymph nodes with neoplastic cells that are variable, but most commonly medium- to large-sized cells with irregular, pleomorphic nuclei and prominent nucleoli. Vascular proliferation in the lymph node is common, and often a mixed inflammatory reaction is prominent, including eosinophils, plasma cells, small lymphocytes, and epithelioid histiocytes. Multinucleated cells resembling Reed-Sternberg cells and "clear cells" with very pale cytoplasm may be present. Two rare subtypes are the T-zone and lymphoepithelioid cell variants. The former has small- to medium-sized neoplastic cells in intact follicles. The latter has small cells and numerous clusters of epithelioid histiocytes.

Anaplastic Large-Cell Lymphoma

This disorder causes about 3% of adult non-Hodgkin lymphoma and about 10% to 30% in childhood. The usual clinical features are generalized lymph node enlargement and constitutional symptoms, including fever. The disease is commonly widespread at the time of diagnosis, typically involving such extranodal sites as skin, bone, lung, and liver. The neoplastic cells are pleomorphic, but despite this lymphoma's having three variants—common, lymphohistiocytic, and small-cell—all cases include some characteristic cells called "hallmark cells" because they are present in all types. These have eccentric nuclei shaped like horseshoes or kidneys, sometimes with a perinuclear eosinophilic area. They are usually, but not always, large. In the *common variant*, which accounts for about 70% of cases, large hallmark cells typically predominate, and they possess abundant cytoplasm that is clear, basophilic, or eosinophilic. Multiple nuclei may occur, the chromatin usually is dispersed, and nucleoli are prominent. Sometimes, the hallmark cells are less numerous than the large neoplastic cells with rounded nuclei. In the *lymphohistiocytic variant*, which constitutes about 10% of cases, the numerous histiocytes coexist with and may outnumber the neoplastic cells, which may be smaller than in the common variant and tend to aggregate around vessels. The histiocytes may demonstrate erythrophagocytosis. In the *small-cell variant*, which accounts for about 5% to 10% of cases, the major neoplastic cells are small to medium in size and have irregular nuclei. Hallmark cells tend to aggregate around blood vessels. Neoplastic cells are rarely visible in the peripheral blood film, where they are large and pleomorphic. On bone marrow aspirates, they are also usually sparse. Bone marrow biopsies may show the large, pleomorphic, and sometimes multinucleated lymphoma cells in an interstitial, focal, or diffuse pattern.

HODGKIN LYMPHOMA

Hodgkin lymphomas constitute about 30% of all lymphomas. The characteristic tumor cells, which have single (Hodgkin cells) or multiple nuclei (Reed-Sternberg cells), intermingle with inflammatory cells and other non-neoplastic cells. The WHO classification divides this disorder into two major categories: nodular lymphocyte–predominant Hodgkin lymphoma and classical Hodgkin lymphoma, which has four subtypes—nodular sclerosis, mixed-cellularity, lymphocyte-rich, and lymphocyte-depleted Hodgkin lymphoma.

Hodgkin lymphoma is classified according to Stages I through IV.

- Stage I: Single lymph node region or lymphoid organ (spleen, thymus, Waldeyer ring) is involved.
- Stage II: ≥ 2 lymph node regions involved on same side of diaphragm, with number of anatomic sites indicated by suffix (e.g., II_3).
- Stage III: Lymph node regions or structures involved on both sides of the diaphragm:
  - III_1: with or without splenic, hilar, celiac, or portal nodes
  - III_2: with paraaortic, iliac, or mesenteric nodes
- Stage IV: Involvement of extranodal sites beyond those designated E.
- E: Involvement of a single extranodal site or contiguous with or proximal to nodal diseases site.

Other qualifying designations include the presence or absence of specific constitutional symptoms: A: no symptoms; B: fever, drenching sweats, or weight loss. The presence of bulky disease, X, is defined by greater than one-third mediastinal widening at T5–T6 or a nodal mass >10 cm.

The neoplastic cells rarely appear in the peripheral blood smear. Even with marrow involvement, they are also uncommon in the bone marrow aspirate, where they appear as large cells with two nuclei and prominent nucleoli. On bone marrow biopsy, neoplastic cells are present in about 10% of cases and usually exist in a mixture of small lymphocytes, eosinophils, and macrophages. The pattern can be either focal or diffuse. Variations include the presence of numerous Reed-Sternberg cells with few other cells, a fibrotic marrow with few neoplastic cells, and a hypocellular marrow with scattered foci of neoplastic and reactive cells.

Nodular Lymphocyte–Predominant Hodgkin Lymphoma

This monoclonal B-cell disorder accounts for about 5% of Hodgkin lymphoma and typically occurs in adults 30 to 50 years of age, with males more commonly affected than are females. It usually causes localized lymph node enlargement in cervical, axillary, and inguinal lymph nodes. These nodes are replaced partly or completely by a nodular or diffuse infiltrate of small lymphocytes, histiocytes, and large neoplastic cells that are variants of Reed-Sternberg cells, known as popcorn or L&H (lymphocytic and histiocytic) cells. These usually have a single, large nucleus that often is folded or multilobulated, with several basophilic nucleoli, and sparse cytoplasm.

Classical Hodgkin Lymphoma

This group accounts for 95% of cases of Hodgkin lymphoma and tends to occur in two age groups: between 15 and 35 years and a second, smaller group in the sixth decade. Most patients present with localized lymph node enlargement affecting cervical, mediastinal, axillary, or para-aortic regions. The spleen often is affected, but primary extranodal involvement is rare, as is bone marrow infiltration, except in advanced disease. The diagnosis requires finding neoplastic cells. One type is Reed-Sternberg cells, which are large with multiple nuclei or nuclear lobes and prominent eosinophilic nucleoli, at least two in two separate nuclear lobes to be diagnostic. Similar, but mononuclear, cells are called Hodgkin cells. These cells are thought to originate nearly always from mature B cells in the germinal center. Rarely, they derive from peripheral T cells. Accompanying and far outnumbering these neoplastic cells are reactive, non-neoplastic cells, whose identity varies according to the histologic subtype.

Nodular Sclerosis Hodgkin Lymphoma

This type accounts for about 70% of classical Hodgkin lymphoma, with a median age of 28 and equal gender distribution. Most patients present with stage II disease, and about 40% have B symptoms. The most common site of involvement is the mediastinum. The affected lymph nodes demonstrate the presence of collagen bands that divide the lymphoid tissue into nodules. The neoplastic cells, which occur in a mixture of small lymphocytes, plasma cells, eosinophils, and macrophages, tend to have nuclei with more lobules and smaller nucleoli than in other types of classical Hodgkin lymphoma. In formalin-fixed tissue sections, a clear space surrounds these Reed-Sternberg cells because of cytoplasmic retraction, giving them the name of *lacunar cells*, because they seem to rest in lacunae.

Mixed-Cellularity Hodgkin Lymphoma

This type accounts for about 25% of cases of classical Hodgkin lymphoma, is more common in males, sometimes occurs in patients with HIV infection, and has evidence of genomes of Epstein-Barr virus in the tissue in at least 70% of cases. The average age is about 35 to 40 years. Patients commonly have advanced disease and B symptoms, with widespread enlargement of peripheral lymph nodes. The spleen is involved in 30% of patients. The internal structure of the lymph nodes is effaced by diffuse infiltration with a combination of small lymphocytes, plasma cells, eosinophils, macrophages, and numerous neoplastic cells, including both Reed-Sternberg cells and mononuclear variants.

Lymphocyte-Rich Classical Hodgkin Lymphoma

In this disease, which constitutes about 5% of classical Hodgkin disease, peripheral lymph node enlargement is the main feature, and patients usually have stage I or II disease without B symptoms. About 70% of patients are males. The lymph nodes can show a diffuse or nodular pattern with numerous small lymphocytes, no neutrophils or eosinophils, and scattered neoplastic cells that can either be characteristic Reed-Sternberg and Hodgkin cells or resemble L&H cells. About 40% have evidence of infection with Epstein-Barr virus.

Lymphocyte-Depleted Classical Hodgkin Lymphoma

This type, which accounts for <5% of classical Hodgkin lymphoma, often is associated with HIV infection. The median age is 37 years, and about 75% of patients are male. Peripheral lymph nodes are less commonly involved than are retroperitoneal lymph nodes, abdominal organs, and bone marrow. Most patients have advanced disease with B symptoms. The lymph nodes have a relative paucity of lymphocytes compared with neoplastic cells. Sometimes, diffuse fibrosis is present, and the neoplastic cells may be pleomorphic. Evidence of Epstein-Barr infection is common.

Table 5.1

World Health Organization classification of lymphoproliferative disorders

B-cell Neoplasms

Precursor B-cell neoplasm

Precursor B-lymphoblastic
  leukemia/lymphoma

Mature B-cell neoplasms

Chronic lymphocytic leukemia/small
  lymphocytic lymphoma

B-cell prolymphocytic leukemia

Lymphoplasmacytic lymphoma

Splenic marginal-zone B-cell lymphoma

Hairy cell leukemia

Plasma cell myeloma

Monoclonal gammopathy of
  undetermined significance

Solitary plasmacytoma of bone

Extraosseous plasmacytoma

Primary amyloidosis

Heavy-chain diseases

Extranodal marginal zone B-cell
  lymphoma of mucosa-associated
  lymphoid tissue

Nodal marginal zone B-cell lymphoma

Follicular lymphoma

Mantle cell lymphoma

Diffuse large B-cell lymphoma

Mediastinal (thymic) large B-cell
  lymphoma

Intravascular large B-cell lymphoma

Primary effusion lymphoma

Burkitt lymphoma/leukemia

**B-cell proliferations of uncertain
  malignant potential**

Lymphomatoid granulomatosis

Posttransplant lymphoproliferative
  disorder, polymorphic

T-cell and NK-cell Neoplasms

Precursor T-cell neoplasm

Precursor T-lymphoblastic
  leukemia/lymphoma

Mature T-cell and NK-cell neoplasms

T-cell prolymphocytic leukemia

T-cell large granular lymphocytic leukemia

Aggressive NK-cell leukemia

Adult T-cell leukemia/lymphoma

Extranodal NK-/T-cell lymphoma, nasal type

Enteropathy-type T-cell lymphoma

Hepatosplenic T-cell lymphoma

Subcutaneous panniculitis-like T-cell
  lymphoma

Mycosis fungoides

Sézary syndrome

Primary cutaneous anaplastic large cell
  lymphoma

Anaplastic large cell lymphoma

Angioimmunoblastic T-cell lymphoma

Peripheral T-cell lymphoma, unspecified

**T-cell proliferation of uncertain malignant
  potential**

Lymphomatoid papulosis

**Neoplasm of uncertain lineage and stage of
  differentiation**

Blastic NK-cell lymphoma

Hodgkin lymphoma

Nodular lymphocyte predominance

Classical

  Nodular sclerosis

  Lymphocyte-rich

  Mixed cellularity

  Lymphocyte depletion

NK, natural killer.
Adapted with permission from *Wintrobe's Clinical Hematology*, 11th Edition, page 2304.

Table 5.2

Selected antibodies that are useful in immunophenotypic analysis of non-hodgkin lymphomas

Clusters of Differentiation (CD)

Number	Antibodies	Reactivity
CD1	Leu-6, T6, and OKT6	Thymocytes, dendritic cells, and epidermal Langerhans cells
CD2	Leu-5, T11, and OKT11	T cells and natural killer cells
CD3	Leu-4, T3, OKT3, UCHT-1, and poly-CD3	T cells
CD4	Leu-3, T4, and OKT4	Helper and inducer T cells, monocytes, and macrophages
CD5	Leu-1, T1, OKT1, and UCHT-2	T cells and B-cell subset
CD7	Leu-9 and 3A1	T cells and natural killer cells
CD8	Leu-2, T8, OKT8, and UCHT-4	T-cytotoxic and -suppressor cells and natural killer cells
CD10	CALLA, J5, and BA-3	Progenitor B lymphocytes and B-cell subset (follicular center cells)
CD11b	Leu-15 and Mo-1	Granulocytes, monocytes, natural killer cells, T-cell subset
CD11c	Leu-M5 and Ki-M1	Monocytes and macrophages, granulocytes, natural killer cells, and B-cell subset (hairy cell leukemia and monocytoid B cells)
CD14	Leu-M3, Mo2, MY4, and UCHM-1	Monocytes, granulocytes, and epidermal Langerhans cells
CD15	Leu-M1 and MY1	Granulocytes, monocytes, Reed-Sternberg cells, activated lymphocytes, and some epithelial cells
CD16	Leu-11	Natural killer cells, granulocytes, macrophages, and T-cell subset
CD19	Leu-12 and B4	B cells
CD20	Leu-16, B1, and L26	B cells
CD21	B2	B-cell subset and follicular dendritic cells
CD22	Leu-14	B-cell subset
CD23	Leu-20 and B6	Activated B cells and follicular mantle B cells
CD24	BA-1	B cells and granulocytes
CD25	IL2R and Tac	Activated T and B cells and activated macrophages
CD30	Ki-1 and Ber-H2	Activated T and B cells and Reed-Sternberg cells
CD38	Leu-17 and T10	Plasma cells, thymocytes, and activated T cells

Table 5.2

Selected antibodies that are useful in immunophenotypic analysis of non-hodgkin lymphomas (continued)

Cluster of Differentiation (continued)

CD43	Leu-22, MT1, and DFT1	T cells, B-cell subset, granulocytes, and monocytes and macrophages
CD45	T29/33, HLe-1, and T200	Leukocytes
CD45RA	Leu-18 and 4KB5	B cells, T-cell subset, granulocytes, and monocytes
CD45RB	LCA and PD7/26/16	B cells, T-cell subset, granulocytes, and monocytes and macrophages
CD45RO	UCHL1 and A6	T cells, B-cell subset, granulocytes, and monocytes and mocrophages
CD56	Leu-19 and NKH1	Natural killer cells and T-cell subset
CD57	Leu-7 and HNK1	Natural killer cells and T-cell subset
CD68	KP1, Ki-M6, and KiM7	Monocytes and macrophages
CD71	T9 and OKT9	Activated T and B cells, macrophages, and proliferating cells
CD74	LN2	B cells, monocytes and macrophages, and Reed-Sternberg cells
CDw75	LN1	B cells and some epithelial cells
CD79a	mb-1	B cells
CD103	HML-1	Intestinal intraepithelial T cells
CD138	Syndecan	Plasma cells and plasmablasts
	IgG, A, M, D, and E	Immunoglobulin heavy chains
	κ, λ	Immunoglobulin light chains
	Anti-TCR $\alpha\beta$, βF1	$\alpha\beta$ T cells
	Anti-TCR $\gamma\sigma$	$\gamma\sigma$ T cells
	HLA-DR and LN3	Activated T and B cells, monocytes, and macrophages
	Anti-TdT	Lymphoblasts and some myeloblasts
	Anti-lysozyme	Monocytes, macrophages, and granulocytes
	MAC 387	Macrophage subset
	EMA	Epithelial cells, plasma cells, and some lymphoid neoplasms, including lymphocyte predominant Hodgkin lymphoma and anaplastic large cell lymphoma
	Ki-67, PCNA	Nuclear proliferation antigens
	Antiperforin, antigranzymes A, B, and C; and anti-TIA-1	Cytolytic granule-associated proteins in natural killer cells and cytotoxic T cells

Table 5.3

Staging of non-hodgkin lymphoma

Staging System	Stage	Definition		
Ann Arbor	I	Involvement of a single lymph node region or a single extranodal organ or site (stage I_E).		
	II	Involvement of two or more node regions on the same side of the diaphragm or localized involvement of an extranodal site or organ (stage II_E) and one or more lymph node regions on the same side of the diaphragm.		
	III	Involvement of lymph node regions on both sides of the diaphragm that may also be accompanied by localized involvement of an extranodal organ or site (stage III_E) or spleen (stage III_S), or both (stage III_{SE}).		
	IV	Diffuse or disseminated involvement of one or more distant extranodal organs with or without associated lymph node involvement.		
	B symptoms	Fever >38°C, night sweats, or weight loss >10% of body weight in the 6 mo preceding admission, or a combination of these, is defined as a systemic symptom.		
National Cancer Institute Modified Staging System	I	One or two nodal sites or one extranodal site of disease without poor prognostic features.		
	II	More than two nodal sites of disease or one or more localized extranodal sites plus draining nodes with none of the following poor prognostic features: performance status ≤70, B symptoms, any mass >10 cm in diameter (particularly abdominal), serum lactate dehydrogenase >500 IU/dl, bone marrow involvement, three or more extranodal sites of disease.		
	III	Stage I or II plus any poor prognostic features.		
International Prognostic Index		Adverse factors	Risk group	Number of factors
		Performance status ≥2[a]	Low	0, 1
		Lactate dehydrogenase > normal[a]	Low-intermediate	2
		Extranodal sites ≥2	High-intermediate	3
		Stage III and IV disease[a]	High	4, 5
		Age >60 yr		

[a]Age-adjusted factors.
Reprinted with permission from *Wintrobe's Clinical Hematology*, 11th Edition, page 2374.

Table 5.4

Pathologic features in the differential diagnosis of small B-cell lymphomas

	Growth Pattern	Cytology	Immunophenotype			Surface Ig	Cytogenetics
			CD5	CD23	CD10		
B-cell chronic lymphocytic leukemia/small lymphocytic lymphoma	Diffuse effacement with proliferation centers	Small round nuclei, scant cytoplasm	+	+	−	Weak IgM and IgD	Trisomy 12 dels: 17p13, 11q22, 13q14
Lymphoplasmacytic lymphoma	Diffuse or interfollicular	Small lymphocytes, plasma cells, and plasmacytoid lymphocytes	−	−	−	Moderate IgM	t(9;14) (p13;q32)
Mantle cell lymphoma	Diffuse or vaguely nodular	Irregular nuclei, scant cytoplasm, and few large cells	+	−	−	Moderate IgM and IgD Lambda > kappa	t(11;14) (q13;q32)
Follicular lymphoma	Follicular	Irregular cleaved nuclei (centrocytes) and admixed large cells (centroblasts)	−	−	+	Bright IgM > IgG > IgA	t(14;18) (q32;q21) >85%
Nodal marginal zone B-cell lymphoma	Interfollicular and perisinusoidal	Small, round, and folded nuclei and abundant cytoplasm ± plasma cells	−	−	−	Moderate IgM	Trisomy 3
Extranodal marginal zone B-cell lymphoma of mucosa-associated lymphoid tissue	Diffuse	Small, round, and folded nuclei and abundant cytoplasm ± plasma cells	−	−	−	IgM	Trisomy 3 t(11;18) (q21;q21)

Ig, immunoglobulin; +, positive; −, negative.
Adapted with permission from *Wintrobe's Clinical Hematology*, 11th Edition, page 2304.

Table 5.5

Immunophenotype of CLL and other chronic B-cell disorders

Condition	smIg	CD5	CD10	CD11c	CD19	CD20	CD22	CD23	CD25	CD43	CD79b	CD103	FMC7
Chronic lymphocytic leukemia	Dim	++	−	−/+	++	Dim	−/+	++	+/−	+	−	−	−/+
Waldenström macroglobulinemia	++	−	−	−/+	++	++	+	−	−/+	+/−	+	−	+
Prolymphocytic leukemia	+++	−/+	−/+	−/+	++	+++	++	++	−/+	+	++	−	+
HCL	+++	−	−	++	+++	+++	+++	−	+++	+	+	+++	+++
HCL variant	+++	−	−	++	+++	+++	+++	−	−	+	+	+++	+++
Splenic lymphoma with villous lymphocytes	++	−/+	−/+	+/−	++	++	++	+/−	−/+	+	++	−/+	++
Marginal-zone B-cell lymphoma	++	−	−	+/−	++	++	+/−	+/−	−	−/+	++	−	+
Mantle cell lymphoma	++	++	−/+	−	++	++	++	−	−	+	++	−	++
Follicular lymphoma	++	−/+	++	−	++	++	++	−/+	−	−	++	−	++

−, not expressed; −/+, usually is not expressed; +/−, usually is expressed; + to +++, varying degrees of strength of expression; HCL, hairy cell leukemia; smIg, surface membrane immunoglobin.
Reprinted with permission from *Wintrobe's Clinical Hematology*, 11th Edition, page 2438.

Diagram 5.1

Oncoproteins targeted by chromosomal translocations in children and adult B-cell lymphoproliferative disorders

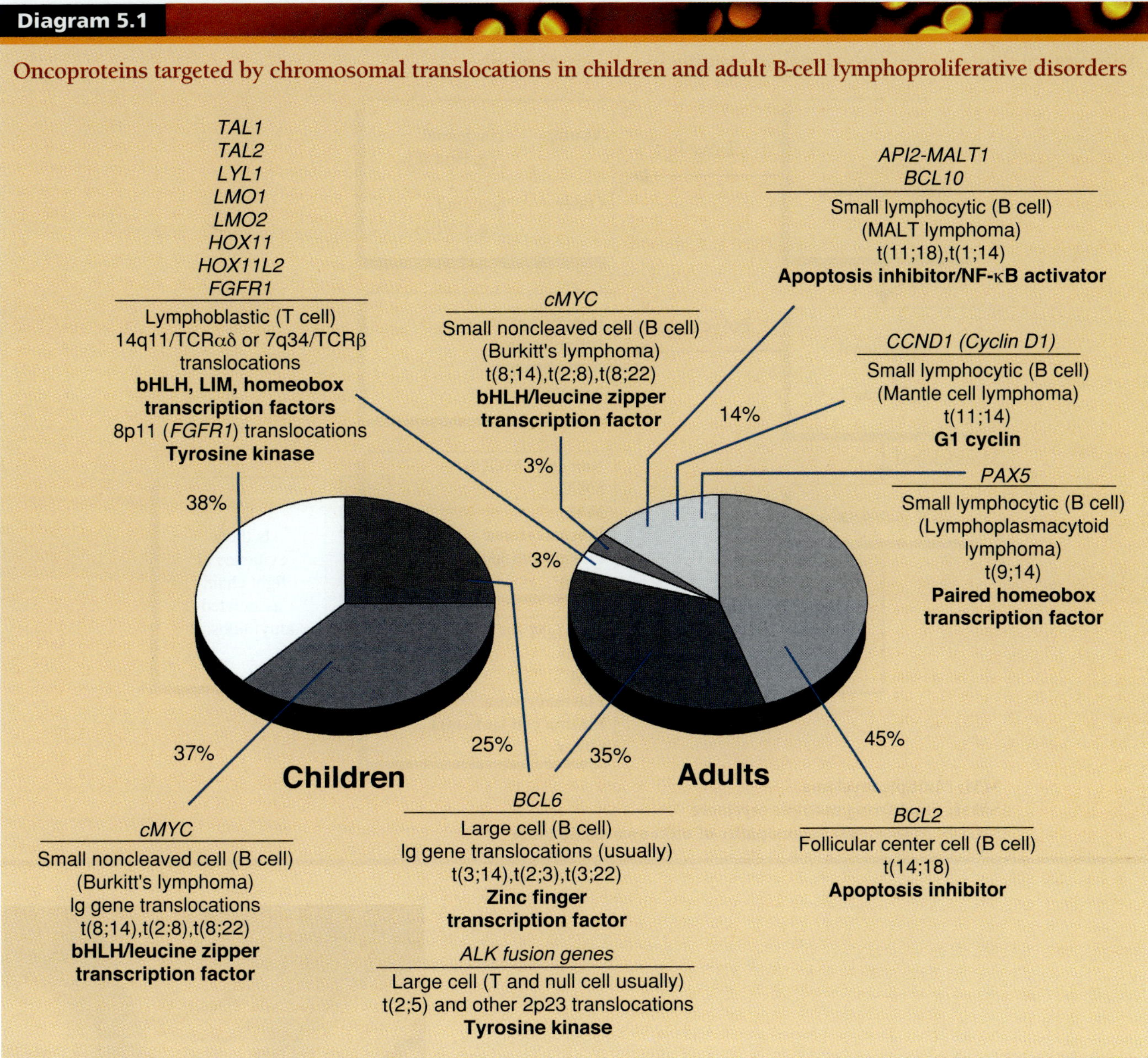

Reprinted with permission from *Wintrobe's Clinical Hematology*, 11th Edition, page 2327.

Diagram 5.2

Differential diagnoses of polyclonal and monoclonal gammopathies

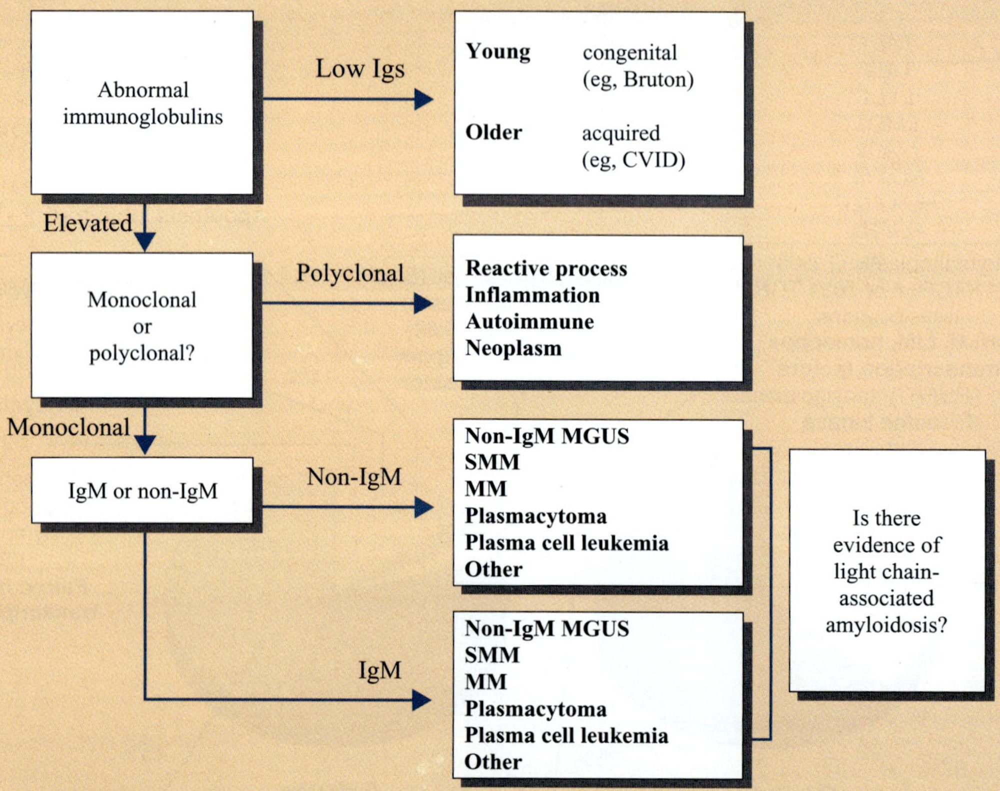

Abnormal immunoglobulins

— Low Igs →

Young congenital (eg, Bruton)

Older acquired (eg, CVID)

↓ Elevated

Monoclonal or polyclonal?

— Polyclonal →

Reactive process
Inflammation
Autoimmune
Neoplasm

↓ Monoclonal

IgM or non-IgM

— Non-IgM →

Non-IgM MGUS
SMM
MM
Plasmacytoma
Plasma cell leukemia
Other

— IgM →

Non-IgM MGUS
SMM
MM
Plasmacytoma
Plasma cell leukemia
Other

Is there evidence of light chain-associated amyloidosis?

MM: Multiple myeloma
SMM: Smoldering multiple myeloma
MGUS: Monoclonal gammopathy of unknown significance

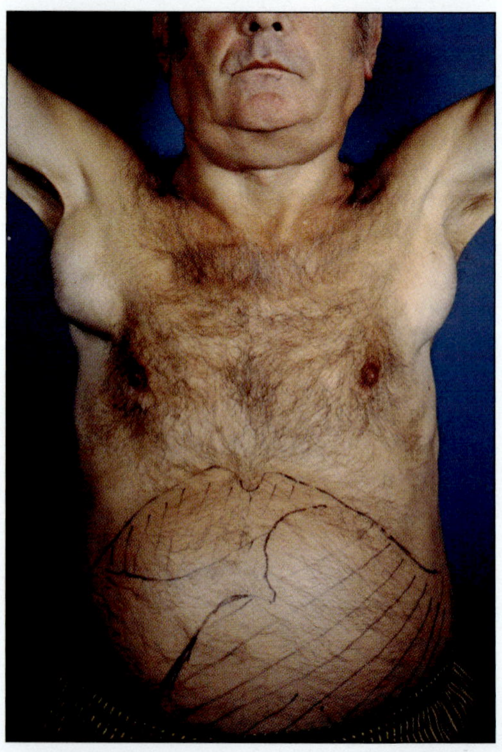

Figure 5.1 Generalized lymphadenopathy in chronic lymphocytic lymphoma/small lymphocytic lymphoma (CLL/SLL). Bilateral axillary lymphadenopathy and hepatosplenomegaly are present in a patient with advanced stage CLL/SLL. (Courtesy Dr. D. Amato.)

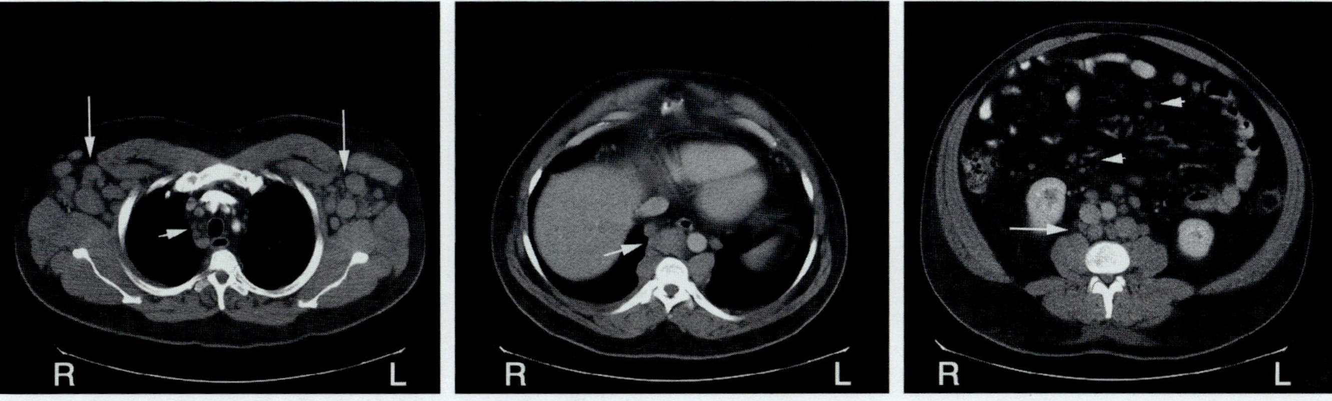

Figure 5.2 Generalized lymphadenopathy in CLL/SLL. Axial computed tomography (CT) scans from a case of CLL/SLL. *Left panel:* Upper thorax shows prominent bilateral axillary lymphadenopathy (*long arrows*) and some small mediastinal lymph nodes (*short arrow*). *Middle panel:* Lower thorax/upper abdomen reveals prominent retrocrural lymphadenopathy (*arrow*). Enlarged retroperitoneal (*long arrow*) and multiple prominent mesenteric lymph nodes (*short arrows*) are present in the right panel.

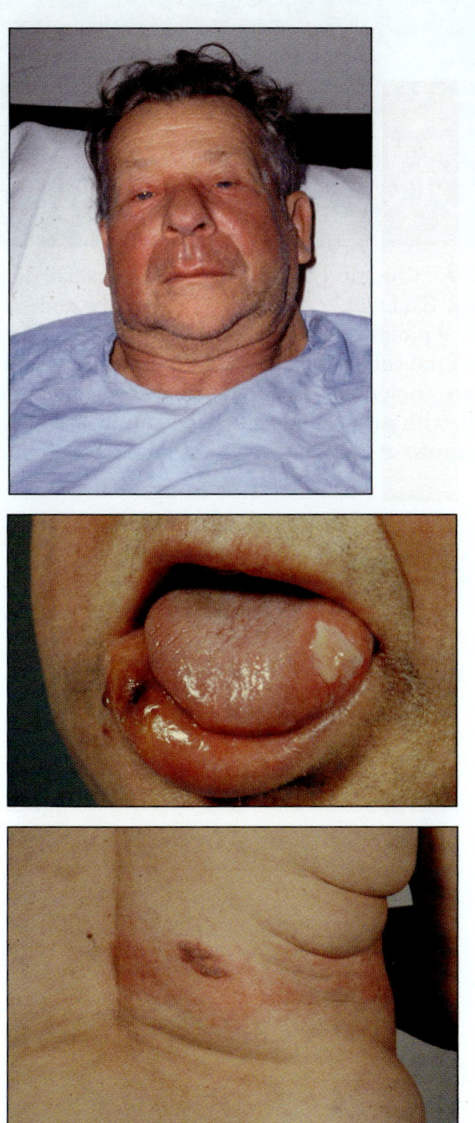

Figure 5.3 *Top panel:* Erysipelas in a patient with CLL. (Courtesy Dr. P. Galbraith.) Herpes Simplex I gingivostomatitis (*middle panel*) and varicella-zoster shingles (*bottom panel*) in two patients with CLL. (Courtesy Dr. I. Quirt.)

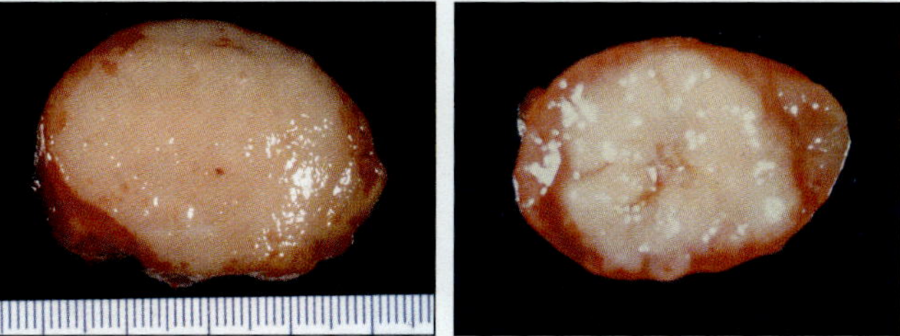

Figure 5.4 Enlarged lymph nodes. Gross lymph nodes specimens have been cut to show characteristic homogenous pattern ("fish flesh" appearance) of a lymph node diffusely involved by CLL/SLL on the left, as compared with the nodular, heterogeneous appearance of a lymph node involved with metastatic cancer on the right.

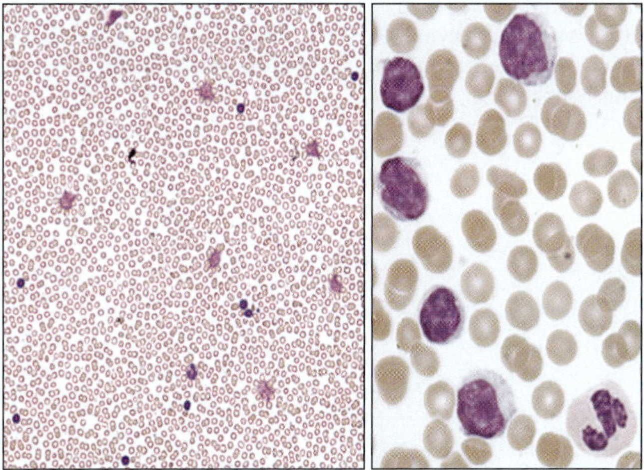

Figure 5.5 CLL in blood smear. A low-power view of a blood smear shows lymphocytosis with smudge cells (*left panel*). A higher-power view demonstrates the typical appearance of the CLL cell: a small mature lymphocyte with condensed, clumpy chromatin pattern ("soccer ball" pattern) and regular nuclear contours (*right panel*). CLL cells can be difficult to distinguish from normal circulating lymphocytes.

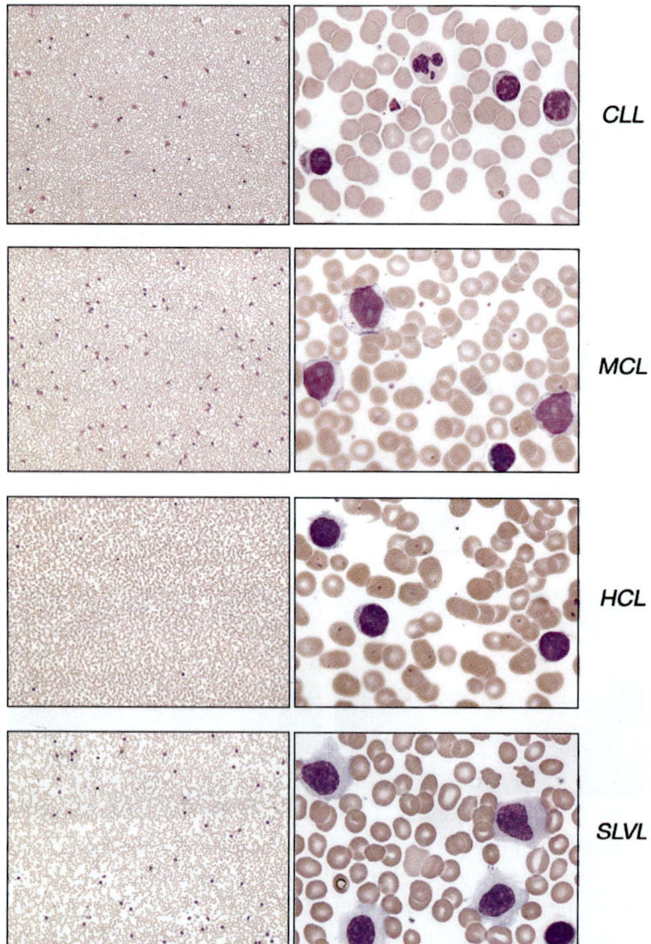

Figure 5.6 Mature B-cell neoplasms in peripheral blood. Low- and high-power views on the left and right sides of the figure, respectively, show the four common mature B-cell lymphoproliferative disorders in blood: CLL, chronic lymphocytic leukemia; MCL, Mantle cell lymphoma; HCL, hairy cell leukemia; SLVL, splenic lymphoma with villous lymphocytes (splenic marginal zone lymphoma).

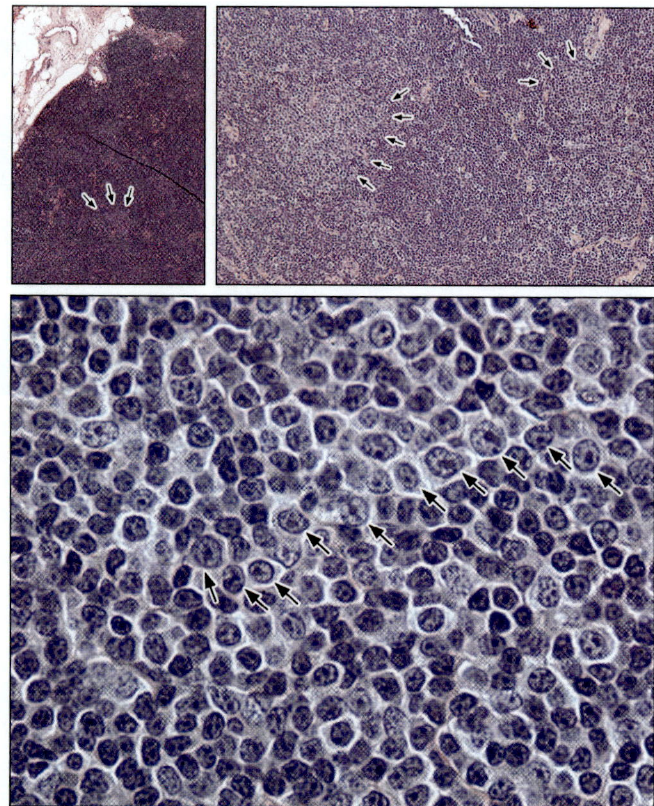

Figure 5.7 Chronic lymphocytic leukemia/small lymphocytic lymphoma (CLL/SLL). An internal mammary node is diffusely effaced by a proliferation of small, mature lymphocytes with high N:C ratios and condensed chromatin. Inconspicuous proliferation centers are composed of prolymphocytes and immunoblasts— larger cells with paler-staining nuclei and nucleoli, which are delineated by arrows at the boundary of the proliferation centers.

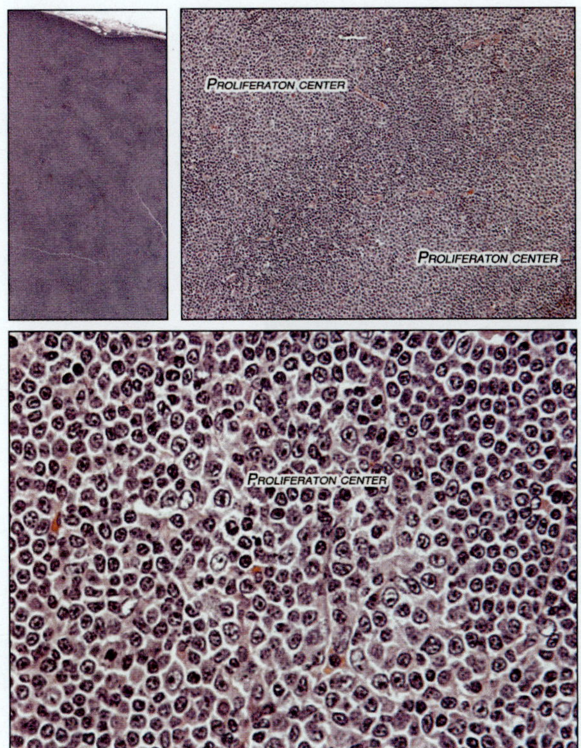

Figure 5.8   CLL/SLL. The lymph node is diffusely replaced by small mature lymphocytes with high N:C ratios and condensed chromatin. Coalescent proliferation centers consisting of prolymphocytes and immunoblasts surround the smaller, mature-appearing CLL cells.

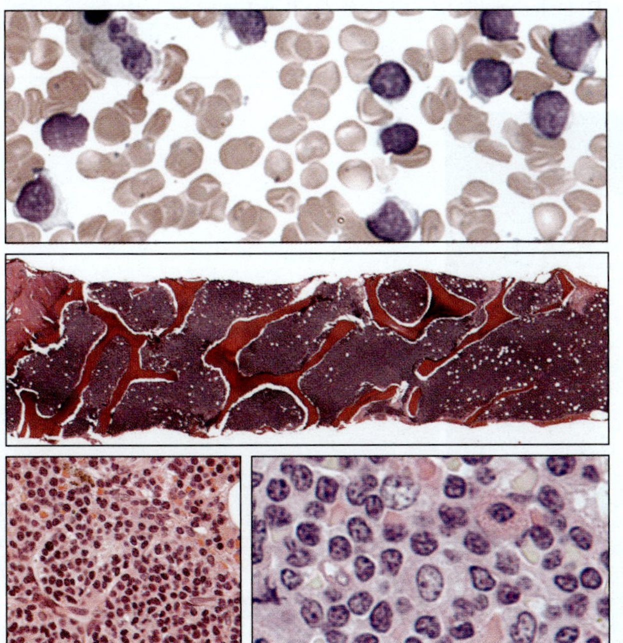

Figure 5.9   Diffuse marrow involvement by CLL/SLL. A blood smear demonstrates mature lymphocytosis (*upper panel*) and various magnified views of a marrow biopsy are shown (*lower panels*). The biopsy shows a diffuse pattern of involvement of marrow by CLL, with total effacement of the architecture by small, mature lymphoid cells possessing regular nuclear contours.

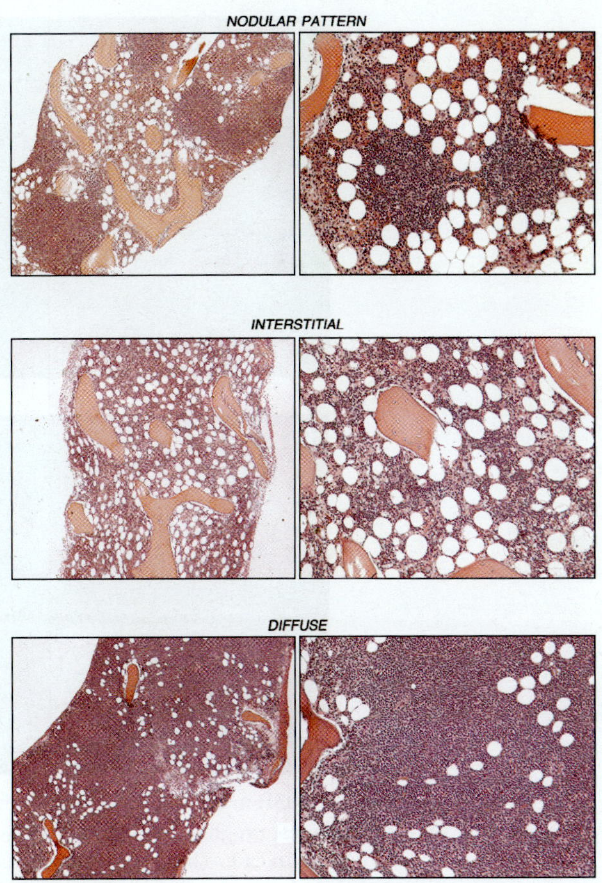

Figure 5.10   Patterns of marrow involvement by CLL. Low- and higher-power views of bone marrow biopsies are shown on the left and right, respectively, demonstrating the three patterns commonly seen in marrow involvement by CLL: nodular, interstitial, and diffuse. Nodular infiltration indicates the presence of foci of lymphoma cells separated by unaffected bone marrow and is typically distributed in a mid-paratrabecular pattern in CLL (*upper panels*). Interstitial infiltration is marked by diffuse, patchy bone marrow invasion by individual CLL cells interspersed between hematopoietic and fat cells. Diffuse infiltration, associated with a poorer prognosis, involves complete effacement of bone marrow architecture by sheets of lymphoma cells.

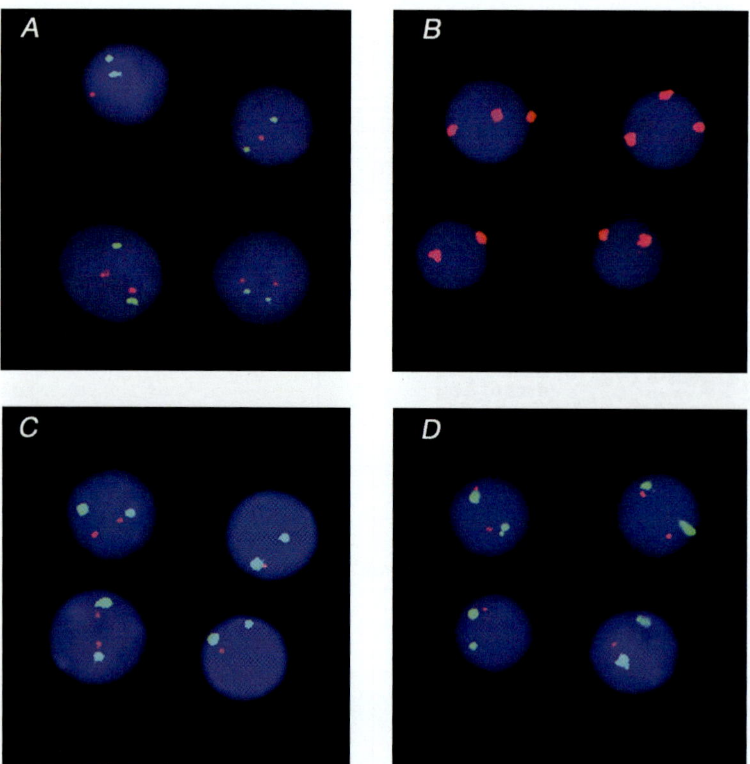

Figure 5.11 FISH in CLL. Cytogenetic abnormalities such as del(17)(p13.1) and del(11)(q22) portend rapid disease progression and poor survival, whereas del(13)(q14.3) as the sole abnormality has good prognosis in CLL. The significance of trisomy 12 is undetermined. The loss of p53 function predicts poor survival in this disease. This slide shows results from an interphase FISH panel performed on CLL cells. **A.** Deletion of the ATM gene (*red*) at 11q22.3 compared with a centromere 11 control (*green*). **B.** Trisomy 12 as indicated by three centromere 12 signals. **C.** Deletion of the 13q14.3 region (*red*) as compared to the LAMP1 gene (*green*) at 13q34. **D.** Deletion of the p53 gene (*red*) at 17p13 as compared with a centromere 17 control (*green*).

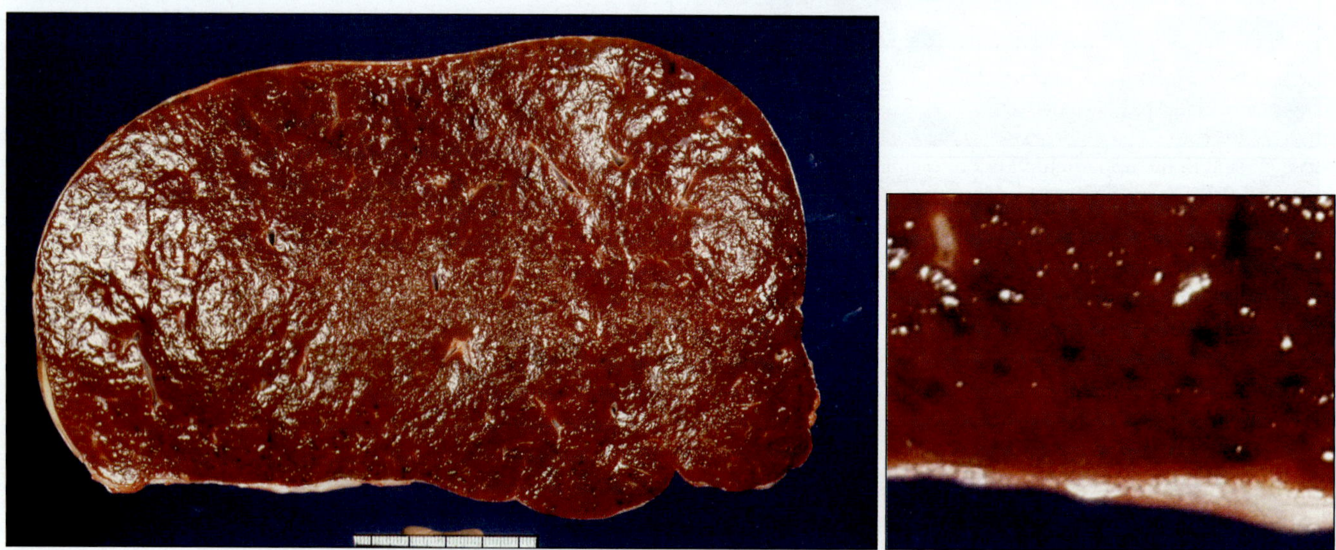

Figure 5.12 Spleen in CLL. CLL involvement of organs is often diffusely infiltrative, but with retention of the underlying architecture. In this gross specimen, the spleen is homogeneously enlarged by diffuse infiltration of the red pulp.

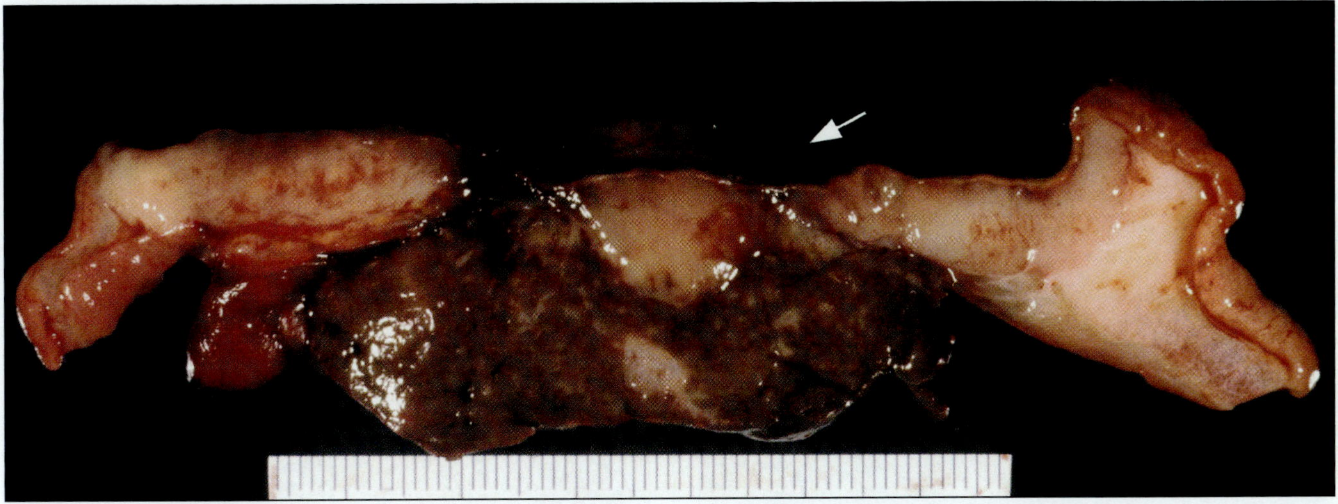

Figure 5.13   CLL in the stomach. This figure is an example of CLL causing stomach ulceration (*arrow*) and diffusely infiltrating the stomach wall and extending into the adjacent liver. Note the small nodules of CLL in the hepatic parenchyma.

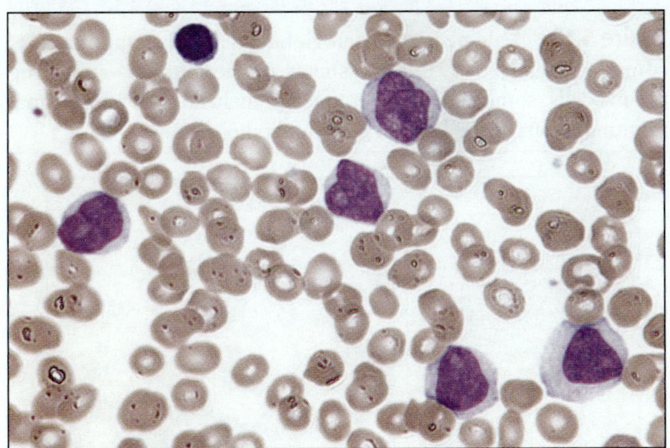

Figure 5.14   Prolymphocytic leukemia (PLL). A blood smear demonstrates large, nucleolated lymphoid cells in a case of PLL transformed from CLL. For comparison, a normal small lymphocyte is present in the upper left corner of the figure.

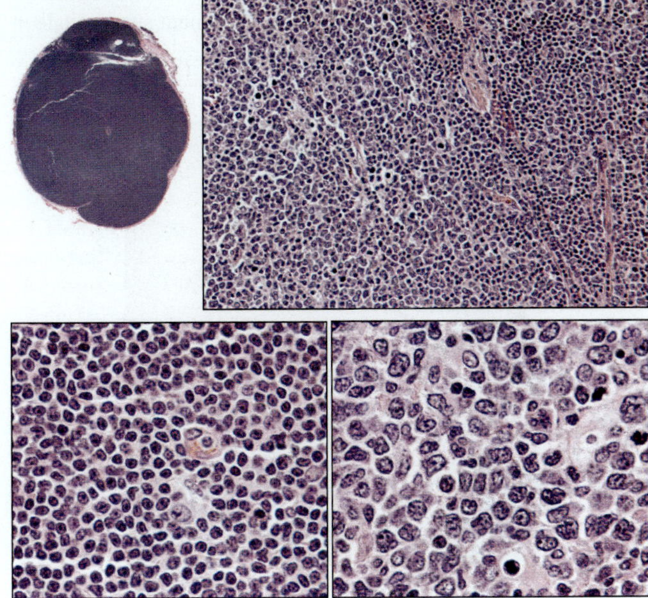

Figure 5.15   Richter syndrome. This lymph node is diffusely effaced by a dual population of small CLL/SLL and large B-lymphoma cells. Different areas of the lymph node are composed exclusively of either the smaller CLL/SLL or larger B-cell lymphoma cells as shown in the left and right lower panels, respectively.

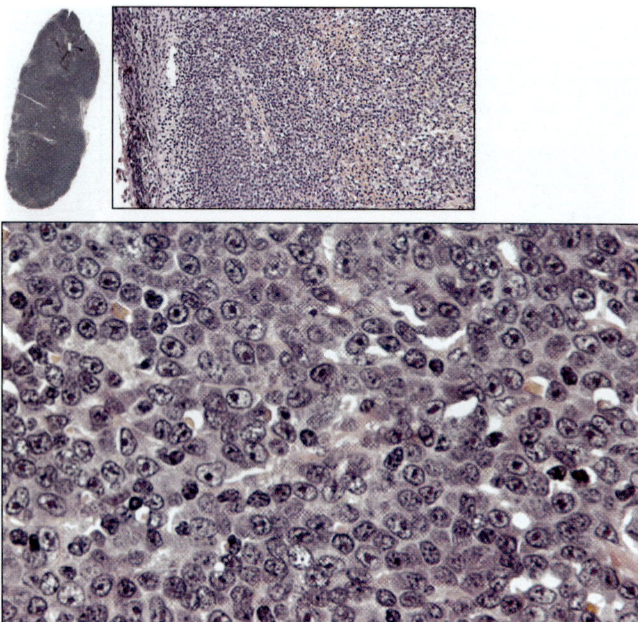

Figure 5.16 B-cell prolymphocytic lymphoma (PLL). Sheets of monomorphic large lymphoid cells with prominent single nucleoli diffusely efface a lymph node.

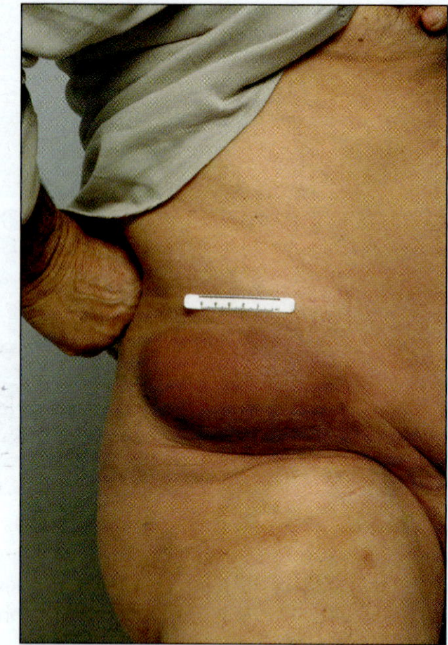

Figure 5.17 Lymphoplasmacytic lymphoma (LPL). This figure demonstrates a right flank mass in a patient suffering from recurrent Waldenström macroglobinemia.

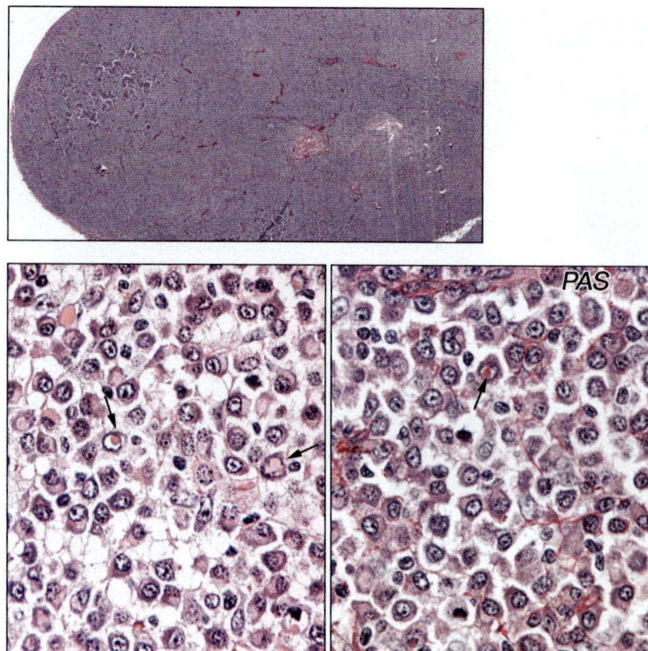

Figure 5.18 Waldenström macroglobinemia. This lymph node is completely effaced by diffuse sheets of monotonous-appearing plasma cells, some showing intranuclear inclusions of monoclonal immunoglobin in the form of Dutcher bodies (*arrows*).

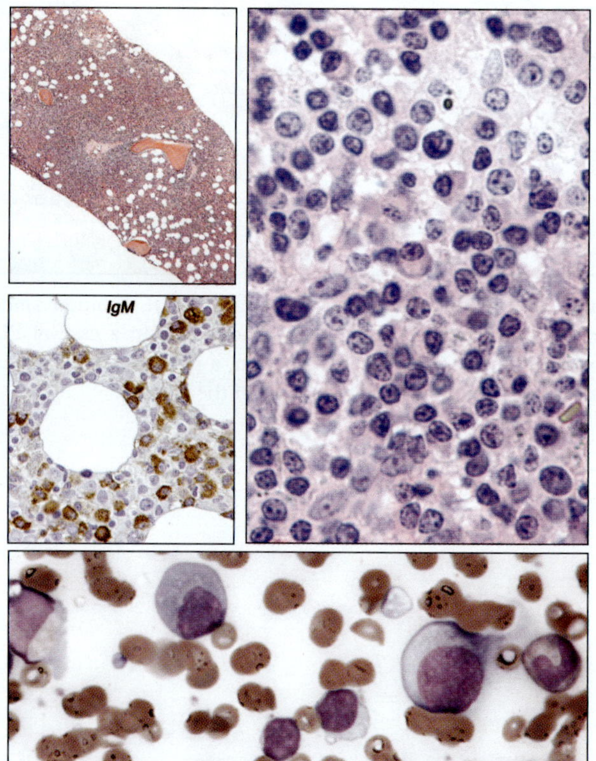

Figure 5.19 Waldenström macroglobinemia. Bone marrow biopsy sections in the upper three panels show diffuse replacement of the marrow by a small lymphocytic/plasma cell population that exhibits restricted IgM expression by immunohistochemistry. The bottom panel demonstrates a mixed population of lymphocytic/plasmacytoid cells in a marrow aspirate smear.

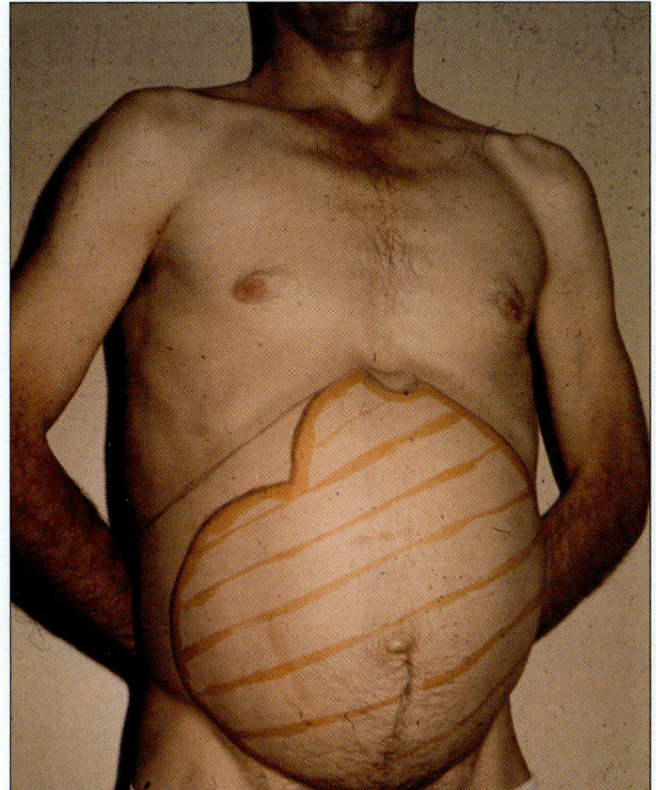

Figure 5.20 Massive splenomegaly in a patient with hairy cell leukemia. (Courtesy of The Crookston Collection.)

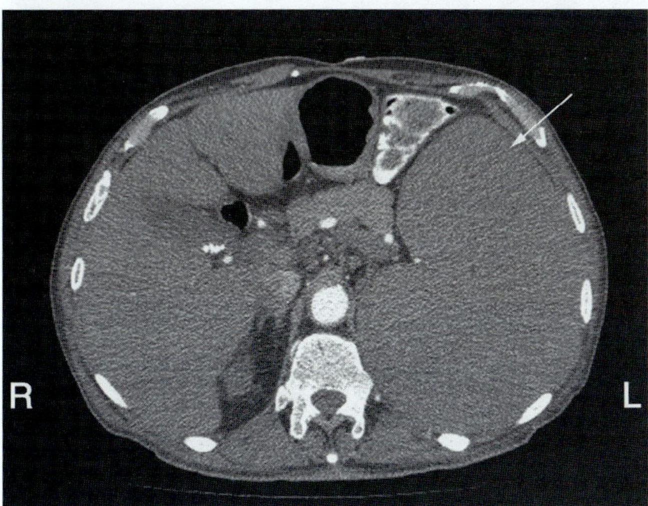

Figure 5.21 Splenomegaly in HCL. An axial CT scan with oral and intravenous contrast shows prominent splenomegaly with no focal lesions in a case of HCL.

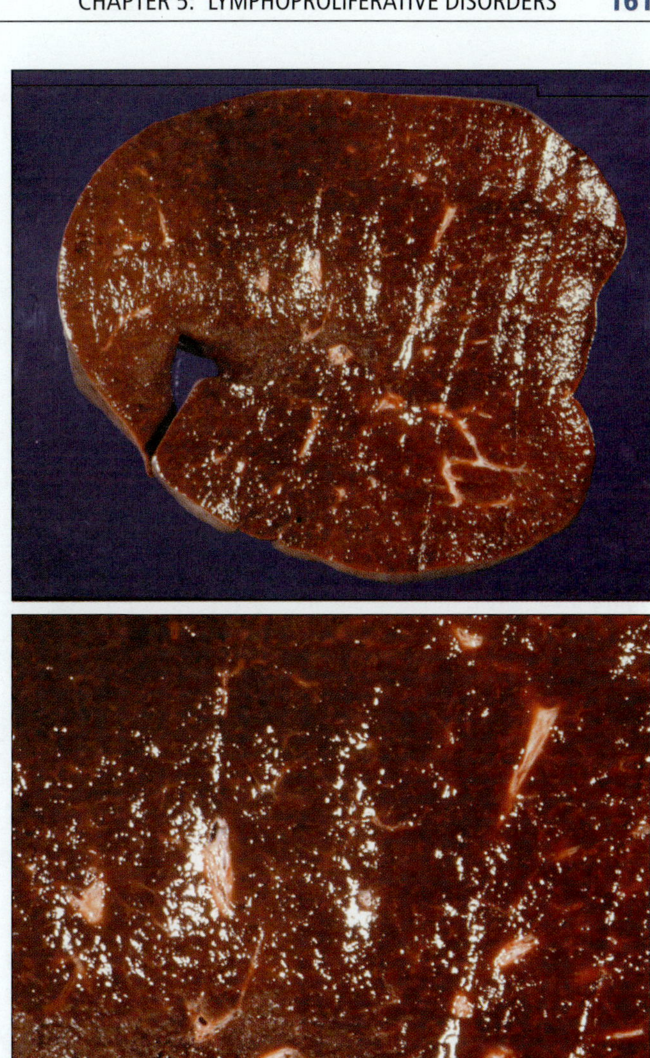

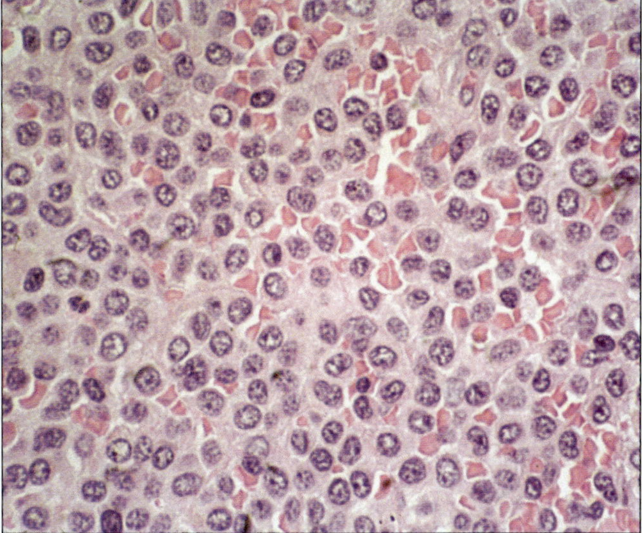

Figure 5.22 Spleen in HCL. The spleen is diffusely enlarged, and the red pulp is infiltrated, by uniformly, well-spaced lymphoid cells possessing regular nuclear contours and condensed chromatin. (Courtesy Dr. D. Amato.)

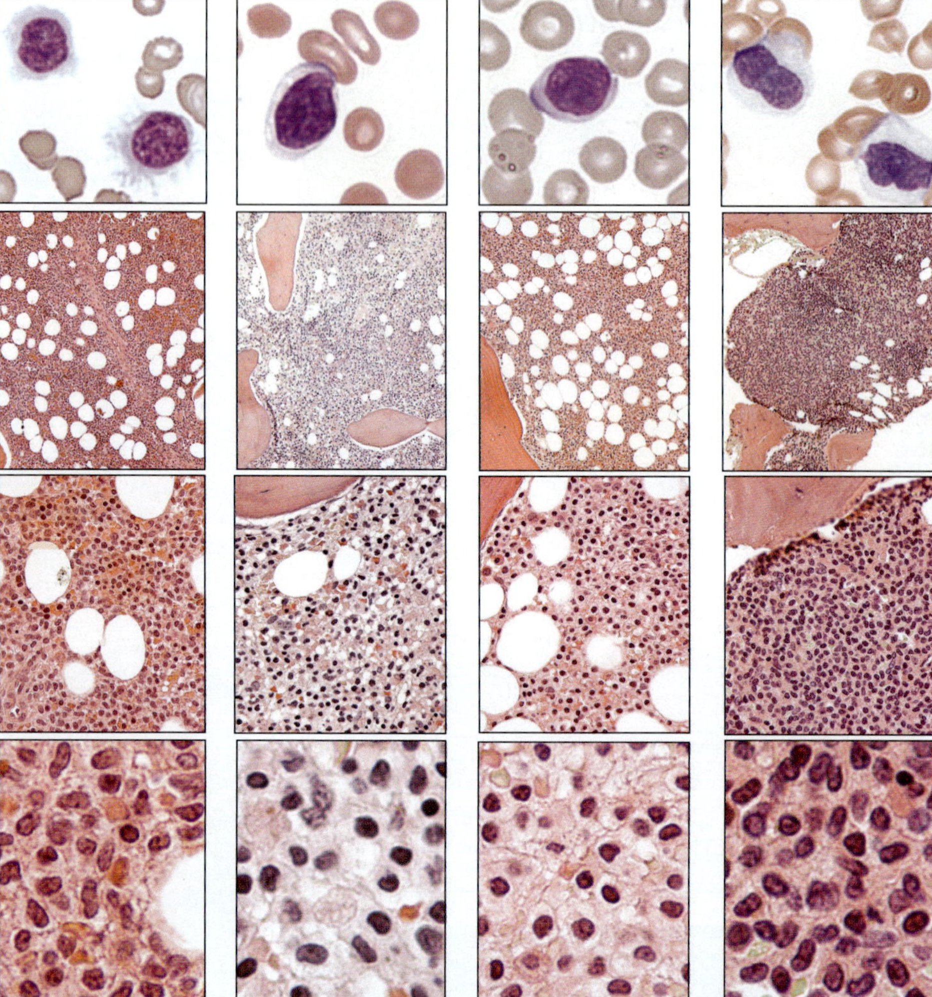

Figure 5.23 HCL in blood smears and bone marrow biopsies. This is a composite figure from four cases of HCL. These examples illustrate the variability in the appearance of HCL cells in blood smear (*top panels*). HCL cells are small to medium in size with mature chromatin and display ample, neutral-staining cytoplasm that may form hair-like villous projections. The distinctive "fried egg" appearance of HCL in biopsy specimens is shown in the bottom panels. HCL usually is associated with extensive reticulin fibrosis that results in failed attempts to obtain cellular aspirate smears (dry taps).

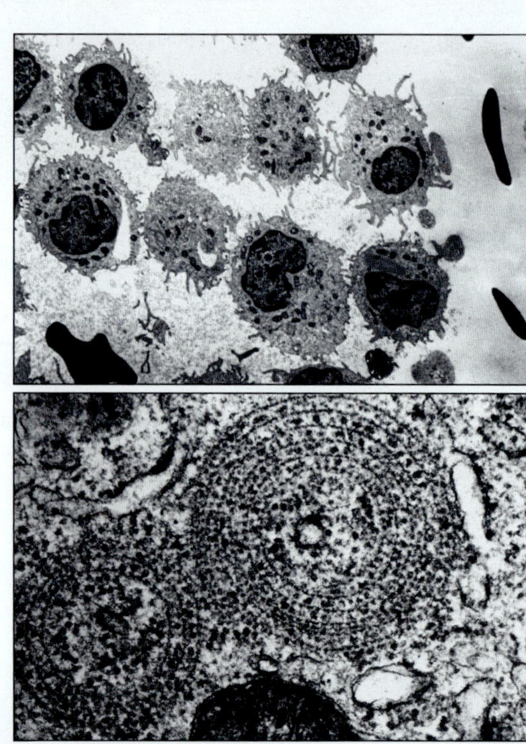

Figure 5.24 Electron micrographs of HCL. Transmission electron micrographs of cells from a case of hairy cell leukemia show numerous cytoplasmic villous projections at low magnification (*top panel*), and at higher power (*lower panel*), the characteristic ribosomal-lamella complexes composed of concentrically arranged sheets of membranes alternating with rows of ribosomes are seen.

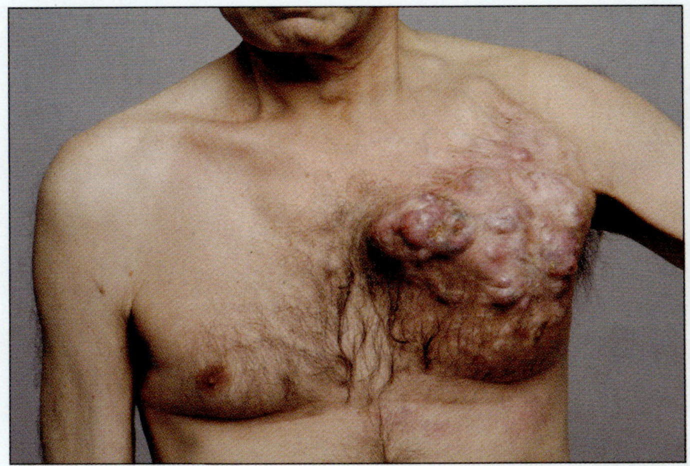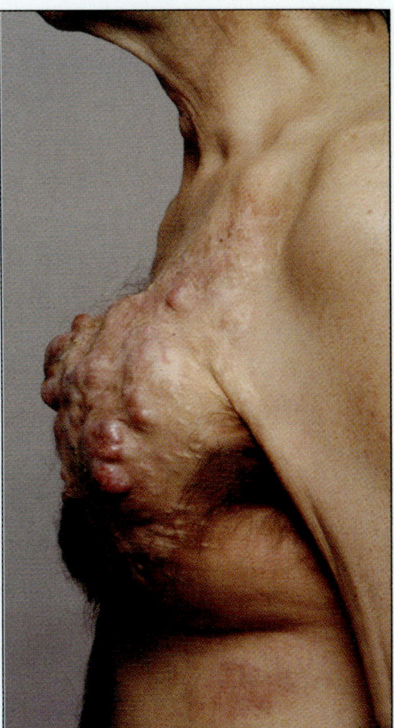

Figure 5.25 Multiple myeloma. An unusually advanced case of myeloma shows the anterior extension of a rib tumor into subcutaneous tissues, forming a large nodular mass.

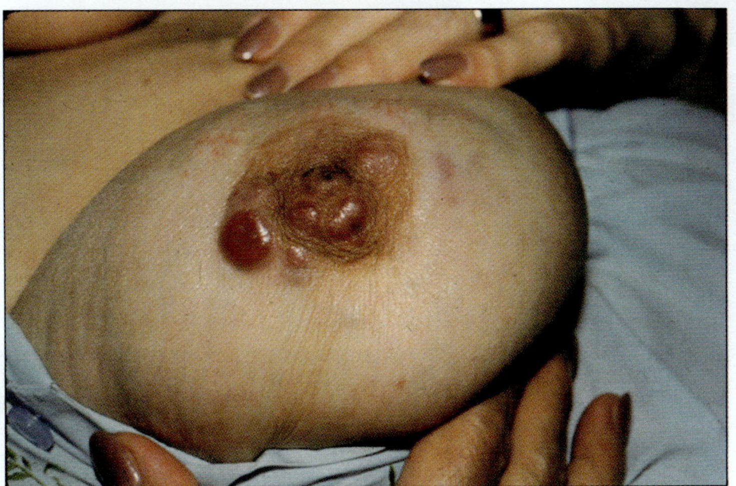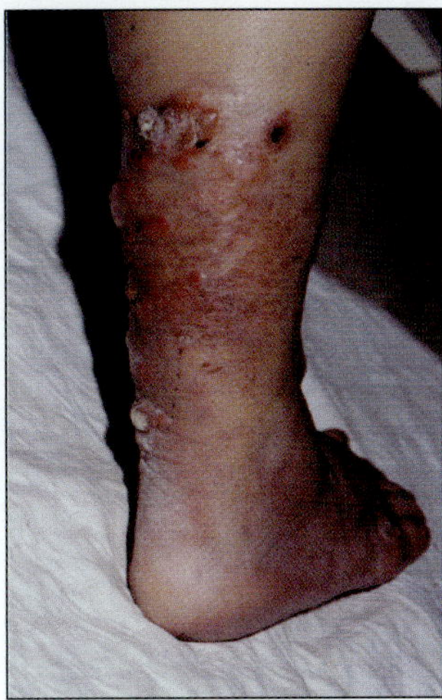

Figure 5.26 Multiple myeloma involving the skin. This figure shows two cases of myeloma involving the skin. Extramedullary sites of involvement at diagnosis or during the course of multiple myeloma are rare.

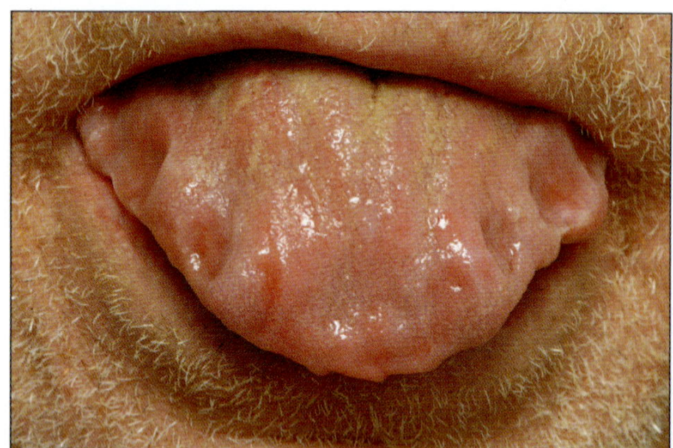

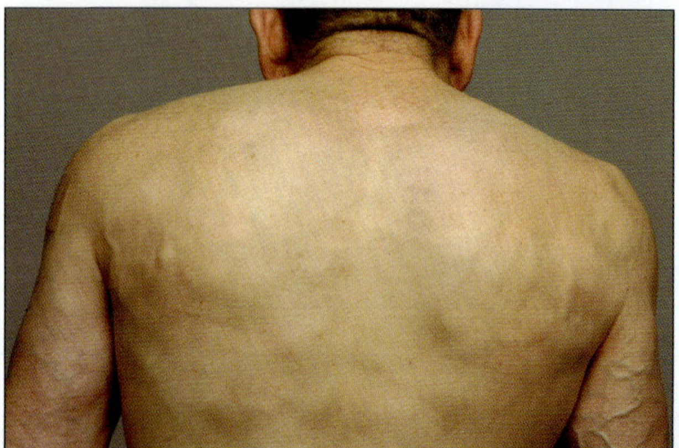

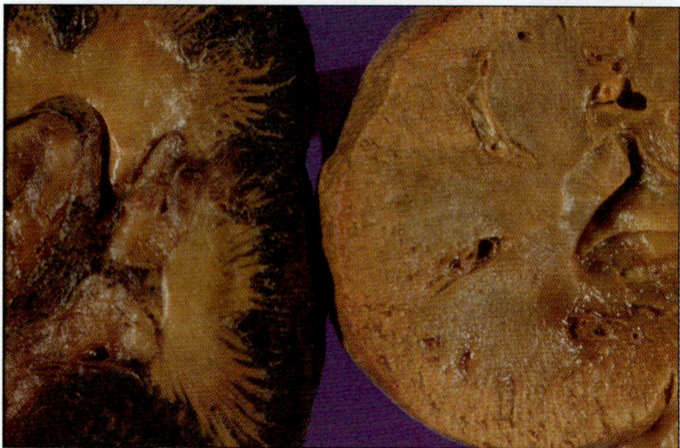

Figure 5.27 AL type of amyloidosis. Amyloidosis occurs in approximately 5% to 10% of patients with myeloma and is related to the deposition of monoclonal immunoglobulin light-chain components that are synthesized by neoplastic plasma cells. This form of amyloidosis mainly affects the heart, kidneys, gastrointestinal tract, liver, and central nervous system. Skin involvement occurs in about 30% to 40% of patients. Amyloid of the tongue can cause it to become enlarged, woody, and indurated (*top panel*, courtesy Dr. I. Quirt). Direct skin infiltration with amyloid can produce the featureless tightening and thickening appearance of scleroderma (*middle panel*). Amyloid is identified grossly by a staining reaction with iodine similar to that of starch (hence the term "amyloid," meaning "starch-like"). Autopsy kidneys stained with iodine are shown in the lower panel, with an amyloid kidney on the left and a normal kidney on the right. (Courtesy Dr. I. Wanless.)

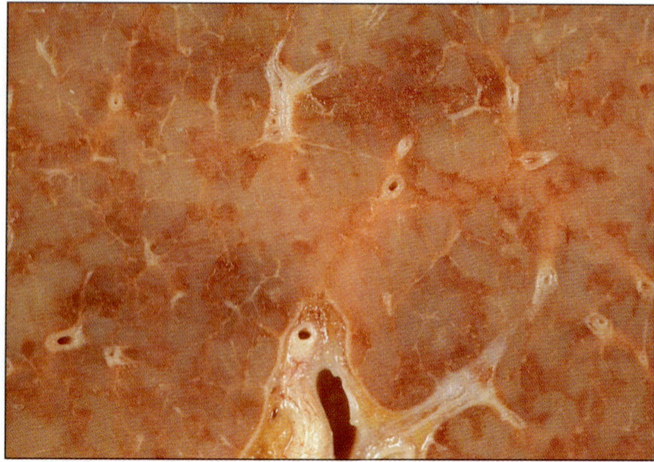

Figure 5.28 Amyloidosis of spleen. A freshly cut splenectomy specimen displaying the wax-like appearance of amyloid deposits. (Courtesy Dr. D. Driman.)

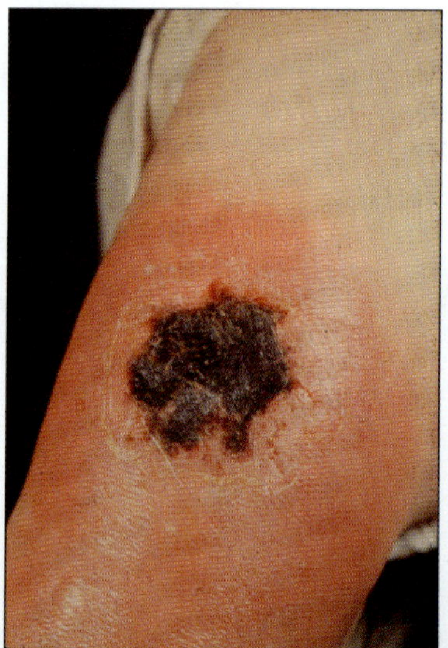

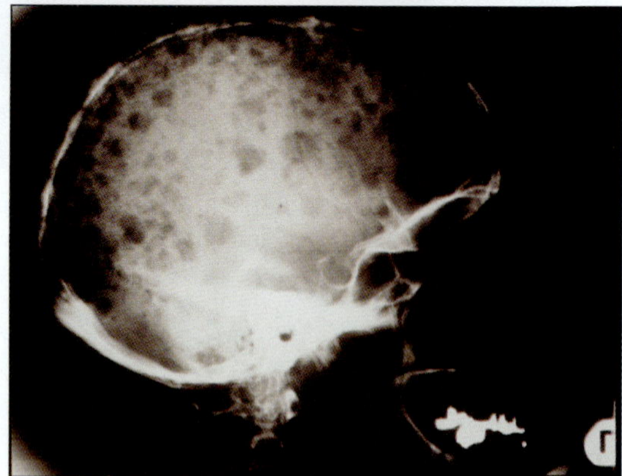

Figure 5.29 *Top panel:* Post-vaccination necrosis in a myeloma patient. Vaccinations with live attenuated viruses are contradicted in patients suffering from myeloma and other conditions leading weakened immune systems. Widespread skin necrosis at the vaccination site (progressive vaccinia/vaccinia necrosum) may occur, as in this patient. (Courtesy Dr. I. Quirt.) Skull radiograph showing multiple punched out lesions affecting the skull, from a patient with multiple myeloma (*bottom panel*, courtesy Dr. P. Galbraith).

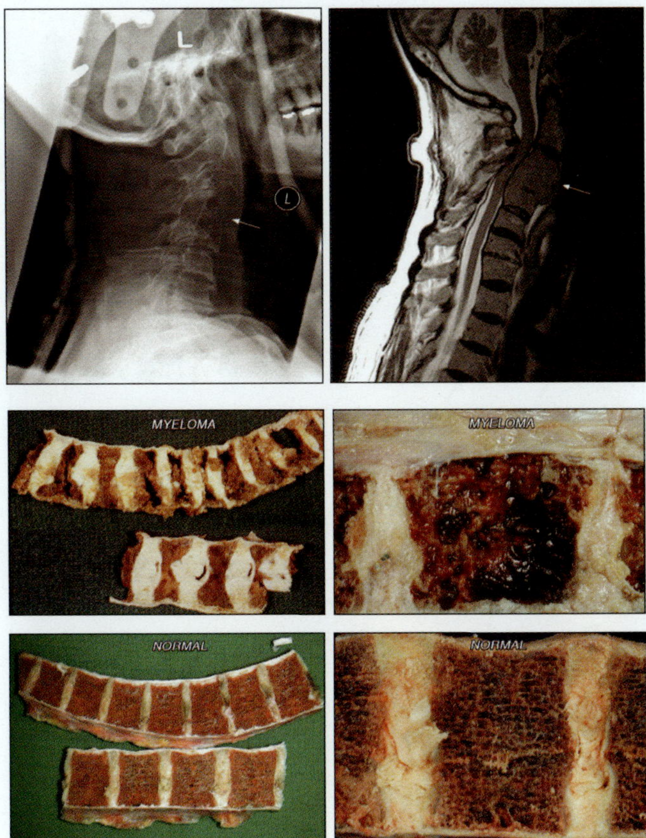

Figure 5.30 Lytic boney lesions in myeloma. This lateral view of the cervical spine shows lytic lesions mainly involving the vertebral bodies of the cervical spine in case of myeloma (*arrow, left upper panel*). Sagittal MRI of the cervical spine in same patient discloses myeloma replacing mid-cervical vertebral bodies (*arrow*) causing anterior spinal cord compression (*right upper panel*). Gross specimens of vertebral columns with multiple, punched-out, hemorrhagic, lytic lesions from myeloma (*middle panels*) are compared to normal (*lower panels*).

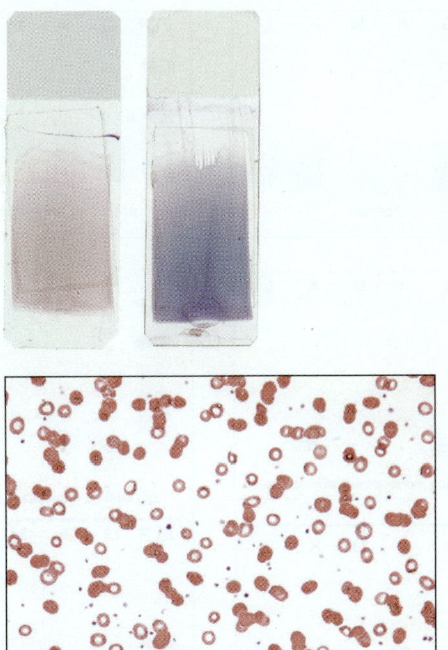

Figure 5.31 Background staining and rouleaux formation in myeloma. The excessive immunoglobins produced by the neoplastic plasma cells in myeloma are acidic and take up the basophilic stains used in blood smears. The consequence is an increase in background bluish staining in blood smears in myeloma patients (slide on *right in upper panel*) compared with normal (slide on *left*). The abnormal immunoglobulins also cause the RBCs to adhere. This resulting rouleaux ("stacking of coins") formation may be visible on those portions of the smear where erythrocytes are normally apart (*lower panel*).

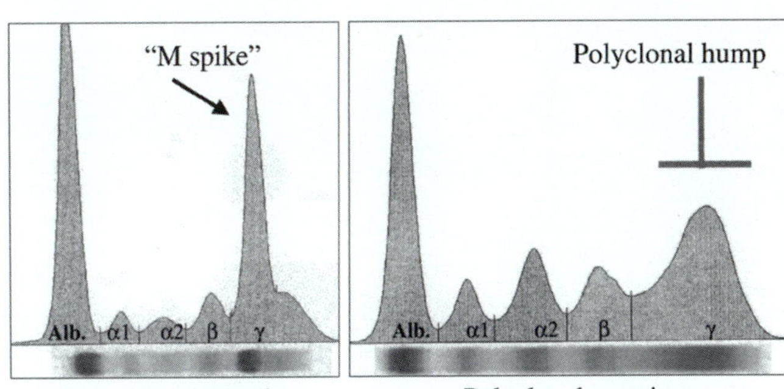

Figure 5.32 Serum electrophoresis. Albumin (Alb.) is the largest peak and closest to the positive electrode and the next peaks are globulins: α-1, α-2, β, and γ. The γ-peak is closest to the negative electrode. The presence of a monoclonal protein is characterized by a sharp, well-defined "M spike" with a single heavy chain and a similar band with a κ- or λ-light chain. A broad diffuse band with one or more heavy chains and κ- and λ-light chains characterizes a polyclonal protein.

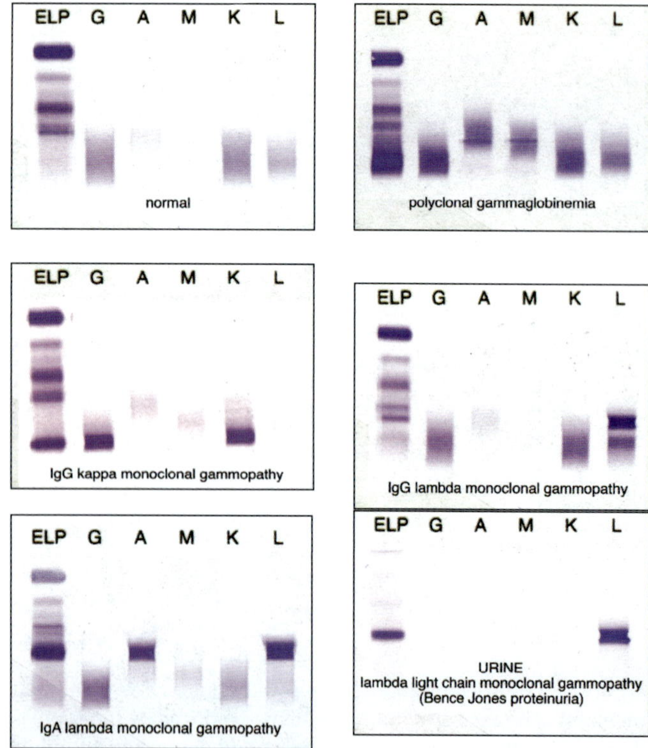

Figure 5.33 Serum and urine electrophoresis with immunofixation. The composition of monoclonal abnormalities (M spikes) are analyzed by immunofixation to determine the identities of the heavy-chain and light-chain types. Several examples of normal and abnormal results from immunofixation electrophoresis are shown here. (Courtesy Dr. P. Y. Wong.)

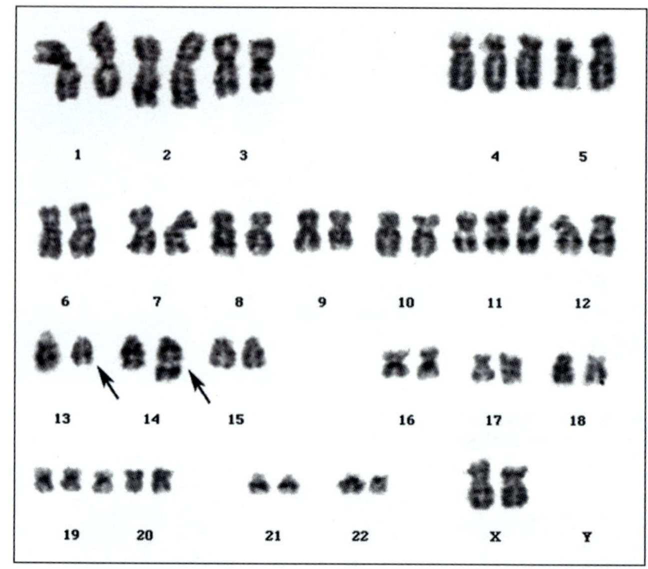

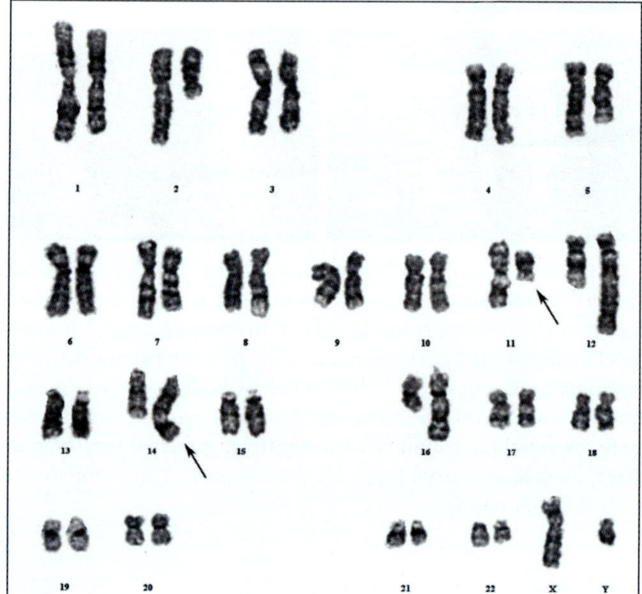

Figure 5.34 Cytogenetics in myeloma. Certain cytogenetic abnormalities are associated with poor prognosis in myeloma. These include translocations involving the IgH locus on 14q32: t(11;14), t(4;14), t(14;16); chromosome 13 deletions that are detected by conventional cytogenetics; and loss of 17p13 demonstrated best by interphase FISH. A multiple myeloma karyotype with del(13)(q14;q22) and a derivative 14 chromosome from a t(11;14)(q13;q32), along with other trisomies is shown in the upper panel. The lower panel illustrates another myeloma case with t(11;14)(q13;q32) along with other structural aberrations.

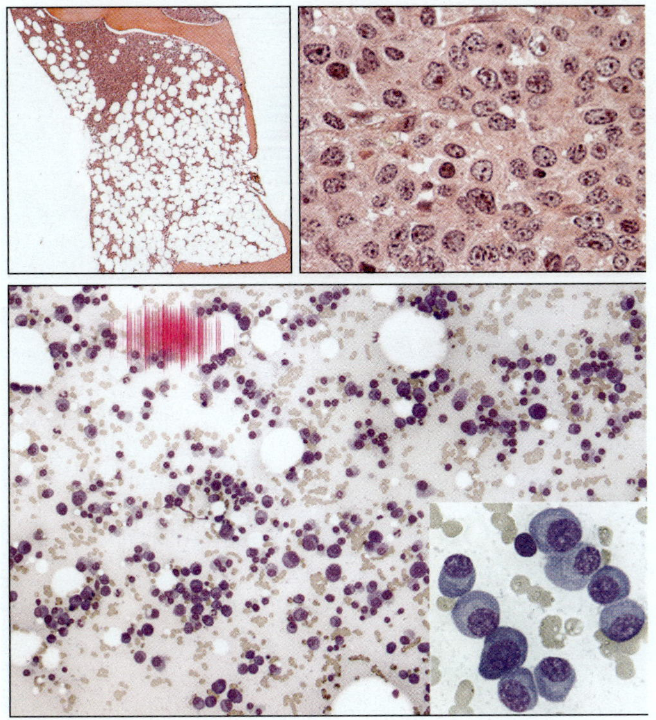

Figure 5.35 Bone marrow morphology in myeloma. Myeloma usually involves the bone marrow in a widespread, but patchy manner. A low- and high-power view of a biopsy is shown in the upper two panels, showing focal involvement by myeloma. The lower panel shows an aspirate smear composed almost exclusively of plasma cells.

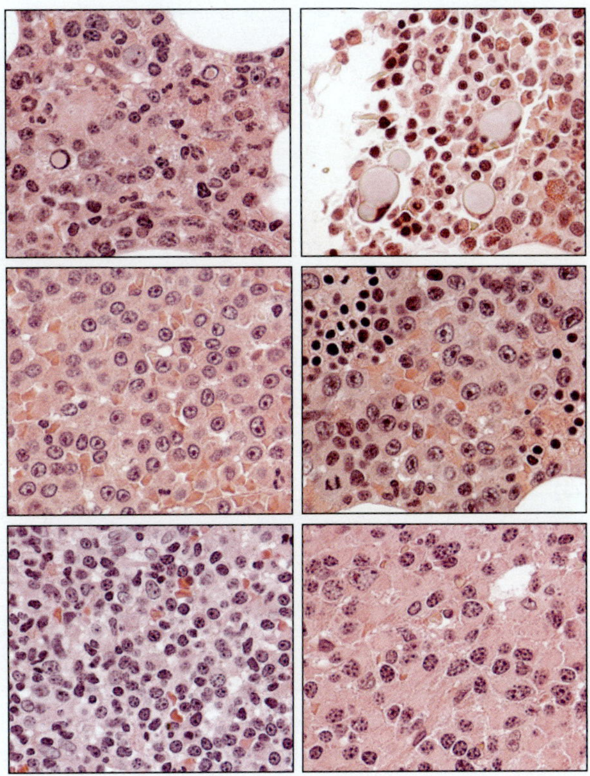

Figure 5.37 Appearance of myeloma on bone marrow biopsy. High-power views of biopsy specimens from six different cases of myeloma cases are shown here. Intranuclear (Dutcher bodies) and intracytoplasmic (Mott cells) inclusions of abnormal immunoglobin appear in neoplastic plasma cells in the left and right upper panels, respectively.

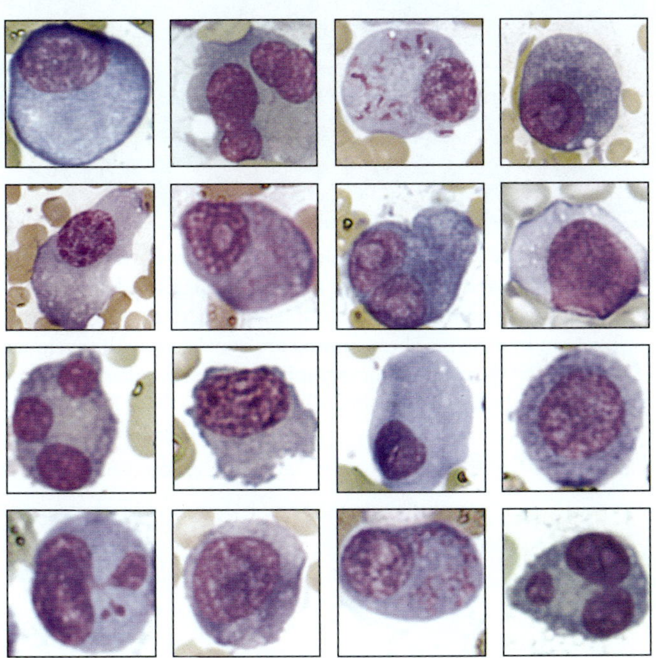

Figure 5.36 The diverse morphology of myeloma. Plasma cells, from 16 different cases of myeloma, are displayed here.

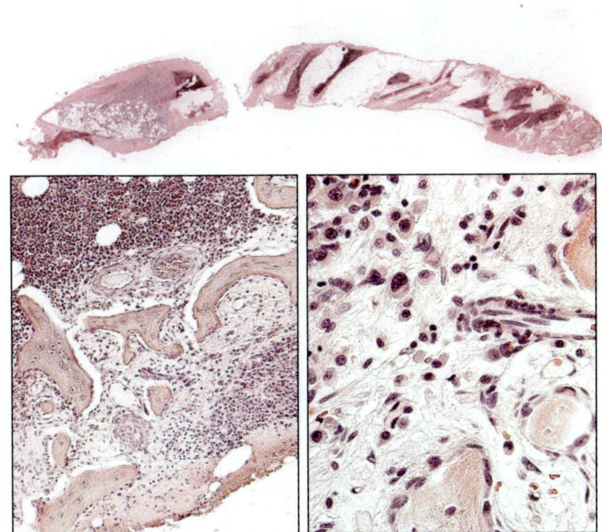

Figure 5.38 Myeloma and bone formation. *Upper panel:* A low-power view of a marrow biopsy shows areas of thickened bone associated with a hypercellular focus of myeloma (*left side* of biopsy core). The bottom two panels display foci of new bone formation associated with irregular lamellar bone and increased numbers of osteoblasts. The latter are easily confused with plasma cells.

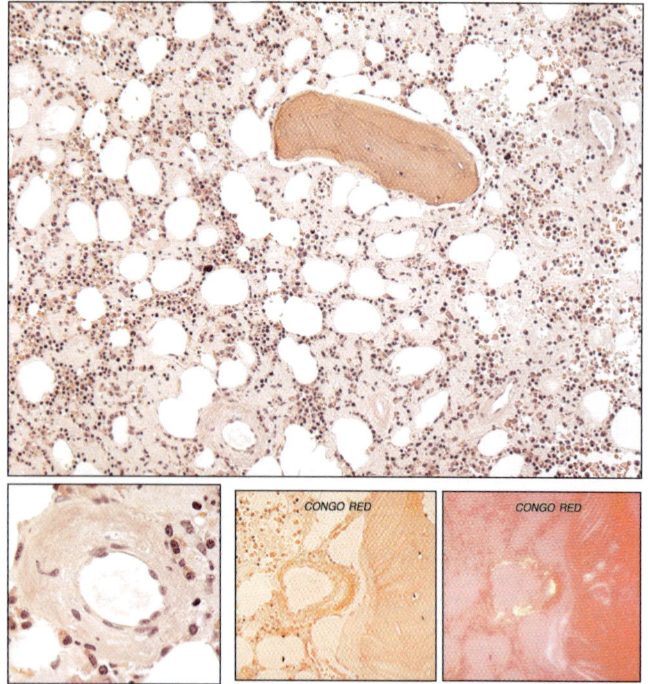

Figure 5.39 Amyloid in marrow. A bone marrow biopsy is diffusely infiltrated by eosinophilic, proteinaceous material that accumulates in and around blood vessels. The characteristic apple-green birefringence can be demonstrated after Congo-red staining.

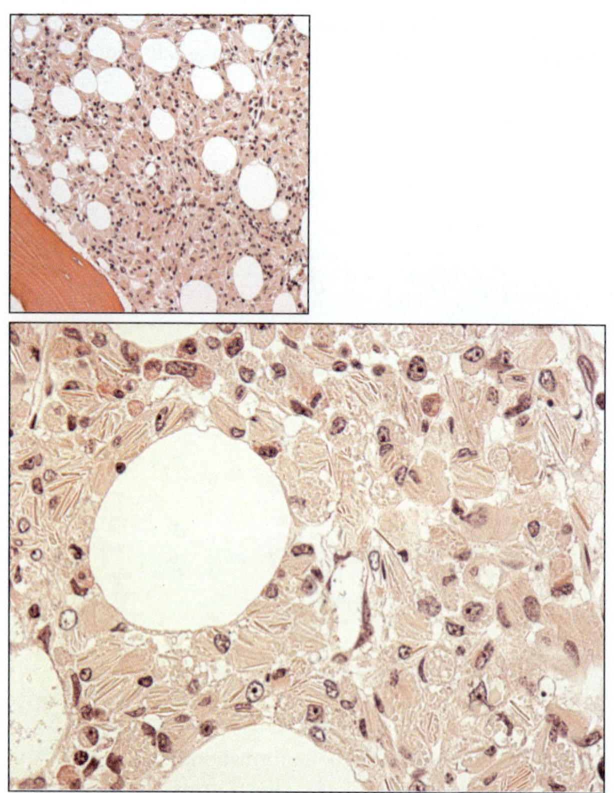

Figure 5.40 Crystal-storing histiocytosis in myeloma. Abnormal proteins can precipitate and form crystals in myeloma and other hematopoietic malignancies, such as lymphoplasmacytic lymphoma and granulocytic sarcoma.

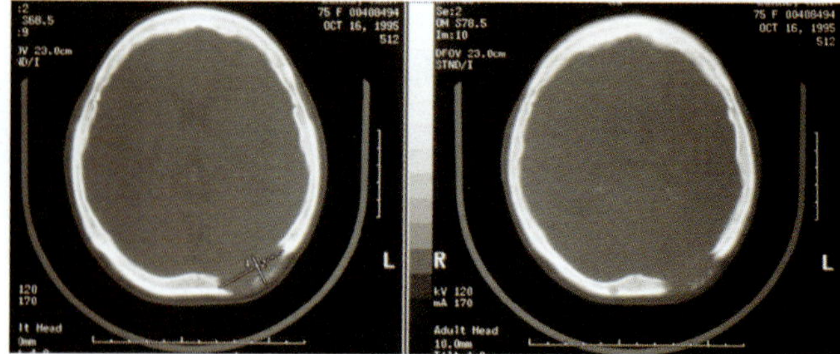

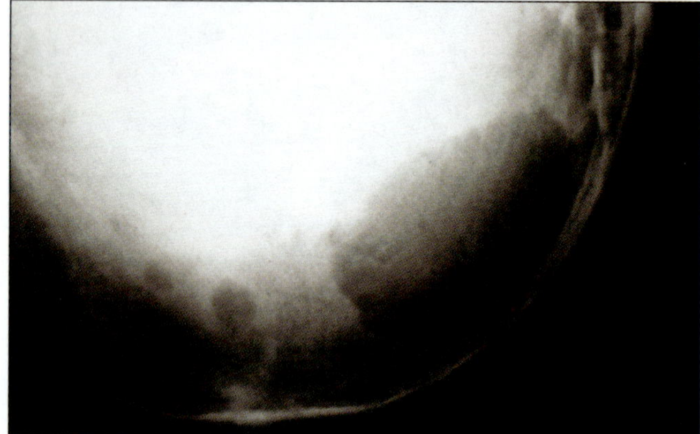

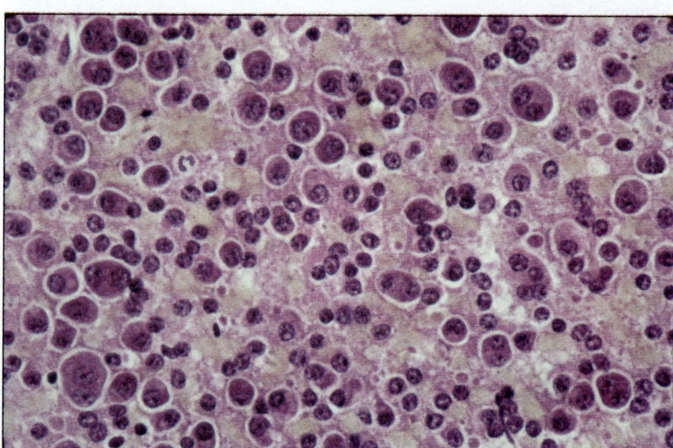

Figure 5.41 Myeloma of the skull. A CT scan of the head with bone windows and a radiograph (*upper two panels* and *middle panels,* respectively) showing lytic skull lesions, with the largest measuring 4 cm by 1.8 cm. These finding are consistent with myeloma. The lower panel is a photomicrograph from a biopsy demonstrating sheets of highly atypical plasma cells. (Courtesy Dr. J. Bilbao.)

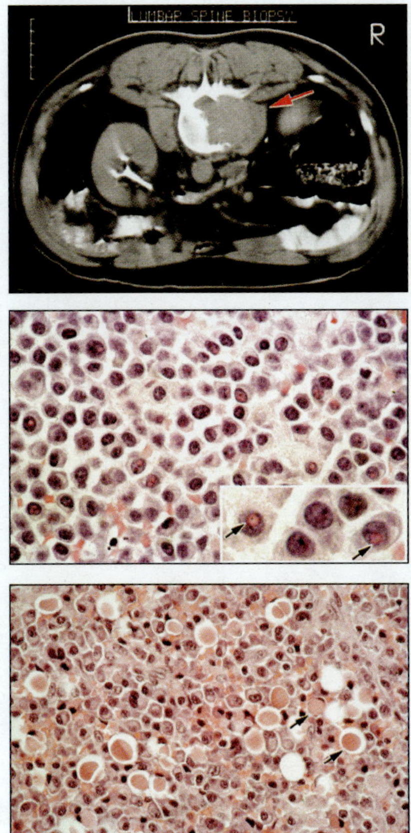

Figure 5.42   Myeloma of the spine. A contrast-enhanced CT scan of the abdomen for image-directed biopsy of a lytic vertebral lesion discloses destruction and soft-tissue replacement of the right aspect of the vertebral body, extending into the vertebral canal (*red arrow*). The other panels contain photomicrographs of the biopsy consisting exclusively of plasma cells with both intranuclear Dutcher bodies (*arrows, middle panel*) and cytoplasmic (Mott cells, *arrows, lower panel*) inclusions of monoclonal immunoglobin. (Courtesy Dr. J. Bilbao.)

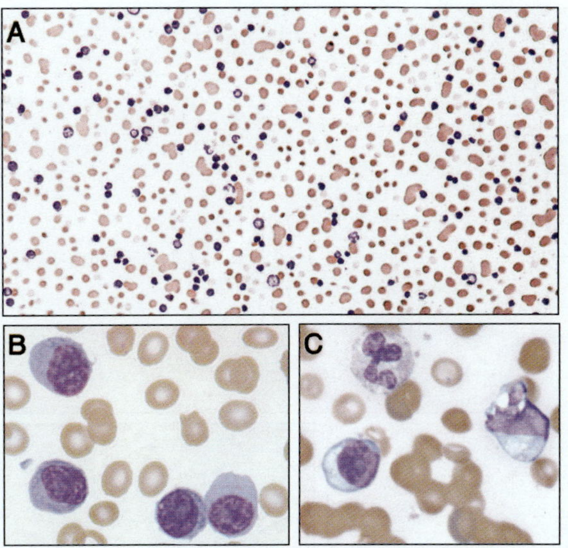

Figure 5.43   Plasma cell leukemia. **A.** Low-power examination of blood smear shows leukocytosis and rouleaux formation. **B.** Higher-power view shows that the leukocytosis is due exclusively to circulating plasma cells. The "atypical" appearance of normal circulating lymphocytes associated with high levels of serum immunoglobins is shown in **C.** Cytoplasmic vacuolation and the resulting appearance of the nucleus pushed to one side can lead to mistaking this for plasma cell leukemia.

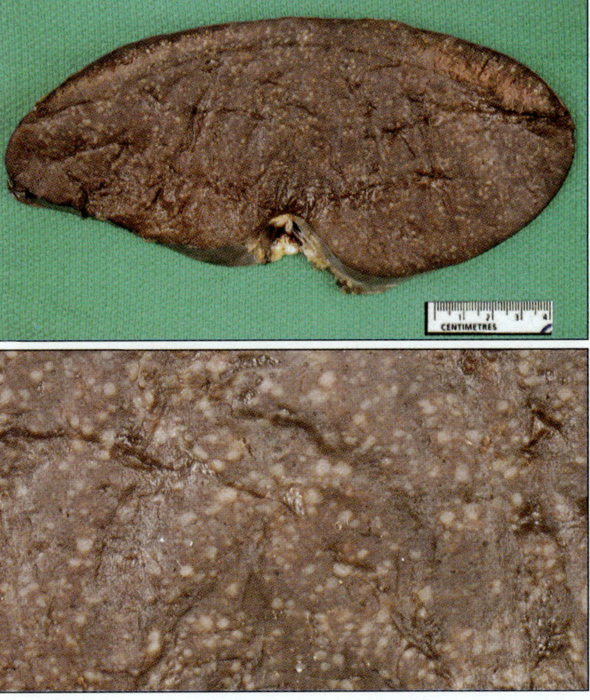

Figure 5.44   Splenic marginal zone lymphoma (SMZL). This figure demonstrates the gross appearance of a splenectomy specimen from a case of SMZL. Multiple small (1 to 3 mm) discrete nodules of expanded white are diffusely distributed throughout the splenic parenchyma.

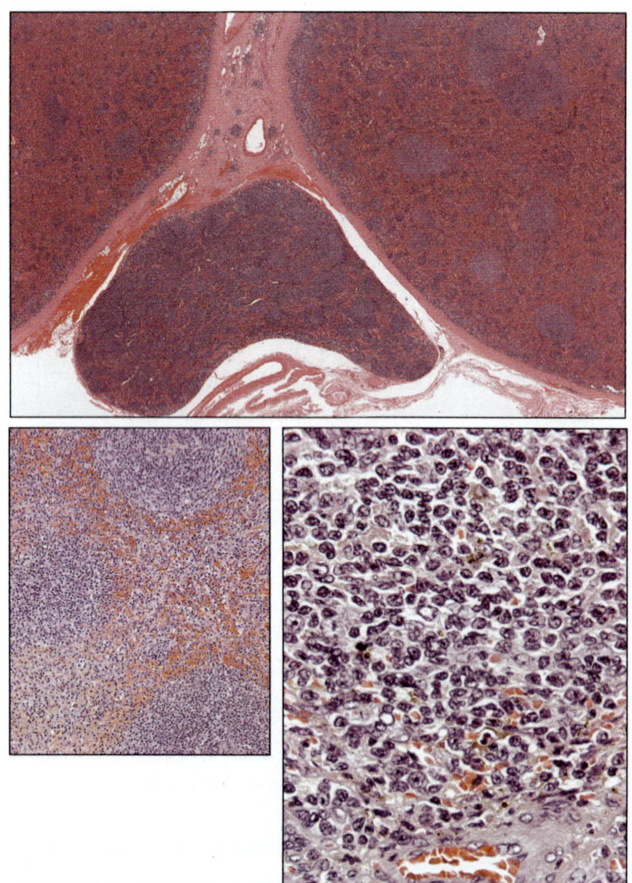

Figure 5.45 Splenic marginal-zone lymphoma with hilar lymph node involvement. The spleen is diffusely infiltrated by macroscopically visible nodular expansions of white pulp. Perivascular nodules made up of monotonous-appearing, well-spaced, medium-sized lymphoid cells are shown.

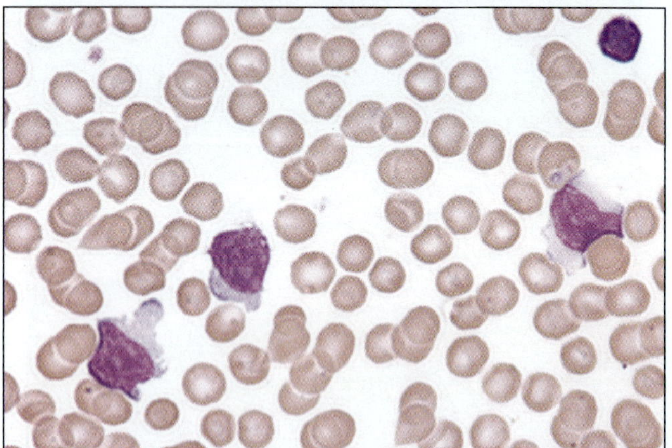

Figure 5.46 SMZL in blood smear. The typical cells in this disease are mature-appearing, medium-sized lymphocytes with ample cytoplasm that forms villous projections. A normal small lymphocyte is seen in the right upper corner.

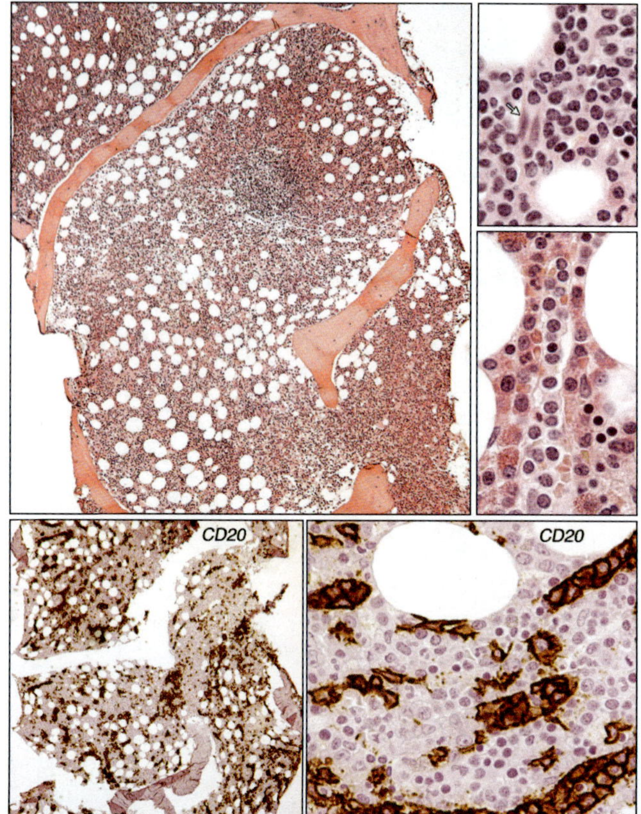

Figure 5.47 Marrow involvement SMZL. Marrow biopsies show a mostly sinusoidal pattern of marrow involvement by lymphoma. High-power views show small-sized lymphoma nuclei (compared with the larger endothelial nucleus, *arrow in right upper figure*), which possess a condensed chromatin pattern and regular nuclear contours. Low- and high-power views of CD20 immunostained biopsy sections accentuate the sinusoidal pattern of marrow involvement characteristic of this lymphoma.

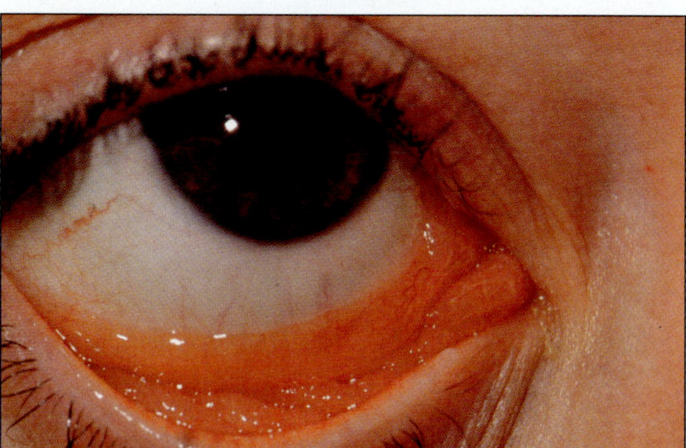

Figure 5.48 MALT lymphoma of sclera. Clinical photograph of eye showing fleshy "salmon-color patch" of the superficial ocular surface.

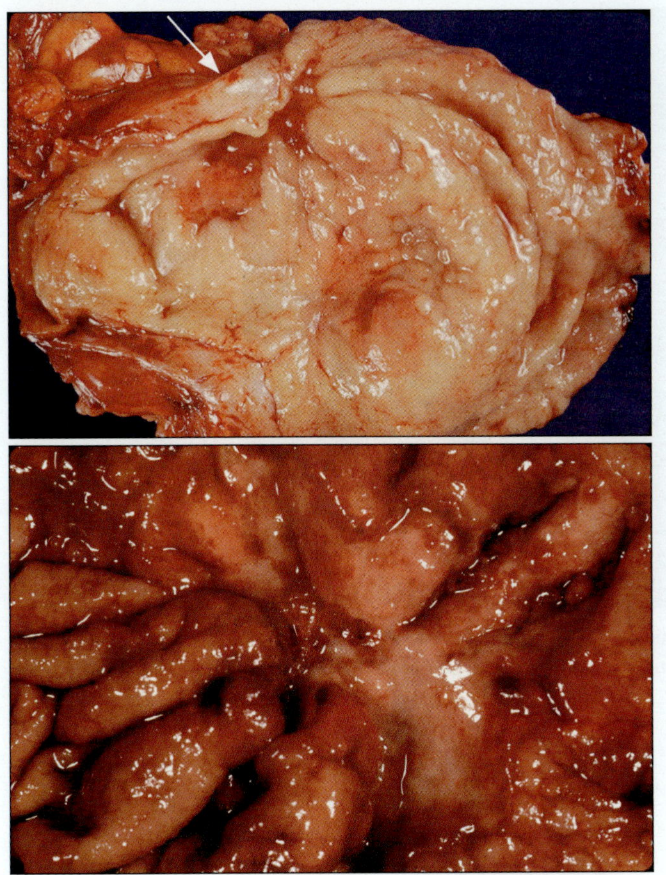

Figure 5.49 This gastrectomy specimen shows a thickened stomach wall (*arrow*) from MALT lymphoma with a well-demarcated ulcer (*bottom panel*).

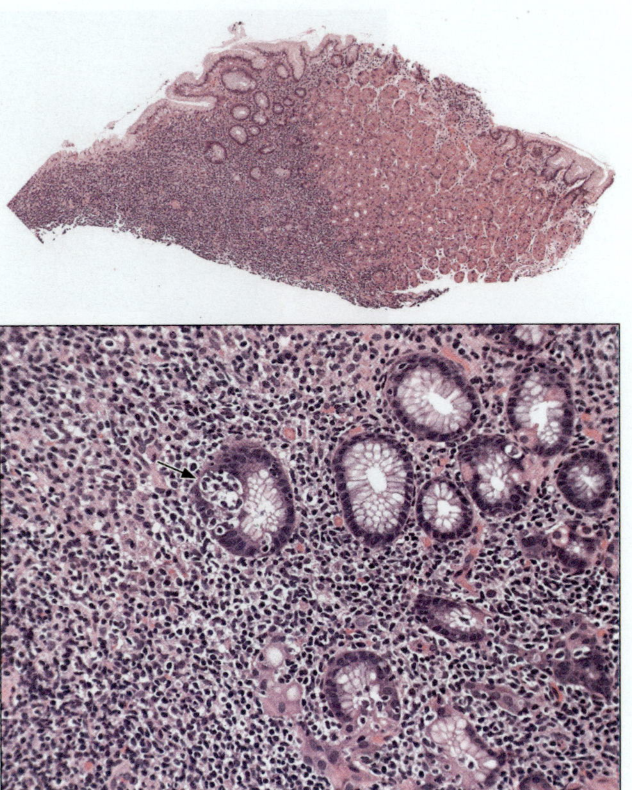

Figure 5.50 Extranodal marginal-zone B-cell lymphoma of mucosa-associated lymphoid tissue (MALT lymphoma). This gastric biopsy demonstrates extensive involvement by well-spaced, medium-sized lymphoid cells that invade and destroy glands to form lymphoepithelial lesions.

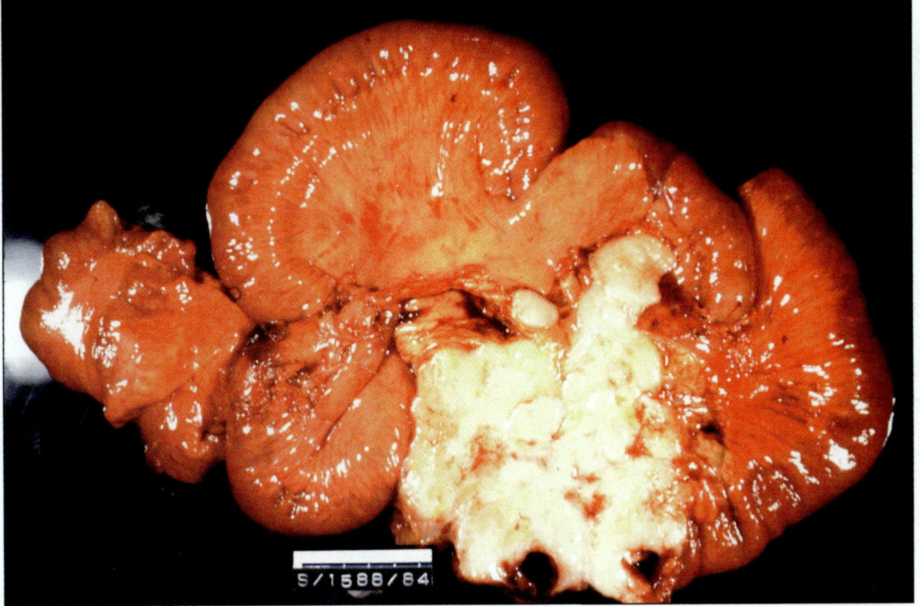

Figure 5.51 MALT lymphoma of small bowel mesenteric lymph nodes. This gross specimen from a small bowel resection shows a large (20 cm) obstructing mass involving numerous small-bowel mesenteric lymph nodes.

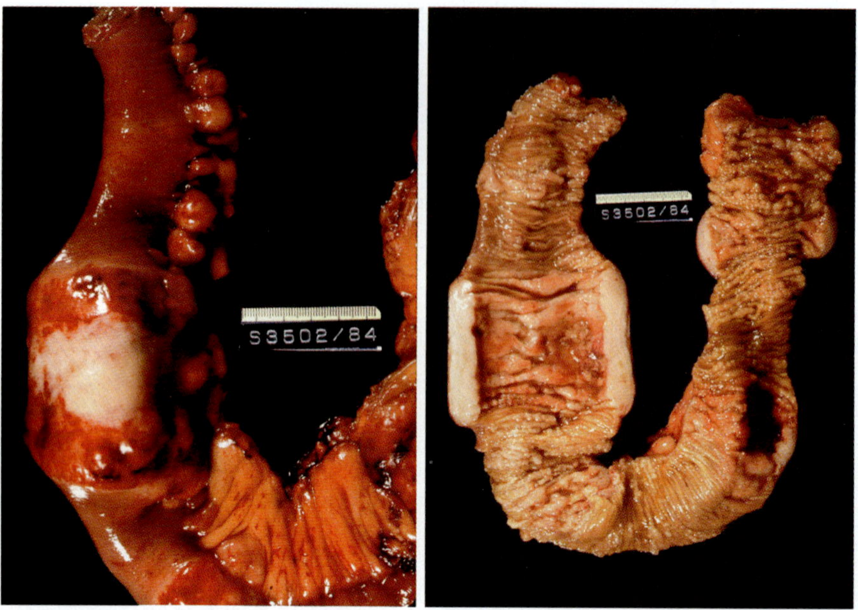

Figure 5.52 MALT lymphoma of small bowel. This MALT lymphoma involves a very well-defined segment of small bowel. Note the circumferential and transmural involvement of the bowel wall.

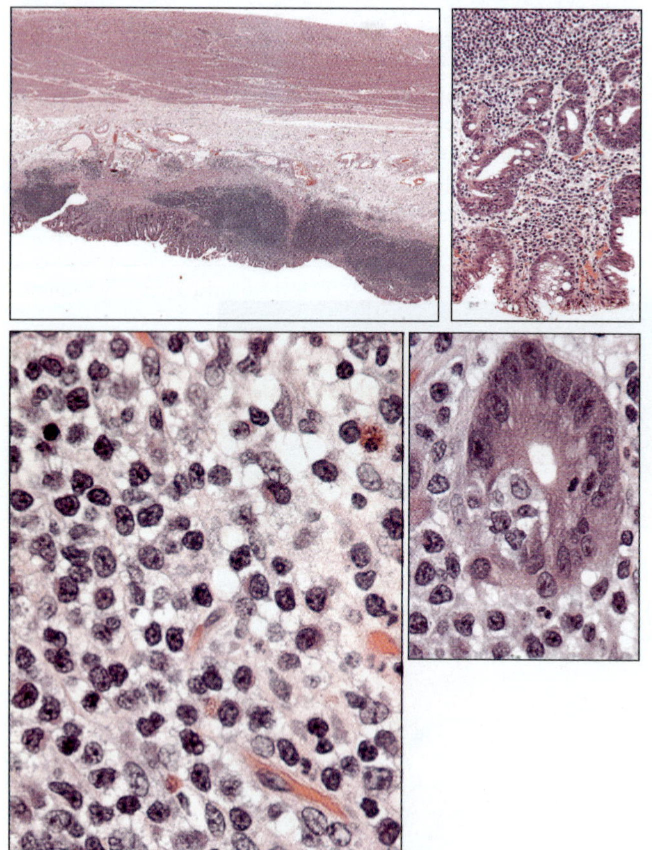

Figure 5.53 Extranodal marginal-zone B-cell lymphoma of mucosa-associated lymphoid tissue (MALT lymphoma). This partial gastrectomy specimen demonstrates a MALT lymphoma ulcerating through the muscularis mucosae. Uniformly, well-spaced, medium-sized lymphoid cells invade and destroy glands to form lymphoepithelial lesions (*right lower panel*).

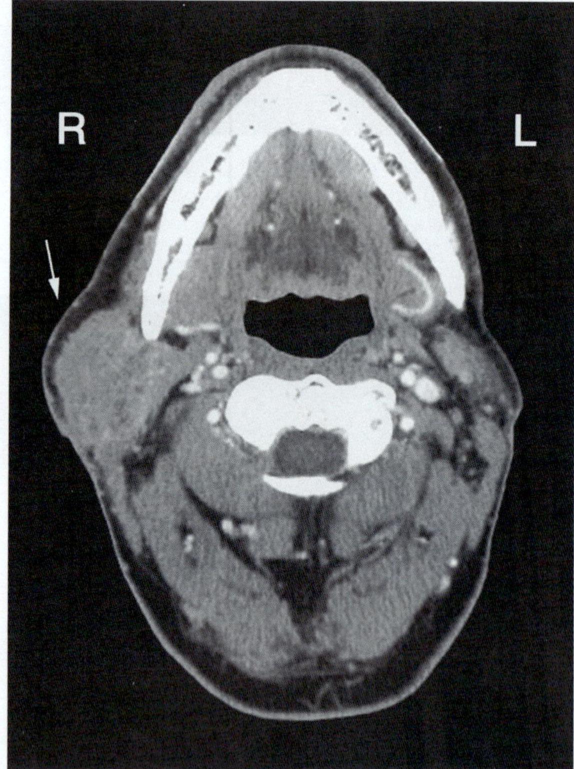

Figure 5.54 MALT lymphoma of right parotid gland. An axial CT scan through the lower jaw reveals an enhancing soft-tissue mass in the region of the right parotid gland.

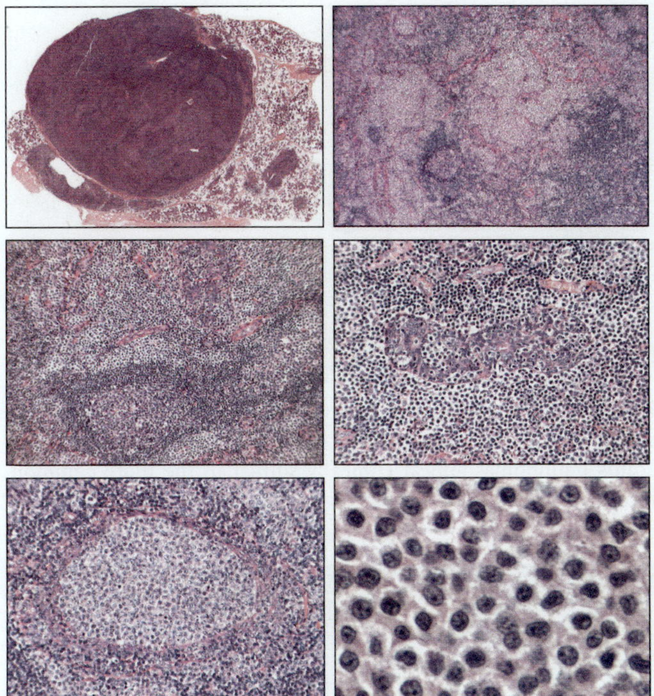

Figure 5.55 Extranodal MALT lymphoma of parotid gland. A lymph node and subjacent parotid gland demonstrate a vaguely nodular proliferation of well-spaced monocytoid lymphocytes invading germinal centers (*left middle panel*) and glandular structures to form lymphoepithelial lesions (*right middle panel*). Nodules of MALT lymphoma are seen filling sinuses (*left lower panel*), and these exhibit a characteristic uniformly well-spaced pattern reminiscent of the so-called "fried egg" appearance of hairy cell leukemia involving the bone marrow (*right lower panel*).

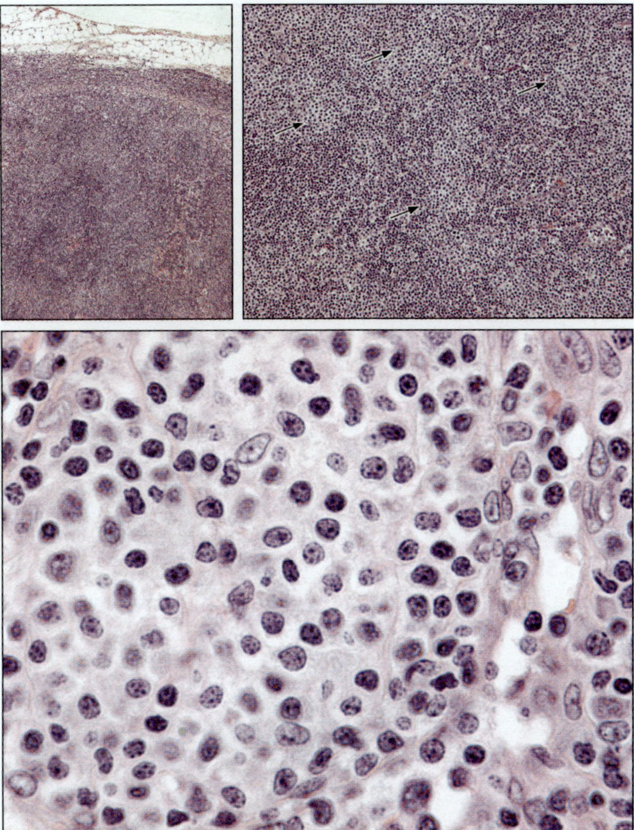

Figure 5.57 Lymph node involvement by extranodal marginal-zone B-cell lymphoma of mucosa-associated lymphoid tissue (MALT lymphoma). A cervical lymph node from a case of MALT lymphoma of the parotid gland shows diffuse involvement by uniformly well-spaced, medium-sized lymphoid cells. Islands of MALT lymphoma are visible in the medium-power photomicrograph in the right upper corner (*arrows*).

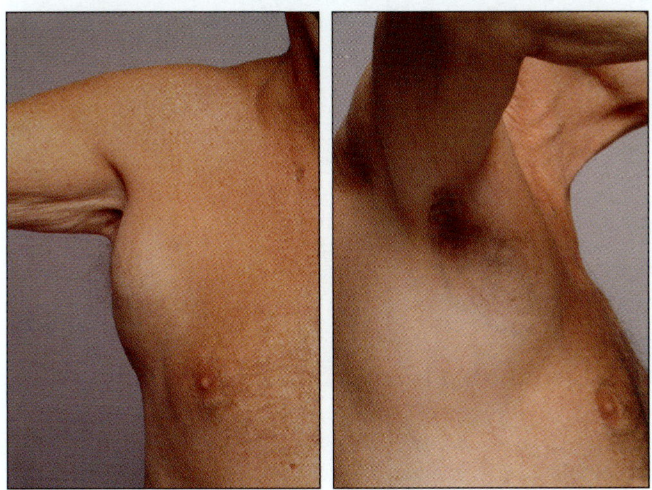

Figure 5.56 Axillary lymphadenopathy in a case of extranodal MALT lymphoma.

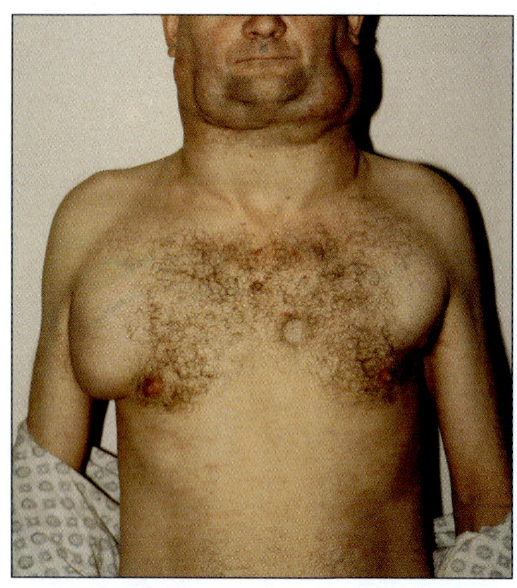

Figure 5.58   Extensive bilateral cervical and axillary lymphadenopathy in a patient with advanced-stage follicular lymphoma at presentation.

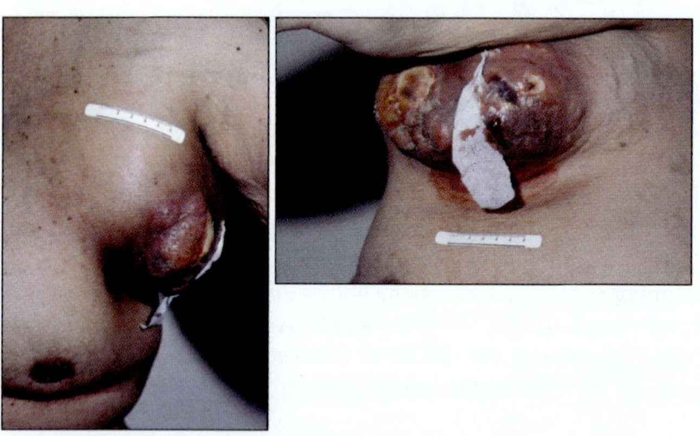

Figure 5.59   Ulcerating, enlarged axillary lymph nodes with follicular lymphoma.

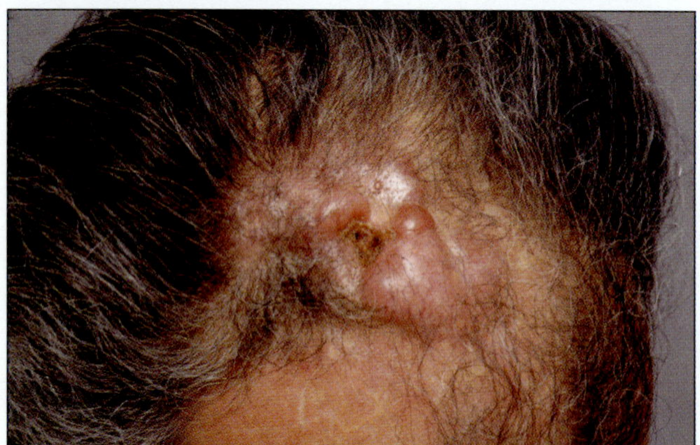

Figure 5.60   Follicular lymphoma involving the scalp.

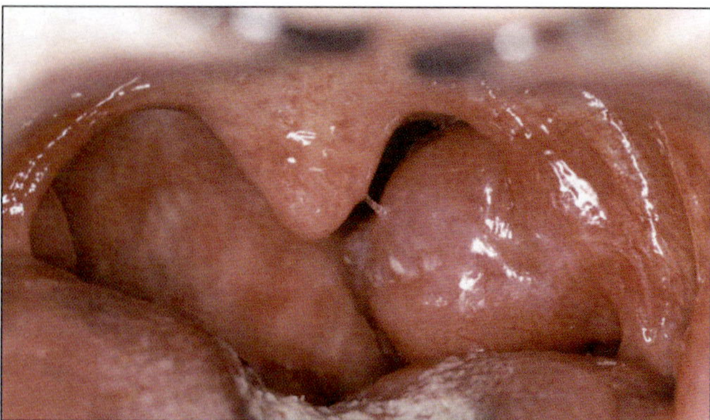

Figure 5.61   Follicular lymphoma of the left tonsil. Lymphoma is the most common tumor of the tonsils in children; however, in adults lymphomas appear clinically similar to the more common tonsillar tumor, squamous cell carcinoma.

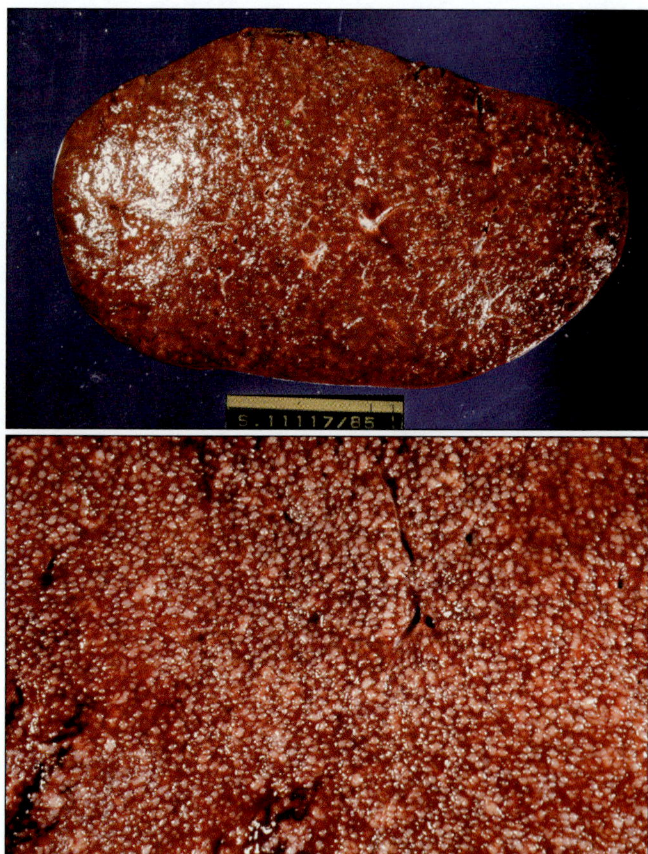

Figure 5.62   Follicular lymphoma in spleen. This gross splenectomy specimen shows tiny macroscopically visible neoplastic nodules of follicular lymphoma diffusely involving the entire spleen.

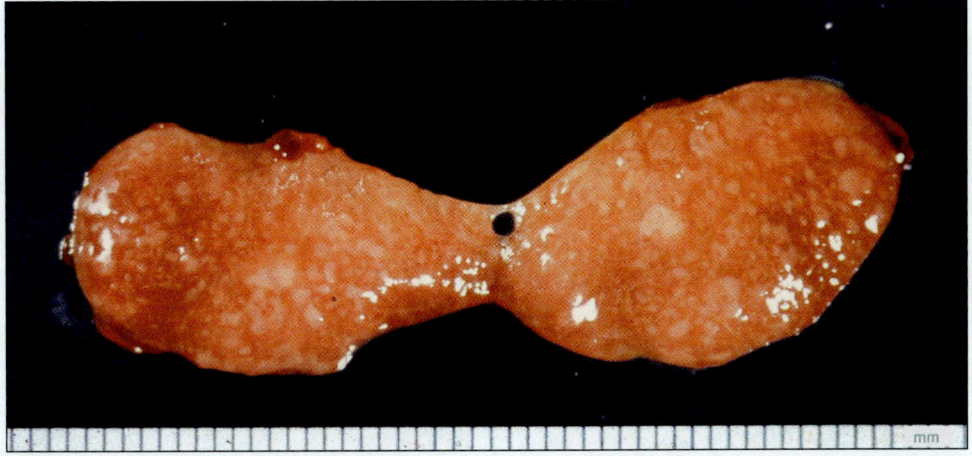

Figure 5.63 Follicular lymphoma. This gross specimen of a freshly resected lymph node is cut to reveal the macroscopically visible neoplastic follicles in follicular lymphoma.

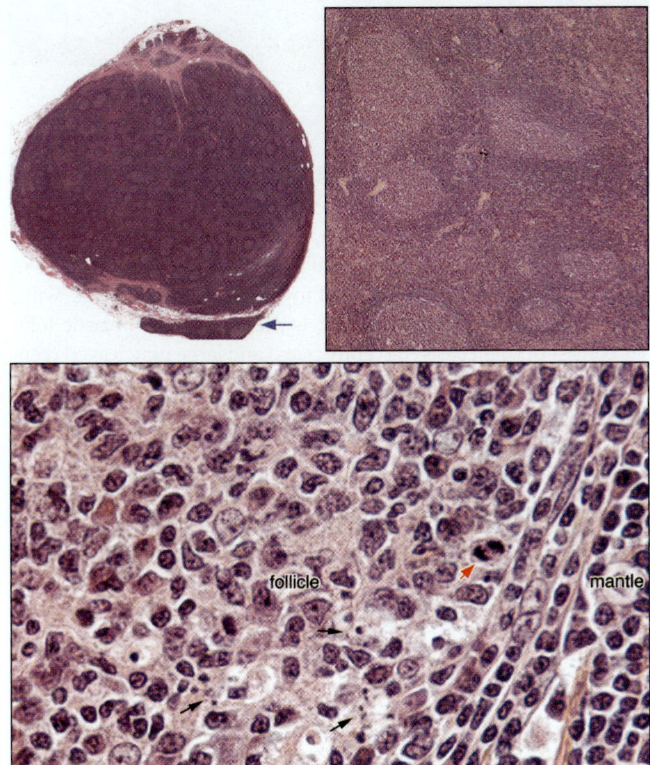

Figure 5.64 Reactive follicular hyperplasia. An enlarged submandibular lymph node shows numerous follicles of varying size that do not appear crowded. Focally (*blue arrow*), the lymphoid tissue extends outside the capsule into adjacent adipose tissue. This extracapsular tissue, however, contains reactive follicles similar to the follicles inside the capsule. The follicles contain prominent, well-defined germinal centers that have a reactive appearance, with frequent tingible body macrophages (*black arrows*) and a brisk mitotic rate (*red arrow*). Undisrupted, well-demarcated, broad mantle zones surround the follicles. Immunohistochemistry was negative for bcl-2 protein.

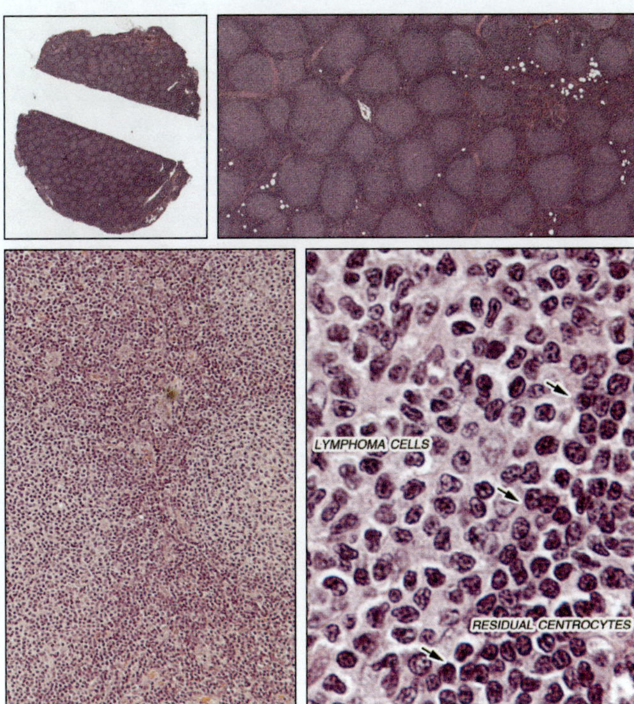

Figure 5.65 Follicular lymphoma, Grade 1. Fibroadipose tissue is involved by crowded, diffusely distributed, uniformly sized aggregates composed almost exclusively of well-spaced centrocytes with cleaved nuclear contours. For comparison, the right corner of the bottom right panel shows benign centrocytes with regularly contoured nuclei and condensed chromatin (*arrows*).

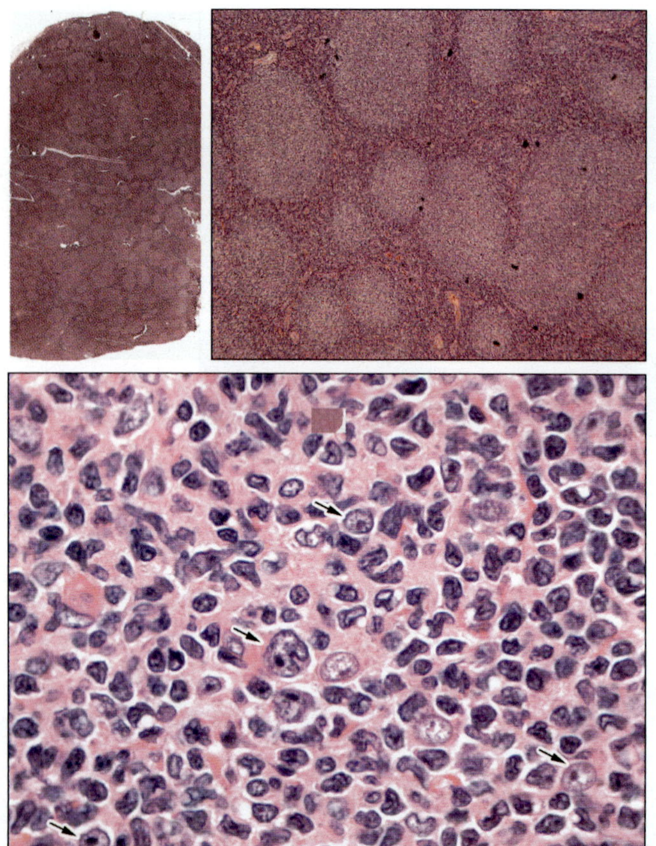

Figure 5.66   Follicular lymphoma, Grade 1. This lymph node is replaced by regularly distributed, uniformly sized aggregates consisting almost exclusively of centrocytes with cleaved nuclear contours. The lymph node appears to be replaced by expanding sheets of monotonous small-cleaved follicular center cells. Only occasional, larger nucleolated cells are seen (*arrows*) in this example of low-grade follicular lymphoma.

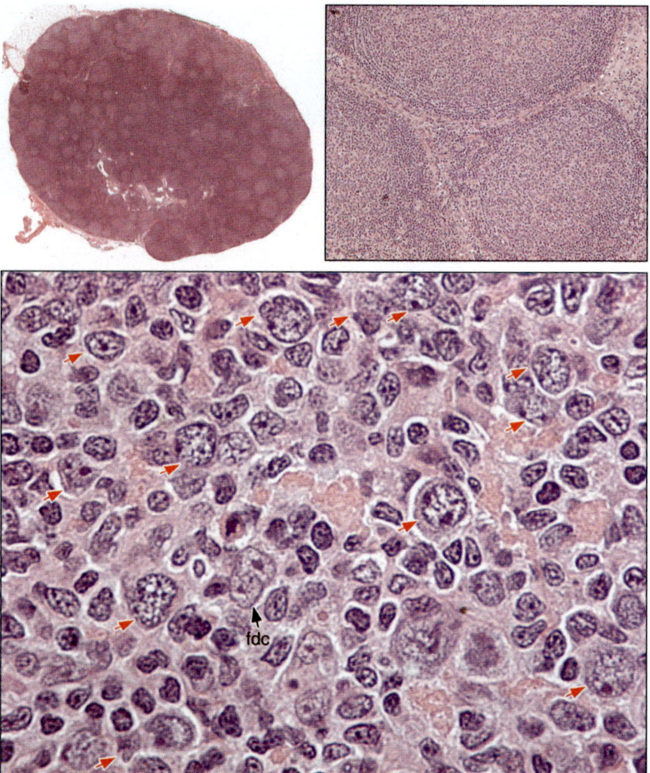

Figure 5.67   Follicular lymphoma, Grade 2. The lymph node architecture is completely effaced by uniform, crowded follicles, some of which merge into each other. Focal invasion into the capsule, without extension into perinodal tissue, is present. The neoplastic follicles consist of small cleaved (centrocytes) and large noncleaved (centroblasts, *red arrows*) cells. An average of nine large noncleaved cells was present in 10 high-power fields. A rare follicular dendritic cell (fdc) is also visible among the lymphoma cells. Immunophenotype (by immunohistochemistry and flow cytometry) of the lymphoma cells revealed: CDs 20$^+$/10$^+$/23$^+$/5$^-$/11c$^-$/bcl2$^+$/ bcl6$^+$. MIB-1 staining showed positivity in approximately 25% of the follicular lymphoma cells. DNA analysis revealed a low S-phase fraction of 1%.

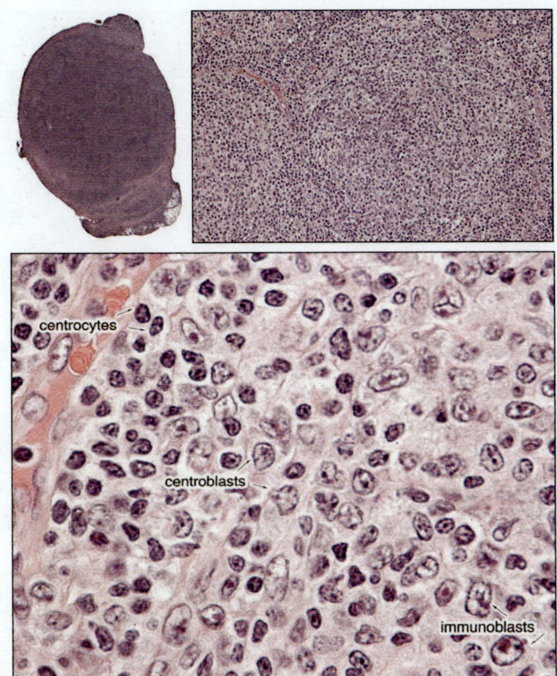

Figure 5.68 Follicular lymphoma, Grade 3. This lymph node shows numerous uniformly spaced and sized nodules composed almost exclusively of large nucleolated centroblasts. Squeezed between the malignant nodules of centroblasts are linear arrays of centrocytes.

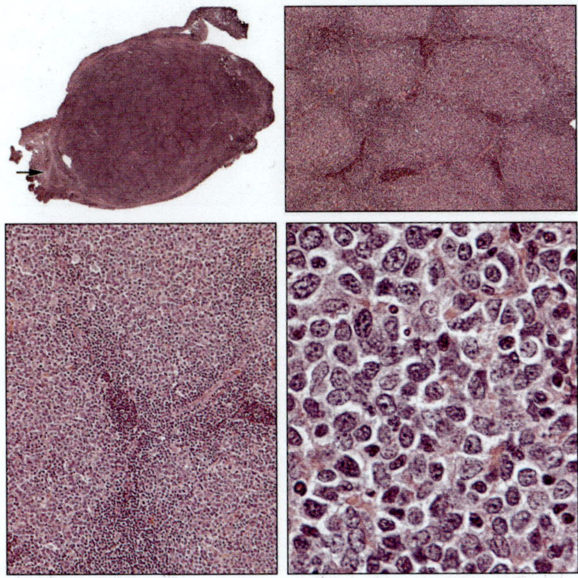

Figure 5.69 Follicular lymphoma, Grade 3 (3b subtype). A retroperitoneal lymph node is replaced by numerous, back-to-back lymphoid follicles that often merge together. The follicles consist of monotonous, intermediate-to-large cells with irregular nuclei, vesicular chromatin, small distinct nucleoli, and scanty, basophilic cytoplasm. The proliferation extends through the lymph node capsule into surrounding adipose tissue (*arrow*). Immunophenotype of the lymphoma cells reveals: CDs $20^+/10^+/20^+/23^+/5^-/11c^-$, and $bcl6^+$. DNA analysis revealed that 60% of lymphoma cells had an aneuploid DNA content, with a DNA index of 1.18 and an S-phase fraction of 10%, the last consistent with intermediate grade.

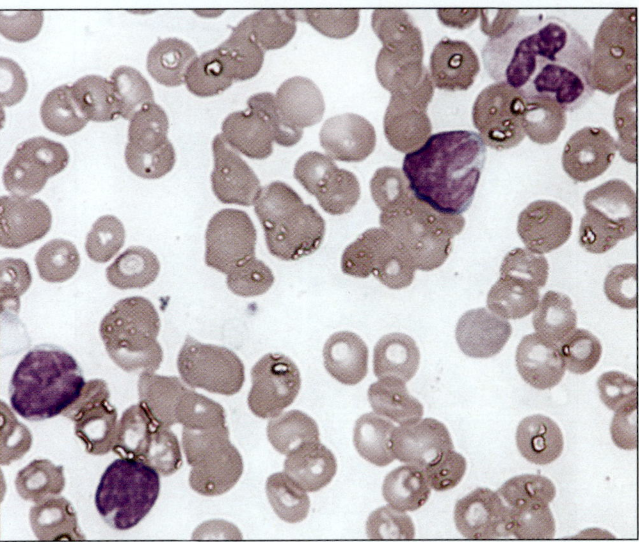

Figure 5.70 Follicular lymphoma cells in aspirate smear. Medium-sized atypical lymphoid cells with cleaved nuclei are present in this aspirate from a marrow replaced by follicular lymphoma.

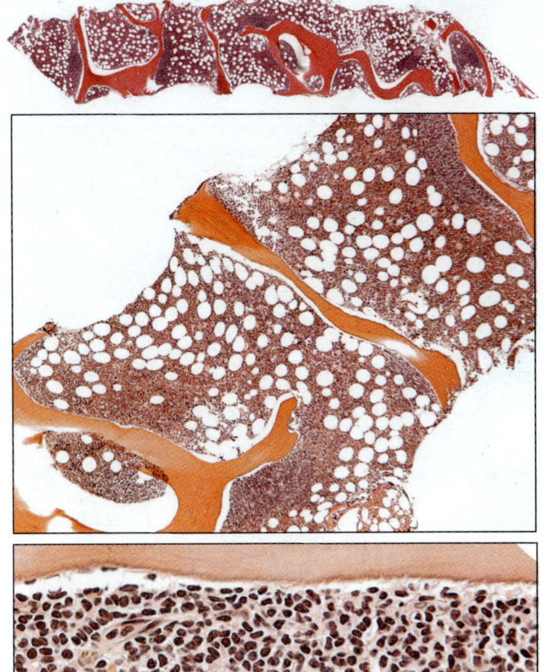

Figure 5.71 Marrow involvement by non-Hodgkin lymphoma (NHL), follicular type. This bone marrow biopsy demonstrates extensive involvement by NHL, follicular type, with the multiple paratrabecular lymphoid aggregates closely hugging bony trabeculae. As shown in the lower panel, closer inspection reveals that the lymphoid infiltrate consists primarily of small lymphocytes with close chromatin pattern and irregular nuclear contours.

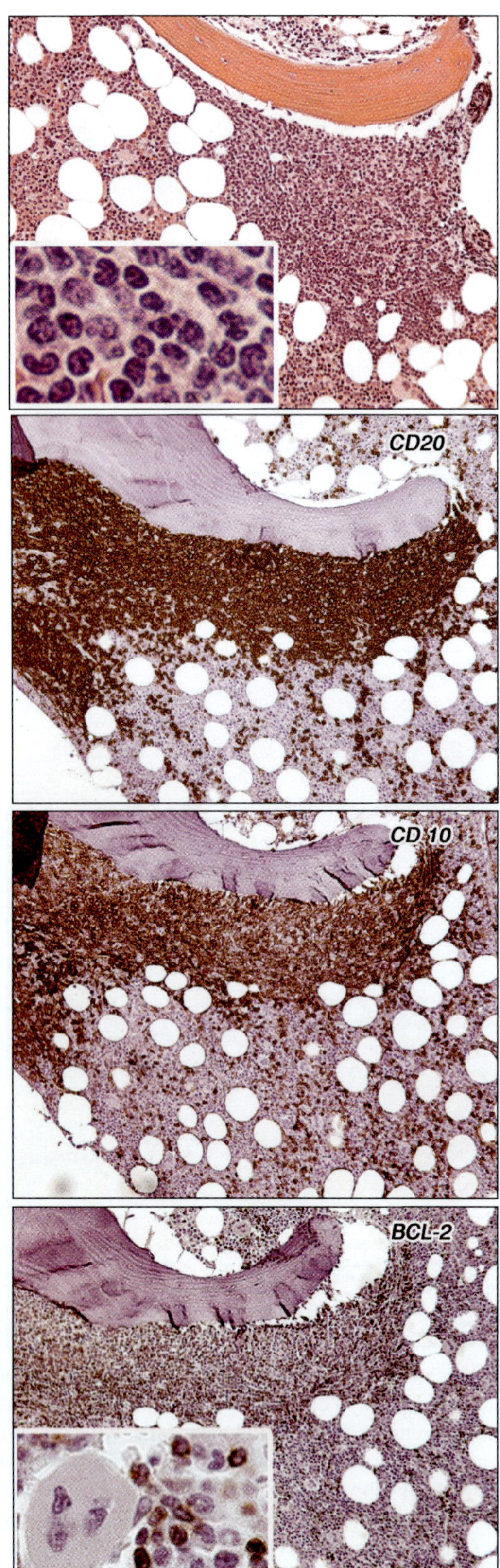

Figure 5.72   NHL, follicular type involving marrow. Medium-power views of biopsy from a case of NHL, follicular type, show the characteristic paratrabecular aggregates. Paratrabecular collections of CD20$^+$/CD10$^+$/bcl2$^+$ small lymphoid cells are typical when this disease affects the bone marrow. Note the nuclear staining pattern for bcl2 (*inset, lower panel*).

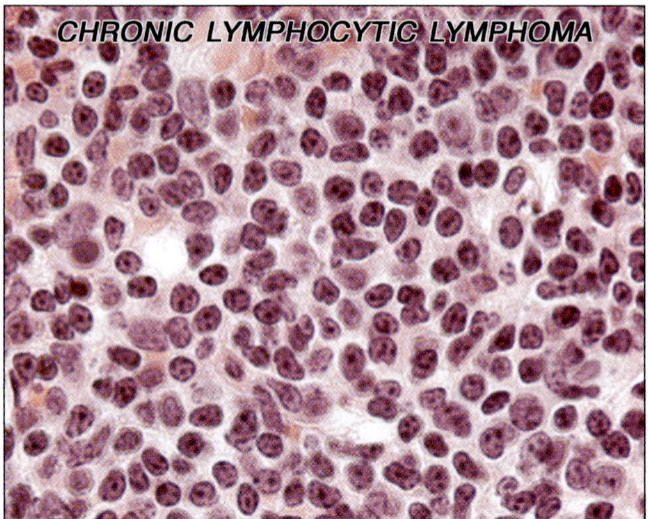

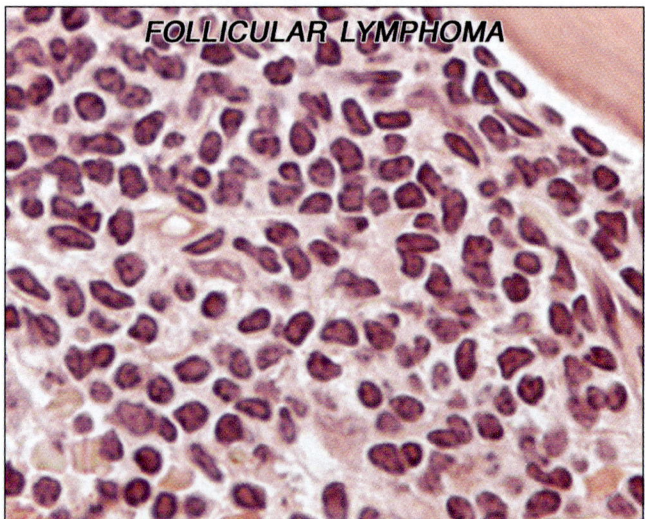

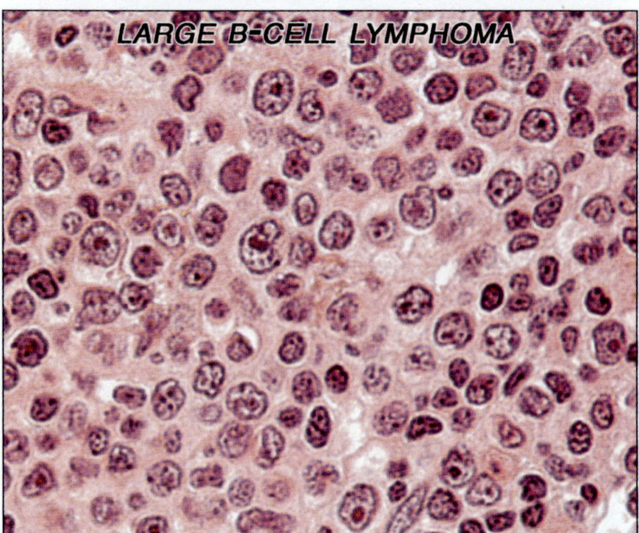

Figure 5.73   Nuclear morphology of CLL, follicular lymphoma, and large B-cell lymphoma cells in biopsy. Although lymphomas should not be classified based on appearance in bone marrow, this composite figure highlights the differences in nuclear morphology among these three different B-cell lymphoproliferative disorders.

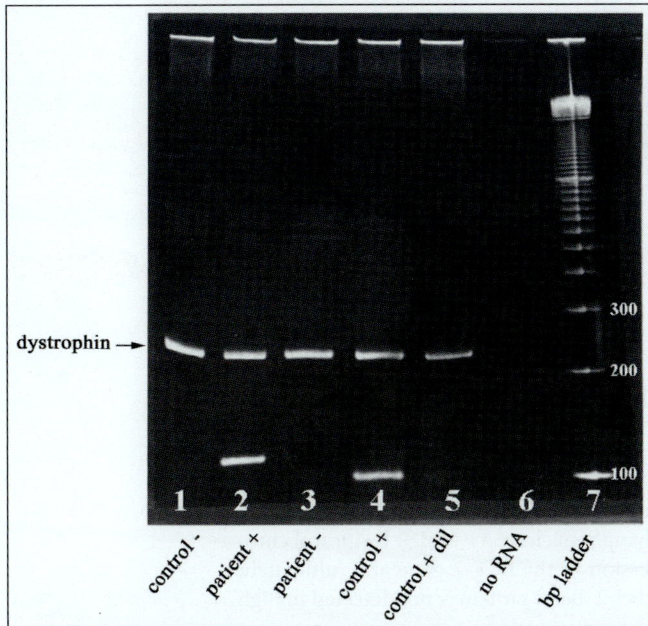

Figure 5.74 Detection of clonal B cells by PCR. Malignant B- or T-cell proliferations are clonal, which helps to distinguish them from reactive polyclonal proliferations. PCR is a sensitive assay used to detect abnormal clonal B- and T-cell populations in which JH primers are used to amplify the V and J regions in the IGH gene. The internal control is a region of the dystrophin gene. Lane 1 is the negative control, 2 is a positive patient, 3 is a negative patient, 4 is positive control, 5 is positive control diluted to 1:1,000, 6 is without input RNA, and 7 is a 100-bp DNA ladder. In a polyclonal population of B cells, a variety of PCR products are produced, resulting in a mixed population of DNA fragments that differ slightly in size and result in a very faint or undetectable smear when run on gels (patient⁻). In B-cell lymphoma, a single PCR product is produced resulting a discrete band (patient⁺ and control⁺ lanes). (Courtesy Dr. S. Kamel-Reid.)

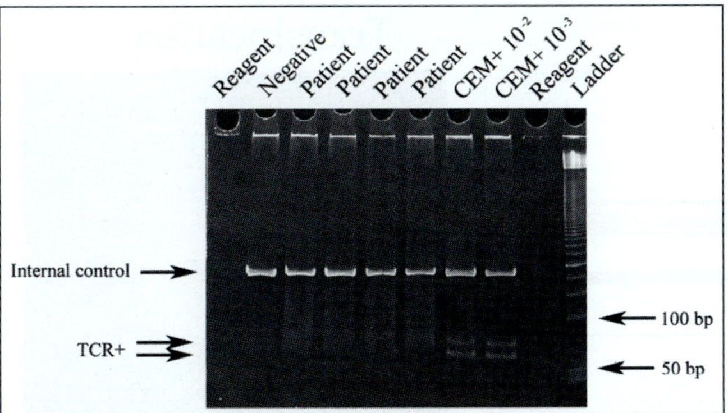

Figure 5.75 Detection of clonal T cells by PCR. The faint DNA smears between the 50- and 100-bp marker on this gel indicates that no clonal T-cell population is detectable in the four patient samples analyzed. Clonal T-cell receptor rearrangement is not lineage specific and not uncommonly detected in B-cell and other neoplasms. (Courtesy Dr. S. Kamel-Reid.)

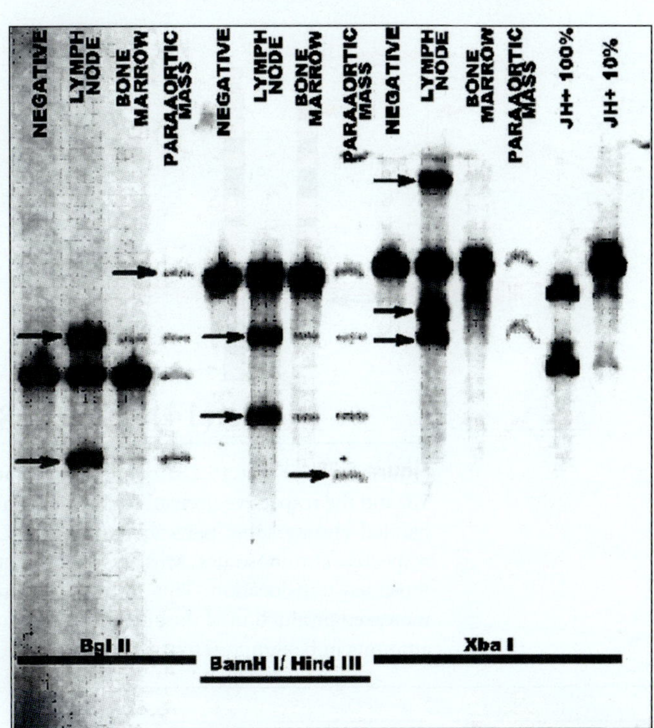

Figure 5.76 Detection of clonal B cells by Southern blot. Southern blot is a specific assay and regarded as the gold standard to detect abnormal clonal B-cell populations. Clonal populations are detected by the appearance of new bands (*arrows*) following digestion of extracted tumor DNA by enzymes (restriction endonucleases) that cleave DNA in a sequence-specific manner. Compared with PCR, Southern blot is a time-consuming test that requires more tissue. (Courtesy Dr. S. Kamel-Reid.)

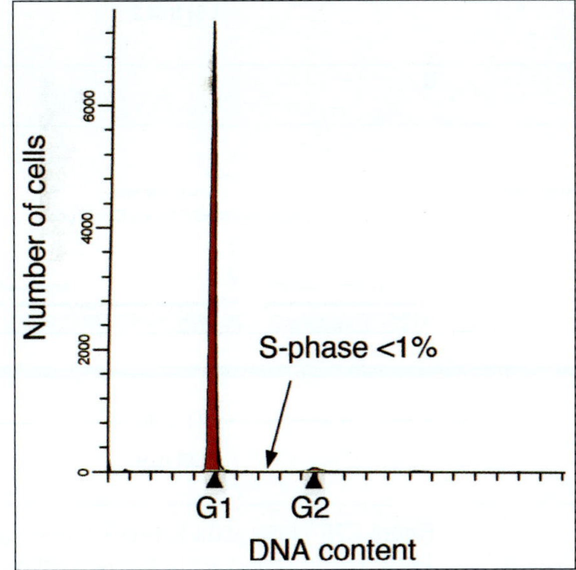

Figure 5.77 Low S-phase fraction in low-grade lymphomas. S-phase fraction, an index of cellular proliferation measured by DNA flow cytometry, of less than 5% is typically seen in low-grade follicular lymphoma. (Courtesy J. Davidson.)

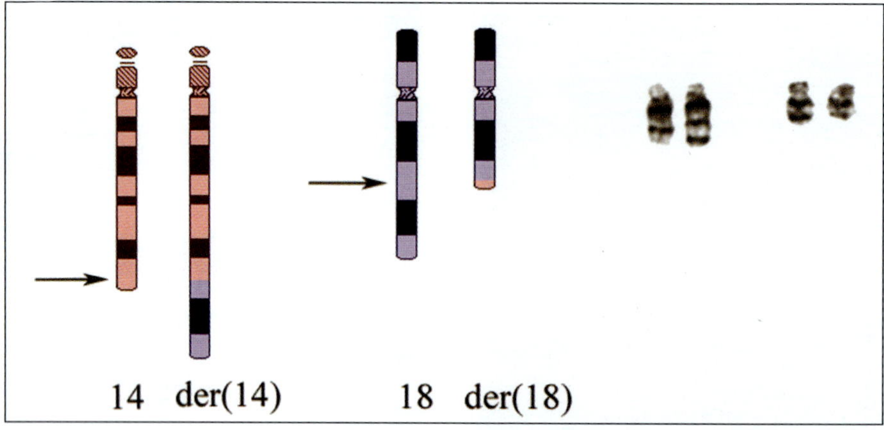

Figure 5.78 The t(14;18)(q32;q21) rearrangement. The ideograms of chromosomes 14, 18, and the respective derivative chromosomes are to the left in color. The corresponding G-banded chromosome pairs are to the right. The arrows indicate the breakpoints on the respective chromosomes. Most cases of follicular lymphoma have a t(14;18) reciprocal chromosomal translocation. This results in overexpression of the BCL-2 gene and, ultimately, increased production of the antiapoptotic protein bcl-2. Bcl-2 protein is not detected in high amounts in benign, reactive germinal-center cells.

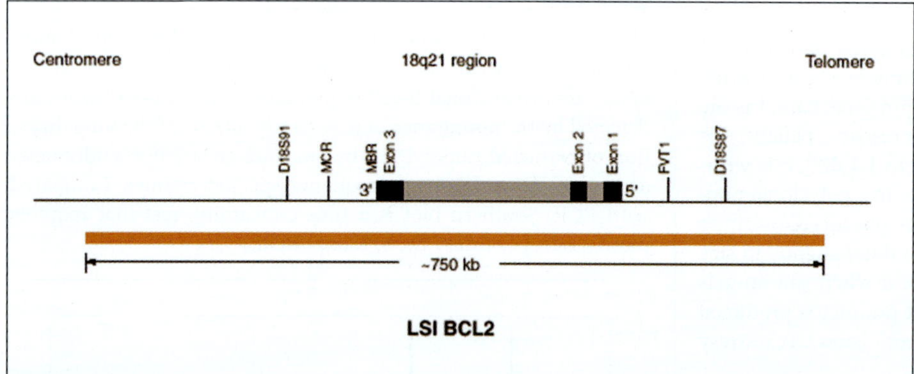

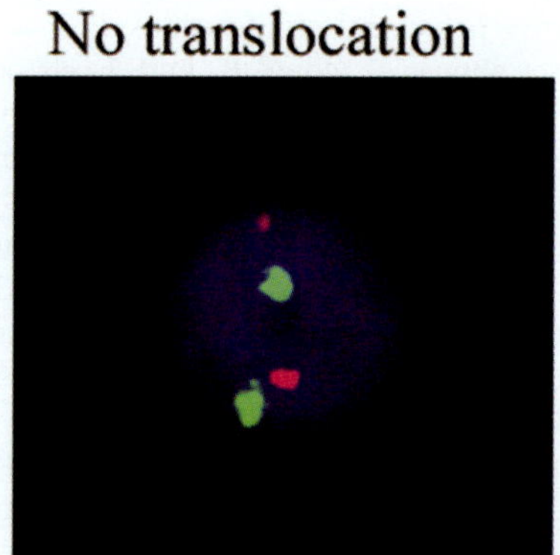

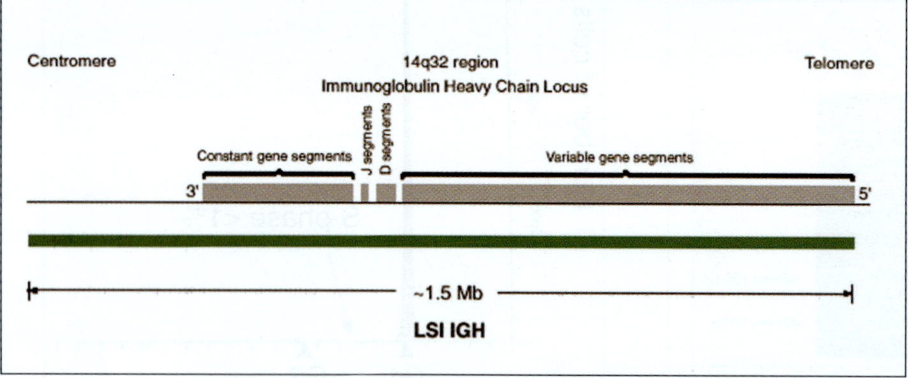

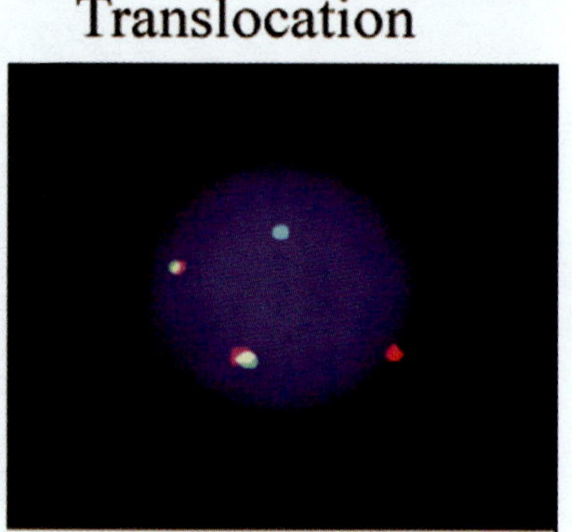

Figure 5.79 FISH of the IGH/BCL2 fusion gene. The BCL2 gene at 18q21 (*red*) and the IGH gene at 14q32 (*green*) co-localize to generate yellow signals, indicating a reciprocal translocation involving these loci.

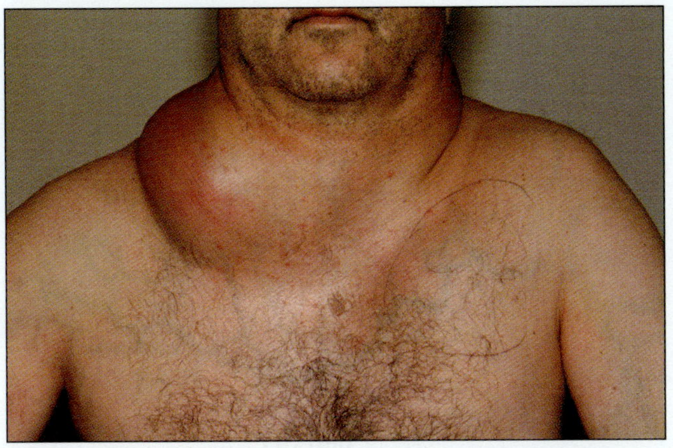

Figure 5.80 Mantle cell lymphoma. This middle-aged man has extensive lymphadenopathy, including prominent right supraclavicular lymph nodes from recurrent Mantle cell lymphoma (MZL).

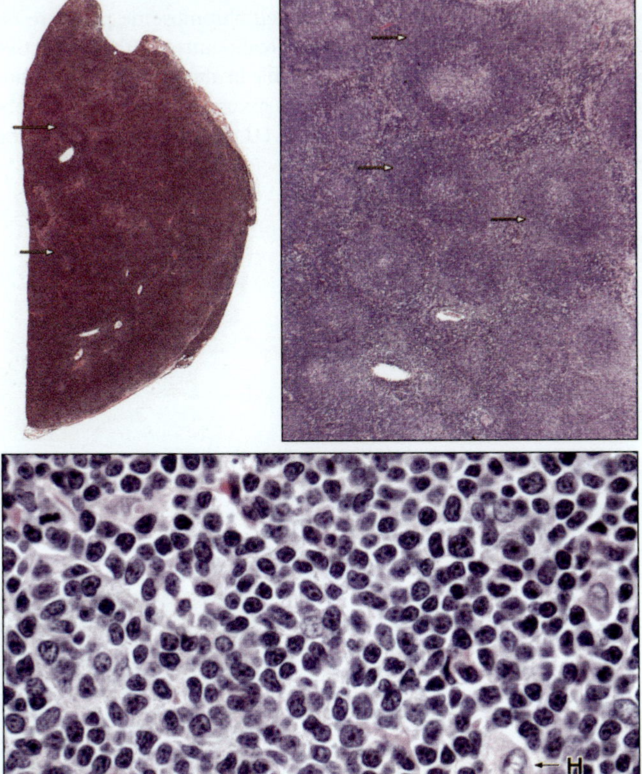

Figure 5.81 Mantle cell lymphoma, nodular type, and mantle-zone pattern. Neoplastic nodules of medium-sized lymphoid cells with slightly irregular nuclear contours efface the lymph node architecture. Some of the nodules retain a distinctly mantle-zone pattern, in which expanded collars of mantle zones surround germinal centers (*arrows*). The high-power view on the bottom panel shows cytologic detail of the mantle lymphoma cells with a histiocyte nucleus (H) for size comparison.

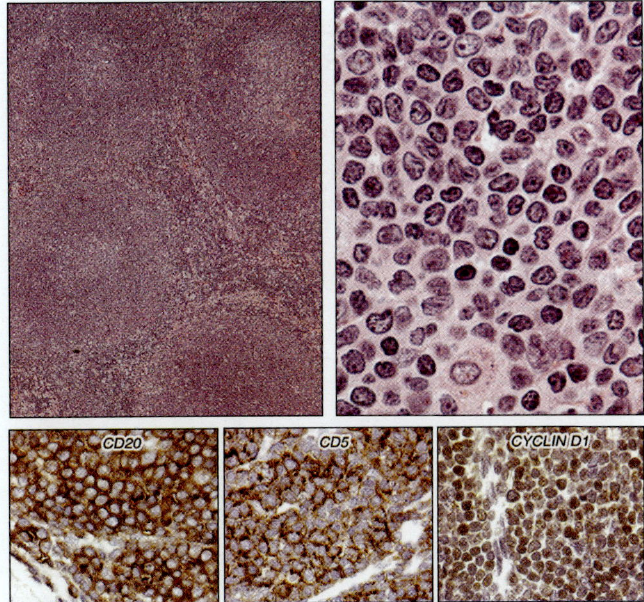

Figure 5.82 Mantle cell lymphoma (multiple lymphomatous polyposis). Sections from the jejunum show widespread polypoid lesions composed of submucosal nodules of small lymphoid cells that were cyclin D1$^+$/CD5$^+$/CD20$^+$ B-cells by immunohistochemistry.

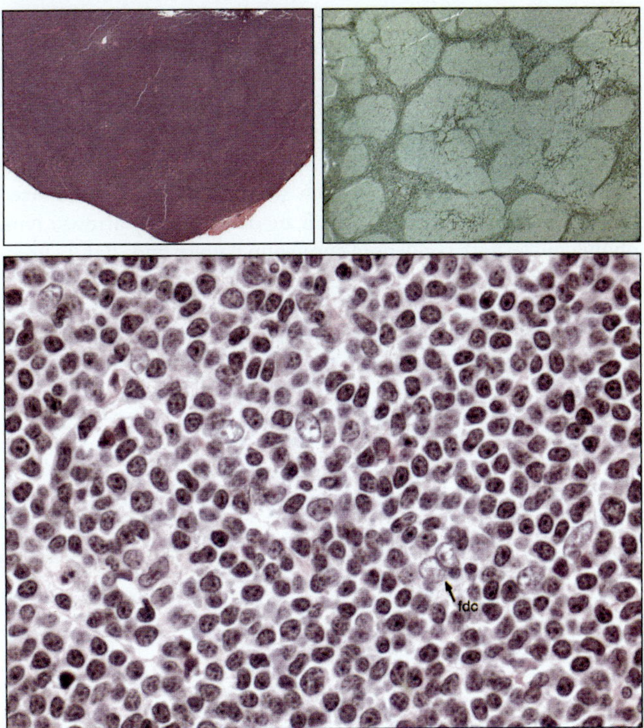

Figure 5.83 Mantle cell lymphoma, nodular type. This lymph node is effaced by a nodular expansion of medium-sized lymphoid cells with a closed chromatin pattern and fairly regular nuclear contours. The low-power view of a reticulin-stained lymph node section in the right upper panel highlights the nodular pattern of involvement. Admixed with the mantle lymphoma cells are occasional follicular dendritic cells, one delineated by an arrow showing classic "kissing" nuclei.

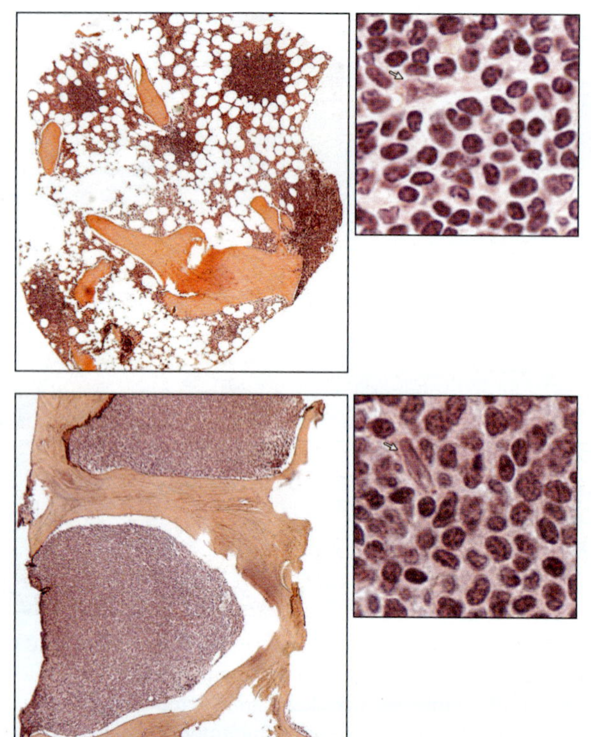

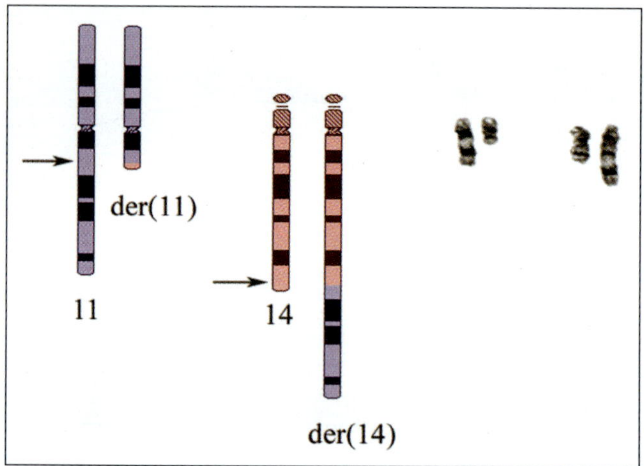

Figure 5.85   The t(11;14)(q13;q32) rearrangement in Mantle cell lymphoma. The diagnostic t(11;14) of Mantle cell lymphoma is depicted here. The ideograms of chromosomes 11, 14, and the respective derivative chromosomes are illustrated on the left in color, and the corresponding G-banded chromosome pairs are on the right. The arrows indicate the breakpoints on the respective chromosomes. The t(11;14) is detectable in almost all cases of Mantle cell lymphomas. This translocation juxtaposes the immunoglobulin heavy chain (IGH) and the cyclin D1 gene (CCND1), resulting in overexpression of cyclin D1.

Figure 5.84   Marrow involvement by non-Hodgkin lymphoma, mantle cell. Low- and high-power views of bone marrow biopsies from two cases of Mantle cell lymphoma are shown here. The pattern of marrow involvement and the cytologic appearance of Mantle cell lymphoma can be quite variable. Two different cases are demonstrated here, with one revealing a nodular pattern of infiltration (*top panels*) and the other displaying a diffuse pattern (*lower panels*). High-power views in both show small- to medium-sized (endothelial nuclei for comparison are delineated by arrows) lymphoma nuclei with condensed chromatin pattern and slightly irregular nuclear contours.

Figure 5.86 FISH of the IGH/CCND1 fusion gene in Mantle cell lymphoma. A standard FISH assay that is used to detect the t(11;14) in either formalin-fixed/ paraffin embedded or fresh tissues is illustrated here. The CCND1 gene at 11q13 (*red*) and the IGH gene at 14q32 (*green*) co-localize to generate yellow signals, indicating a reciprocal translocation involving these loci. The t(11;14)(q13;q32) occurs in 95% of cases by FISH, although it may not be readily detectable by standard cytogenetics.

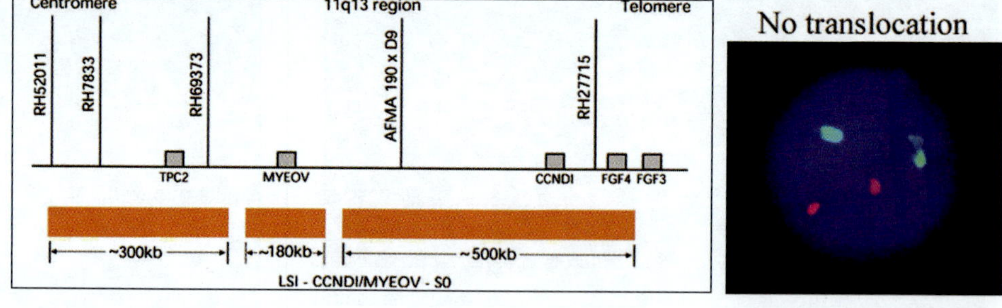

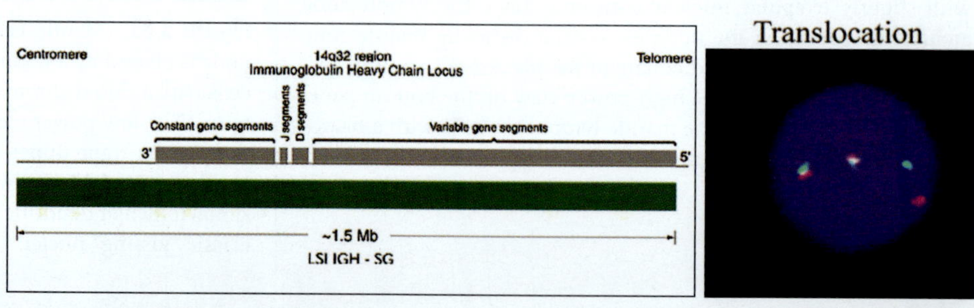

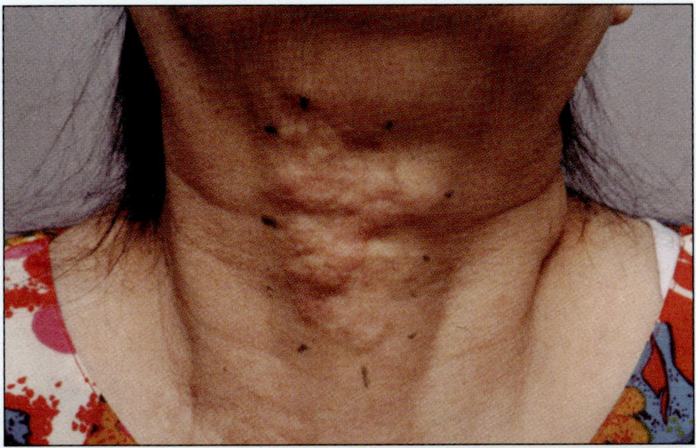

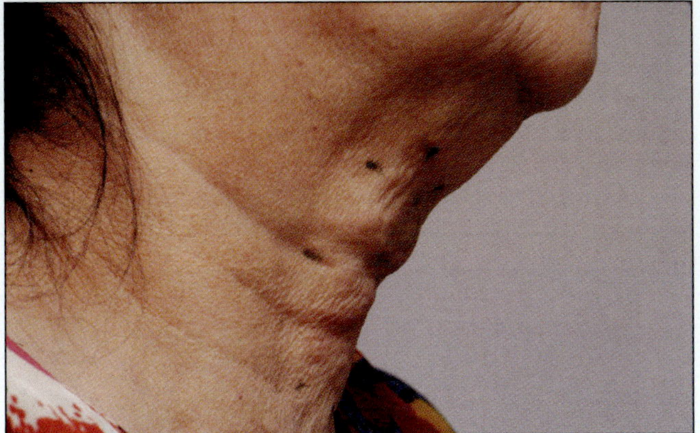

Figure 5.87 Diffuse large B-cell lymphoma (DLBL) of the thyroid. Any extranodal location can be a primary site for diffuse large B-cell lymphoma.

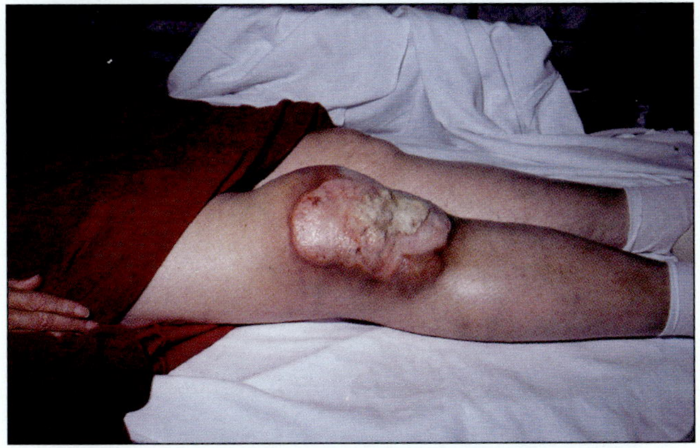

Figure 5.88 Diffuse large B-cell lymphoma involving the skin and subcutaneous tissues of knee.

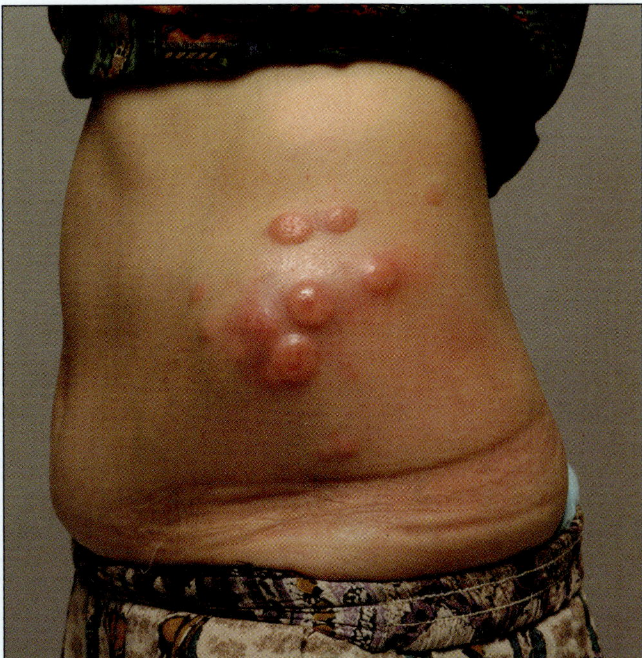

Figure 5.89 Diffuse large B-cell lymphoma involving the skin and subcutaneous tissues of abdominal wall.

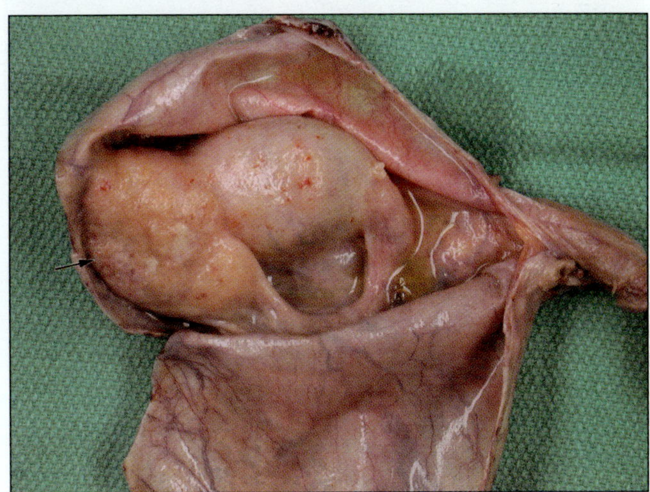

Figure 5.90 Diffuse large B-cell lymphoma involving the inferior aspect of a testis.

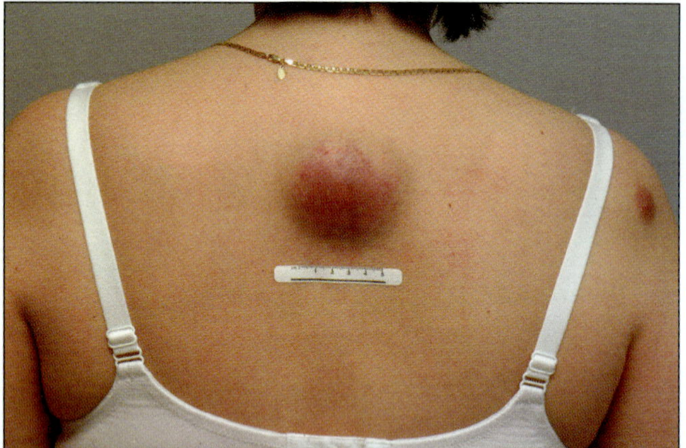

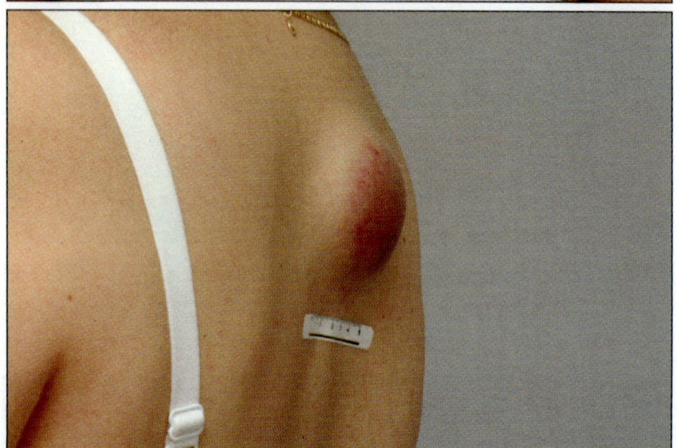

Figure 5.91   Diffuse large B-cell lymphoma involving the skin and subcutaneous tissues of back.

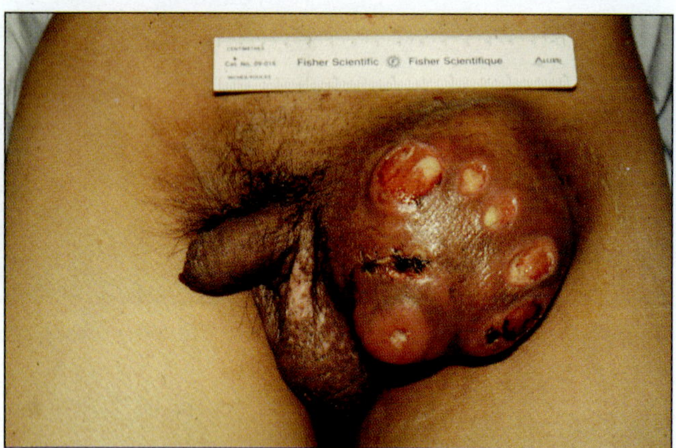

Figure 5.92   Diffuse large B-cell lymphoma involving left inguinal lymph nodes.

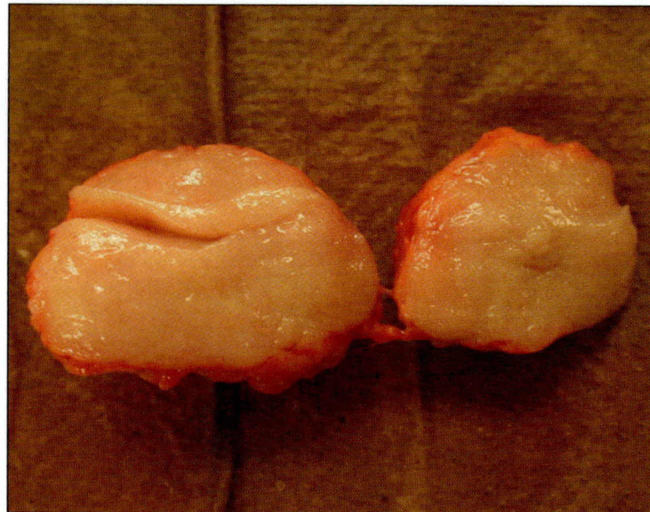

Figure 5.93   Diffuse large B-cell lymphoma involving lymph node. This lymph node shows the homogenous, fish-flesh appearance of lymphoma totally replacing the entire lymph node.

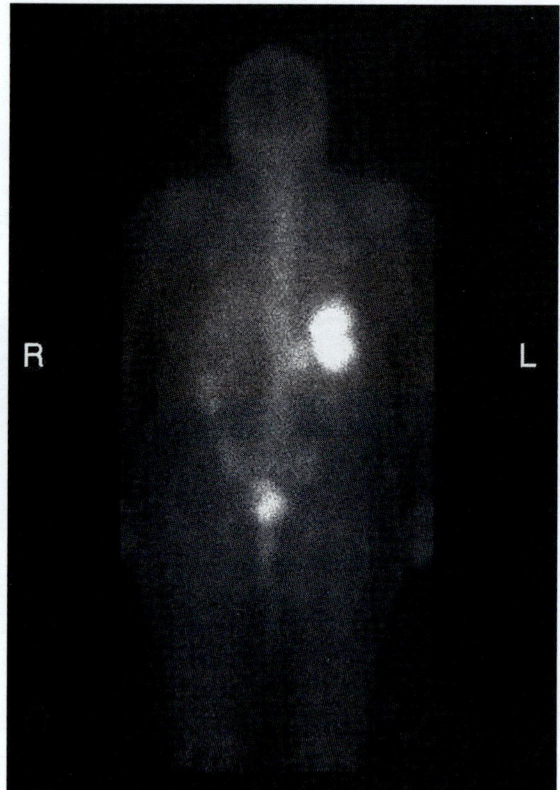

Figure 5.94   Gallium uptake scan showing two prominent discrete areas of increased uptake in the spleen in a case of DLBL extensively involving the spleen.

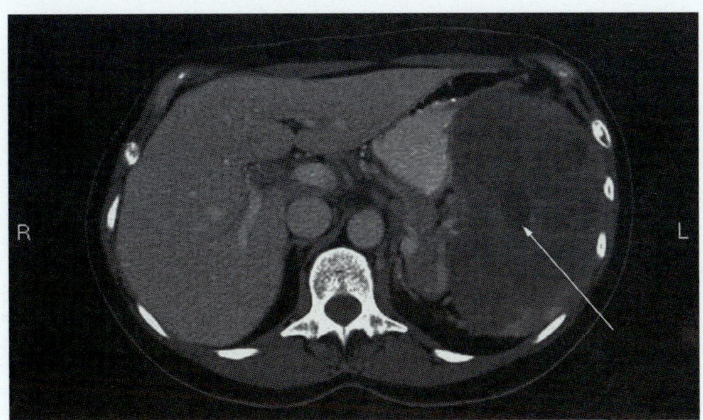

Figure 5.95 An axial CT of abdomen with oral and intravenous contrast. The spleen is enlarged and heterogeneous, with multiple hypodense lesions (*arrow*). The latter may represent necrotic tumor. The large spleen indents the body of the stomach. (Same case as shown in Fig. 5.94.)

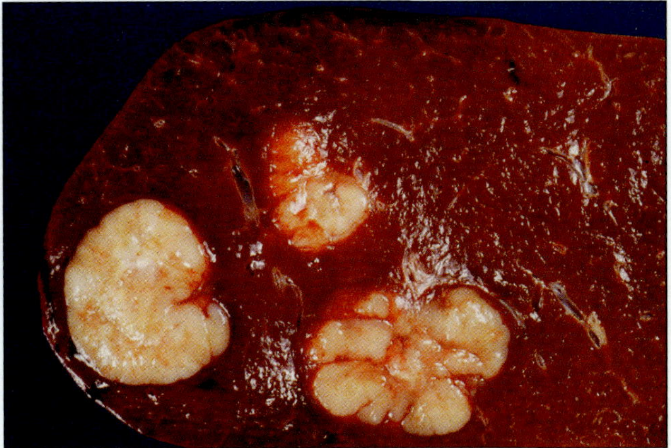

Figure 5.96 Diffuse large B-cell lymphoma involving spleen. Multiple large discrete tumors are visible in this gross splenectomy specimen.

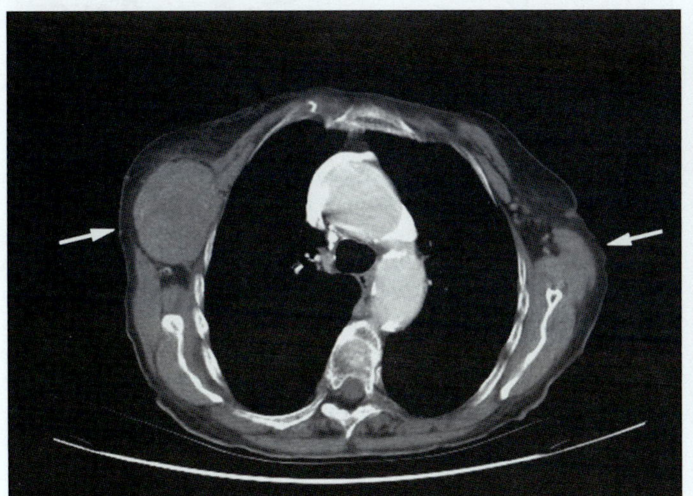

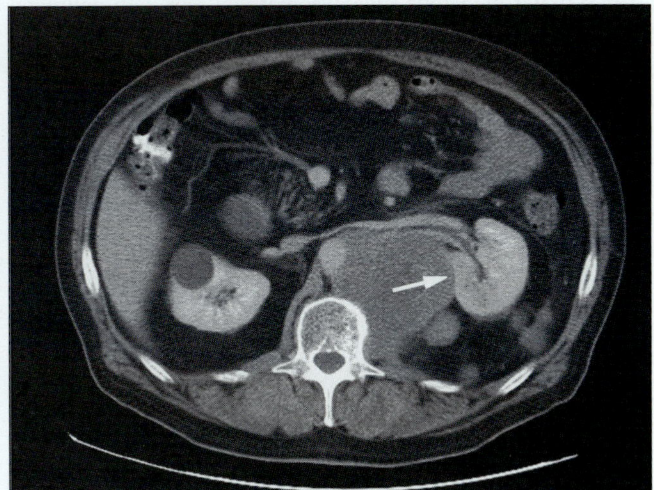

Figure 5.97 Generalized lymphadenopathy from diffuse large B-cell lymphoma. On the left is an axial thoracic CT scan with contrast that reveals soft-tissue masses in the right axillary region at the level just inferior to the aortic arch. On the right is an abdominal CT scan at the level of the left renal vein showing large retroperitoneal soft-tissue masses. The largest mass displaces the left kidney laterally.

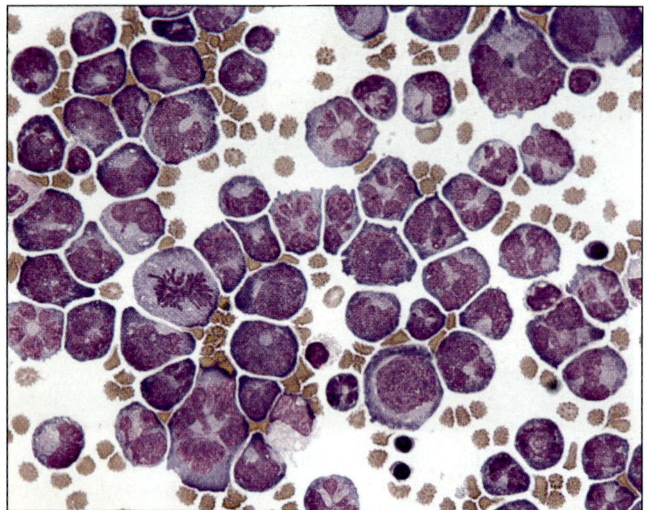

Figure 5.98   Diffuse large B-cell lymphoma involving cerebral spinal fluid (CSF). This CSF sample stained with Wright-Giemsa demonstrates numerous large, pleomorphic cells with multilobulated nuclei and a high mitotic rate.

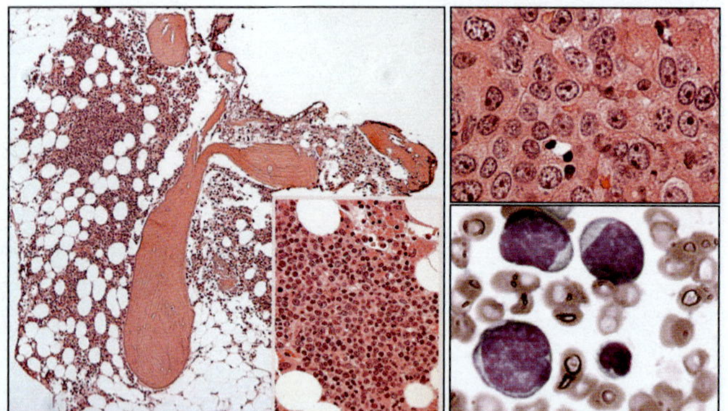

Figure 5.99   Diffuse large B-cell lymphoma involving bone marrow. As with many of the mature B-cell lymphomas, the appearance of DLBL in the marrow is highly variable, and classifying these diseases based solely on the morphologic appearance in the marrow is discouraged. Shown here are mid-trabecular aggregates composed almost exclusively of atypical, large lymphoid cells with the characteristic vesicular (or "glassy") chromatin pattern and one to two prominent nucleoli of DLBL. An aspirate smear from the same case shows a pleomorphic population of highly atypical, large lymphoid cells (*right lower panel*).

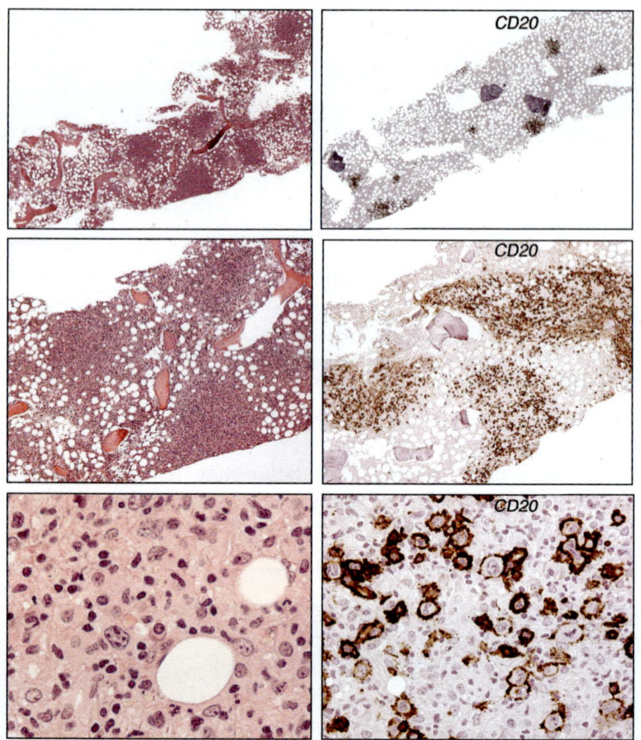

Figure 5.100   Marrow involvement by DLBL, T-cell rich type. Low-, medium-, and high-power views (*top to bottom panels, respectively*) demonstrate numerous large, poorly circumscribed, mid-trabecular aggregates made up of a heterogeneous population of large, atypical lymphoid cells with vesicular nuclei admixed with small mature lymphocytes. CD20-immunostained biopsy sections accentuate the nodular pattern of marrow involvement by the minor subpopulation of large malignant-appearing B cells that are admixed with benign reactive small T cells. This case could be mistaken for marrow involvement by Hodgkin lymphoma.

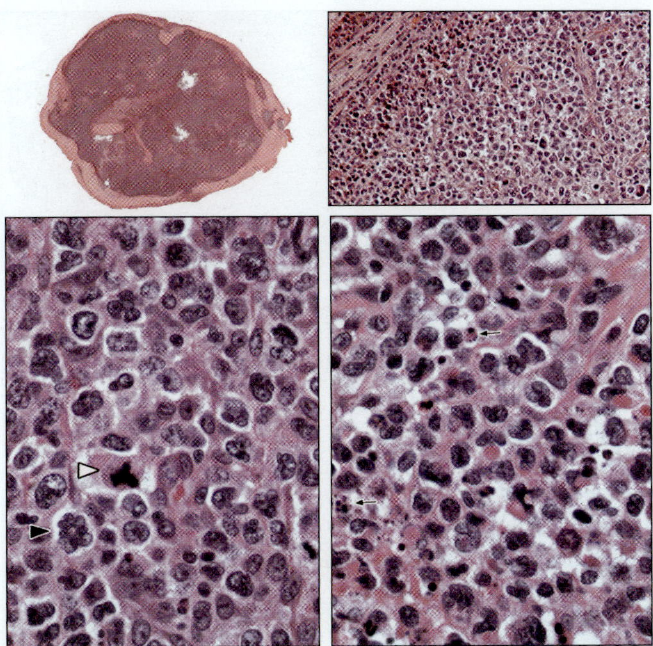

Figure 5.101   Diffuse large B-cell lymphoma (centroblastic, with multilobated cells). This lymph node shows marked sclerotic thickening of its capsule, with complete effacement of the architecture by extensive, noncohesive sheets of monotonous, large cells. A high mitotic rate with tripolar mitotic figure (*white triangle*) and multilobed nuclei (*small black triangle*) is seen, as well as numerous apoptotic bodies (*small arrows, right lower panel*). Immunophenotype of the lymphoma cells by flow cytometry and immunohistochemistry reveals a CDs $20^+/10^+/bcl6^+/kappa^+$ immunophenotype.

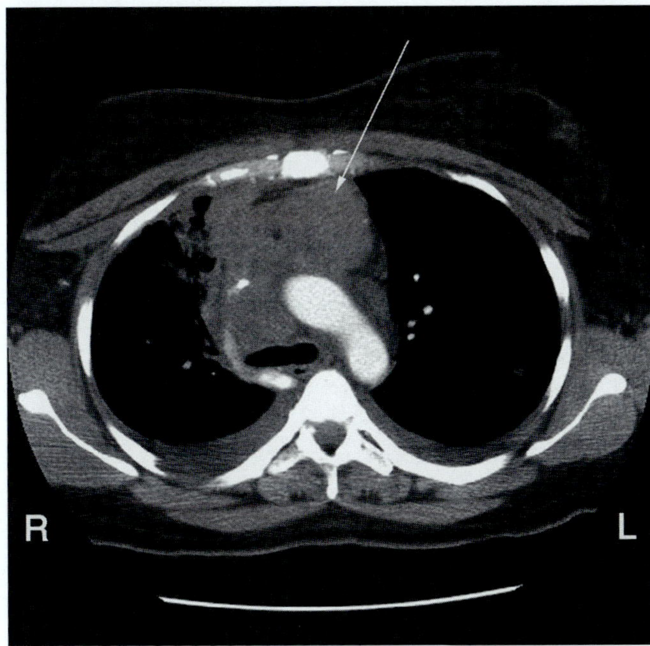

Figure 5.102   Mediastinal large B-cell lymphoma. An axial CT scan through upper thorax at the level of the aortic arch shows a large mass (*arrow*) mostly involving the anterior mediastinum.

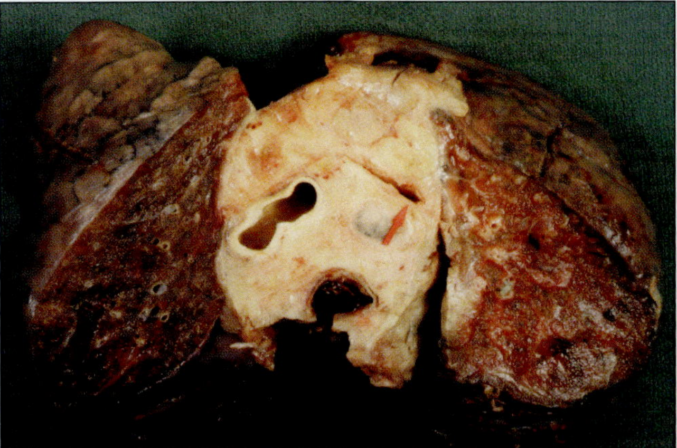

Figure 5.103   Mediastinal large B-cell lymphoma. This autopsy specimen with transversely cut lungs and mediastinum at the level of the aortic arch demonstrates a large infiltrative mass encasing the entire aortic arch and extending into adjacent lung.

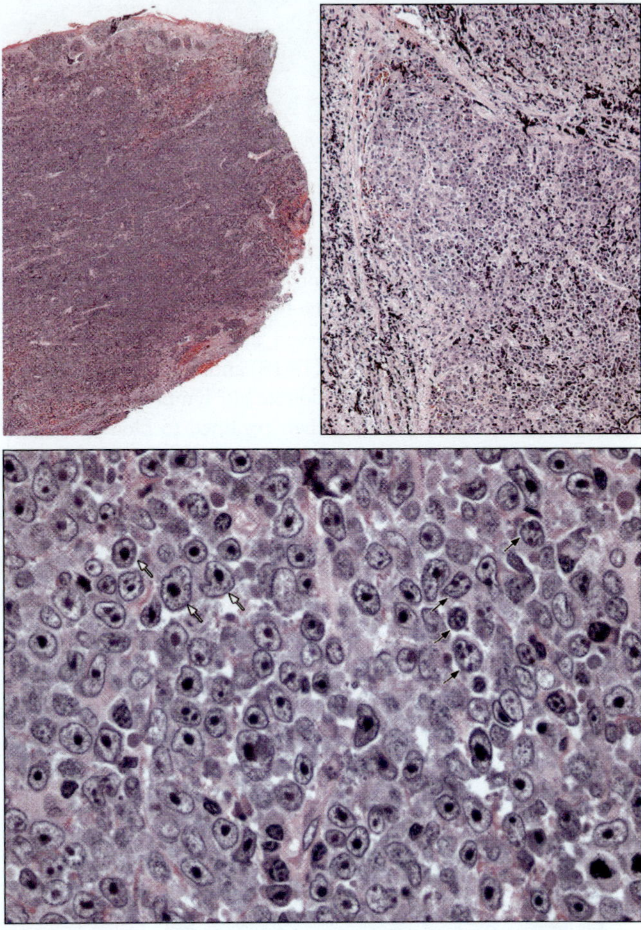

Figure 5.104   Diffuse large B-cell lymphoma (immunoblastic and centroblastic). A biopsy from the base of the tongue shows necrosis and extensive infiltration of tissue with atypical large lymphoid cells composed of immunoblasts with large, single, central nucleoli (*open arrows*) and centroblasts with multiple smaller nucleoli situated near the nuclear membrane (*closed arrows*).

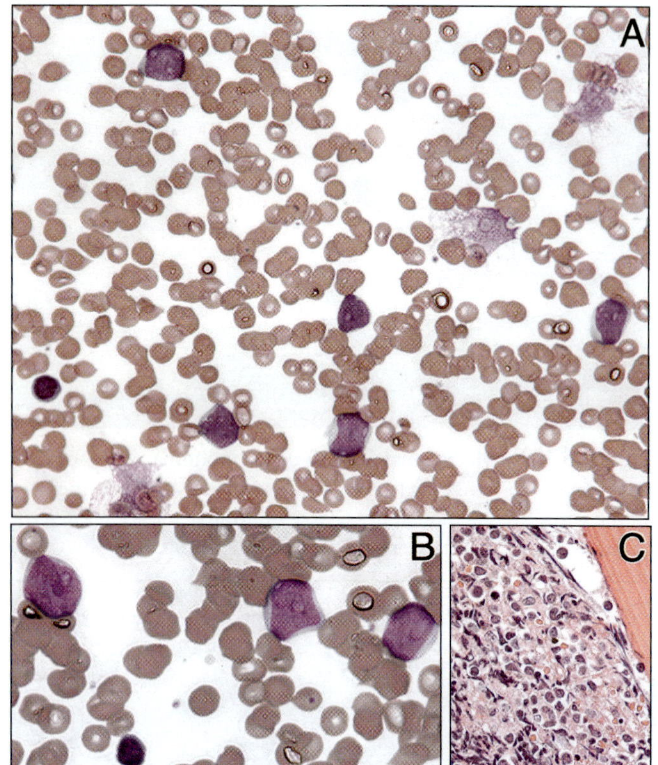

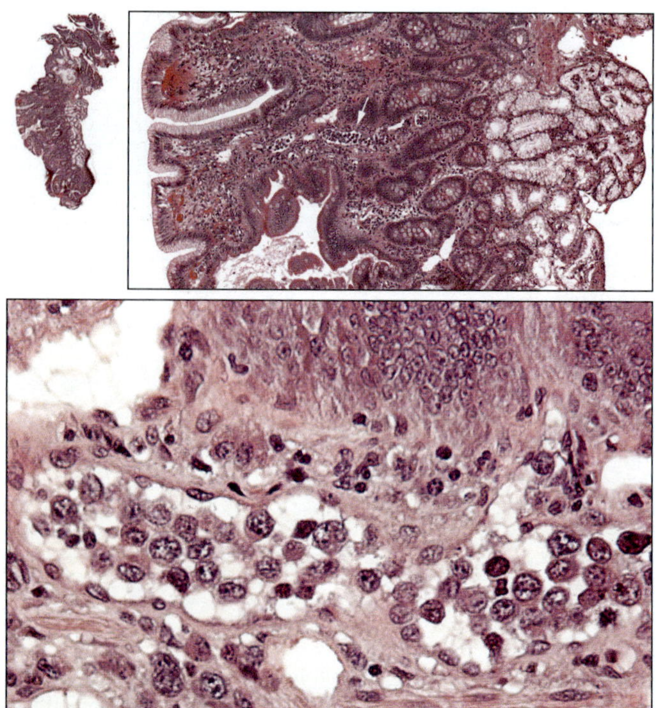

Figure 5.105   **A** and **B.** B-cell NHL associated with t(14;18) and t(8;14), leukemic phase. These blood smears show circulating, large nucleolated blasts, some with clefted nuclear contours. For comparison, mature small lymphocytes are present near the lower left corners of both figures. **C.** The bone marrow biopsy is totally replaced by sheets of poorly preserved, malignant cells that display extensive crush artifact. FISH for (14;18) and c-myc rearrangement were positive in this case. These "double hit" lymphomas, as well as diffuse large B-cell lymphoma, when confined to blood and marrow; at time of diagnosis, are easily misdiagnosed as precursor B-cell lymphoblastic leukemia/lymphoma.

Figure 5.106   Intravascular large B-cell lymphoma. This gastric biopsy from a 45-year-old man shows normal overall architecture, but higher magnification in lower panel reveal a vessel filled with highly atypical large CD20$^+$ B-cell lymphoma cells.

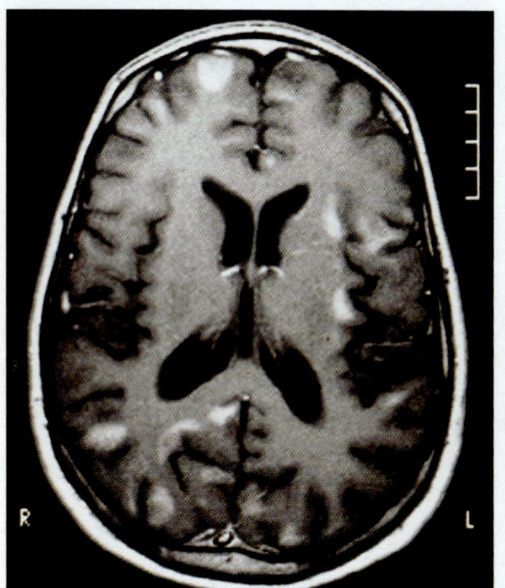

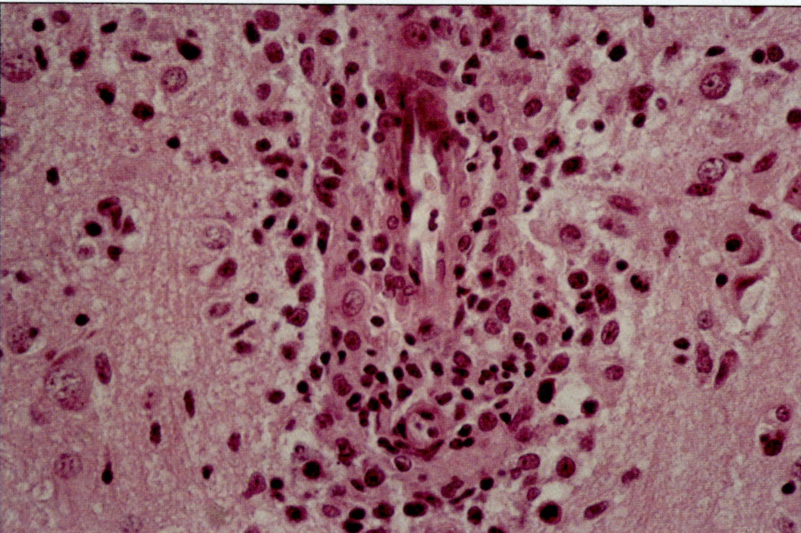

Figure 5.107   Angiocentric diffuse large B-cell lymphoma (lymphomatoid granulomatosis). The left panel is a magnetic resonance image (MRI) axial T1-weighted image with intravenous contrast showing multiple enhancing lesions at the gray–white junctions of the cerebral cortex. The figure on the right is from the autopsy brain of the same case, showing atypical lymphoid cells invading cerebral blood vessels and causing fibrinoid necrosis. (Courtesy Dr. J. Bilbao.)

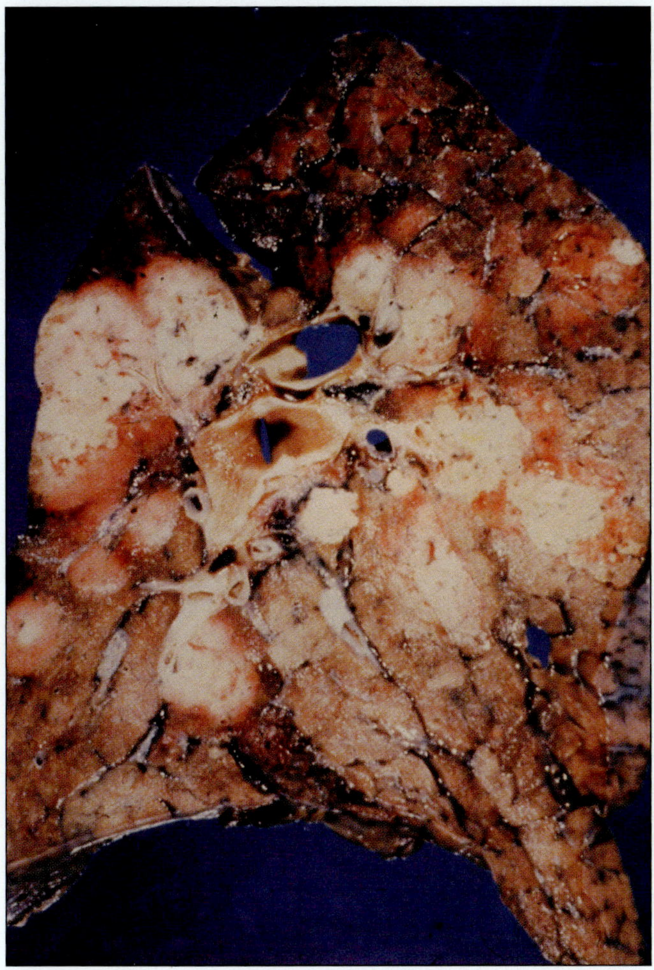

Figure 5.108 Angiocentric diffuse large B-cell lymphoma (lymphomatoid granulomatosis). An autopsy lung from a patient with lymphomatoid granulomatosis reveals extensive involvement with multiple necrotizing lesions.

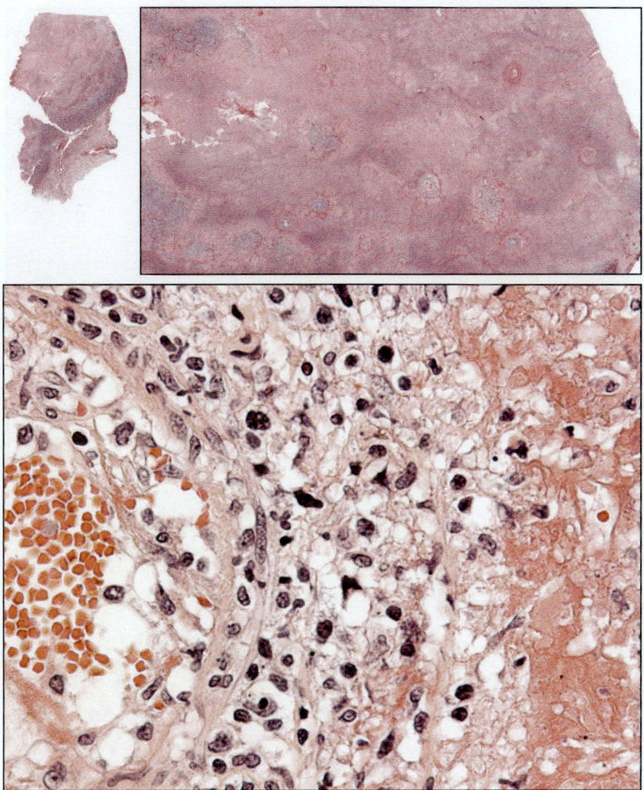

Figure 5.109 Angiocentric diffuse large B-cell lymphoma (lymphomatoid granulomatosis), grade 3/3. Lung biopsy showing large lymphoid cells restricted to blood vessels and displaying a vasculitic pattern of involvement, with fibrinoid necrosis and angioinvasion. Commonly EBV-positive, this large B-cell lymphoma variant often is accompanied with a predominant T-cell background and usually manifests as pulmonary or paranasal sinus involvement.

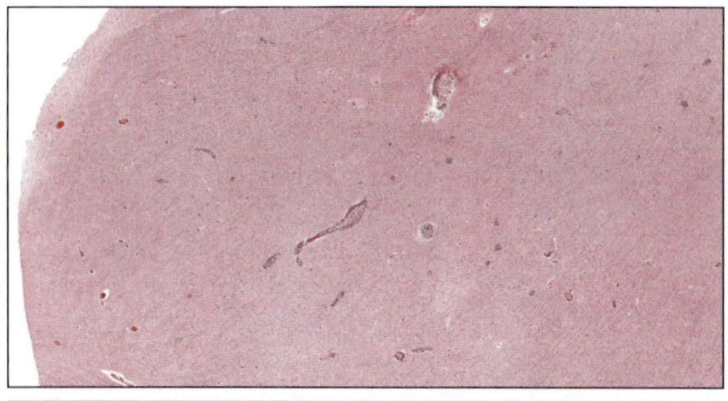

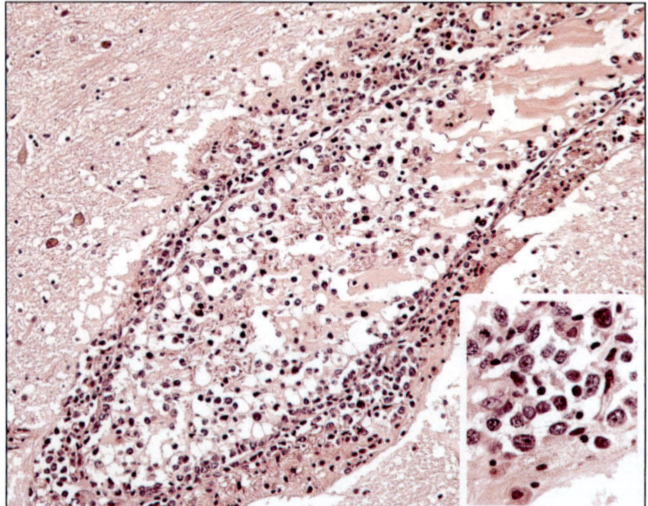

Figure 5.110 Intravascular large B-cell lymphoma. Sections of cerebrum from autopsy brain specimen reveal widespread involvement of small vessels by large atypical lymphoid cells, that by immunostains are CD20$^+$ B cells. The lymphoma cells extend through the walls of the vessels but do not invade brain parenchyma. Other names for this disease are *malignant angioendotheliomatosis* and *angiotropic large-cell lymphoma*.

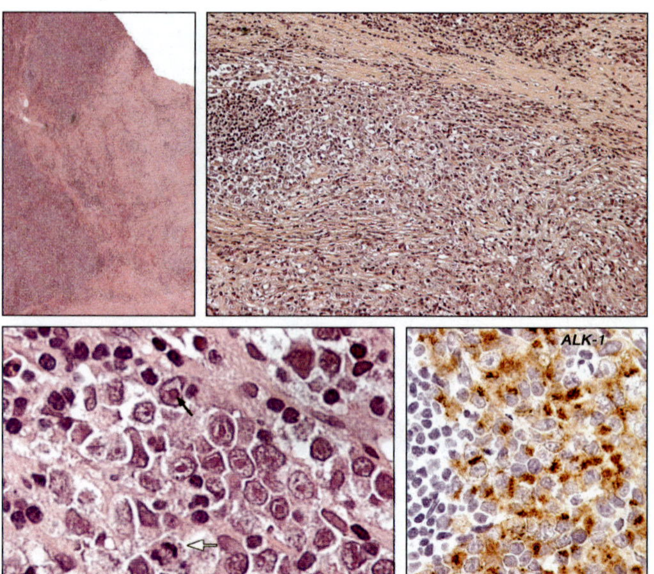

Figure 5.111 Diffuse large B-cell lymphoma, ALK-positive. A supraclavicular lymph node biopsy shows dense fibrous tissue and extensive coagulative tumor necrosis intimately associated with sheets of large, malignant lymphoid cells. The malignant cells have giant-sized, eosinophilic staining nucleoli (*closed arrow*) and a high mitotic rate (*open arrow*). Immunostains for ALK-1 show strong granular staining with focal enhancement in the Golgi region. Additional immunostains revealed the lymphoma cells were CD138$^+$/EMA$^+$ and negative for B-cell and T-cell markers. In this case, approximately 50% of the lymphoma cells were positive for the proliferation marker MIB1.

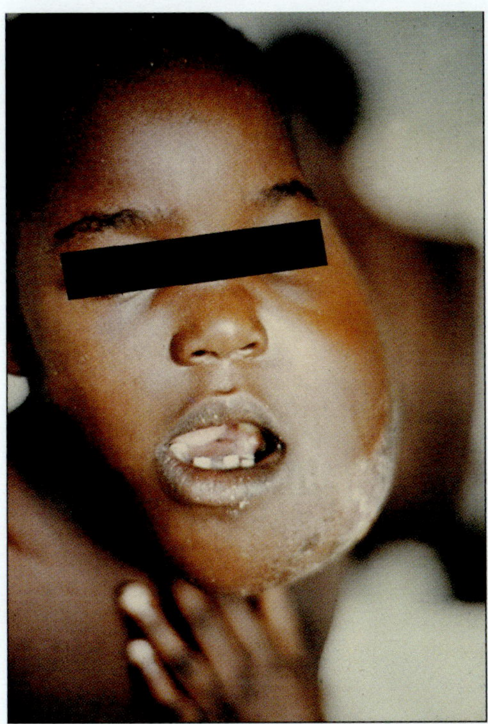

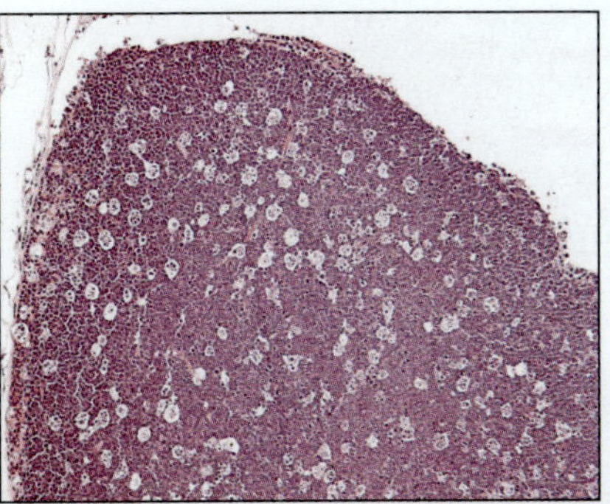

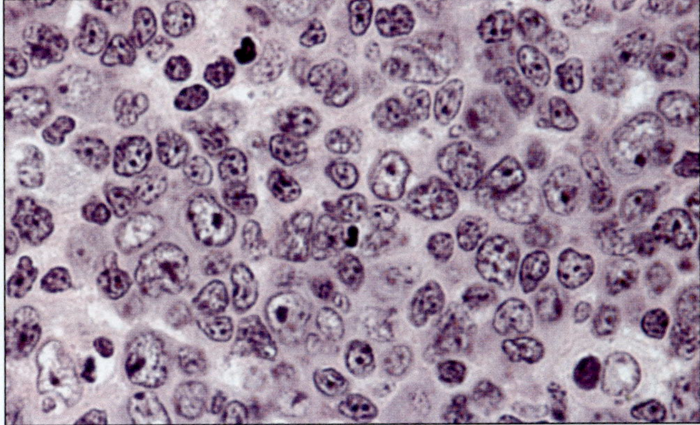

Figure 5.113 Burkitt lymphoma. The biopsy of an abdominal mass shows, at low-power, the classic "starry sky" appearance of rapidly proliferating malignant cells intermixed with larger histo-cytes actively engulfing tumor debris (*upper panel*). The lower panel shows intermediate-sized cells that are uniform in size and shape, with multiple small basophilic nucleoli. FISH for c-myc translocation was positive in this case.

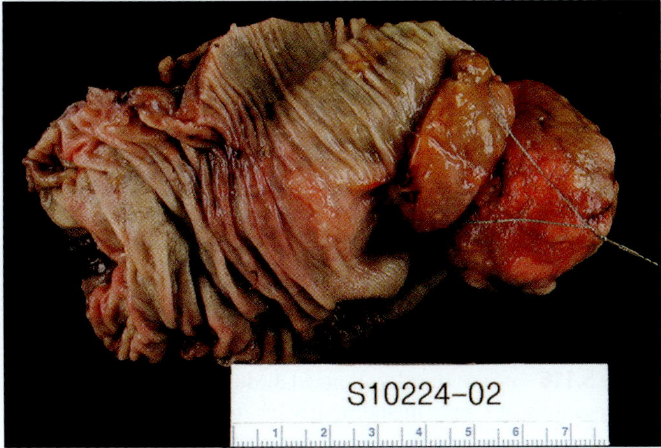

Figure 5.112 *Top panel:* Burkitt's lymphoma, endemic type. A large tumor involves the mandible of a young girl. (Courtesy of The Crookston Collection.) *Bottom panel:* Burkitt's lymphoma of the large intestine, nonendemic type. Burkitt lymphoma presenting as a large polypoid mass of the large intestine. (Courtesy Dr. Bill Geddie.)

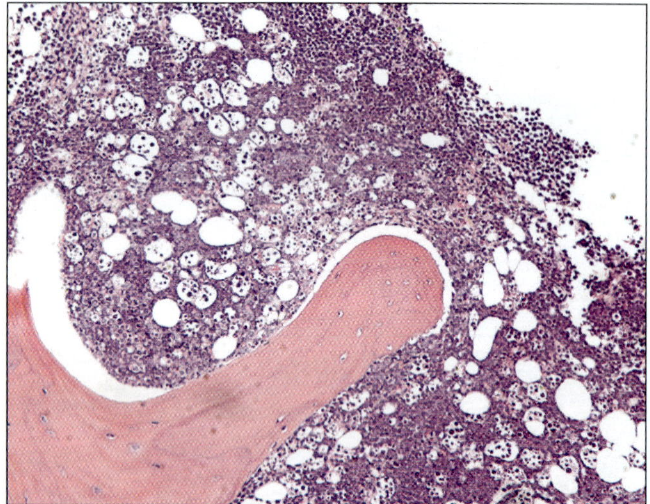

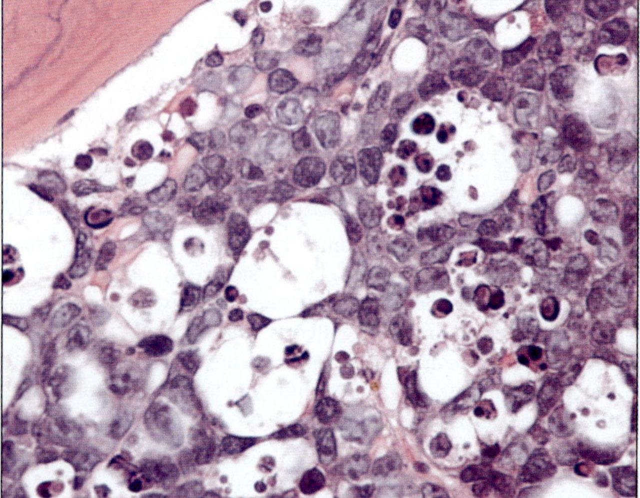

Figure 5.114 Burkitt lymphoma involving bone marrow. This bone marrow biopsy demonstrates total replacement by rapidly growing tumor cells, some of which exhibit apoptosis that are admixed with "starry-sky" histocytes engulfing tumor debris.

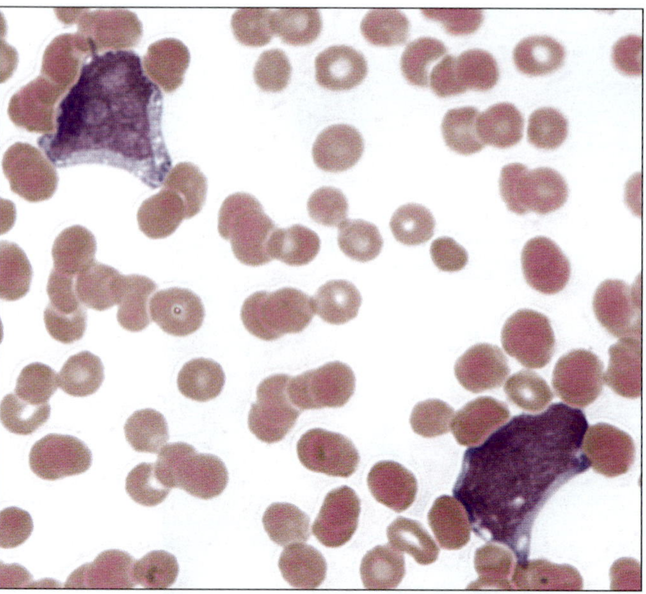

Figure 5.115 Burkitt's leukemia. This blood smear reveals L3-type lymphoblasts with multiple nucleoli and basophilic staining, vacuolated cytoplasm.

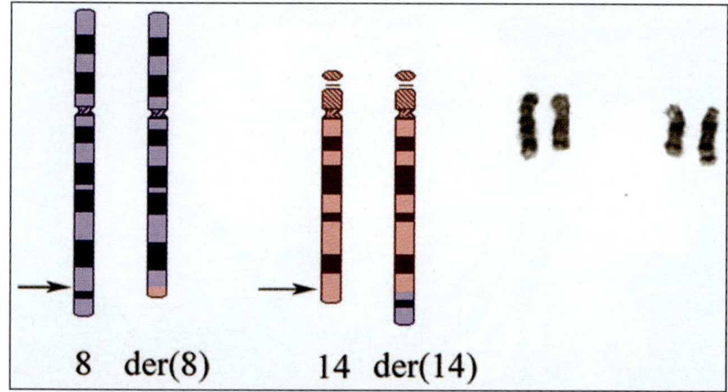

Figure 5.116 c-myc translocations in Burkitt lymphoma/leukemia. Translocations of c-myc including t(8;14), t(2;8), and t(8;22) have been reported in nearly all cases of Burkitt lymphoma. The t(8;14)(q24.1;q32) rearrangement is the most common and is found in 60% to 70% of cases. The ideograms of chromosomes 8, 14, and the respective derivative chromosomes are to the left in color; the corresponding G-banded chromosome pairs are to the right. The arrows indicate the breakpoints on the respective chromosomes.

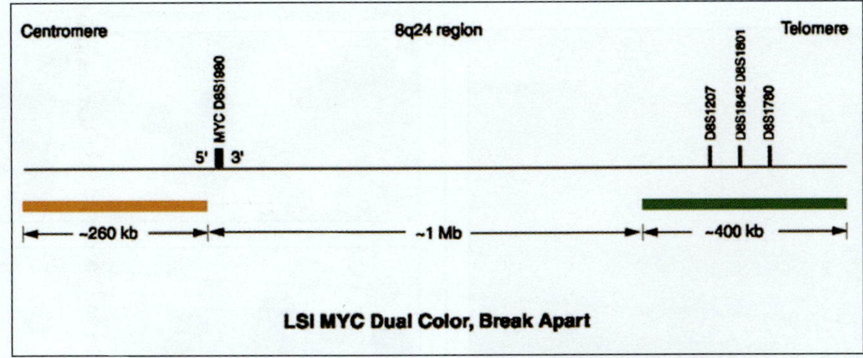

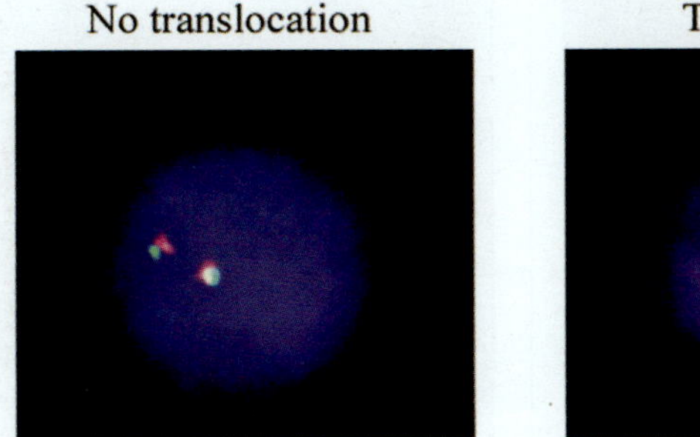

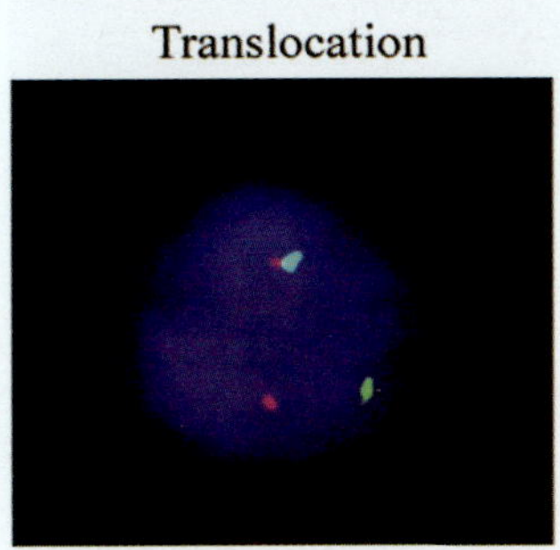

Figure 5.117 FISH for c-myc translocations in Burkitt's lymphoma/leukemia. FISH of a c-MYC rearrangement. The region centromeric to the c-MYC gene is labeled with a red fluor and the region ~ 1 Mb telomeric to the c-MYC gene is labeled with a green fluor. When a translocation occurs involving the c-MYC gene, the red and green signals split apart. A yellow fusion signal indicates an intact c-MYC gene. This approach can detect the t(8;14), t(2;8), and t(8;22) involving the c-MYC locus at 8q24.

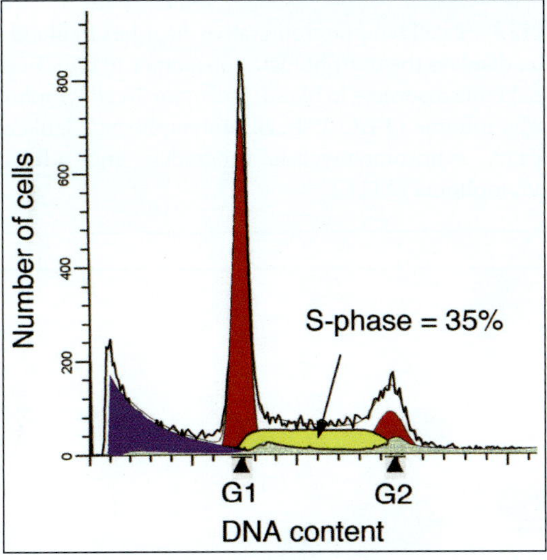

Figure 5.118 DNA content in Burkitt lymphoma. A high S-phase fraction, an index of cellular proliferation measured by DNA flow cytometry, of greater than 20% is typically seen in Burkitt lymphoma. (Courtesy J. Davidson.)

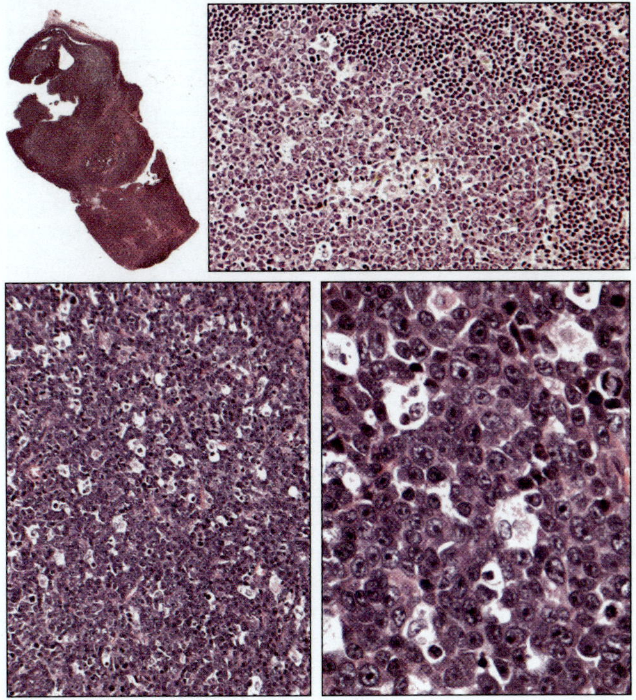

Figure 5.119 Atypical Burkitt/Burkitt-like lymphoma. This breast mass in a 23-year-old woman shows sheets of large, pleomorphic cells infiltrating in a sinusoidal pattern that is associated with necrosis and scattered individual debris-laden macrophages, creating a "starry sky" appearance (*lower panels*). Lymphoma cells are large, display multiple prominent nucleoli, contain moderate amounts of cytoplasm, and have a high mitotic rate. FISH for c-myc translocations are negative.

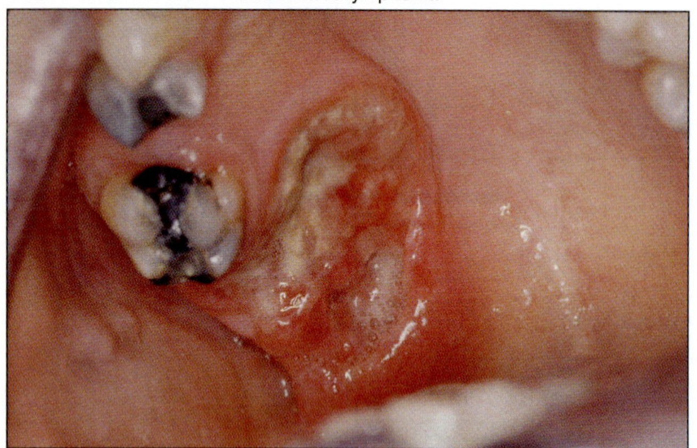

Figure 5.120   Plasmablastic lymphoma involving soft palate.

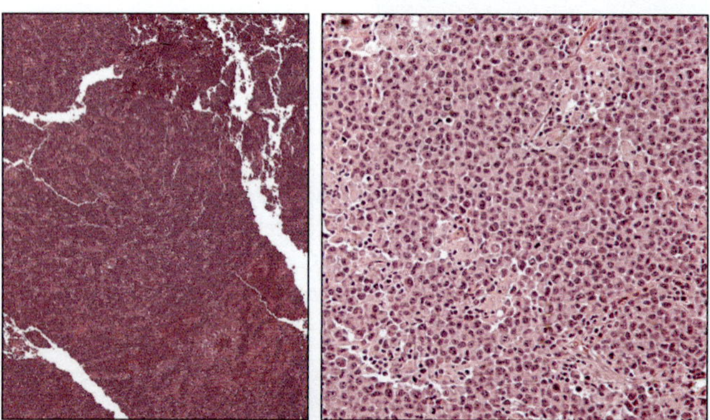

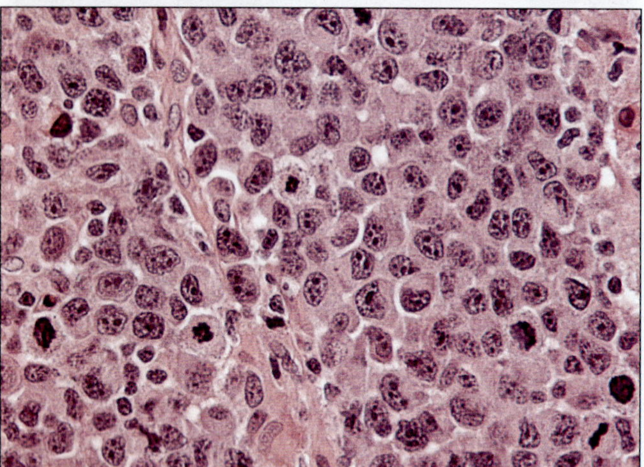

Figure 5.121   Plasmablastic lymphoma. This figure shows fragments of a solitary nasal tumor from an HIV-negative patient with no evidence of paraproteinemia. The tumor contains sheets of atypical plasmacytoid cells with a high mitotic rate.

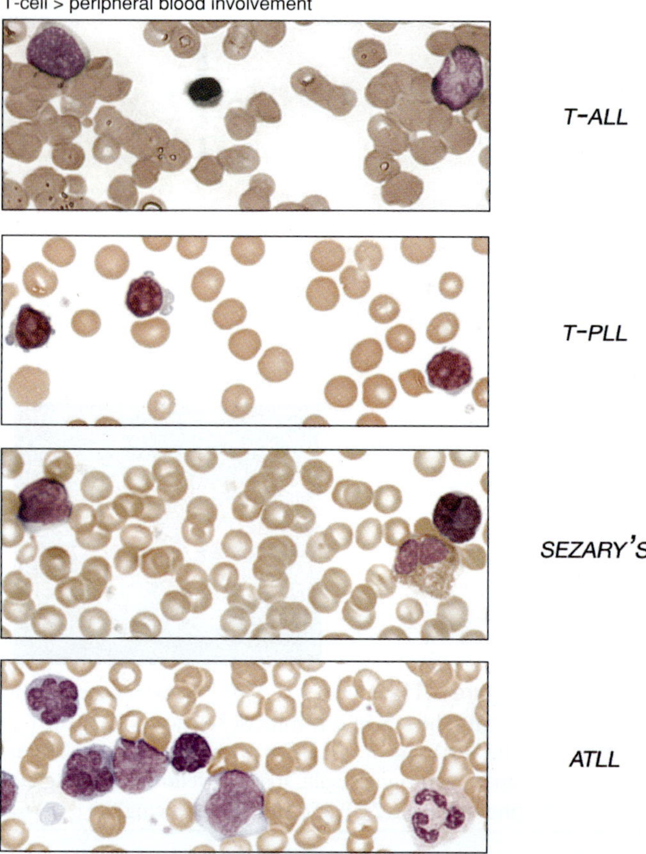

Figure 5.122   T-cell lymphoproliferative disorders in blood smear. This figure displays the morphologic appearance of four T-cell lymphoma/leukemia disorders in blood: precursor T-cell lymphoblastic leukemia/lymphoma (T-ALL); T-cell prolymphocytic leukemia (T-PLL); Sézary syndrome/mycosis fungoides; and adult T-cell leukemia/lymphoma (ATLL).

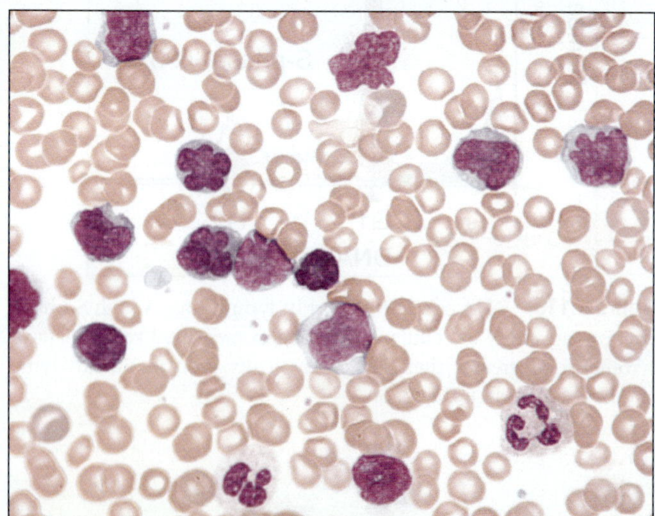

Figure 5.123   Adult T-cell leukemia/lymphoma (ATLL). This blood smear from a case of ATLL shows a pleomorphic population of large cells with polylobated nuclei ("flower cells"). By flow cytometry, these cells were $CD3^+/CD4^+/CD2^+/CD7^-/CD25^+$. Serology for HTLV-1 was positive.

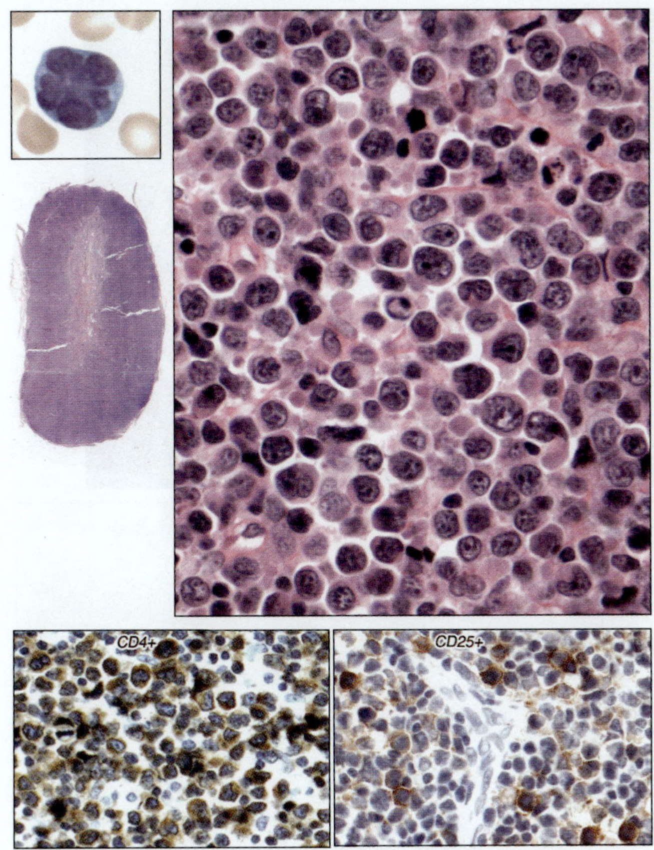

Figure 5.124 Acute adult T-cell leukemia/lymphoma, (ATLL). Large atypical lymphoid cells, "flower cells" with convoluted nuclei, are seen circulating in blood (*top left figure*) and in involved lymph nodes (*all other figures*). ATLL cells are typically CD4$^+$/CD25$^+$ (*bottom two panels*) and Tdt negative.

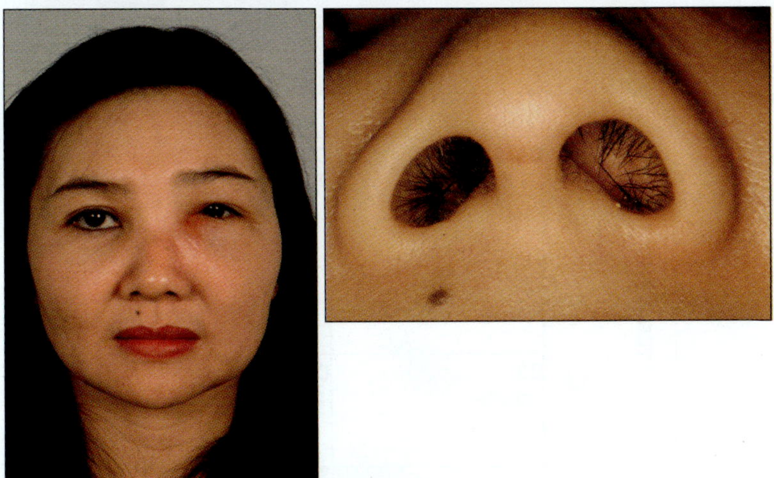

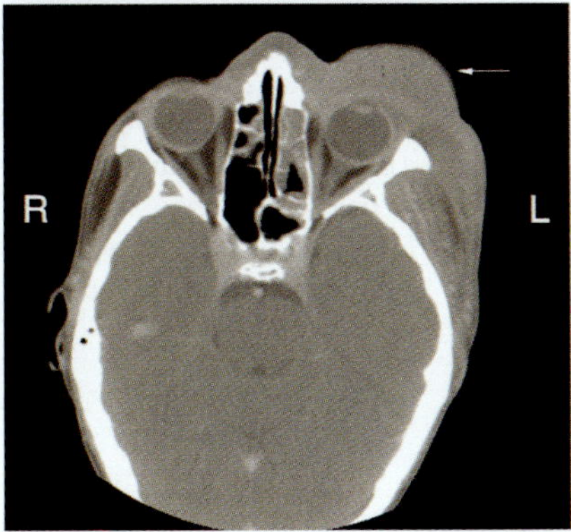

Figure 5.125 Extranodal NK-/T-cell lymphoma, nasal type. A nasal NK-/T-cell lymphoma in a middle-aged women of Asian descent (*top two panels*). An axial CT through the level of the orbit demonstrates increased density in the left ethmoid sinus (*lower panel*). A large soft-tissue mass is present anterior and lateral to the right orbit (*arrow*).

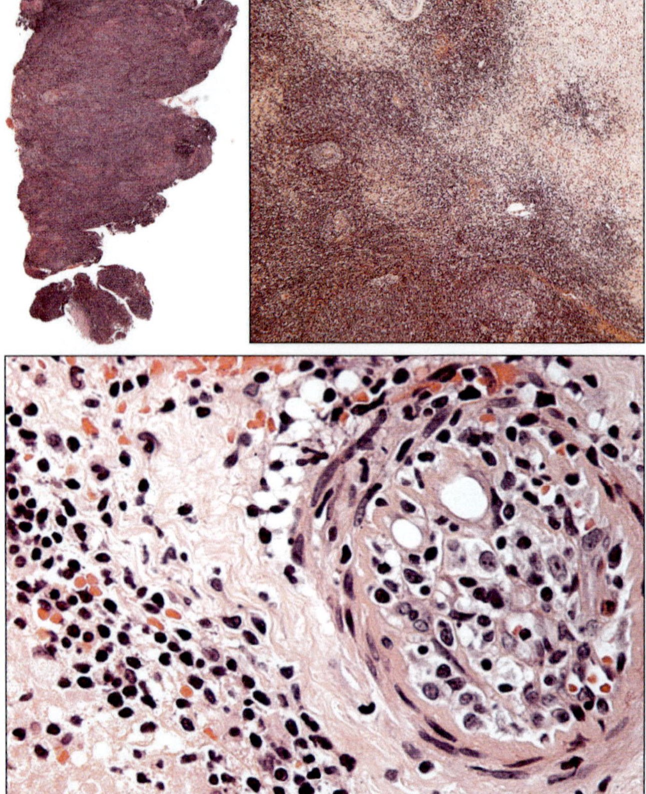

Figure 5.126 Extranodal NK-/T-cell lymphoma, nasal type. Ethmoid sinus tissue fragments from a 38-year-old woman show extensive necrosis and an angiocentric, pleomorphic population of large atypical lymphoid cells mixed with some histiocytes, small lymphocytes, and rare plasma cells. The lymphoma cells were positive for T-cell markers, CD56 and EBV.

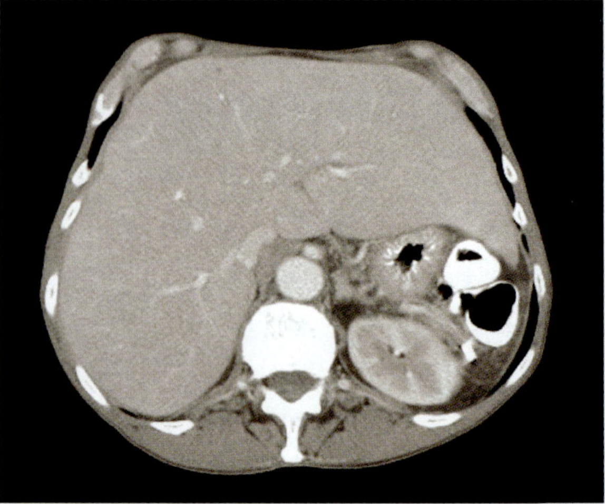

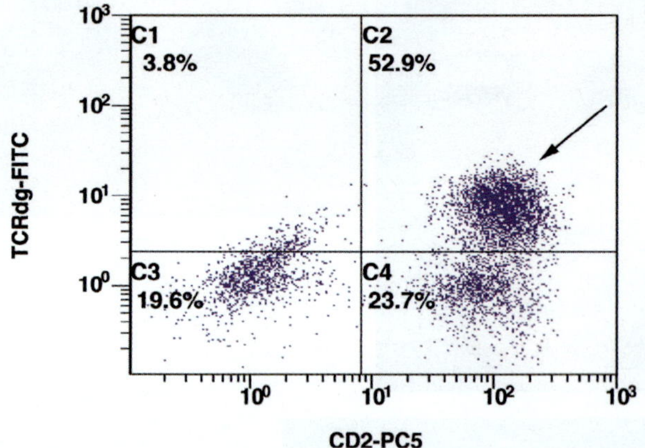

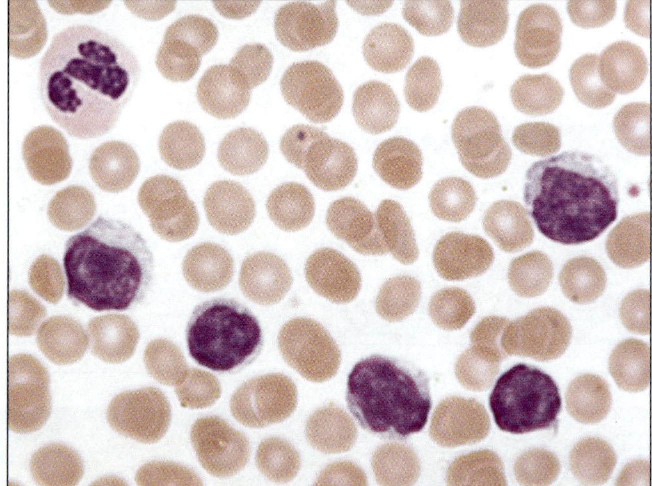

Figure 5.127 Hepatosplenic T-cell lymphoma. *Top panel:* An axial CT scan of the upper abdomen reveals a homogeneously enlarged liver. The spleen is absent. The middle panel is a blood smear showing medium-sized lymphoid cells with pale rims of cytoplasm and slightly irregular nuclear contours. The lymphoma cells typically express the γ/δ T-cell receptor, as shown in the flow cytometric scattergram (*arrow, bottom panel*).

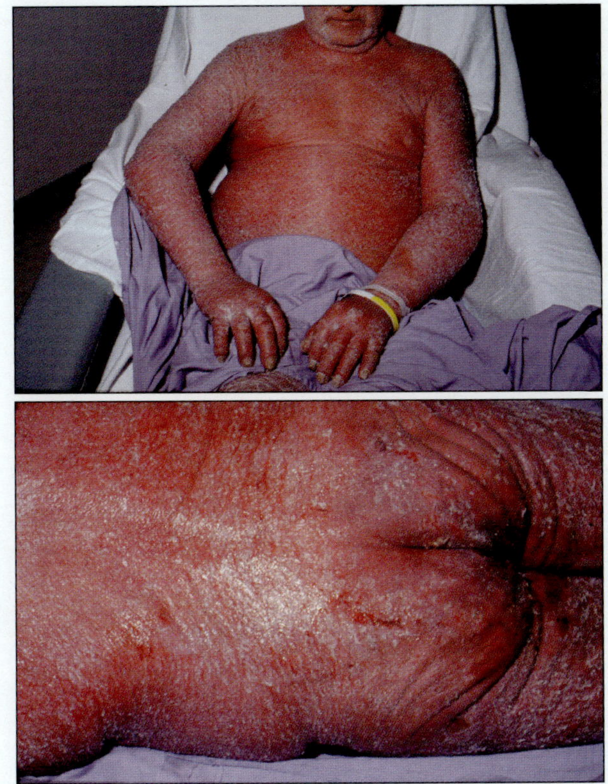

Figure 5.128   Mycosis fungoides. Generalized erythrodermic type.

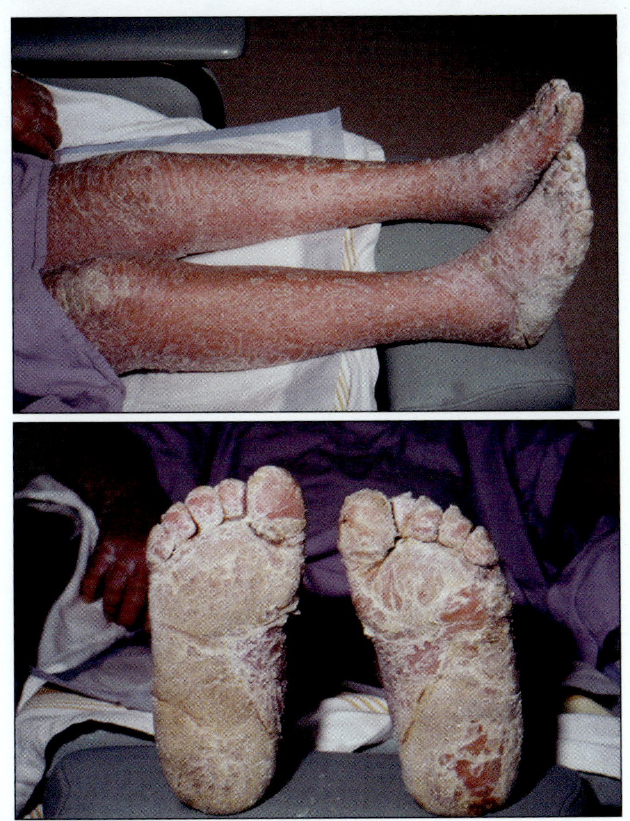

Figure 5.129   Mycosis fungoides involving the lower extremities with hyperkeratosis and fissuring of soles.

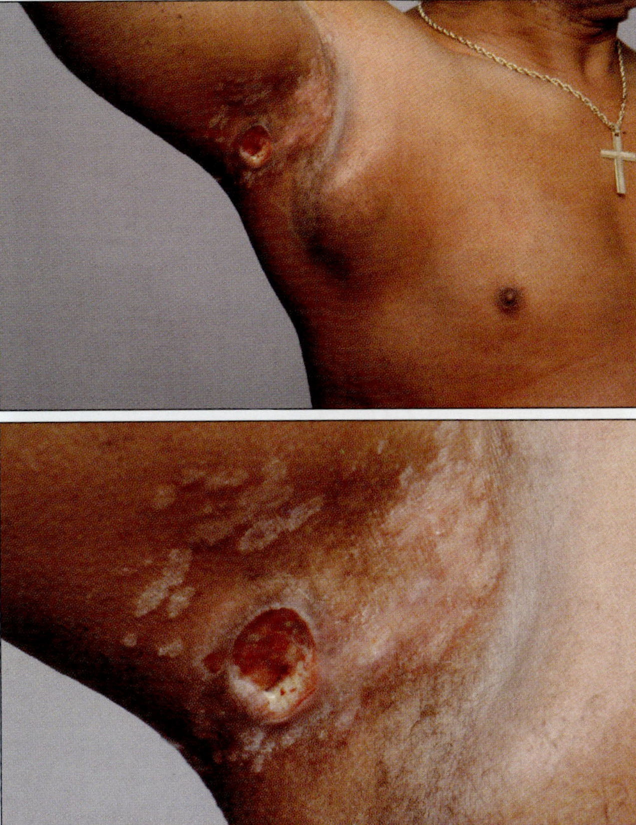

Figure 5.130   Mycosis fungoides and Sézary syndrome. Plaques, ulceration, and lymphadenopathy are present in a case of stage T3 mycosis fungoides with necrotic and ulcerated tumors.

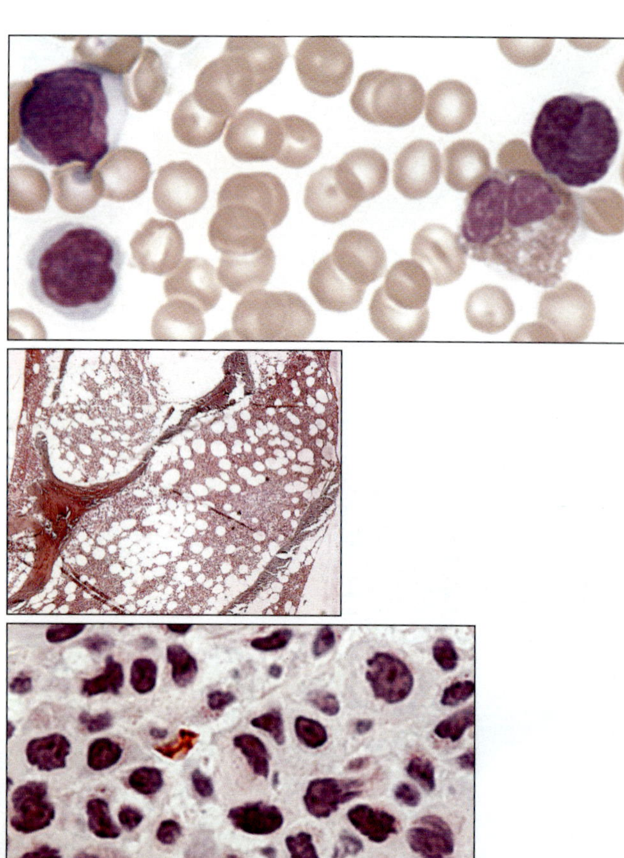

Figure 5.131 Sézary syndrome involving the bone marrow. In the top panel is a blood smear showing large Sézary cells with characteristic convoluted ("cerebriform") nuclei. Poorly defined nodules of Sézary cells are visible in these plastic-embedded bone marrow sections (*bottom two panels*).

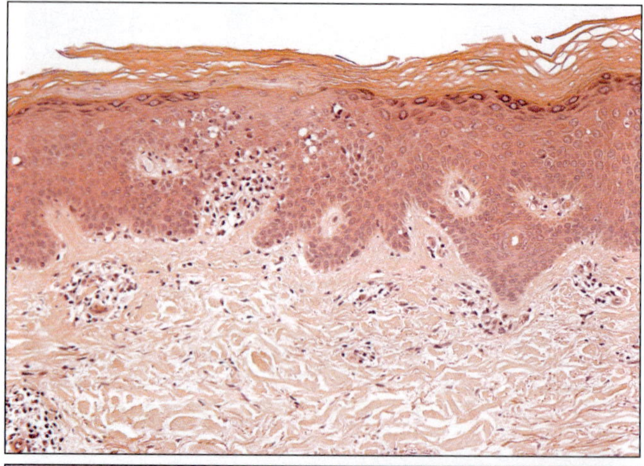

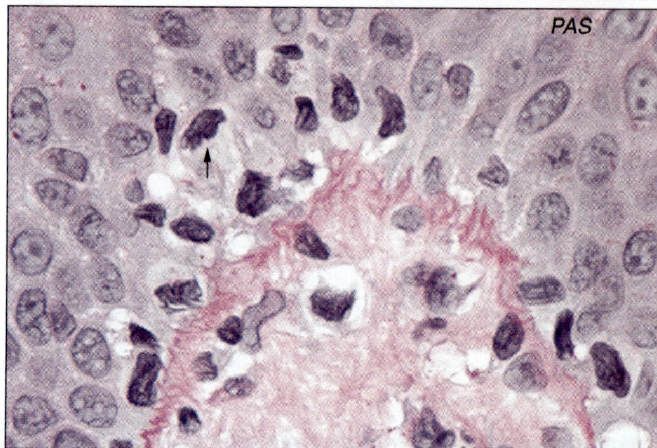

Figure 5.132 Mycosis fungoides. The figure shows epidermal involvement with single-cell exocytosis and individual large, atypical lymphoid cells with convoluted nuclear contours (*arrow*) infiltrating the epidermis (epidermotropism). The lymphoma cells in this particular case by immunohistochemistry, displayed an abnormal T-cell phenotype: CD4$^+$ T-cells with aberrant loss of CD7.

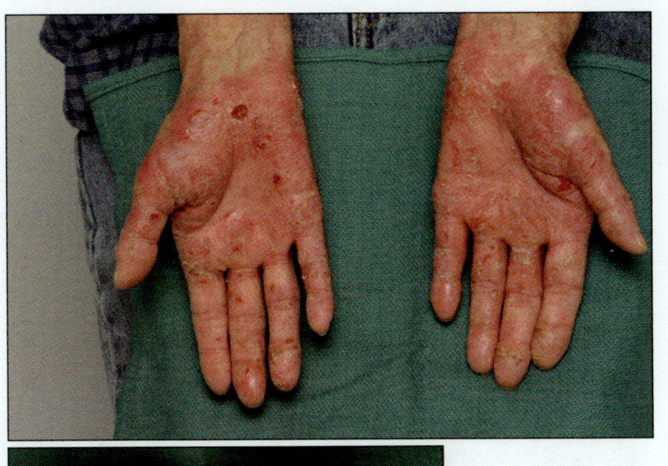

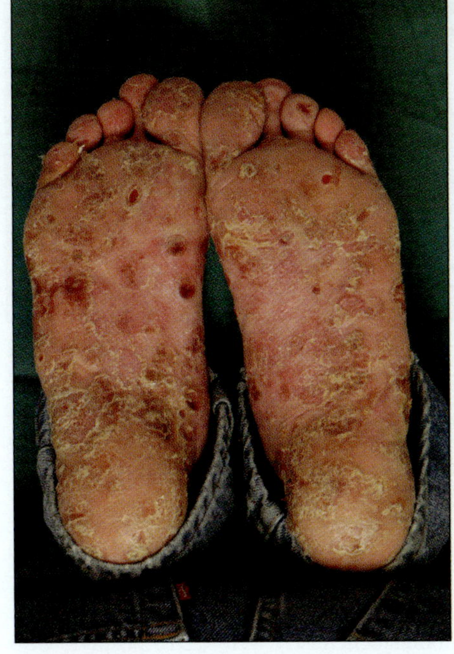

Figure 5.133   Peripheral T-cell lymphoma involving skin of hands and feet.

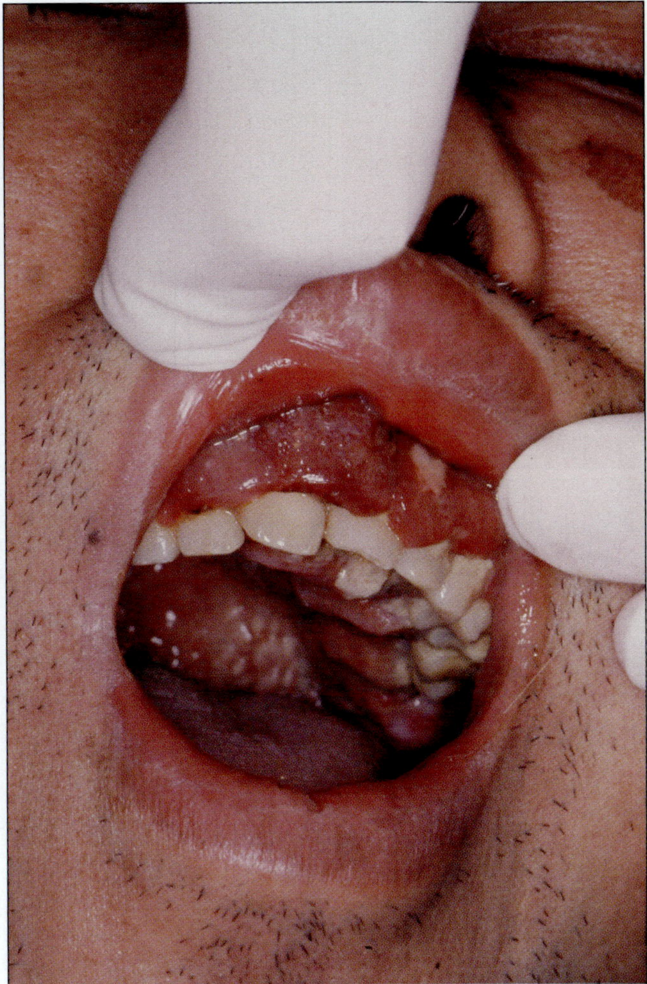

Figure 5.134   Peripheral T-cell lymphoma presenting in gums.

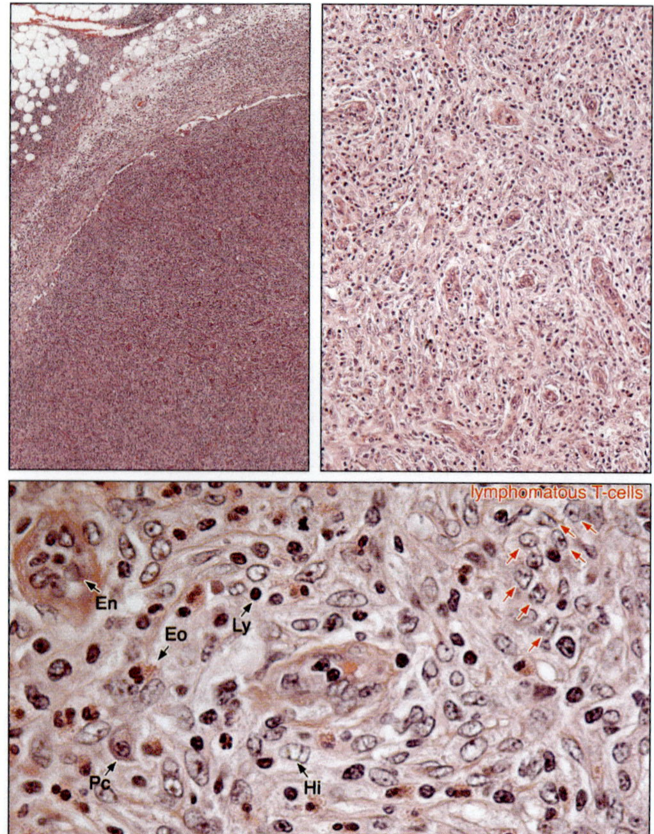

Figure 5.135   Angioimmunoblastic T-cell lymphoma (angioim-munoblastic lymphadenopathy). An enlarged lymph node is com-pletely effaced by a polymorphic proliferation of small lymphocytes (Ly), histiocytes (Hi), eosinophils (Eo), plasma cells (Pc), and transformed nucleolated T-cell lymphoma cells (*red arrows*). This infiltrate is accompanied by a profuse increase in small, thin-walled vessels lined by plump endothelial cells (En). The nucleolated T-cell lymphoma cells expressed an aberrant transformed T-cell phe-notype CDs 3$^+$/5$^-$/7$^-$/38$^+$ and HLADR$^+$ by immunohistochem-istry. Monomorphic sheets of transformed T cells were not present in this case.

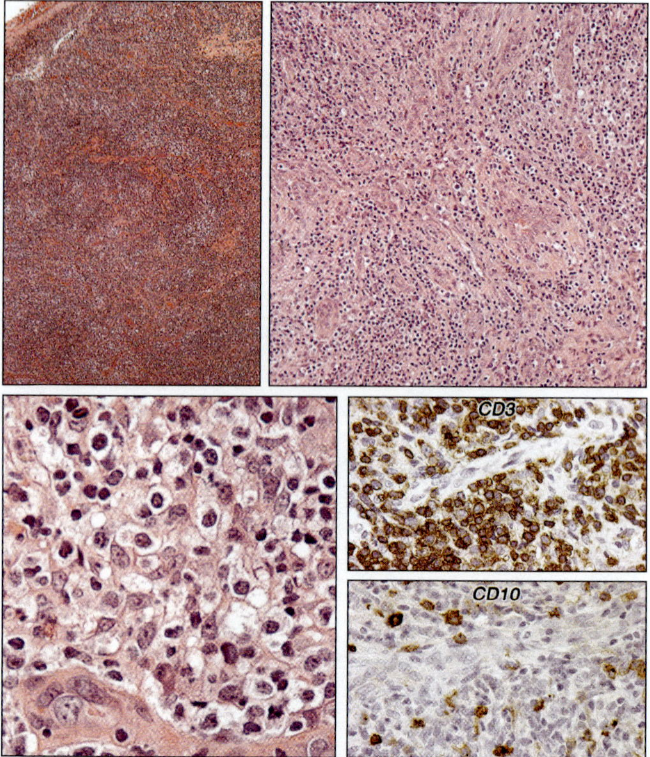

Figure 5.136   Angioimmunoblastic T-cell lymphoma. The normal lymph node architecture is effaced by a mixed-cell infiltrate con-sisting of small lymphocytes, scattered plasma cells, eosinophils, and transformed lymphocytes. The infiltrate is accompanied by a marked increase in arborizing thin-walled blood vessels lined by plump endothelial cells. Clusters of atypical, transformed lympho-cytes with abundant clear cytoplasm are present (*left lower panel*). There is a background increase in CD3$^+$ small T cells (*upper small panel*) with large atypical clear lymphoid cells strongly CD10$^+$ (*lower small panel*). The atypical clear lymphoid cells by flow cytometry and immunohistochemistry were CD10 positive, CD3 positive T cells with loss of CD7. PCR studies were negative for B-cell clonality, Epstein-Barr virus, and Human Herpes Virus 8 in this case.

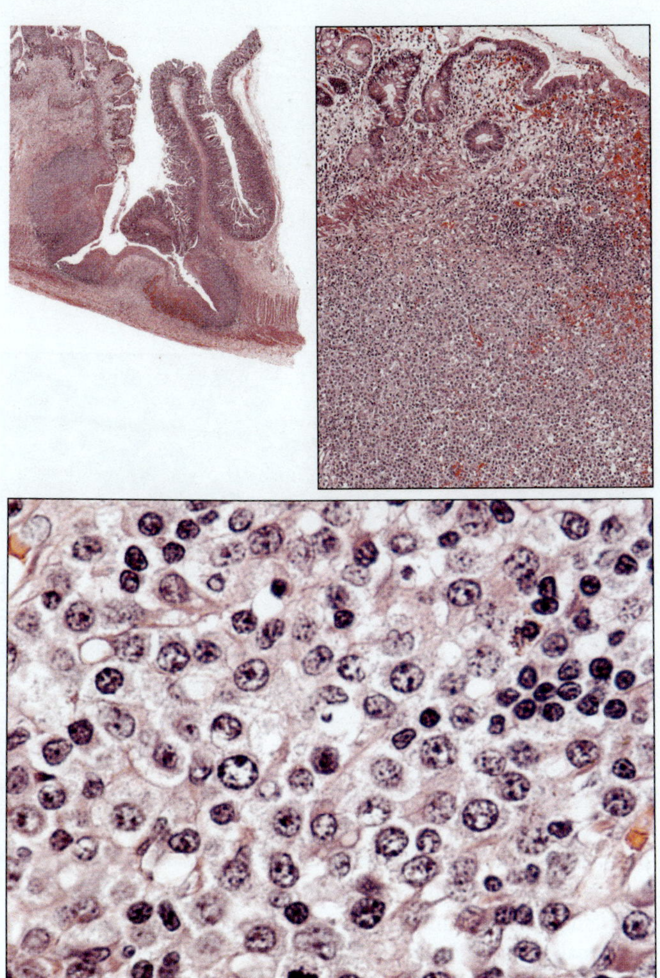

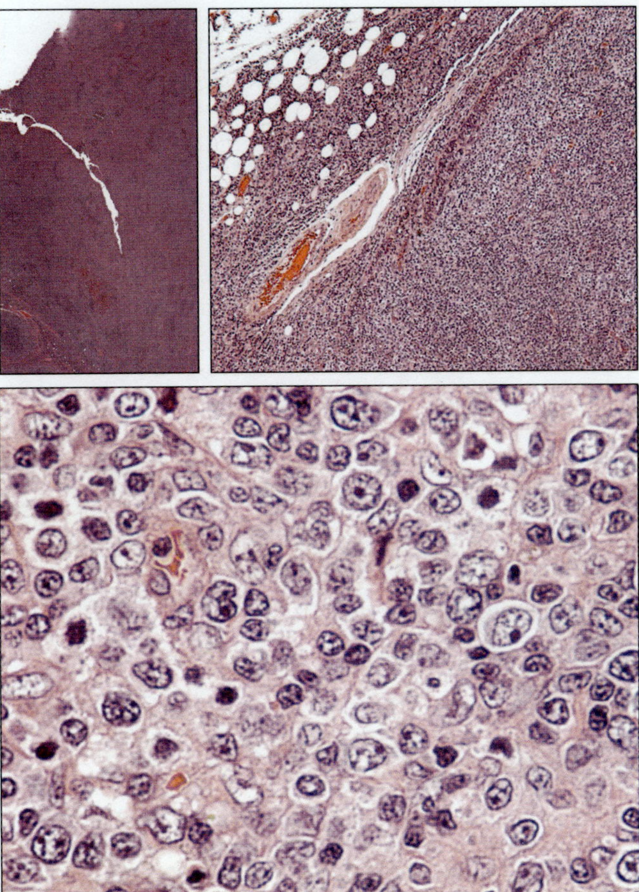

Figure 5.138 Peripheral T-cell lymphoma. The lymph node architecture is disrupted by a diffuse interfollicular proliferation of clusters of "clear" lymphoid cells admixed with centrocytes. The morphologic spectrum for this disease entity is broad, with this particular case composed primarily of large cells.

Figure 5.137 Enteropathy-type T-cell lymphoma. This figure shows sections near a small-bowel fistula from a 53-year-old man with history of celiac disease. A large ulcerating lesion with transmural extension into the surrounding serosa is associated with necrosis and an extensive multifocal infiltrate composed mostly of atypical large lymphoid cells with vesicular nuclei that were positive for T-cell markers CDs 3, 2 and 5 with aberrant loss of CD7 by immunohistochemistry.

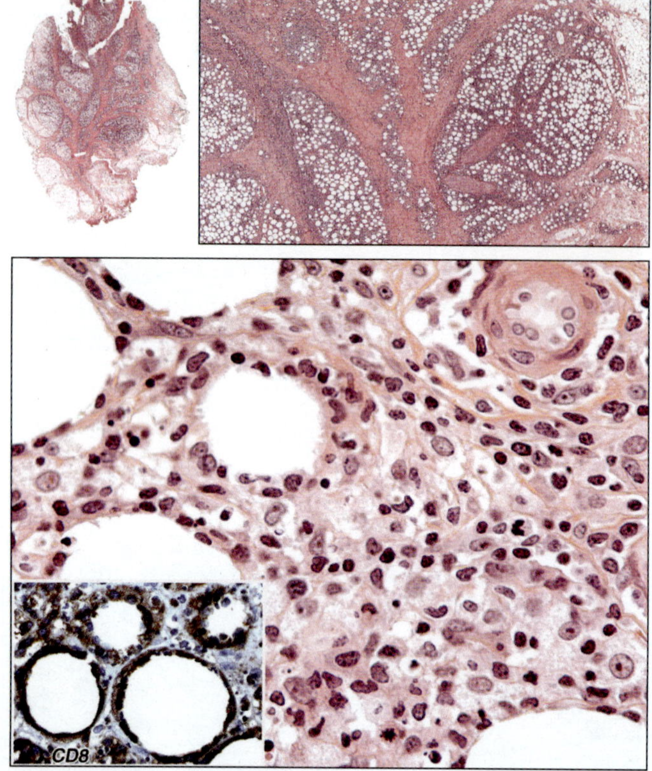

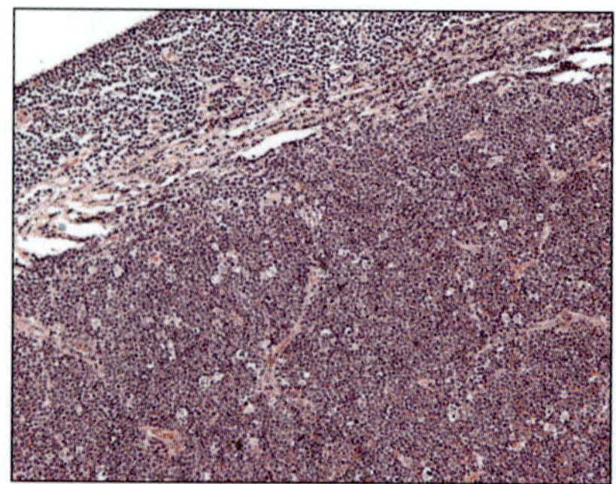

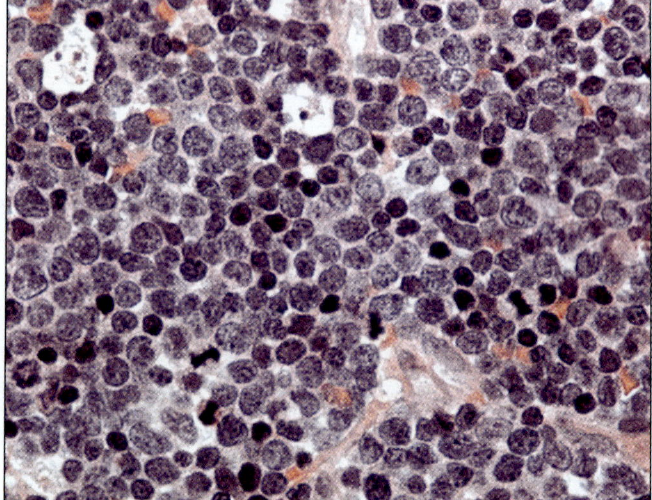

Figure 5.139   Subcutaneous panniculitis-like T-cell lymphoma (large cell variant). A subcutaneous neck nodule shows adipose tissue infiltrated by a heterogeneous population of fibroblasts, histiocytes, and atypical lymphoid cells. The large atypical lymphoid cells stained positively for T-cell markers such as CD8 (*inset of lower panel*).

Figure 5.140   Precursor T-lymphoblastic leukemia/lymphoma. This lymph node is diffusely replaced by sheets of rapidly proliferating malignant cells interspersed by debris-laden histiocytes creating the typical "starry sky" appearance at low-power (*upper panel*). Medium-sized lymphoma cells with high N:C ratios, finely reticulated ("open") chromatin patterns, and high mitotic rate are characteristic of this disease (see Figs. 2.96 and 2.97).

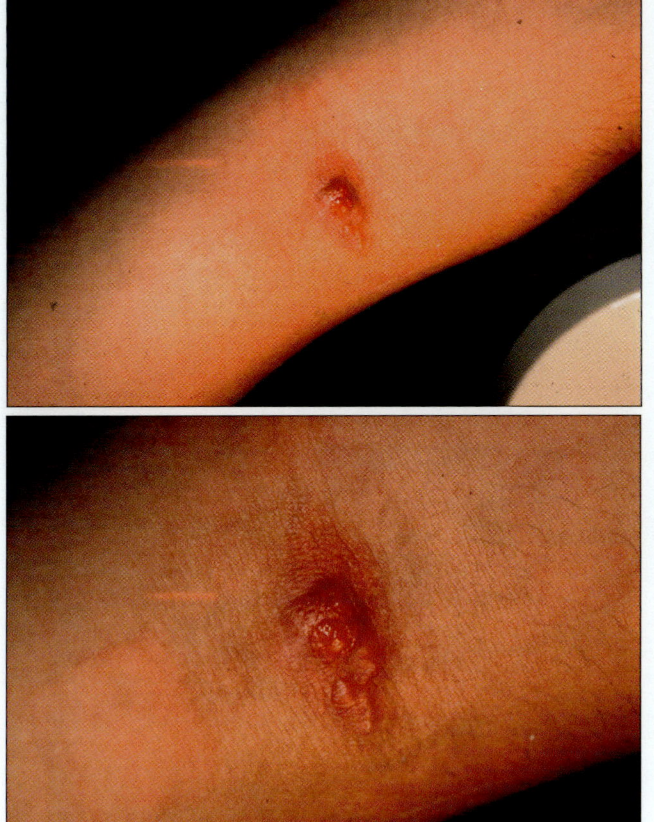

Figure 5.141 Lymphomatoid papulosis on the skin of the fore-arm. The lesions in this case of lymphomatoid papulosis sponta-neously regressed without treatment. Lymphomatoid papulosis and CD30$^+$ cutaneous lymphoma are part of a spectrum of diseases characterized by large CD30$^+$ lymphoma cells. Lymphomatoid papulosis lesions are typically rapidly growing but self-healing nodules, whereas CD30$^+$ cutaneous lymphoma (see Fig. 5.142) can have a similar clinical feature at presentation but does not spon-taneously regress.

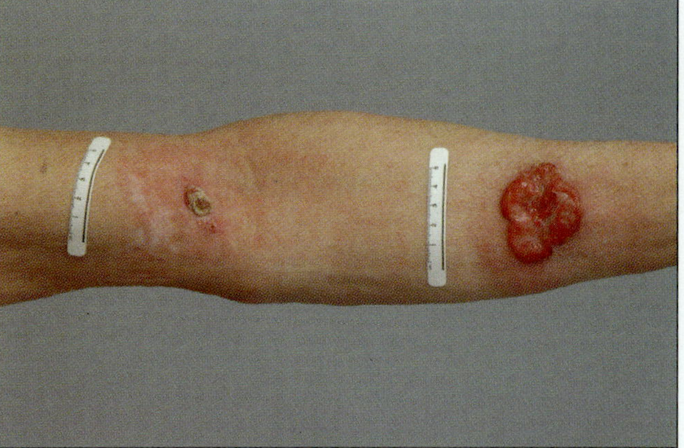

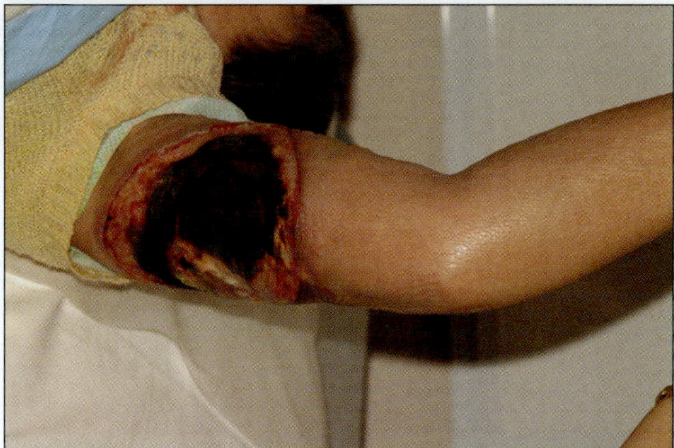

Figure 5.142 Primary cutaneous anaplastic CD30$^+$ large-cell lymphoma. This figure shows two cases involving skin and under-lying tissues of the upper extremity.

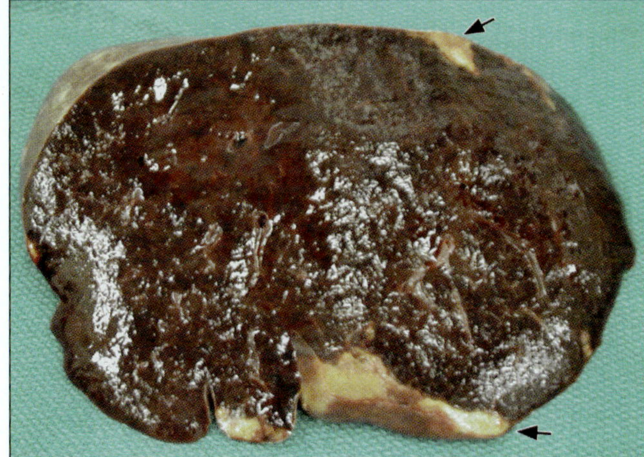

Figure 5.143 Anaplastic CD30$^+$ large-cell lymphoma involving spleen. Nodules of lymphoma are seen near the capsule (*arrows*).

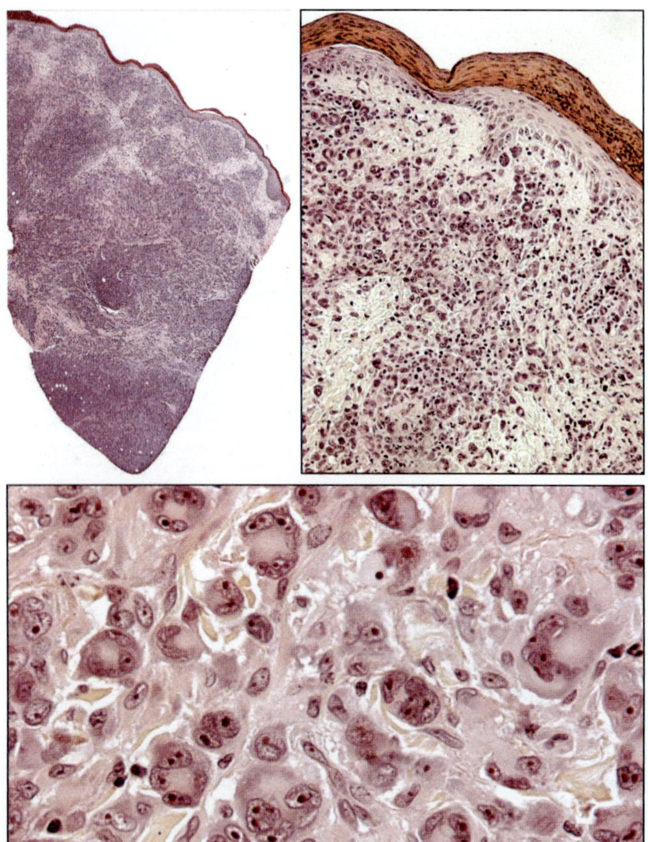

Figure 5.144 Primary cutaneous anaplastic CD30$^+$ large-cell lymphoma. This skin biopsy from the upper arm of a 54-year-old woman reveals deep infiltration into subcutaneous tissue by poorly defined nodules of large, anaplastic cells with multilobulated nuclei. Many of the cells are "hallmark cells," with lobulated nuclei forming horseshoe or wreath-like configurations. Immunostains were positive for T-cell markers and CD30.

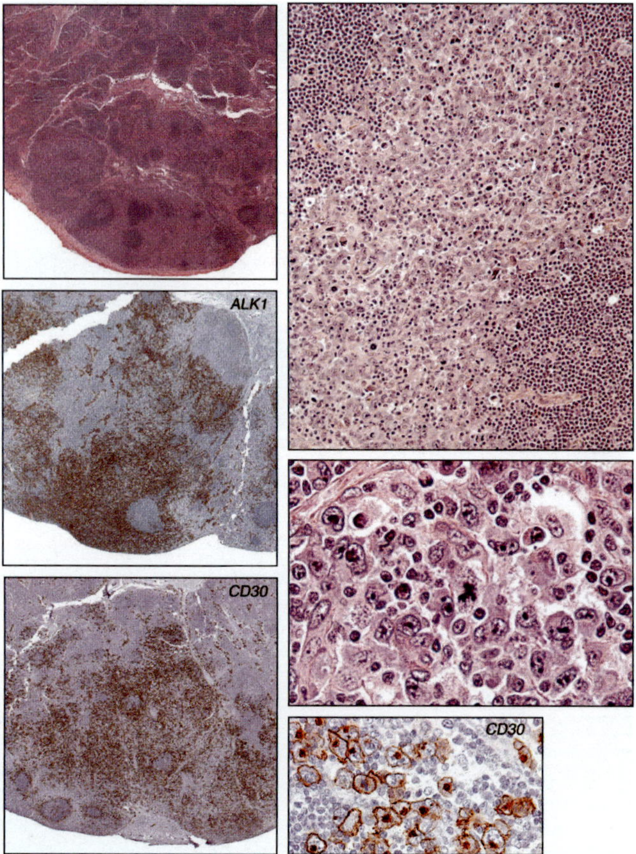

Figure 5.145 Anaplastic CD30$^+$ large-cell lymphoma, ALK-1 positive. This inguinal lymph node from a 19-year-old man displays a sinusoidal pattern of involvement by large pleomorphic CD30$^+$/ALK-1$^+$ T cells. The diffuse pattern of sinusoidal spread, similar to metastatic carcinoma, preserves nodal architecture.

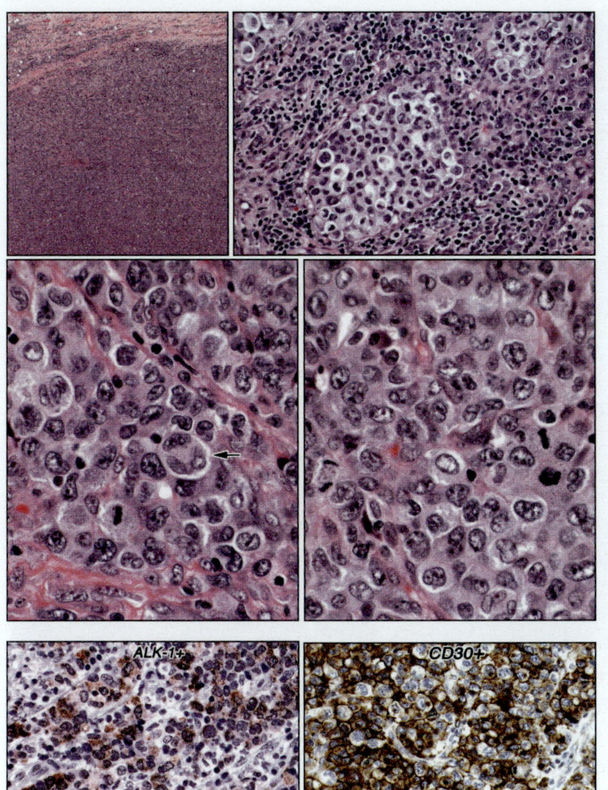
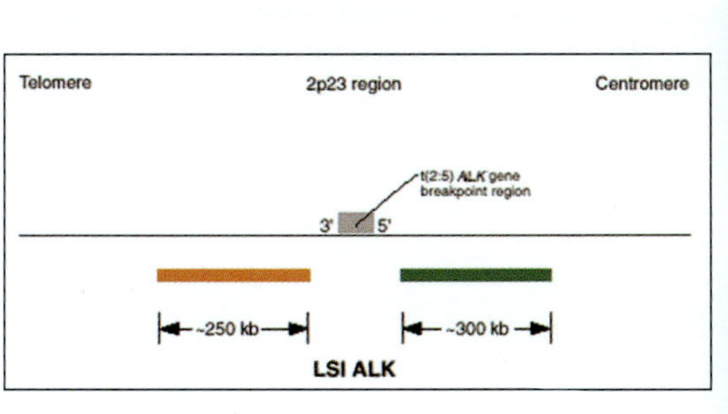

Figure 5.146   Anaplastic CD30$^+$ large-cell lymphoma, ALK-1 positive. Nests of large malignant CD30$^+$/ALK1$^+$ cells fill sinuses throughout this lymph node. The arrow in the left middle panel shows a lymphoma cell with an atypical multilobed or horseshoe-shaped (wreath-like) nucleus. Numerous mitotic figures are present. The t(2;5) associated with anaplastic large-cell lymphoma results in the expression of a ALK-1 fusion protein that can be detected either by immunohistochemistry (*left bottom panel*) or FISH (Fig. 5.147).

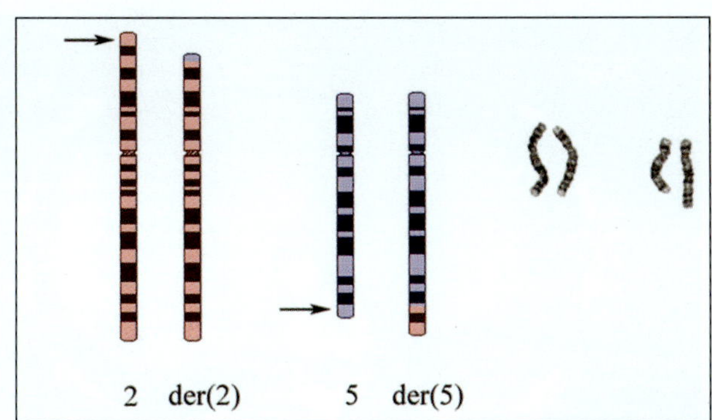

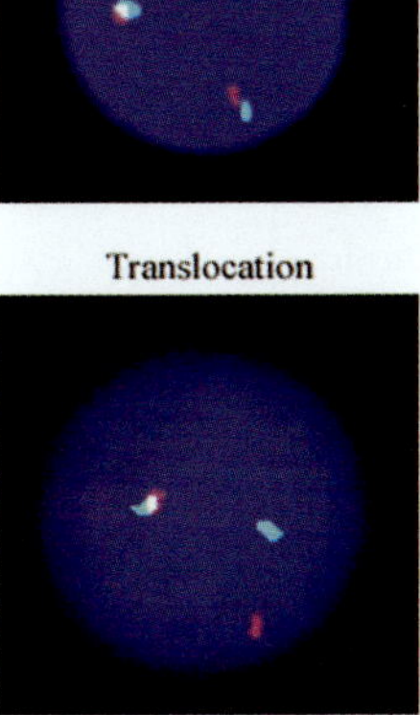

Figure 5.147   t(2;5)(p23;q35) by cytogenetics and FISH in diffuse anaplastic large-cell lymphoma. Approximately one-third of anaplastic CD30$^+$ large-cell lymphomas harbor the t(2;5) which is associated with favorable outcome in this disease. The upper panel shows ideograms of chromosomes 2, 5, and the respective derivative chromosomes are to the left in color. The corresponding G-banded chromosome pairs are to the right. The arrows indicate the breakpoints on the respective chromosomes. *Lower panel:* FISH of an ALK rearrangement. The region telomeric to the ALK gene is labeled with a red fluor, and the region centromeric to the ALK gene is labeled with a green fluor. When a translocation occurs involving the ALK gene, the red and green signals split apart. A yellow fusion signal indicates an intact ALK gene.

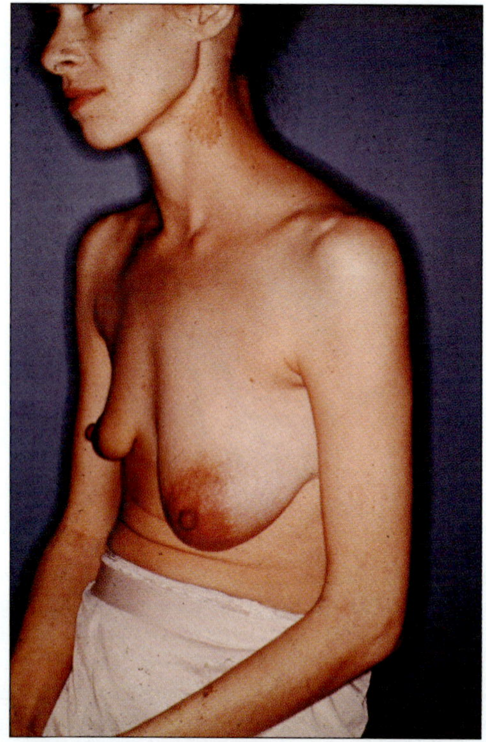

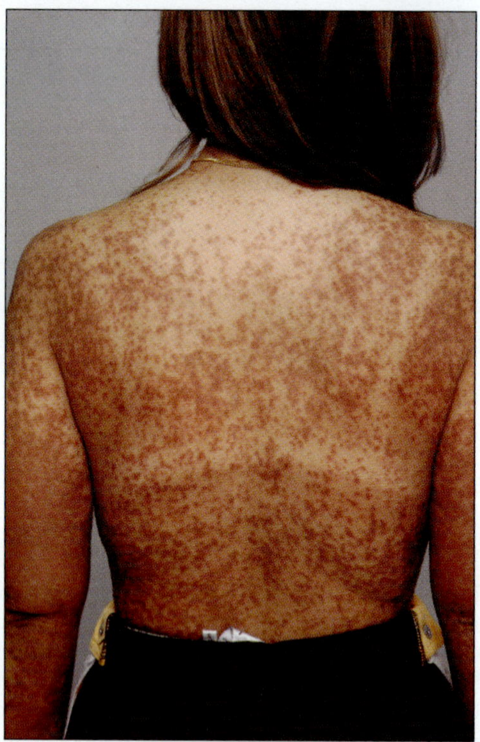

Figure 5.148 Hodgkin lymphoma with axillary lymph node involvement causing edema and enlargement of the right breast (*top panel*, courtesy Dr. P. Galbraith). *Bottom panel*: Rash in Hodgkin lymphoma. Hodgkin lymphoma in this young woman was accompanied by a generalized, pruritic macular papular rash at the time of diagnosis.

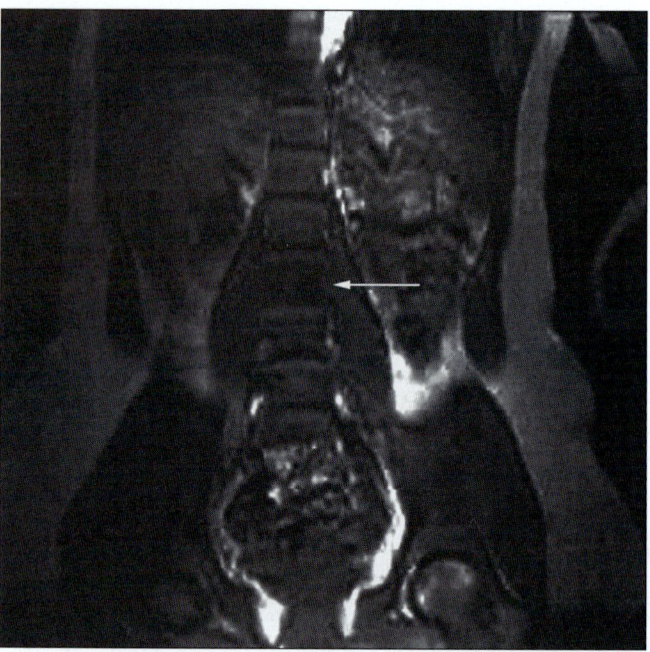

Figure 5.149 Hodgkin lymphoma of spine. A coronal MRI reveals a diffuse low signal through a lumbar vertebral body (*arrow*). This is the MRI equivalent of an "ivory vertebra," a term used to describe isolated, diffuse sclerosis of a vertebral body on radiographs. The differential diagnoses include non-Hodgkin and Hodgkin lymphoma, metastases, and Paget disease.

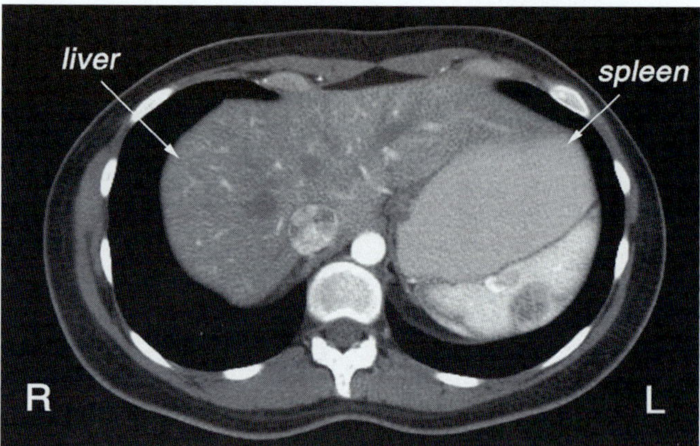

Figure 5.150 Hodgkin lymphoma of spleen. An axial CT scan with intravenous contrast shows a very large spleen with large, complex, hypodense masses. The low-density regions centrally within the masses likely represent areas of necrosis.

Table 5.6

Relative incidence of each stage for each histopathologic subtype of Hodgkin disease

Stage	Histologic subtype			
	Lymphocyte-Predominant (%)	Nodular Sclerosis (%)	Mixed-Cellularity (%)	Lymphocyte-Depleted (%)
IA and IB	47	8	12	9
IIA and IIB	38	52	34	14
IIIA and IIIB	14	29	41	41
IVA and IVB	1	11	13	36
Total	100	100	100	100

Modified from Kaplan HS, Hodgkin's disease, 2nd ed. Cambridge: Harvard University Press, 1980.
Reprinted with permission from *Wintrobe's Clinical Hematology*, 11th Edition, page 2525.

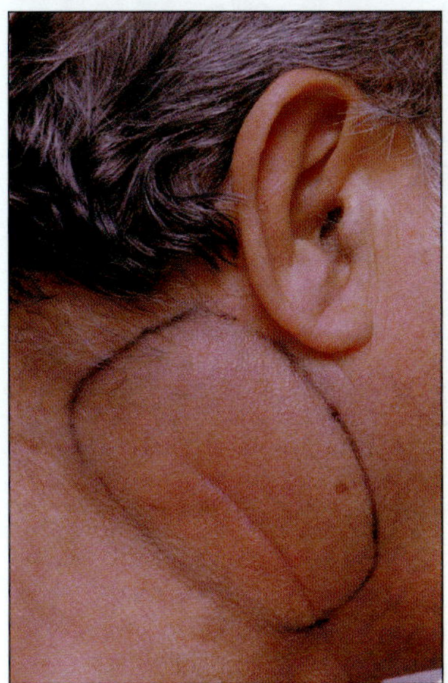

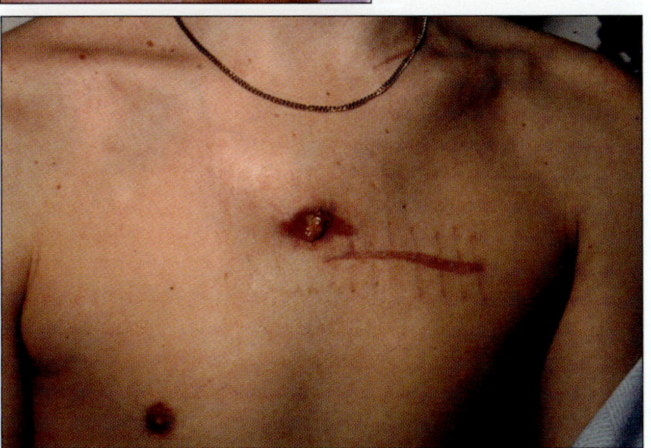

Figure 5.151 Right cervical lymphadenopathy in a case of Hodgkin lymphoma (*top panel*). Recurrent Hodgkin lymphoma of anterior mediastinum eroding through anterior chest wall (*bottom panel*, courtesy Dr. P. Galbraith).

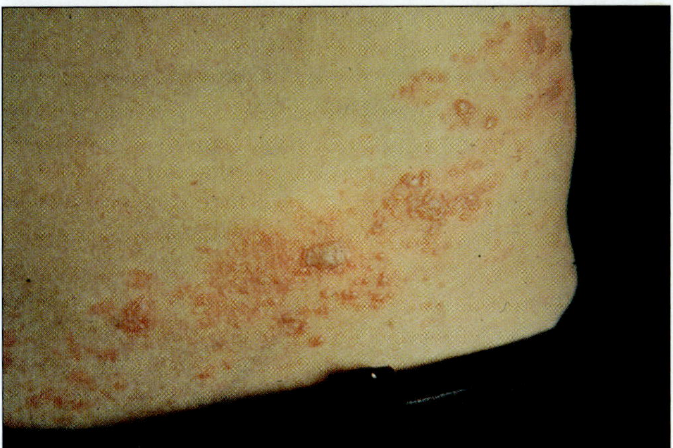

Figure 5.152 Herpes zoster in a patient presenting with Hodgkin lymphoma. (Courtesy Dr. I. Quirt.)

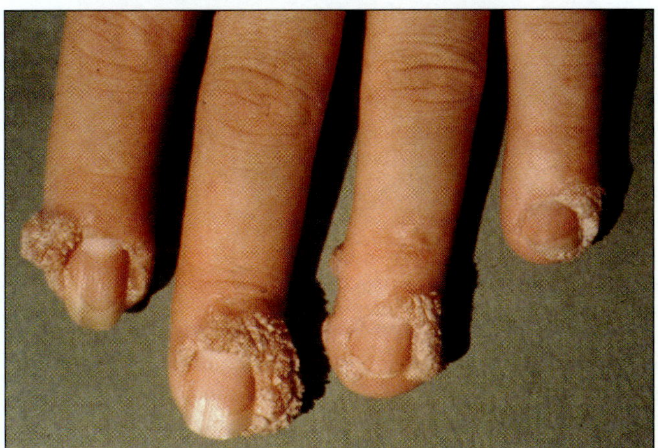

Figure 5.153 Finger warts (verruca simplex) in a patient presenting with Hodgkin lymphoma. (Courtesy of The Crookston Collection.)

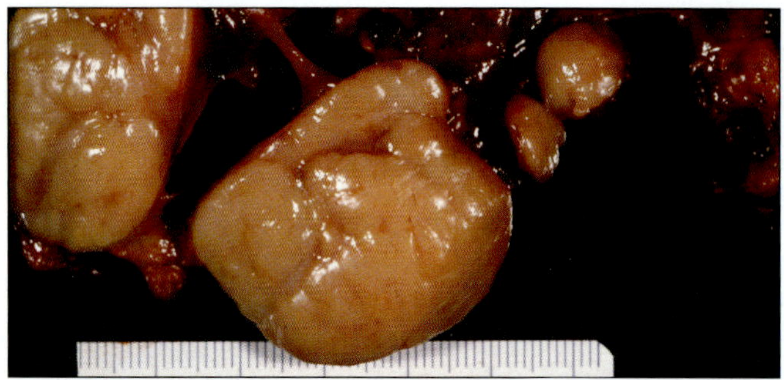

Figure 5.154   Gross appearance of a group of resected lymph nodes matted together by nodular sclerosis Hodgkin lymphoma. A vague nodular appearance can be discerned.

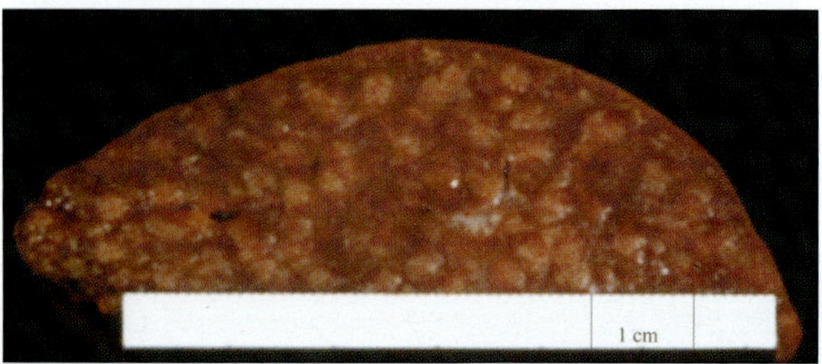

Figure 5.155   Hodgkin lymphoma of spleen. Multiple small nodules of Hodgkin lymphoma are distributed throughout the splenic parenchyma.

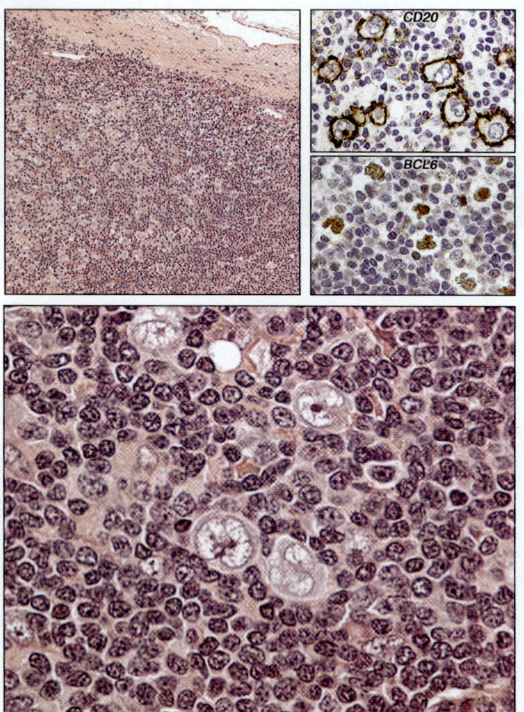

Figure 5.156   Nodular lymphocyte-predominant Hodgkin lymphoma. This lymph node is effaced by a small lymphocyte/histiocyte infiltrate and occasional "L&H" (popcorn) cells that are large cells with multilobulated nuclei and very fine neutral-staining nucleoli (*bottom panel*). In this disease, distinct from classical Hodgkin disease, these cells are typically CD45[+]/CD20[+]/BCL6[+]/CD30[−]/CD15[−].

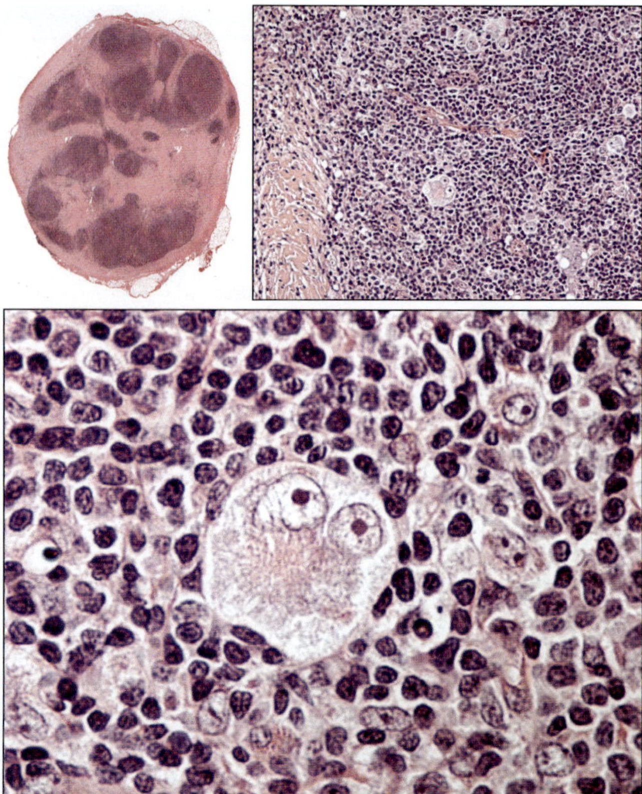

Figure 5.157   Nodular sclerosis Hodgkin lymphoma, grade 1. A spinal accessory node from a 31-year-old woman shows a thickened capsule with the architecture distorted by broad bands of collagenous fibrosis interspersed with nodular aggregates composed primarily of small lymphocytes, scattered histiocytes, occasional eosinophils, plasma cells, and classic Reed-Sternberg cells.

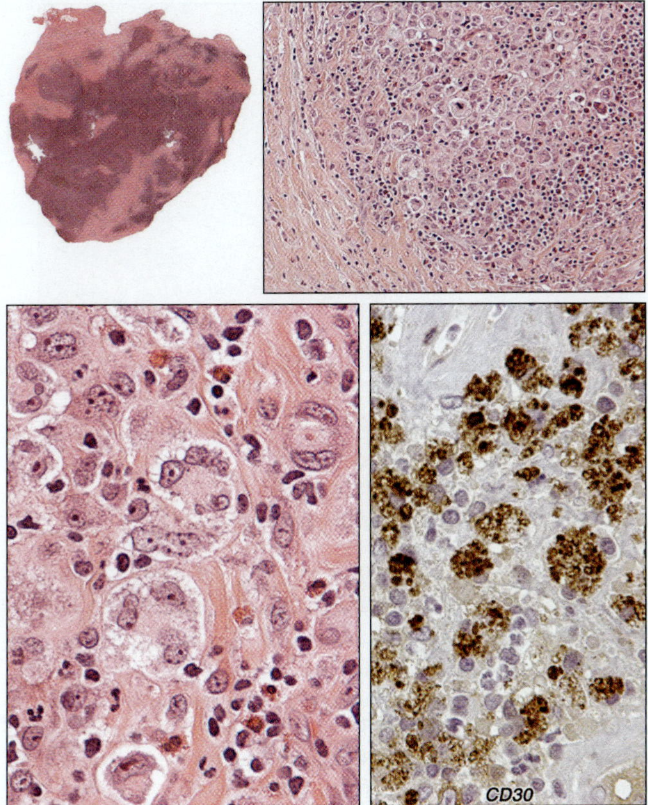

Figure 5.158 Nodular sclerosis Hodgkin lymphoma, grade 2 (syncytial variant). A scalene node from a 32-year-old woman is distorted by wide bands of collagen sclerosis and nodules consisting mostly of highly atypical, large, multinucleated cells that stain positively for CD30 (*right lower panel*) and CD15.

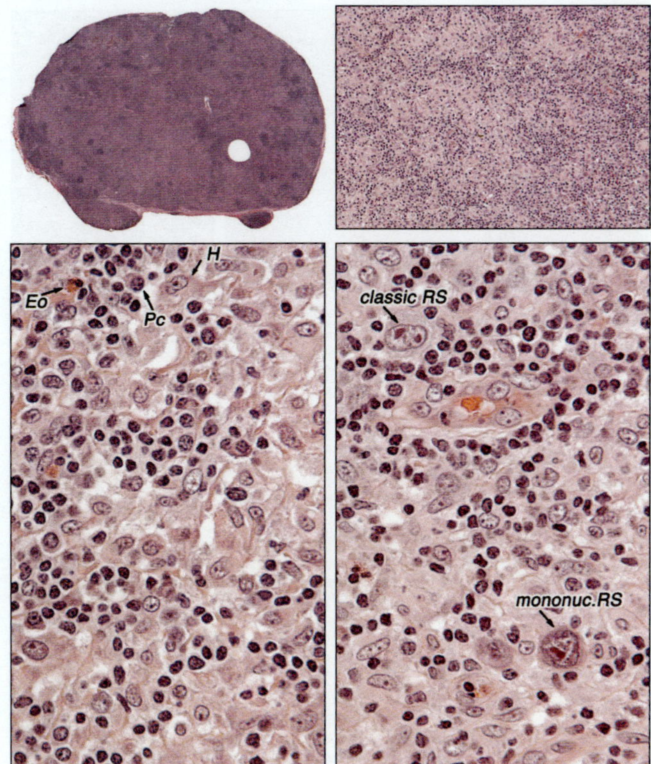

Figure 5.160 Mixed-cellularity Hodgkin lymphoma. This lymph node from 37-year-old woman displays diffuse proliferation of small lymphocytes, eosinophils (Eo), plasma cells (Pc), and histiocytes (H) admixed with occasional classic Reed-Sternberg (RS) cells, which are characterized by a bilobed nucleus, vesicular chromatin, and prominent, dual, eosinophilic nucleoli. In addition, mononuclear RS variants (mononuclear RRS) actually are often easier to find in this and other subtypes of Hodgkin lymphoma.

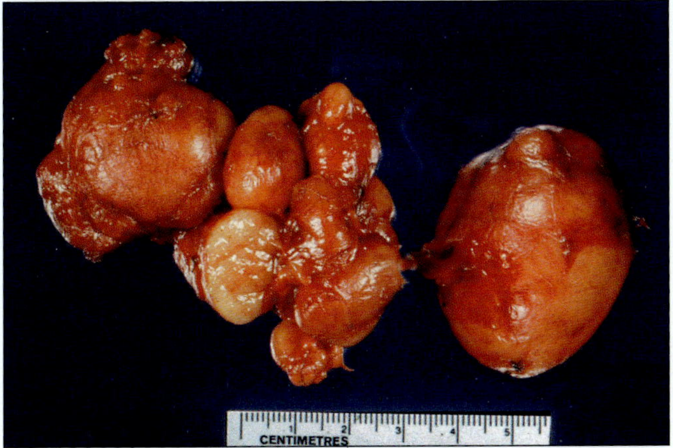

Figure 5.159 Gross appearance of a group of resected lymph nodes contiguously involved by mixed-cellularity Hodgkin lymphoma.

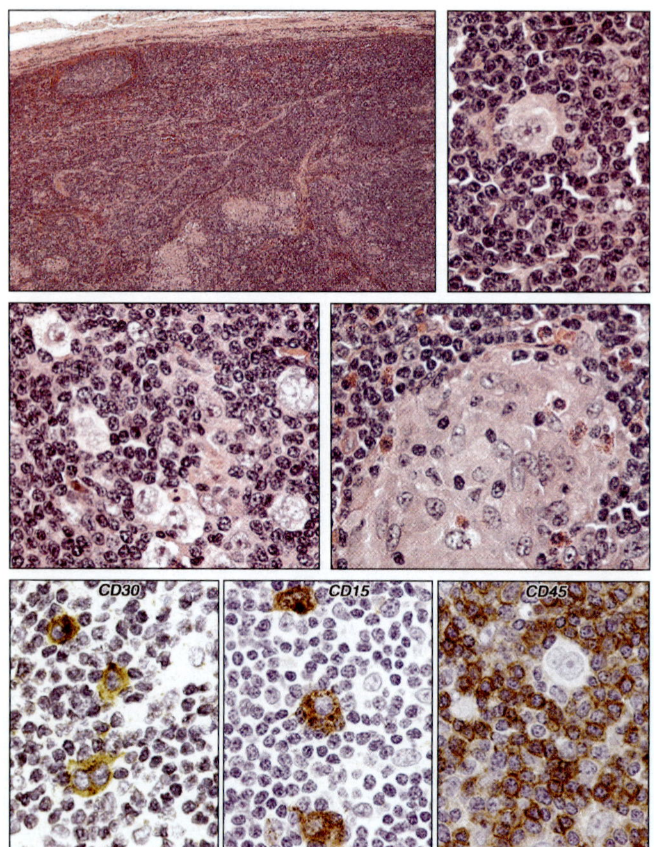

Figure 5.161 Lymphocyte-rich classical Hodgkin lymphoma. An enlarged lymph node is replaced by a vaguely nodular proliferation of small lymphocytes interspersed with classical RS cells (*right upper panel*), L&H cells (*left middle panel*), clusters of histiocytes (*right middle panel*), and immunohistochemistry showing the typical RS phenotype in classical Hodgkin lymphoma, namely positive for CD30 and CD15 and negative for CD45.

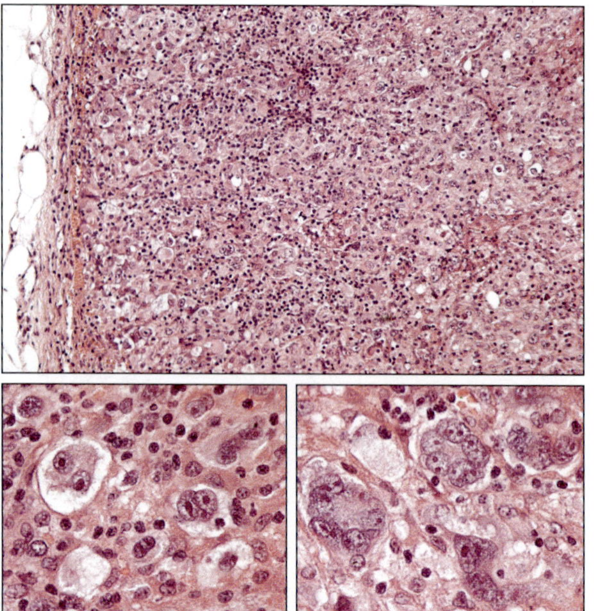

Figure 5.162 Lymphocyte-depleted Hodgkin lymphoma. This axillary lymph node is totally replaced by a primarily large-cell infiltrate accompanied by some small mature lymphocytes. Numerous classic Reed-Sternberg cells (CDs $30^+/15^+/45^-$) were present in addition to bizarre forms with multilobulated nuclei mimicking wreath cells of anaplastic large-cell lymphoma.

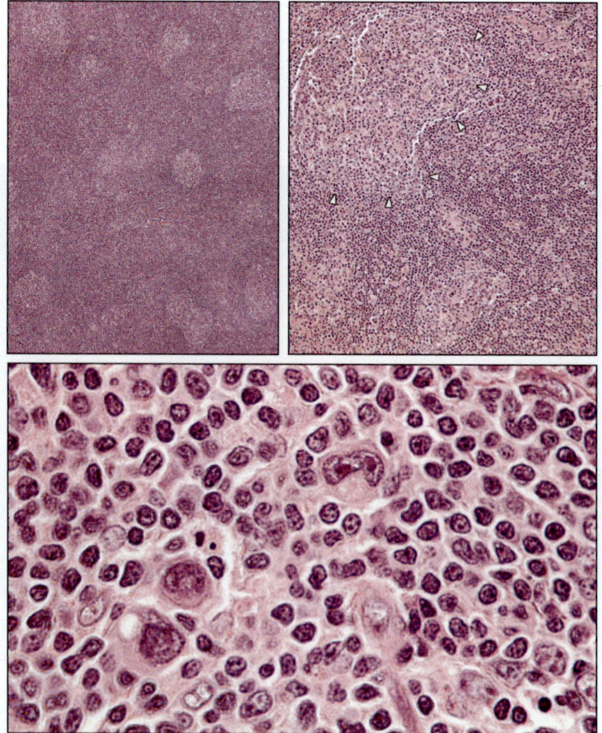

Figure 5.163 Hodgkin lymphoma, interfollicular pattern. An enlarged axillary lymph node from a 39-year-old woman shows expansion of the interfollicular area by nodules invading germinal centers (*triangles*) and composed of a mixture of small lymphocytes, histiocytes, and occasional classic bilobed and mononuclear variants of Reed-Sternberg cells.

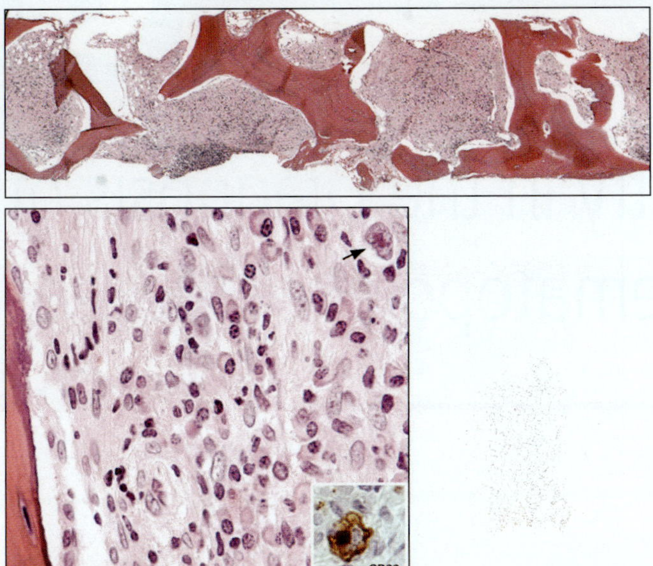

Figure 5.164 Hodgkin lymphoma involving the bone marrow. A dense fibrosclerotic process totally replaces the marrow and is composed of a heterogeneous mixture of inflammatory cells including small lymphocytes, histiocytes, plasma cells, eosinophils and occasional large CD30$^+$ mononuclear Reed-Sternberg cell variants (*arrow and inset*).

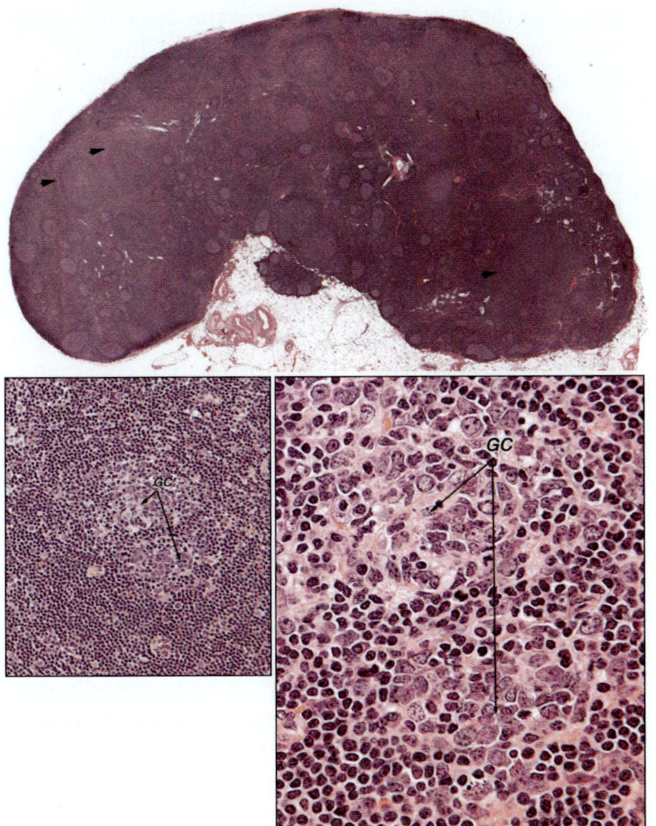

Figure 5.165 Progressive transformation of germinal centers (PTGC). Large, expanded, and partially obliterated follicles (*arrows*) are being invaded by small mantle cells. This condition often is seen in the same lymph nodes involved by nodular lymphocyte-predominant Hodgkin lymphoma.

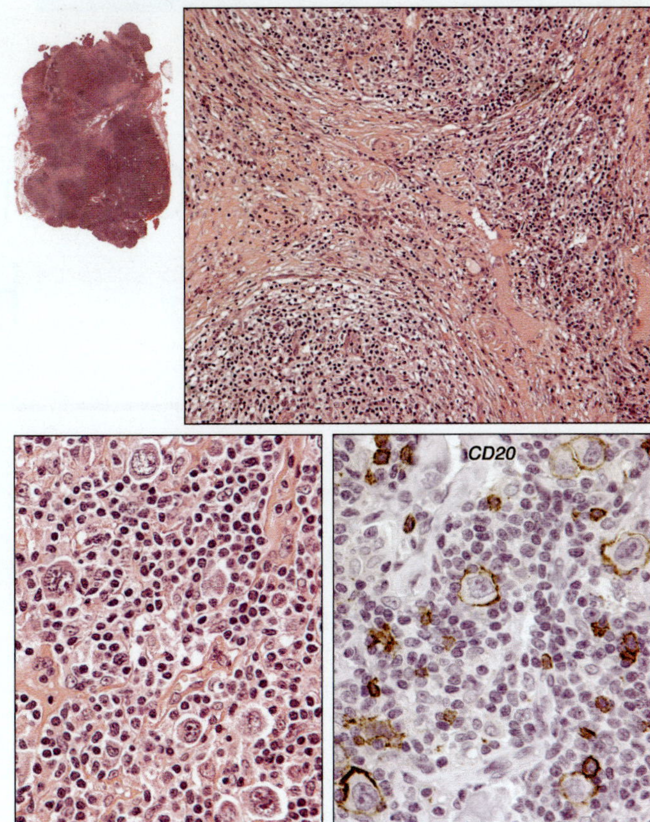

Figure 5.166 Large B-cell lymphoma mimicking nodular sclerosis Hodgkin lymphoma. This retroperitoneal lymph node reveals extensive fibrosis, associated with nodules composed mostly of small mature lymphocytes and occasional large, highly atypical multinucleated large B-cell lymphoma cells. The latter, by immunostains, were CDs 45$^+$/30$^-$/15$^-$/20$^+$. Many displayed bilobed nuclei with a vesicular (open or uncondensed) chromatin pattern, with two eosinophilic staining nucleoli that could easily, in the absence of immunohistochemistry, be confused with Reed-Sternberg cells.

Flow Cytometry in the Diagnosis of Hematopoietic Diseases

Steven J. Kussick, MD, PhD

Flow cytometry is an analytic technique in which cell suspensions created from virtually any type of fresh, unfixed tissue or body fluid, including peripheral blood or bone marrow, are stained with fluorescently labeled antibodies and then subjected to analysis on a highly specialized instrument known as a flow cytometer. Since it was first realized that a wealth of information could be derived by evaluating living cells in suspension, the field of flow cytometry has steadily progressed to the point where flow cytometry alone can now diagnose, or strongly suggest the diagnosis, of a number of benign and malignant hematopoietic diseases. Parallel advances in flow cytometer design, the availability of monoclonal antibodies to a variety of important hematopoietic antigens, and the development of a variety of new fluorescence dyes have been critical to the success of flow cytometry as a diagnostic tool.

The explosion of information about the basic biology of both benign and malignant hematopoietic diseases has been a major contributor to the current prominence of flow cytometry in hematopathology practice. As more and more specific antigens have been associated with specific diagnoses, flow cytometry has emerged as an extremely powerful technique by which such antigens can be identified to facilitate definitive diagnosis. The importance of immunophenotyping in diagnostic hematopathology was first emphasized by the Revised European-American Lymphoma (REAL) classification, and more recently by the World Health Organization (WHO) classification of hematolymphoid neoplasms, in which many myeloid and lymphoid malignancies are defined by the antigenic features of the neoplastic cells.

THE FLOW CYTOMETER

The flow cytometer is a relatively complex analytic device consisting of four major components (see Fig. 6.1 for a schematic illustration of a flow cytometer):

- The fluidics system begins with the various pumps and tubing used to introduce the specimen into the cytometer at a controlled rate. There, the specimen stream is surrounded by a pressurized stream of buffered saline known as sheath fluid, such that the cells assume a roughly single-file position due to the phenomenon of hydrodynamic focusing. The focused stream is then propelled to the flow chamber, where the cells are illuminated by light from one or more lasers. Ultimately, the focused stream is directed to a waste receptacle.
- The optics system includes: (a) the light source, most commonly a laser, used to excite the fluorescence dyes conjugated to the antibodies; (b) the system for conveying the emitted light from the flow chamber to specific detectors; and (c) the specific detectors themselves, which are typically photomultiplier tubes (PMTs) that convert the detected photons to electrical impulses whose magnitude is proportional to the amount of light. In most flow cytometers, the emitted light is conveyed to the PMTs via a combination of dichroic mirrors (which allow light of defined wavelengths to pass, while reflecting light of other wavelengths) and optical filters (which further narrow the wavelengths reaching a PMT, and include short pass, long pass, and band pass filters).
- The electronics system measures the electrical impulses generated by the PMTs and converts these analog measurements to digital information that is gathered and interpreted by the analysis software.
- The associated computer system, which typically consists of a personal computer that directly interfaces with the flow cytometer and controls the functions of the flow cytometer, including the acquisition and analysis of the flow cytometric data.

All four of these flow cytometer components have seen major advances over the past few decades. Fluidics systems are now managed electronically. Optical systems have progressed from utilizing single, relatively inefficient lasers and in-air transmission of emitted light from one or two fluorochromes, to utilizing two or more, highly efficient lasers and, in some instruments, fiberoptic systems for transmitting emitted light to the PMTs. Digital electronic systems have replaced analog systems on many of the newer flow cytometers. Finally, flow cytometry has benefited from the revolution in personal computer technology, in terms of both computer hardware and data acquisition and analysis software. The net result of these technical advances has been steady progression in the number of antigens that can be measured simultaneously by flow cytometry and the quality of the data generated.

CLINICAL INDICATIONS FOR FLOW CYTOMETRY

Four major indications have evolved for the use of flow cytometry in the clinical laboratory in the clinical evaluation of hematopoietic neoplasms. First, flow cytometry has been critical for the diagnosis and classification of hematopoietic neoplasms, especially chronic lymphoproliferative disorders and acute leukemias. Second, with improved understanding of the antigen expression profiles associated with prognostic subgroups in certain diseases (e.g., ZAP-70 expression in chronic lymphocytic leukemia/small lymphocytic lymphoma), flow cytometry has been used increasingly to identify antigens with prognostic significance in hematopoietic neoplasms. Third, with the advent of therapies targeted at specific antigens in hematopoietic neoplasms (e.g., anti-CD20 therapy in B-cell non-Hodgkin lymphomas), flow cytometry can identify potential therapeutic targets in hematopoietic neoplasms. Fourth, flow cytometry has been extensively utilized to monitor response to therapy by looking for residual disease. Such utilization of flow cytometry includes the evaluation for so-called "minimal residual disease," which is invariably defined as submicroscopic disease, and typically represents less than 1% involvement by neoplastic cells. Indeed, by evaluating a sufficiently large number of cells from a specimen (e.g., 500,000 to 1,000,000 cellular events), it is possible to detect minimal residual disease in peripheral blood or bone marrow at a level of 0.01% or less.

SPECIMEN REQUIREMENTS FOR FLOW CYTOMETRY

Although flow cytometric evaluation of DNA content can be performed on isolated nuclei from fixed tissue, flow cytometric immunophenotyping requires fresh, unfixed cells to permit evaluation of surface antigens. In the clinical flow cytometry laboratory, such specimens most commonly derive from peripheral blood, bone marrow, or finely minced lymphoid tissue (e.g., from a lymph node

biopsy or splenectomy). However, body fluids, including paucicellular cerebrospinal fluid (CSF) specimens, as well as disaggregated nonhematopoietic solid tumors such as carcinomas and sarcomas, can be evaluated by flow cytometry. Regardless of the starting tissue type, it is critical that the cells be maintained in an environment that maximizes viability prior to analysis. For tissues and paucicellular body fluids such as CSF, immediate immersion into an ample volume of tissue culture medium, such as RPMI-1640 supplemented with 10% fetal bovine serum, 1% glutamine, and 1% penicillin-streptomycin antibiotics, is a common method for enhancing cell viability. If the specimen is likely to reach the flow cytometry laboratory in 24 hours or less, the cells may be maintained at room temperature. For tissue samples, if delivery to the flow cytometry laboratory is likely to take more than 24 hours, it is reasonable to place the sample container on wet ice prior to shipment, particularly during the summer months. However, cell suspensions should never be subjected to extremes of temperature (below 0°C or above 37°C), and should therefore never be transported on dry ice.

Peripheral blood or bone marrow specimens, as well as other body fluids containing a large amount of peripheral blood contamination, should be anticoagulated prior to transport to the flow cytometry lab. The most common anticoagulants include ethylenediamine tetraacetic acid (EDTA) and heparin, both of which allow adequate flow cytometric evaluation although EDTA may deplete myeloid cells more rapidly than heparin. Note that acid citrate dextrose (ACD) anticoagulation is not recommended for bone marrows, as it may adversely affect cell viability. Peripheral blood, bone marrow, and body fluid specimens are typically transported and stored at room temperature.

THE PROCESS OF FLOW CYTOMETRIC ANALYSIS

Specimen Processing

Specimen processing is summarized in detail elsewhere. All clinical specimens must be handled with universal biohazard precautions. Laboratory coats and gloves should be worn by all personnel who directly manipulate specimens. Specimen processing steps that could potentially release hazardous aerosols, such as mincing lymph node or other tissues to create cell suspensions, should be performed in a biologic safety cabinet or other contained area. Sharp objects, such as scalpels for mincing tissues, must be handled with caution and disposed of properly. After specimens have been incubated with antibodies and washed, but before they are analyzed on the flow cytometer, the specimens should be fixed in 1% paraformaldehyde which both stabilizes antigen-antibody interactions by introducing cross-links and inactivates infectious agents. The addition of bleach to the instrument's waste container, at a final concentration of 10%, as well as daily purging of the cytometer fluidic system with a bleach solution prior to instrument shutdown, further minimize biohazard risks.

A zero-tolerance policy should exist for specimen mix-ups in the flow cytometry laboratory, to minimize the chance that incorrect patient data are reported. Therefore, procedures must be instituted to minimize the chance of such mix-ups occurring. Such procedures can include fastidious labeling and double-checking of all specimens at multiple points during processing and the separate processing of specimens to minimize the risk of cross-contamination. Morphologic evaluation of a smear or cytospin of each specimen, at the time of processing for flow cytometry, is a very useful mechanism for ensuring that the correct specimen is being used, in addition to providing valuable information about specimen cellularity and viability.

In any specimen containing a large amount of peripheral blood, the numerically dominant erythrocyte component should be removed prior to the introduction of the specimen into the flow cytometer. Although density gradient centrifugation with Ficoll-Hypaque historically was used to separate mononuclear cells from other blood elements, this technique suffers from two major shortcomings: Granulocytes are not maintained in the specimen following centrifugation and, even among the mononuclear cell component, selective cell loss may occur. Therefore, most clinical flow cytometry laboratories do not manipulate the leukocytes prior to adding antibodies, but rather lyse the red cells at some point during specimen processing. Bulk lysis of the red cells using either a commercially available reagent, or a homemade ammonium chloride solution, may be performed prior to the incubation of cells with antibodies. Alternatively, antibodies may be incubated with the cells in the presence of erythrocytes, and the erythrocytes lysed at the end of the preparation step (the so-called "whole blood" technique), just prior to evaluation of the cell suspension on the flow cytometer. Note that erythrocyte lysis techniques, when applied to bone marrow specimens, destroy the great majority of the nucleated erythroid precursors, thus significantly compromising the ability to evaluate such precursors by flow cytometry. Therefore, when analysis of nucleated erythroid precursors is desired, erythrocyte lysis must be avoided.

For tissue biopsies, including fine needle aspirates and bone marrow *core* biopsies, cell suspensions should be prepared by mechanical dissociation of the tissue in nutrient medium such as RPMI-1640, followed by removal of larger particles by filtration through 40–50 μm mesh. In this author's experience, enzymatic digestion of tissue is never used to generate a cell suspension.

Although the majority of antigens currently evaluated in diagnostic flow cytometry are cell surface–associated, note that cytoplasmic antigens (e.g., terminal deoxynucleotidyl transferase, or TdT, in lymphoblasts) also can be evaluated by flow cytometry (see Table 6.1 for a list of common antigens evaluated in clinical flow cytometry laboratories). A number of commercially available reagents are available for fixation and permeabilization of cells prior to the addition of antibodies to cytoplasmic antigens. When both cell surface and cytoplasmic antigens are evaluated in the same assay, the surface staining is performed first. The cells then are fixed and permeabilized, then stained for the cytoplasmic antigen(s).

Instrument Configuration and Quality Control

The decision as to how many antigens to evaluate simultaneously is critically dependent on the type of flow cytometer used in the laboratory. Single-laser flow cytometers typically are used to evaluate three or four antigens simultaneously, in addition to the two generic light-scatter properties of forward scatter (which is proportional to cell size) and side scatter (also known as orthogonal or 90-degree light scatter, which is proportional to cytoplasmic complexity and granularity). Two-laser instruments can potentially evaluate six to eight antigens simultaneously, depending on the PMT configuration, whereas three-laser instruments generally are required to evaluate nine or more antigens simultaneously. Although most clinical flow cytometry laboratories utilize three- or four-color flow cytometry for leukemia and lymphoma immunophenotyping, the feasibility of nine- and ten-color flow cytometry for this purpose has been demonstrated. The simultaneous assessment of such a large number of antigens minimizes the number of tubes of cells and antibodies that must be set up, and therefore is of particular benefit for the analysis of scanty specimens, while offering the potential for cost savings.

Regardless of the type of flow cytometer, quality control (QC) measures must be performed on a daily, weekly, and monthly basis to ensure optimal instrument performance. Daily QC measures typically use a stable fluorescence standard, such as brightly fluorescent microbeads, to ensure that the voltages allotted to the individual PMTs are adequate to detect the expected level of fluorescence from these microbeads. PMT voltages are typically set so that the autofluorescence of unstained lymphocytes (that is, the innate fluorescence of the cell due to endogenous biomolecules such as flavins, in the absence of added antibodies) falls within the first decade of the logarithmic scale. On a less frequent basis, the linearity of detected fluorescence should be confirmed by using a series of microbeads having known fluorescence properties ranging from negative to very bright; in addition, acceptably low-levels of cell carryover between specimens must be confirmed.

Antibodies: Compensation and Panel Design

Each of the fluorochromes used in flow cytometry has well-characterized absorption and emission spectra. Because the emission spectrum of each of the commonly-used fluorochromes extends over a range of wavelengths (see Fig. 6.2), the simultaneous use of multiple antibodies conjugated to different fluorochromes invariably results in some degree of spillover, in which a portion of the fluorescence from a given fluorochrome is detected by a PMT whose range of detected wavelengths is targeted for a different fluorochrome. As a result of this spectral overlap, the fluorescence detected by each PMT actually represents the sum of the fluorescence from multiple fluorochromes. Although most of the fluorescence typically comes from the fluorochrome the PMT was designed to detect, significant contributions may occur from other fluorochromes due to spillover. To adjust for the spillover fluorescence from other fluorochromes, a mathematical correction, known as compensation (or color compensation), is applied routinely to all multiparametric flow cytometry data. Although a detailed discussion of compensation is beyond the scope of this chapter, it is important to recognize that proper compensation of flow cytometry data is another critical QC function in the flow cytometry laboratory.

In the clinical flow cytometry laboratory, antibodies typically are used in defined combinations, or panels, to answer specific questions about specific cell populations. For example, most laboratories that perform leukemia and lymphoma immunophenotyping have an acute leukemia panel designed to distinguish acute myeloid leukemia from acute lymphoid leukemia, a lymphoma panel to distinguish benign from malignant lymphoid tissue, and the like (see Table 6.2 for a list of antigens important in the evaluation of specific hematopoietic cell populations). Although a detailed discussion of flow cytometric panel design is beyond the scope of this chapter, suffice it to say that a great deal of thought must go into panel design. At a minimum, antibody panels should measure a sufficient number of antigens to distinguish normal and benign from abnormal and neoplastic cell populations with a high degree of sensitivity and specificity. However, the quality of the flow cytometric data also depends on how antibodies are used in combination. For example, when the detection of a dimly expressed antigen—such as an aberrantly expressed lymphoid antigen on myeloid blasts—is important, conjugation of the relevant antibody to a bright fluorochrome, such as phycoerythrin (PE), can maximize the chance of detecting such aberrant antigen expression. Conversely, it may be unwise to use a bright fluorochrome to detect a brightly expressed antigen, because the bright fluorescence emission from this strategy will likely create compensation problems due to spillover.

When a specimen is received in the flow cytometry laboratory, it is important that the pathologist or flow cytometry technologist consider the underlying clinical question in deciding which antibodies and panels to use in the evaluation. If the clinical question is a limited one, such as whether a bone marrow aspirate from a patient with known B-cell non-Hodgkin lymphoma has any evidence of disease, then it may be appropriate to perform a limited study focused primarily on the cell population in question,

such as the mature B cells in this case. On the other hand, when the clinical question is much broader, for example, when ruling out a hematolymphoid neoplasm in the bone marrow of a patient with pancytopenia and no known malignancy, then a broader evaluation of the myeloid, lymphoid, and plasmacytic lineages is likely to be appropriate. When clinical concern exists for a lymphoproliferative disorder, then it is prudent to evaluate both the B cells and T cells whenever possible. However, because B-cell lymphomas are much more common than are T-cell lymphomas in Western patient populations, if only a minimal amount of specimen is available, it is reasonable to rule out a B-cell malignancy before evaluating the T cells.

Data Acquisition

The actual collection of flow cytometric data, during which time the stained cells are propelled through the flow cytometer, illuminated by the laser(s), and detected by the PMTs, is known as acquisition. The number of cellular events (i.e., individual cells) required for evaluation depends on both the purpose of the flow cytometric evaluation and on the nature of the specimen. For example, if one is evaluating a lymph node that is replaced by lymphoma, acquisition of a relatively low number of events per tube of cells and antibodies (e.g., 10,000 events) may allow adequate characterization of the neoplastic population. In contrast, if one is looking for evidence of very low-level bone marrow or peripheral blood involvement by lymphoma, then a much larger number of cells (e.g., 100,000 to 500,000) should be collected. In the author's practice, if adequate cells are available, then at least 100,000 viable cells are routinely acquired per tube. However, at least 500,000 cells will be acquired when the bone marrow and blood are evaluated in a patient being considered for stem cell harvest for autologous stem cell transplantation, to maximize the chance of identifying an occult neoplastic population capable of contaminating collected stem cells. Assuming that the presence of 50 neoplastic cells in the tube would enable confident identification of this population, then the evaluation of 500,000 cells offers the ability to detect the neoplastic population at a frequency of 1 in 10,000 cells, or 0.01%.

A potential artifact in the evaluation of flow cytometric data is carryover from one tube to the next, in which stained cells from previously acquired specimens accumulate in the tubing of the instrument and are released in relatively small numbers as subsequent acquisition occurs. The hazard in carryover is that certain combinations of bound fluorochromes on the contaminating cells could lead to interpretation as a small abnormal cell population, suggesting the possibility of malignancy despite the fact that no such cell population truly exists in the specimen at hand. Most clinical flow cytometers have manufacturer specifications guaranteeing no more than 1% carryover, and these instruments frequently demonstrate much less carryover in practice. However, if one is looking for minimal residual disease then one should make every effort to eliminate carryover altogether. One way to accomplish this is to run plain sheath fluid through the instrument between tubes of cells and antibodies and to monitor the data generated by such a procedure to ensure that no increase occurs in the number of cellular events beyond the usual background level for the instrument.

Data Analysis

The analysis of the acquired flow cytometric data requires specialized computer programs designed for this purpose. Such programs are available for both PC and Macintosh platforms and ideally permit adequate evaluation of both QC and specimen data. At a minimum, such programs should be able to perform compensation, generate two-dimensional histograms (also known as two-parameter dot plots or scatter plots) of the data that can be adjusted to define abnormal cell populations, and enumerate the various cell populations of interest for reporting purposes.

The process of targeting the analysis to the cell population(s) of interest is known as gating. In this process, greater and greater numbers of extraneous cellular events are excluded from the analysis in a sequential manner, to maximize the likelihood of identifying an abnormal cell population.

An early gating step in virtually all flow cytometric evaluation is the exclusion of nonviable cells from the analysis. Because nonviable cells typically have a marked decrease in forward scatter as a result of membrane damage secondary to cellular degeneration, forward (FS) versus side scatter (SS) gating (Fig. 6.3, left) is a simple technique for excluding the nonviable cells. Forward versus side scatter gating also will exclude many residual, unlysed erythrocytes due to their small size. An alternative method for removing nonviable cells from the analysis is the addition of a viability dye, such as 7-amino-actinomycinD (7-AAD), to the cell suspension just prior to data acquisition on the flow cytometer. 7-AAD penetrates the damaged plasma membranes of nonviable cells, but is excluded from viable cells. Therefore, cells demonstrating the characteristic fluorescence of 7-AAD, are excluded from further evaluation by gating.

The second step in the gating process frequently separates complex cell mixtures, such as blood or bone marrow, into their constituent cell populations. Because lymphocytes, monocytes, and granulocytes typically show reproducible differences in their forward and side scatter characteristics, FS versus SS gating can be used effectively to separate these three cell populations in peripheral blood (see Fig. 6.3, left). This gating strategy becomes somewhat less effective when applied to bone marrow, because one particularly important bone marrow population—the blasts—have FS versus SS characteristics that overlap both the lymphocytes and monocytes. Given the limitations of FS versus SS gating as applied to bone marrow, most clini-

cal flow cytometry laboratories now include an antibody to the leukocyte common antigen, or CD45, in all tubes used to evaluate bone marrow, so that CD45 versus SS gating can be used to separate the various bone marrow cell populations, including the blasts (see Fig. 6.3, right).

A third gating strategy that can be applied to the viable cells, which is particularly useful when one is looking for a mature B-cell or T-cell lymphoproliferative disorder, is lineage-specific gating (Fig. 6.4). In this gating strategy, staining with an antibody to a pan–B-cell antigen such as CD19, or to a pan–T-cell antigen such as CD3, is employed to restrict the analysis to these lymphoid populations.

A variety of antigenic abnormalities may be observed during the flow cytometric evaluation of malignant hematopoietic cell populations. These abnormalities typically contrast with the very regular and reproducible patterns of antigen expression one sees in benign hematopoietic cell populations and include:

- Abnormal increases or decreases in the levels of expression of antigens normally on the cells of interest, including complete loss of expression (e.g., aberrant loss of CD7 on the neoplastic CD4$^+$ T cells of mycosis fungoides or Sézary syndrome)
- Abnormally homogeneous expression of antigens that normally show variable expression in a population of interest (e.g., abnormally homogeneous expression of CD34 and CD38 on myeloid blasts in myelodysplasia or acute myeloid leukemia; light chain restriction among B cells or plasma cells)
- Asynchronous antigen expression, in which the timing of antigen expression during a maturational process is abnormal (e.g., asynchronous expression of CD13 and CD16 during neutrophil maturation in myelodysplasia)
- Aberrant expression of nonlineage antigens (e.g., aberrant expression of the T-cell–associated antigen CD7 on leukemic myeloid blasts)

To appreciate these abnormalities, the flow cytometrist must have a thorough prior understanding of the normal patterns of antigen expression in the cell populations of interest.

Data Reporting

Although some attempts have been made to standardize the reporting of clinical leukemia and lymphoma immunophenotyping data, no such standardization has yet been achieved. Simply reporting the percentage of cells in the population of interest that is considered positive for each of the antigens evaluated is not adequate and should be avoided. Although such lists of antigens do indicate how broad the flow cytometric evaluation was, and do provide information needed for billing purposes, these lists do not provide a unifying description of the salient features of any abnormal cell populations in the specimen. Therefore, it is strongly recommended that the immunophenotype of each abnormal cell population, including the proportion each abnormal population represents of the total viable cells, be described in a free-text format in the flow cytometry report. Descriptions of the fluorescence intensities of diagnostically-relevant antigens are useful; commonly used values, such as CD4:CD8 and κ:λ ratios, may also be included. Finally, the addition of key two-dimensional histograms to the report can provide a very useful snapshot of a neoplastic immunophenotype that can be of great help in following the patient's disease when subsequent specimens are received.

BENIGN HEMATOPOIETIC DISORDERS IDENTIFIABLE BY FLOW CYTOMETRY

Human Immunodeficiency Virus (HIV) and Other Immunodeficiency States

Flow cytometry can be very helpful in evaluating immunodeficiency states. The most widely used test for this purpose is T-cell subset analysis in HIV-infected individuals. In HIV-positive patients who are not receiving highly active antiretroviral therapy (HAART), the CD4:CD8 ratio typically shows progressive decline over time, and this ratio can be used to assess the progression of disease.

Two different methods have been used to evaluate T-cell subsets in peripheral blood specimens from HIV-infected patients. In two-platform tests, the percentages of $CD4^+$ and $CD8^+$ T cells are determined among the lymphocytes or total leukocytes by flow cytometry, and these percentages then are applied to the absolute lymphocyte or total leukocyte count determined by routine complete blood count (CBC) analysis to produce a final absolute $CD4^+$ T-cell count on a per microliter basis. In single platform tests, for which a number of kits are now commercially available, the absolute $CD4^+$ T-cell count is determined entirely by flow cytometry. These kits invariably use fluorescent microbeads of known quantity to determine the absolute $CD4^+$ T-cell count and require very careful pipetting techniques for the counts to be valid.

In addition to HIV disease, congenital immunodeficiency syndromes can be identified and/or monitored by flow cytometry. For example, the flow cytometric evaluation of peripheral blood in patients with common variable immunodeficiency (CVID) typically reveals decreased numbers of B cells, particularly memory B cells and an inverted CD4:CD8 ratio. Patients with congenital X-linked agammaglobulinemia (Bruton disease) typically have a marked decrease in circulating mature B cells. Severe combined immunodeficiency (SCID) patients generally show significant decrease in the absolute numbers of both B and T cells. Patients with the autoimmune lymphoproliferative syndrome characteristically show abnormal expansion of dual $CD4^-/CD8^-$ α/β T cells.

Evaluation of the Immune Response in Sepsis

Although sepsis is a clinical diagnosis, flow cytometry can be used to evaluate the immune response in the setting of sepsis. In particular, neutrophils typically show activation in a setting of sepsis, with increased expression of CD64. Monocytes also can show variable amounts of activation, with increased CD16. Decreased expression of HLA-DR on monocytes in the setting of sepsis has been shown to be a poor prognostic sign by some studies, but not all.

Feto-Maternal Hemorrhage

Because of the potential need to initiate anti-D therapy following feto-maternal hemorrhage in the setting of an Rh-negative (D^-) mother and Rh-positive (D^+) father, quantitative evaluation of fetal red cells in maternal circulation is an important application of flow cytometry. Flow cytometry enables this evaluation to be done in a more rapid and reproducible manner than the *manual* Kleihauer-Betke test, the traditional morphologic method for this determination. In the flow cytometric assay, antibodies to fetal hemoglobin are incubated with permeabilized red blood cells from a maternal peripheral blood specimen. The proportion of fetal hemoglobin-positive cells identified by flow cytometry is used as a measure of the contaminating fetal erythrocytes in the maternal circulation. Based on the absolute number of fetal cells present, anti-D dosing will be adjusted accordingly.

MYELOID NEOPLASMS IDENTIFIABLE BY FLOW CYTOMETRY

Low-Grade Myelodysplastic Syndromes (MDS) and Chronic-Phase Myeloproliferative Disorders (CMPD)

Over the past ten years, multiple studies have demonstrated that cases of MDS and CMPD frequently manifest abnormal antigen expression on the myeloid blasts and/or the maturing granulocytes and monocytes. In clinical flow cytometry laboratories in which the normal patterns of antigen expression during myeloid maturation in the bone marrow are well-understood (see Fig. 6.5), abnormalities in these patterns can be used to support the diagnosis of MDS or MPD in patients suspected of having these diagnoses based on clinical and morphologic grounds. This additional information can be particularly helpful in morphologically equivocal cases in which cytogenetic studies fail to detect a clonal karyotypic abnormality. In the example shown (Fig. 6.6), the constellation of antigenic abnormalities among the myeloid blasts and maturing granulocytes is consistent with the diagnosis of MDS, despite the relatively low blast percentage ($<5\%$ by both morphology and flow cytometry, consistent with the WHO entity known as refractory cytopenia with multilineage dysplasia).

Importantly, in all cases of MDS or MPD, clinical, morphologic, and cytogenetic correlation are required to render a specific diagnosis.

Acute Myeloid Leukemia with the t(8;21)(q22;q22)

In addition to a markedly expanded myeloid blast population identified by CD45 versus side-scatter gating, this AML typically shows a relatively prominent population of maturing granulocytes, reflecting the underlying maturation characteristic of this entity, which is considered a form of AML M2 under the French-American-British (FAB) classification (Fig. 6.7). CD34 typically is expressed brightly, frequently in combination with aberrant CD15, which is normally a more mature myeloid antigen not expressed on blasts. The pan-myeloid antigen CD33 typically is expressed weakly, whereas HLA-DR and the myeloid-associated antigens CD13 and myeloperoxidase (the latter is a cytoplasmic protein) generally are bright. There is characteristic aberrant expression of the B-cell–associated antigen CD19, and CD56 and TdT also may be aberrantly expressed.

Acute Myeloid Leukemia with inv(16)(p13;q22) or t(16;16)(p13;q22)

This leukemia, which is known as AML M4eo under the FAB classification, typically shows a prominent CD34$^+$ myeloblast population with evidence of both monocytic and granulocytic differentiation by CD45 versus side-scatter gating. The myeloid blast population commonly shows aberrant coexpression of CD15 and, based on evaluation of CD45 versus SS, generally forms a maturational continuum with both the monocytes and granulocytes. The monocytic component shows relatively strong expression of CD33, CD64, and HLA-DR (Fig. 6.8) and acquisition of CD14 on the more mature forms, whereas the granulocytic component expresses relatively weak CD33 and CD64, without HLA-DR. A variably expanded eosinophil population, with relatively bright CD45 and increased side scatter, but without the CD16 expression characteristic of neutrophils, also is present.

Acute Myeloid Leukemia with the t(15;17)(q22;q12)

This entity, which is also known as acute promyelocytic leukemia (APL, also known as AML M3 under the FAB classification), is a leukemic proliferation of promyelocytes, characteristically expressing CD13, CD33, and CD117 (c-kit), with loss of HLA-DR (Fig. 6.9). In most cases, CD34 is absent on the leukemic promyelocytes. However, in the hypogranular form of APL (approximately 30% of cases), low-level CD34 on a minority of the promyelocytes is not uncommon. The mature myeloid-associated antigen CD15 is expressed more weakly on neoplastic promyelocytes than on normal promyelocytes. Aberrant CD56 and/or CD2

expression may be seen, particularly in hypogranular form. Importantly, while morphology and flow cytometry suggest this diagnosis, FISH or cytogenetic documentation of the t(15;17) or variant translocation is required to confirm the diagnosis.

Acute Myeloid Leukemia, Not Otherwise Categorized

Flow cytometry can be helpful in subclassifying AMLs *without* recurrent cytogenetic abnormalities. For example, the diagnosis of AML, minimally differentiated under the WHO classification (AML M0 under the FAB classification), which by definition lacks myeloperoxidase reactivity by cytochemistry, depends on flow cytometry to establish myeloid lineage via the identification of myeloid-associated antigens such as CD13, CD33, and CD117. In those occasional cases of acute myelomonocytic or monocytic or monoblastic leukemia showing unexpectedly little nonspecific esterase reactivity by cytochemistry, flow cytometry can confirm the presence of monocyte-associated antigens such as CD64, CD36, CD11b, CD4, and CD14. Finally, flow cytometric identification of platelet- and megakaryocyte-associated antigens, such as CD41 (glycoprotein IIb) or CD61 (glycoprotein IIIa) on the blasts provides important support for the diagnosis of acute megakaryoblastic leukemia.

Acute Biphenotypic Leukemia

The definition of acute biphenotypic leukemia has been fraught with ambiguity prior to the WHO classification of hematolymphoid neoplasms, which defines this acute leukemia as "characterized by blasts which coexpress myeloid and T or B lineage-specific antigens or concurrent B and T lineage antigens. Rarely the blasts in this case coexpress markers for all three lineages." Figure 6.10 illustrates a case satisfying this definition, with a single blast population expressing the B-lymphoblast–associated antigens CD19 and TdT, and the myeloid blast-associated antigens CD13 and CD117. The WHO classification contrasts this entity with acute bilineal leukemias, because the latter include two or more discrete blast populations, each of which retains the features of a single lineage. In cases in which surface antigen evaluation is ambiguous for lineage, cytoplasmic antigen evaluation frequently is helpful. In this context, specific B-lymphoid–associated markers include cytoplasmic CD79a, cytoplasmic IgM, and cytoplasmic CD22. The most specific T-lymphoid–associated antigens include membranous or cytoplasmic CD3 or the T-cell receptor, whereas cytoplasmic myeloperoxidase is considered the most specific myeloid-associated antigen. Because no well-defined immunophenotype exists in acute biphenotypic leukemia, these cases must be evaluated on a case-by-case basis. Finally, both acute biphenotypic leukemia and acute bilineal leukemia should be distinguished from undifferentiated acute leukemia. According to the WHO classification, the latter is characterized by an *absence* of lineage-specific antigens. Nonlineage-specific antigens expressed in undifferentiated leukemias include HLA-DR, CD34, and CD38, with a subset of cases expressing TdT and CD7. Note that CD7 is not considered to be T lymphoid specific if only expressed at low levels, in the absence of other T-cell–associated antigens.

Paroxysmal Nocturnal Hemoglobinuria (PNH)

The flow cytometric hallmarks of this clonal myeloid stem cell abnormality reflect the acquired loss of glycosylphosphatidylinositol (GPI)-linked proteins—due to acquired mutation of the pigA gene—that is the defining feature of PNH, and leads to abnormal susceptibility to complement-mediated lysis. Specific antigenic abnormalities reflect the loss of GPI-linked proteins, and include loss of CD55 or CD59 on erythrocytes, loss of CD14 on mature monocytes, and loss of CD16 and CD66b on mature neutrophils (Fig. 6.11). Because of the heterogeneity of CD14, CD16, and CD66b expression among immature monocytes and neutrophil precursors in the bone marrow, PNH evaluation is best performed on peripheral blood, where only mature forms of these cell lineages are expected to occur. Note that serial evaluation of the size of the PNH-like monocyte and neutrophil populations in the peripheral blood may be used to monitor the extent of marrow involvement by the PNH clone. Evaluation of CD55$^-$ or CD59$^-$ erythrocyte populations is less useful for this purpose, because affected erythrocytes appear to be more sensitive to complement-mediated lysis than are leukocytes; therefore, the size of the CD55$^-$ or CD59$^-$ erythrocyte population in the blood tends to underestimate the size of the PNH clone in the bone marrow.

B-LYMPHOID NEOPLASMS

B-lymphoid neoplasms are best understood in the context of normal B-cell maturation, which is illustrated schematically in Figure 6.12. Precursor B-cell neoplasms correspond to the pro-B cell and pre-B cell, or B-lymphoblast, stages. Mature B-cell neoplasms correspond to the early (naïve), activated (including CD10$^+$ germinal center B cells, which are not shown), and memory B-cell stages. Plasma cell neoplasms correspond to the terminal stage of B-cell maturation.

Precursor B-Cell Neoplasms

Precursor B-cell neoplasms are referred to generically as precursor B-lymphoblastic leukemias/lymphomas (pre–B-ALL) under the WHO classification. The large majority of cases present as leukemias involving the bone marrow and blood, whereas lymphomatous presentation is rare. Pre–B-ALLs include subtypes with a favorable prognosis, such as cases bearing the t(12;21)(p12;q22) or hyperdiploidy with greater than 50 chromosomes, and subtypes with an unfavorable prognosis, such as cases bearing the t(9;22)(q34;q11), the t(1;19)(q23;p13), or the t(4;11)(q21;q23). Virtually all pre–B-ALLs express the B-cell–associated antigen CD19, in addition to HLA-DR and the lymphoblast-associated antigen TdT (Fig. 6.13). Most pre–B-ALLs express CD10, the common acute lymphoblastic leukemia antigen (CALLA), and most lack surface light chains. CD45 expression is typically low to occasionally negative. Certain karyotypes do have characteristic immunophenotypes. The t(12;21) is associated with no CD20 expression, and relatively low-level CD9. Hyperdiploid cases frequently lack CD45. The t(9;22) is associated with aberrant expression of myeloid antigens, such as CD13 and CD33, and occasional lack of CD45. The t(1;19)(q23;p13) is associated with lack of CD34, whereas the t(4;11) is associated with loss of CD10 expression (CALLA-negative pre–B-ALL), lack of CD20, and frequent aberrant expression of the myeloid-associated antigen CD15. Pre-B-ALLs associated with the t(4;11), like other acute leukemias associated with MLL rearrangements, typically express the chondroitin sulfate molecule NG2, which is recognized by monoclonal antibody 7.1.

Mature B-Cell Neoplasms

Neoplastic mature B-cell populations are readily distinguished from benign/reactive B-cell populations by flow cytometry.

Almost all mature B-cell neoplasms express CD19 and the mature B-cell antigen CD20 at some level, and show restricted expression of κ- or λ-light chains, which allows clonality to be confirmed by flow cytometry. In most mature B-cell neoplasms, evaluation of cell surface light chains demonstrates clonality. However, in a minority of cases, a loss of cell surface light chain expression occurs, requiring the evaluation of cytoplasmic light chains to provide formal proof of clonality. Cytoplasmic light-chain evaluation may not be essential to prove malignancy in cases in which the remainder of the surface immunophenotype is unequivocally abnormal. However, in cases with apparent loss of surface light-chain expression but an otherwise normal surface immunophenotype, formal proof of clonality should be obtained from cytoplasmic light-chain evaluation, because benign B-cell populations, particularly germinal center B cells, occasionally down-regulate surface light-chain expression to such an extent that they appear surface light chain-negative. On rare occasion, typically in young patients with localized lymph node or tonsillar enlargement, clonal follicle center B-cell populations can be identified in the absence of clinical or histologic evidence of lymphoma.

Because CD20 is now such an important therapeutic target in the treatment of B-cell malignancies, formal evaluation of CD20 expression should be incorporated in any flow cytometric evaluation of the B cells. Note that in patients recently treated with anti-CD20 antibodies, flow cytometry typically fails to identify a CD20+ cell population, due to therapeutic antibody coating of CD20 on B cells, so an alternative B-cell antigen such as CD19 should be used to identify the B cells.

Chronic Lymphocytic Leukemia/Small Lymphocytic Lymphoma (CLL/SLL)

A major feature of CLL/SLL is aberrant coexpression of the T-cell–associated antigen CD5, and the T-cell/myeloid-associated antigen CD43, on the neoplastic B cells, along with the B-cell–associated antigens CD19 and CD20 (Fig.6.14). Characteristic diminished expression occurs (compared with normal mature B cells) of a variety of mature B-cell–associated antigens, including surface light chains, CD20, CD22, and CD79b. However, some cases show an atypical or "activated" phenotype with higher levels of these antigens. Typically, moderate to bright CD23 is present, with little or no expression of the FMC7 antigen (FMC7 is believed to represent an epitope of the CD20 molecule). Cases bearing unmutated immunoglobulin genes, a feature associated with an adverse prognosis, frequently express CD38 and/or cytoplasmic ZAP-70 (see Fig.6.14). Because CLL/SLL is such a common disease, occasional patients show two different CLL/SLL clones, which are readily separated in Figure 6.15 by virtue of the different surface light chains that the two clones express. Note that, in CLL/SLL progression, the expanded component of larger cells often shows a relative decrease in CD5 and CD23 expression and a relative increase in surface light chain, CD20, CD22, CD79b, and FMC7 expression.

Follicular Lymphoma

The majority of follicular lymphoma cases coexpress the germinal-center–associated antigen CD10 along with the pan–B-cell antigens CD19 and CD20 (Fig.6.16), and clonally restricted light chains. CD19 often is expressed at abnormally low levels. Surface light-chain expression is often brighter than in CLL/SLL, although a subset of cases show aberrant loss of surface light-chain expression; in the latter cases, cytoplasmic light-chain restriction typically can be identified. The neoplastic cells typically overexpress cytoplasmic bcl-2, which is highlighted when these cells are compared to benign, background B cells or T cells in the same specimen. Low-grade follicular lymphomas (grades 1 and 2 out of 3 in the WHO system) tend to show relatively small cell size by forward and side scatter light characteristics, whereas grade 3 follicular lymphomas tend to show a spectrum of larger size.

Hairy Cell Leukemia

Hairy cells show increased side scatter, reflecting their relatively abundant cytoplasm, and relatively bright CD19 and CD20 compared with any benign B cells in the background. The key to making the diagnosis of hairy cell leukemia (HCL) is identifying expression of CD103 on the neoplastic cells, typically in association with CD25 and bright CD22 and CD11c (Fig. 6.17). However, a subset of cases commonly referred to as *hairy cell variants* may lack expression of CD25, with an otherwise characteristic hairy cell leukemia phenotype. CD10 occasionally is expressed by hairy cells. Associated monocytopenia is another characteristic finding in HCL, although this finding can be obscured when the hairy cell population encroaches on the monocyte region of a CD45 versus side scatter plot. Note that, because of its very distinctive immunophenotype, HCL often can be detected at levels less than 0.1% of the leukocytes if a sufficient number of cells is analyzed.

Mantle Cell Lymphoma

Mantle cell lymphoma (MCL), like CLL/SLL, is characterized by the coexpression of the T-cell–associated antigen CD5, and the T-cell/myeloid–associated antigen CD43 on the neoplastic B cells, along with the B-cell–associated antigens CD19 and CD20 and clonally restricted light chains (Fig. 6.18). In contrast to CLL/SLL, MCL shows moderate to bright expression of a variety of B-cell–associated antigens, including surface light chains, CD20, CD22, and CD79b, and typically expresses FMC7, with little or no CD23. Rare cases express low CD10. Flow cytometric evaluation of nuclear cyclin D1 expression, the protein overexpressed as a result of the characteristic t(11;14)(q13;q32) of MCL, is not in common clinical usage, so the diagnosis of MCL is currently confirmed by cyclin D1 immunohistochemistry or t(11;14) FISH in most hematopathology laboratories.

Diffuse Large B-Cell Lymphoma

Diffuse large B-cell lymphoma (DLBCL) generally shows increased cell size based on forward and side-scatter characteristics (Fig. 6.19). Highly variable levels of CD19, CD20, and clonally restricted light chains are present; these antigens are generally moderate to bright, but occasionally can be unusually low, as with decreased CD20 in immunoblastic lymphomas due to the plasmacytoid differentiation in these cases. Variable expression of CD10 occurs, and, when present, suggests a germinal-center immunophenotype of the neoplastic cells. At present, the evaluation Bcl-6 and Mum-1 expression, which also is helpful in establishing if a DLBCL is of germinal-center immunophenotype, is performed by immunohistochemistry rather than flow cytometry. Certain subtypes of diffuse large B-cell lymphoma recognized by the WHO classification have distinctive immunophenotypes, such as relatively common CD5 coexpression by the neoplastic B cells in intravascular large B-cell lymphoma, a prominent benign background T-cell population with relatively few neoplastic large B cells in T-cell–rich large B-cell lymphoma, relatively common loss of HLA-DR and both surface and cytoplasmic light-chain expression in primary mediastinal large B-cell lymphoma, and loss of B-cell–associated antigens such as CD19 and CD20 with expression of activation antigens such as CD30 and CD38, in primary effusion lymphoma.

Burkitt Lymphoma

Burkitt lymphoma typically demonstrates intermediate, rather than large, cell size based on the light-scatter properties, with a prominent nonviable population due to the very high apoptotic rate among these cells. Moderate to bright expression of CD19, CD20, and clonally restricted light chains occurs, as well as expression of CD10 without bcl-2, in contrast to most follicular lymphomas (Fig. 6.20).

PLASMA CELL NEOPLASMS

Plasma cells characteristically express very bright CD38 (brighter than any other cell in the bone marrow) and increased cell size, making them relatively easy to identify by flow cytometry. Some laboratories also use expression of CD138 (syndecan-1) to aid in identifying the plasma cells. In almost all cases, plasma cell neoplasms express restricted cytoplasmic light and heavy chains identifiable by flow cytometry in permeabilized specimens; in practice, many clinical flow cytometry laboratories that evaluate plasma cell clonality including the author's, examine immunoglobulin light chain expression alone, without evaluating heavy chain expression. In rare cases, neoplastic plasma cells express restricted surface light chains at very low level, or show aberrant loss of light-chain expression altogether. In addition, the majority of cases of plasma cell myeloma demonstrate abnormal surface immunophenotypes, with decreased to absent levels of CD19 and CD45, frequent coexpression of CD56, and occasional aberrant coexpression of CD117/c-kit or other antigens (Fig. 6.21).

T-LYMPHOID/NK-CELL NEOPLASMS

T-lymphoid neoplasms, like B-lymphoid neoplasms, can be understood in the context of normal T-cell maturation, which is illustrated schematically in Figure 6.22. Precursor T-cell neoplasms correspond to the pro–T-cell and thymocyte stages. Mature T-cell neoplasms usually are derived from "single positive" (i.e., CD4$^+$ or CD8$^+$) T cells expressing α-β T-cell antigen receptors, although rare γ-δ T-cell malignancies also occur. NK cells represent a lymphoid lineage distinct from T cells and do not have rearranged T-cell antigen receptors.

Precursor T-Cell Neoplasms

As with the precursor B-cell neoplasms, precursor T-cell neoplasms are grouped under a single overarching diagnostic category under the WHO classification: precursor T-lymphoblastic lymphoma/leukemia (pre-T-ALL). Compared to pre–B-ALL, pre–T-ALL is much more likely to present with soft-tissue involvement, particularly in the anterior mediastinum and thymus. Like pre–B-ALL,

pre–T-ALL consists of a number of genetically distinct entities, many of which are thought to derive from different stages of early T-cell maturation; all these stages typically express TdT and CD7. The least mature pre–T-ALLs are thought to derive from prothymocytes, which express TdT, HLA-DR, CD34, and CD7. Somewhat more mature pre–T-ALLs may correspond to the immature thymocyte stage, at which time HLA-DR and CD34 are lost, and CD2, CD5, and cytoplasmic CD3 are acquired (Fig. 6.23). Pre–T-ALLs of the common thymocyte stage typically show dual expression of CD4 and CD8, and express the common thymocyte antigen CD1a (Fig. 6.24). Finally, occasional pre–T-ALLs have a mature thymocyte immunophenotype, with single positivity for CD4 or CD8 and acquisition of surface CD3.

Because thymoma is always in the differential diagnosis of mediastinal pre–T-ALL, the identification of immunophenotypic aberrancy in thymocytes, such as abnormally homogeneous expression of normal immature T-cell antigens or aberrant expression of myeloid-associated antigens, can be very helpful in distinguishing mediastinal pre–T-ALL from thymoma. Importantly, the immature T cells in thymoma typically show a normal maturational spectrum of antigen expression. If any uncertainty exists about distinguishing pre–T-ALL from thymoma in a mediastinal mass, immunohistochemical evaluation of cytokeratin expression should be performed on paraffin-embedded tissue, because the neoplastic cells of thymoma are cytokeratin-positive epithelial cells, whereas few, if any, cytokeratin-positive cells will be seen in the background of pre–T-ALL.

Mature T-Cell and NK-Cell Neoplasms

With the exception of γ-δ T-cell lymphomas and NK-cell lymphomas, the entities discussed in this section involve α-β T cells. Being composed of mature T cells, these neoplasms all lack expression of CD34, TdT, and CD1a. Historically, the presence of abnormal increases or decreases in the levels of expression of T-cell–associated surface antigens has been used as a surrogate for clonality documentation in the evaluation of T-cell neoplasms; in this approach, care must to taken to avoid overinterpreting changes in surface antigen expression, because certain benign or reactive T-cell populations show characteristic decreases in surface antigen expression. For example, both benign and malignant large granular lymphocytes (LGLs) of the (CD8$^+$) T-cell type characteristically show a decreased level of CD5 compared with other CD8$^+$ T cells, such that mildly decreased CD5 among a subset of the CD8$^+$ T cells is not sufficient to make the diagnosis of T-LGL leukemia. Similarly, CD4$^+$ memory T cells characteristically show variably diminished CD7 expression compared with other T cells.

Over the past few years, the commercial availability of fluorescently-labeled antibodies to a large number of the TCR-beta isoforms – typically representing about 70% of the total TCR-beta usage among normal alpha-beta T cells

– has enabled the flow cytometric indentification of clonality among alpha-beta T-cell populations of interest. For the majority of alpha-beta T-cell neoplasms, restriced expression of 1 of these isoforms can be proven, while in a minority of cases the abnormal T cells will not react with any of the available TCR-beta isoform-specific antibodies, which allows clonality to be inferred rather than formally proven. In the author's experience, TCR-beta antibodies are optimally used with antibodies to 2 or more additional T-cell-associated antigens, to enable the abnormal T-cell population to be distinguished from all benign T cells during data analysis. Importantly, because clonal T-cell expansions can be seen in benign immunologic reactions, flow cytometric demonstration of T-cell clonality must be interpreted in the overall context of the case before a diagnosis of T-cell malignancy is made. In laboratories not using this antibody kit, proof of T-cell clonality typically relies on polymerase chain reaction methodology.

Note that the majority of the mature T-cell malignancies express CD52, an important target in salvage therapy of these tumors. Expression of CD25 and CD30, which are other potential therapeutic targets, is less consistent in T-cell neoplasms.

T-Cell Prolymphocytic Leukemia (T-PLL)

T-PLL cases typically express CD2, CD3, CD5, and CD7, although one or more of these may be expressed at abnormal levels, including weak surface CD3 (Fig.6.25). Sixty percent of cases are CD4[+] and CD8[−], 25% of cases coexpress CD4 and CD8, and 15% of cases are CD8[+] and CD4[−]. The coexpression of CD4 and CD8 is relatively restricted to T-PLL among mature T-cell neoplasms and helps to distinguish it from other mature T-cell neoplasms of small to intermediate cell size. CD52, which is typically expressed in T-PLL, represents a therapeutic target.

T-Cell Large Granular Lymphocytic Leukemia (T-LGLL)

The large majority of T-LGLL cases are CD3[+], CD8[+] neoplasms showing variable loss of CD5 (most commonly) and CD7 (somewhat less commonly; see Fig 6.26). CD57 expression is common in these cases. Rare T-LGLL variants express CD4, occasionally together with CD8. Patients may show profound neutropenia by flow cytometry, and/or morphology.

Mycosis Fungoides (Sézary Syndrome) (MF/SS)

The neoplastic cells in MF/SS are typically CD3[+], CD4[+] T cells (Fig. 6.27) showing loss of CD7 and CD26 expression; rare cases may be positive for CD8. Transforming cases may express CD30.

Peripheral T-Cell Lymphoma, Unspecified (PTCL)

No consistent immunophenotypic pattern exists in PTCLs, although most cases are CD4[+] T-cell neoplasms, and aberrant loss or gain of one or more T-cell–associated antigens is common. Relatively rare cases express CD8, or coexpress CD4 and CD8. A subset of PTCL cases will express variable CD30.

Adult T-Cell Leukemia/Lymphoma (ATLL)

The neoplastic cells in ATLL are typically CD4[+] T cells expressing CD25 and showing aberrant loss of CD7 (Fig. 6.28). Proteins produced by the causative agent of ATLL, human T-lymphotropic virus-1 (HTLV-1), currently are not being assayed in clinical flow cytometry.

Angioimmunoblastic T-Cell Lymphoma (AILT)

The neoplastic cells in AILT are typically CD4[+] T cells that often demonstrate aberrant loss of surface CD3 and, on at least a subset, CD7. In the majority of cases, the neoplastic cells show aberrant coexpression of CD10, a unique feature among T-cell malignancies. In a subset of cases, a simultaneous clonal B-cell population may be detected, presumably as a consequence of the underlying immunologic dysregulation and reactivation of Epstein-Barr virus in B cells that occurs in AILT.

Hepatosplenic γ-δ T-Cell Lymphoma (HSTCL)

The neoplastic cells in this disorder are CD3[+] T cells expressing the γ-δ form of the T-cell receptor, without the α-β form. The neoplastic cells typically lack CD4, CD5, and CD8, but do express CD2 and CD7, with frequent coexpression of CD56; in contrast, benign γ-δ T cells usually express variable low-level CD5 and CD8. Because these cells do not express the α-β T-cell receptor, they cannot be identified as clonal using antibodies to T-cell β-receptor isoforms. Formal proof of clonality in these cases therefore requires molecular evaluation of the TCR-γ or δ chains.

Anaplastic Large-Cell Lymphoma (ALCL)

The neoplastic cells in ALCL are typically large to very large in size, and may require gating strategies including the maximal FS and SS values in two-dimensional dot plots. Moderate to bright CD30 typically is seen by flow cytometry, as is expression of CD45 and the T-cell–associated activation antigens CD25 and HLA-DR (Fig. 6.29). Surface CD2 and CD4 may be identified by flow cytometry, although the cells are frequently negative for surface CD3, CD5, and CD7. Aberrant CD13 expression appears to be relatively common.

Note that the systemic and cutaneous forms of ALCL, although being biologically distinct entities, would be predicted to have relatively similar immunophenotypes by flow cytometry. Therefore, clinical and immunohistochemical criteria, including evaluation of ALK expression, are required to distinguish between these entities.

Aggressive NK-Cell Leukemia/Nasal-Type Extranodal NK-Cell Lymphoma

Although the clinical settings in which aggressive NK-cell leukemia and nasal-type NK-cell lymphoma occur are different, the immunophenotypic features of the neoplastic cells are virtually identical in these two aggressive malignancies. The neoplastic cells typically show an aberrant NK-cell immunophenotype, with the characteristic lack of surface CD3 expression, and frequent loss of one or more NK-cell–associated antigens, including CD2, CD7, CD8, CD16, and/or CD56 (Fig. 6.30). Some studies have suggested that NK-cell clonality can be assessed by flow cytometric evaluation of the killer inhibitory receptor (KIR) antigens, which were initially thought to be expressed in a mutually exclusive manner on NK cells, similar to the TCR genes in T cells. In benign or polyclonal NK-cell populations, flow cytometric evaluation of the 3 KIRs p158a, p158b, and p158e/KIR p70 typically reveals the combined expression of one of these antigens in 50% to 80% of the NK cells. Therefore, restricted KIR expression, or a complete lack of KIR expression, may suggest clonality among an NK-cell population. However, as with the flow cytometric identification of T-cell clonality, the flow cytometric identification of NK-cell clonality does not prove malignancy, and the flow cytometric findings must be interpreted in the overall context of the case before a diagnosis of NK-cell malignancy is made.

CONCLUSIONS

The central importance of immunophenotyping in the current diagnosis and classification of hematolymphoid disease makes an understanding of antigen expression patterns in both benign and neoplastic settings imperative for any pathologist who diagnoses these diseases, and important for any hematologist or oncologist who treats these diseases. Because flow cytometry plays a central role in the immunophenotyping of hematopoietic cell populations, an understanding of both the advantages and the potential pitfalls of this technique is likewise important for all physicians involved in the diagnosis and treatment of these diseases. Although flow cytometry is currently used primarily in hematologic diagnosis and disease monitoring, as more and more potential therapeutic targets are identified by basic research on hematopoietic disease, flow cytometry will almost certainly assume greater importance in therapeutic decision-making.

Suggested Readings

1. Adriaansen HJ, te Boekhorst PA, Hagemeijer AM, van der Schoot CE, Delwel HR, van Dongen JJ. Acute myeloid leukemia M4 with bone marrow eosinophilia (M4Eo) and inv(16)(p13q22) exhibits a specific immunophenotype with CD2 expression. *Blood* 1993;81: 3043–3051.

2. Ahmad E, Kingma DW, Jaffe ES, et al. Flow cytometric immunophenotypic profiles of mature gamma delta T-cell malignancies involving peripheral blood and bone marrow. *Cytometry B Clin Cytom* 2005;67:6–12.

3. Ansari MQ, Dawson DB, Nador R, et al. Primary body cavity-based AIDS-related lymphomas. *Am J Clin Pathol* 1996;105:221–229.

4. Bagwell CB, Adams EG. Fluorescence spectral overlap compensation for any number of flow cytometry parameters. *Ann NY Acad Sci* 1993;677:167–184.

5. Bene MC, Bernier M, Casasnovas RO, et al. The reliability and specificity of c-kit for the diagnosis of acute myeloid leukemias and undifferentiated leukemias. The European Group for the Immunological Classification of Leukemias (EGIL). *Blood* 1998;92:596–599.

6. Bergeron M, Faucher S, Ding T, Phaneuf S, Mandy F. Evaluation of a universal template for single-platform absolute T-lymphocyte subset enumeration. *Cytometry* 2002;50:62–68.

7. Bleesing JJ, Brown MR, Straus SE, et al. Immunophenotypic profiles in families with autoimmune lymphoproliferative syndrome. *Blood* 2001;98:2466–2473.

8. Borowitz MJ, Bray R, Gascoyne R, et al. U.S.-Canadian Consensus recommendations on the immunophenotypic analysis of hematologic neoplasia by flow cytometry: data analysis and interpretation. *Cytometry* 1997;30:236–244.

9. Borowitz MJ, Hunger SP, Carroll AJ, et al. Predictability of the t(l;19)(q23;p13) from surface antigen phenotype: implications for screening cases of childhood acute lymphoblastic leukemia for molecular analysis: a Pediatric Oncology Group study. *Blood* 1993;82(4):1086–1091.

10. Borowitz MJ, Rubnitz J, Nash M, Pullen DJ, Camitta B. Surface antigen phenotype can predict TEL-AML1 rearrangement in childhood B-precursor ALL: a Pediatric Oncology Group study. *Leukemia* 1998;12:1764–1770.

11. Braylan RC, Atwater SK, Diamond L, et al. U.S.-Canadian Consensus recommendations on the immunophenotypic analysis of hematologic neoplasia by flow cytometry: data reporting. *Cytometry* 1997;30:245–248.

12. Caldwell CW. Quality control and quality assurance in immunophenotyping. In: Keren DF, McCoy JP, Carey JL, eds. *Flow Cytometry in Clinical Diagnosis*, 3rd ed. Chicago: ASCP Press, 2001;117–156.

13. Chen JC, Davis BH, Wood B, Warzynski MJ. Multicenter clinical experience with flow cytometric method for fetomaternal hemorrhage detection. *Cytometry* 2002;50:285–290.

14. Chen W, Kesler MV, Karandikar NJ, McKenna RW, Kroft SH. Flow cytometric features of angioimmunoblastic T-cell lymphoma. *Cytometry B Clin Cytom* 2006;70:142–148.

15. Chen YH, Tallman MS, Goolsby C, Peterson L. Immunophenotypic variations in hairy cell leukemia. *Am J Clin Pathol* 2006;125:251– 259.

16. Cheung MM, Chan JK, Wong KF. Natural killer cell neoplasms: a distinctive group of highly aggressive lymphomas/leukemias. *Semin Hematol* 2003;40:221–232.

17. Crespo M, Bosch F, Villamor N, et al. ZAP-70 expression as a surrogate for immunoglobulin-variable-region mutations in chronic lymphocytic leukemia. *N Engl J Med* 2003;348:1764–1775.

18. Dahmoush L, Hijazi Y, Barnes E, Stetler-Stevenson M, Abati A. Adult T-cell leukemia/lymphoma: a cytopathologic, immunocytochemical, and flow cytometric study. *Cancer* 2002;96:110–116.

19. Damle RN, Wasil T, Fais F, et al. Ig V gene mutation status and CD38 expression as novel prognostic indicators in chronic lymphocytic leukemia. *Blood* 1999;94:1840–1847.

20. Davis BH, Bigelow NC. Comparison of neutrophil CD64 expression, manual myeloid immaturity counts, and automated hematology analyzer flags as indicators of infection or sepsis. *Lab Hematol* 2005;11:137–147.

21. Davis BH, Foucar K, Szczarkowski W, et al. U.S.-Canadian Consensus recommendations on the immunophenotypic analysis of hematologic neoplasia by flow cytometry: medical indications. *Cytometry* 1997;30:249–263.

22. Farrant J, Spickett G, Matamoros N, et al. Study of B and T cell phenotypes in blood from patients with common variable immunodeficiency (CVID). *Immunodeficiency* 1994;5:159–169.

23. Glencross D, Scott LE, Jani IV, Barnett D, Janossy G. CD45-assisted Pan*Leuco*gating for accurate, cost-effective dual-platform CD4+ T-cell enumeration. *Cytometry* 2002;50(2):69–77.

24. Hans CP, Weisenburger DD, Greiner TC, et al. Confirmation of the molecular classification of diffuse large B-cell lymphoma by immunohistochemistry using a tissue microarray. *Blood* 2004;103: 275–282.

25. Harris NL, Jaffe ES, Stein H, et al. A revised European-American classification of lymphoid neoplasms: a proposal from the International Lymphoma Study Group. *Blood* 1994;84:1361–1392.

26. Jaffe ES, Harris NL, Stein H, Vardiman JW. *World Health Organization Classification of Tumours: Pathology and Genetics of Tumours of Haematopoietic and Lymphoid Tissues.* Lyon: IARC Press, 2001.

27. Johansson B, Moorman AV, Haas OA, et al. Hematologic malignancies with t(4;ll)(q21;q23)—a cytogenetic, morphologic, immunophenotypic and clinical study of 183 cases. European 11q23 Workshop participants. *Leukemia* 1998;12:779–787.

28. Juco J, Holden JT, Mann KP, Kelley LG, Li S. Immunophenotypic analysis of anaplastic large cell lymphoma by flow cytometry. *Am J Clin Pathol* 2003;119:205–212.

29. Kalman L, Lindegren ML, Kobrynski L, et al. Mutations in genes required for T-cell development: IL7R, CD45, IL2RG, JAK3, RAG1, RAG2, ARTEMIS, and ADA and severe combined immunodeficiency: HuGE review. *Genet Med* 2004;6:16–26.

30. Khoury H, Dalal BI, Nevill TJ, et al. Acute myelogenous leukemia with t(8;21)—identification of a specific immunophenotype. *Leuk Lymphoma* 2003;44:1713–1718.

31. Kilo MM, Dorfman DM. The utility of flow cytometric immunophenotypic analysis in the distinction of small lymphocytic lymphoma/chronic lymphocytic leukemia from mantle cell lymphoma. *Am J Clin Pathol* 1996;105:451–457.

32. Kussick SJ, Wood BL. Using 4-color flow cytometry to identify abnormal myeloid populations. *Arch Pathol Lab Med* 2003;127:1140–1147.

33. Li S, Juco J, Mann KP, Holden JT. Flow cytometry in the differential diagnosis of lymphocyte-rich thymoma from precursor T-cell acute lymphoblastic leukemia/lymphoblastic lymphoma. *Am J Clin Pathol* 2004;121:268–274.

34. Lucio P, Parreira A, van den Beemd MW, et al. Flow cytometric analysis of normal B cell differentiation: a frame of reference for the detection of minimal residual disease in precursor-B-ALL. *Leukemia* 1999;13:419–2779.

35. Matutes E, Brito-Babapulle V, Swansbury J, et al. Clinical and laboratory features of 78 cases of T-prolymphocytic leukemia. *Blood* 1991;78:3269–3274.

36. Matutes E, Owusu-Ankomah K, Morilla R, et al. Immunological profile of B-cell disorders and proposal of a scoring system for the diagnosis of CLL. Leukemia 1994;8:1640–1645.

37. Morice WG, Katzmann JA, Pittelkow MR, el-Azhary RA, Gibson LE, Hanson CA. A comparison of morphologic features, flow cytometry, TCR-Vbeta analysis, and TCR-PCR in qualitative and quantitative assessment of peripheral blood involvement by Sezary syndrome. *Am J Clin Pathol* 2006;125:364–374.

38. Morice WG, Kimlinger T, Katzmann JA, et al Flow cytometric assessment of TCR-Vbeta expression in the evaluation of peripheral blood involvement by T-cell lymphoproliferative disorders: a comparison with conventional T-cell immunophenotyping and molecular genetic techniques. *Am J Clin Pathol* 2004;121:373–383.

39. Morice WG, Kurtin PJ, Leibson PJ, Tefferi A, Hanson CA. Demonstration of aberrant T-cell and natural killer-cell antigen expression in all cases of granular lymphocytic leukaemia. *Br J Haematol* 2003;120:1026–1036.

40. Nonoyama S, Tsukada S, Yamadori T, et al. Functional analysis of peripheral blood B cells in patients with X-linked agammaglobulinemia. *J Immunol* 1998;161:3925–3929.

41. Orfao A, Chillon MC, Bortoluci AM, et al. The flow cytometric pattern of CD34, CD15 and CD13 expression in acute myeloblastic leukemia is highly characteristic of the presence of PML-RAR alpha gene rearrangements. *Haematologica* 1999;84:405–412.

42. Ray S, Craig FE, Swerdlow SH. Abnormal patterns of antigenic expression in follicular lymphoma: a flow cytometric study. *Am J Clin Pathol* 2005;124:576–583.

43. Richards SJ, Rawstron AC, Hillmen P. Application of flow cytometry to the diagnosis of paroxysmal nocturnal hemoglobinuria. *Cytometry* 2000;42:223–233.

44. San Miguel JF, Gutierrez NC, Mateo G, Orfao A. Conventional diagnostics in multiple myeloma. *Eur J Cancer* 2006;42:1510–1519.

45. Shapiro HM. *Practical Flow Cytometry.* 4th ed. Hoboken, NJ: John Wiley & Sons, 2003.

46. Stelzer GT, Marti G, Hurley A, McCoy P Jr, Lovett EJ, Schwartz A. U.S.-Canadian Consensus recommendations on the immunophenotypic analysis of hematologic neoplasia by flow cytometry: standardization and validation of laboratory procedures. *Cytometry* 30:214–230.

47. Stetler-Stevenson M, Arthur DC, Jabbour N, et al. Diagnostic utility of flow cytometric immunophenotyping in myelodysplastic syndrome. *Blood* 2001;98:979–987.

48. Stewart CC, Behm FG, Carey JL, et al. U.S.-Canadian Consensus recommendations on the immunophenotypic analysis of hematologic neoplasia by flow cytometry: selection of antibody combinations. *Cytometry* 1997;30:231–235.

49. Terstappen LW, Huang S, Picker LJ. Flow cytometric assessment of human T-cell differentiation in thymus and bone marrow. *Blood* 1992;79:666–677.

50. Terstappen LW, Loken MR. Myeloid cell differentiation in normal bone marrow and acute myeloid leukemia assessed by multidimensional flow cytometry. *Ann Cell Pathol* 1990;2:229–240.

51. Vidriales MB, San-Miguel JF, Orfao A, Coustan-Smith E, Campana D. Minimal residual disease monitoring by flow cytometry. *Best Pract Res Clin Haematol* 2003;16:599–612.

52. Wood BL. 9-Color and 10-Color Flow Cytometry in the Clinical Laboratory. *Arch Pathol Laboratory Med* 2006;130:680–690.

Table 6.1

Antigens commonly evaluated in diagnostic flow cytometry

Antigen	Key Hematopoietic Cell Type
CD1a	Immature T cells (common thymocytes), Langerhans cells
CD2	Pan–T-cell, NK cells
CD3	Pan–T-cell
CD4	Helper/inducer T cells
CD5	Pan–T-cell, subset of B cells
CD7	Pan–T-cell, NK cells, subset of AMLs
CD8	Cytotoxic/suppressor T cells
CD9	B cells, platelets, and megakaryocytes
CD10	Immature and germinal center B cells, mature granulocytes
CD11b	Maturing myeloid cells (both monocytes and granulocytes)
CD11c	Hairy cell leukemia, some marginal zone lymphomas
CD13	Pan-myeloid
CD14	Maturing monocytes
CD15	Maturing myeloid cells, especially granulocytes
CD16	NK cells, maturing granulocytes
CD19	Pan–B-cell, including plasma cells
CD20	Immature and mature B cells
CD22	Immature (subset) and mature B cells
CD23	Activated B cells, CLL/SLL
CD25	Activated T and B cells, hairy cell leukemia
CD33	Pan-myeloid
CD34	Myeloid and lymphoid blasts, stem cells
CD38	Plasma cells (bright), B-lymphoblasts and myeloblasts (moderate)
CD41	Glycoprotein IIb/IIIa, platelets, and megakaryocytes
CD45	Leukocyte common antigen (nonerythroid hematopoietic cells)
CD56	NK cells, some stem-cell disorders, some activated T cells
CD57	Subset of cytotoxic/suppressor T cells
CD61	Platelets, and megakaryocytes
CD64	Monocytes, activated granulocytes
CD103	Hairy cell leukemia
CD117	Myeloid blasts, promyelocytes proerythroblasts, mast cells
Bcl-2	Naïve B cells, most T cells, most follicular lymphomas
HLA-DR	Myeloid blasts, B cells, activated T cells
FMC7	B-cell lymphoma other than CLL/SLL
κ-light chain	Mature B cells
λ-light chain	Mature B cells
TdT	Immature T cells, immature B cells
Zap-70	T/NK cells, subsets of CLL/SLL and other B-NHLs

Table 6.2

Useful antigens in the evaluation of specific hematopoietic cell populations

Myeloid Blasts	Granulocytes & Monocytes	Immature B Cells	Mature B Cells	Plasma Cells	Immature T Cells	Mature T/NK Cells
CD34	CD4	CD10	CD19	CD19	CD1a	CD2
CD38	CD10	CD19	CD20[c]	CD38	CD2	CD3
CD45	CD11b	CD20[c]	CD10	CD45	CD3	CD4
CD117	CD13	CD34	CD38	Cyto[d]κ	CD4	CD5
CD2[a]	CD14	CD38	CD45	Cyto[d]λ	CD5	CD7
CD5[a]	CD15	CD45	κ	CD56[a]	CD7	CD8
CD7[a]	CD16	HLA-DR	λ		CD8	CD10
CD56[a]	CD33	κ	CD5[a]		CD10	CD16
	CD38	λ	CD11c[b]		CD34	CD45
	CD45	TdT	CD22[b,c]		CD38	CD56
	CD64	CD13[a]	CD23[b]		HLA-DR	TCR-α/β
	HLA-DR	CD33[a]	CD25[b]		TdT	TCR-γ/δ
	CD56[a]		CD52[b]		CD13[a]	CD25[c]
			CD103[a,b]		CD33[a]	CD30[c]
			FMC7[b]		CD117[a]	CD52[c]
			ZAP-70[a]			

[a] Denotes aberrantly expressed, nonlineage antigen.
[b] Denotes additional antigens to help classify mature lymphoid neoplasms.
[c] Denotes antigens of potential therapeutic value.
[d] Denotes cytoplasmic antigens.

Figure 6.1 Schematic illustration of a flow cytometer. A major feature is the complex routing of the emitted light after it leaves the flow cell. At that time, wavelengths are directed to specific detectors, or photomultiplier tubes (PMT), by a series of dichroic lenses/mirrors (DL), which reflect light of shorter wavelength to the appropriate PMT and allow light of longer wavelength to pass through to the next detector. The configuration of a four-color/six-parameter flow cytometer is shown, in which the detectors FL1 to FL4 record light of progressively longer wavelengths emitted by the bound antibodies on cells, while the FS and SS sensors measure 488-nm light emitted by the cell itself, in a pattern determined by the cell's overall size (FS) and cytoplasmic complexity/granularity (SS).

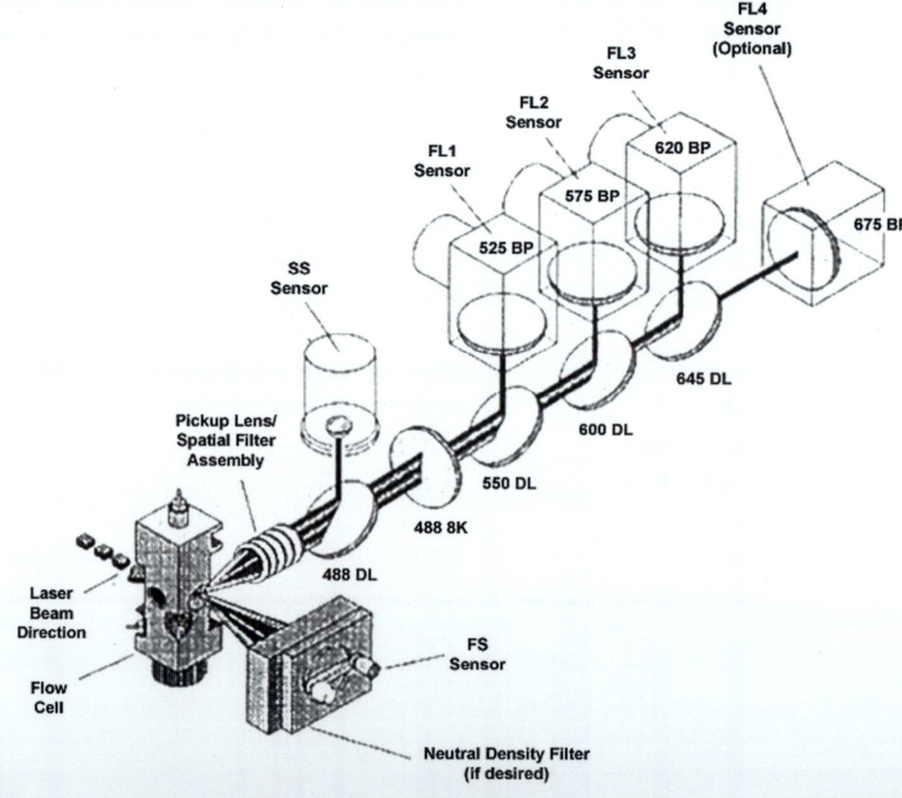

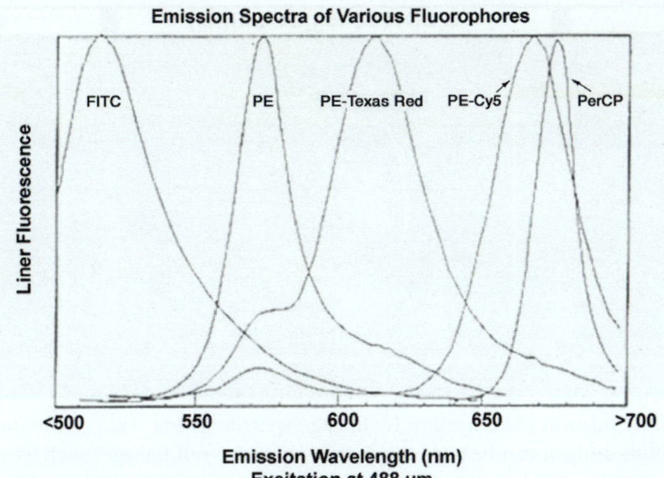

Figure 6.2 Emission spectra of five common fluorophores (fluorochromes). Note the significant overlap of many of these emission spectra, particularly among "adjacent" fluorochromes, necessitating the analytical technique of compensation to guarantee that each detector primarily measures the emission of a single fluorochrome. FITC, fluorescein isothiocyanate; PE, phycoerythrin; PE-Texas Red, Texas Red-PE conjugate; PE-Cy5, Cyanine 5-PE conjugate; Per Cp, Peridinin chlorophyll protein.

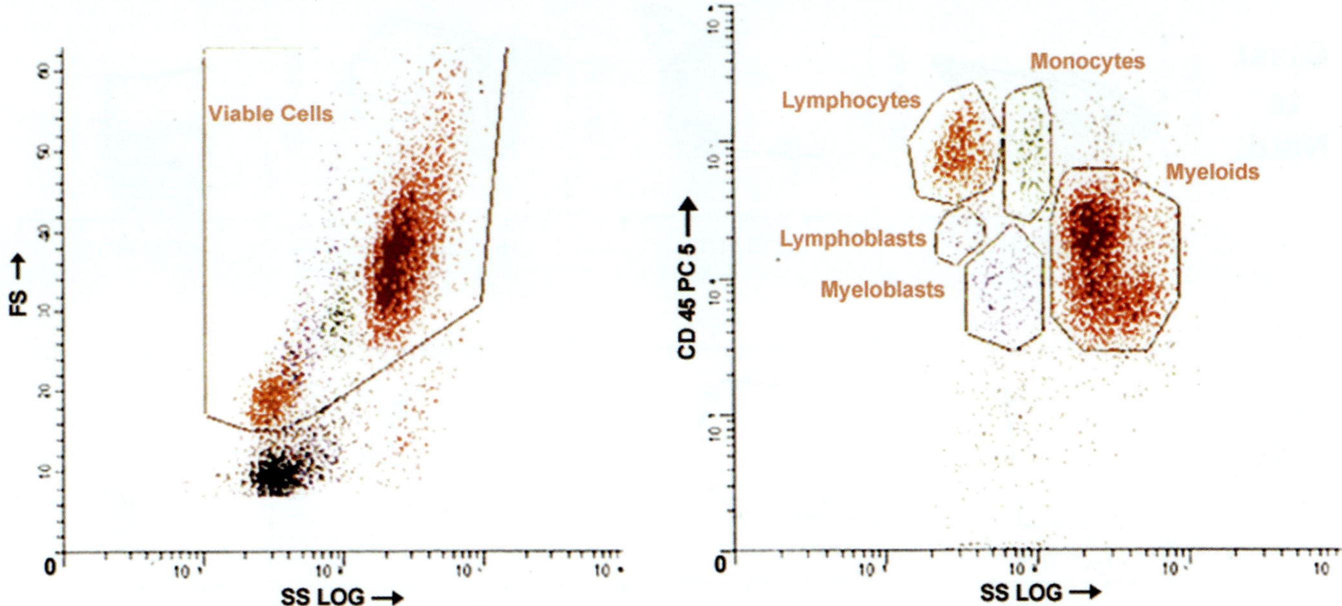

Figure 6.3 Cell population identification by forward versus side scatter (FS/SS) gating in normal peripheral blood (*left*), and by CD45 expression versus side scatter (45/SS) gating in normal bone marrow. FS typically is measured on a linear scale. SS can be measured on linear (not shown) or logarithmic scales. Measuring the dark red, high-SS neutrophils on a log scale enables a more compressed view of the data than does SS measurement on a linear scale. Antibody-specific fluorescence typically is measured on a log scale. Although the constituents of low- to moderate-complexity specimens, such as blood or lymph node, can be adequately separated for analysis using FS versus SS gating, CD45 versus SS gating is more effective for a high-complexity specimen such as bone marrow, enabling more reliable identification of the blasts.

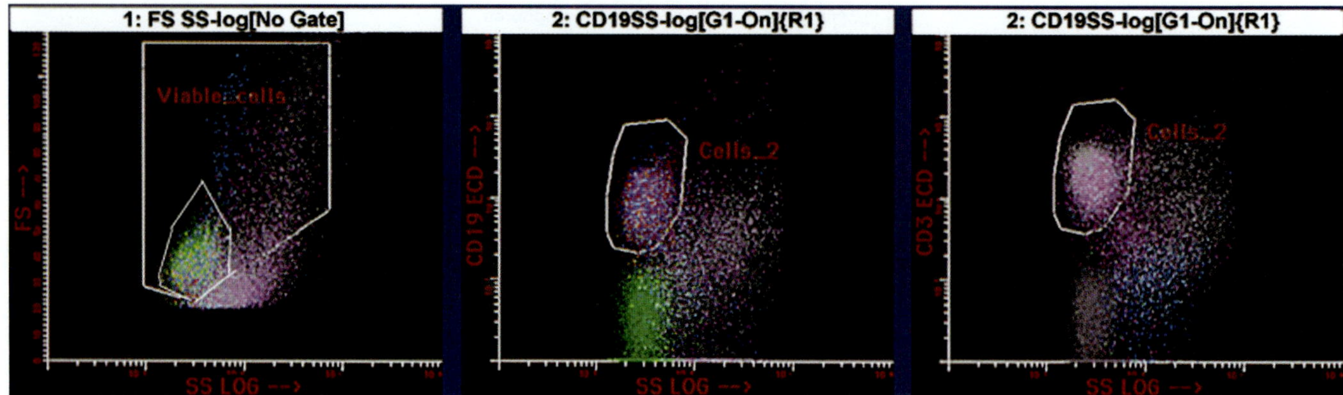

Figure 6.4 Cell population identification by lineage-specific gating. This technique is particularly useful when a single antigen can be used to identify an entire cell lineage, such as surface CD3 for mature T cells and surface CD19 for B cells and plasma cells. One caveat to this approach is that neoplastic cells with abnormally decreased expression of the gating antigen may not be identified by this strategy, necessitating an alternative gating strategy to ensure that such cells will be detected. The leftmost figure shows conventional forward versus side scatter gating of the lymphocyte population in a lymph node biopsy specimen.

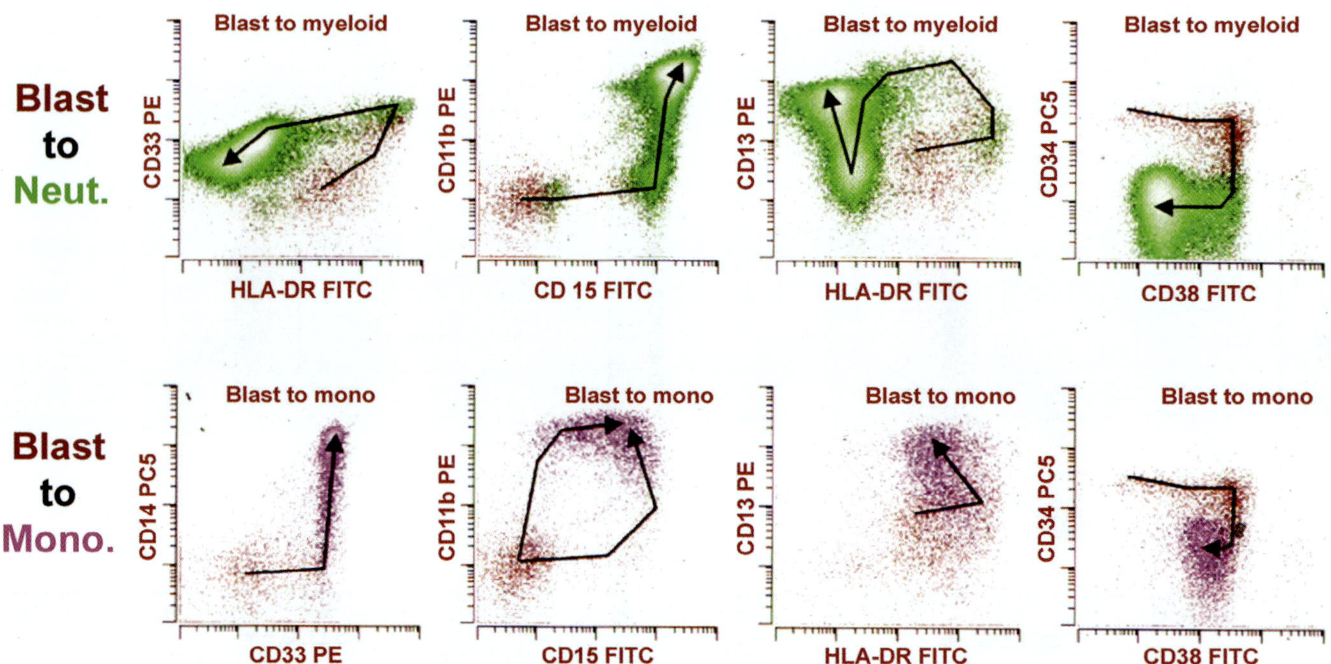

Figure 6.5 Normal maturation of neutrophil lineage and monocytic lineage cells in the bone marrow, showing progression from myeloid blasts (*red*) to neutrophils (*green*) or monocytes (*lavender*). Arrows indicate the normal maturational progression from blasts to mature elements. Note that these patterns are highly reproducible across normal bone marrow specimens.

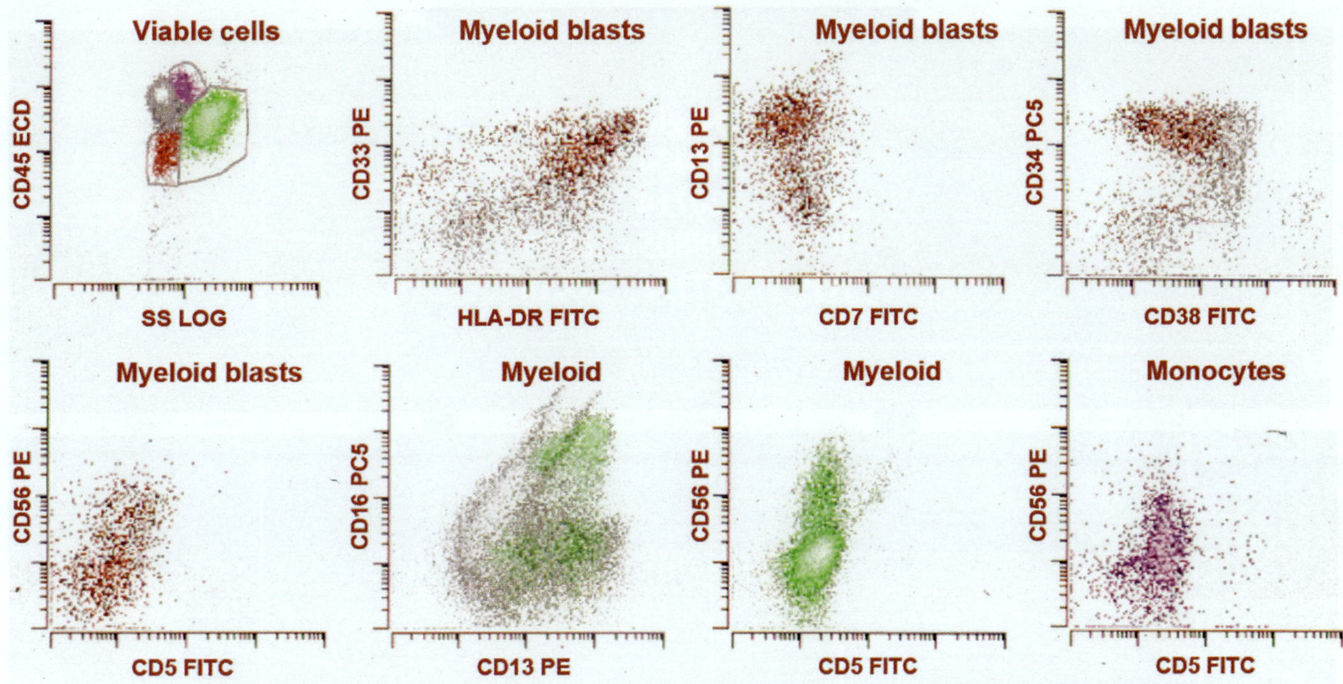

Figure 6.6 Low-grade myelodysplasia showing aberrant antigen expression by flow cytometry. This is an example of refractory cytopenia with multilineage dysplasia. The cell lineages are colored as in Figure 6.5, and the normal patterns of maturation are shown greyish in the background of several of the plots. Despite the low blast count, the presence of multiple immunophenotypic abnormalities—including aberrant CD56 expression on the blasts, granulocytes, and monocytes—and of abnormally homogeneous antigen expression among the blasts strongly suggests a myeloid stem-cell neoplasm. Flow cytometry represents a useful adjunct to morphology and cytogenetics in the diagnosis of low-grade myelodysplasia.

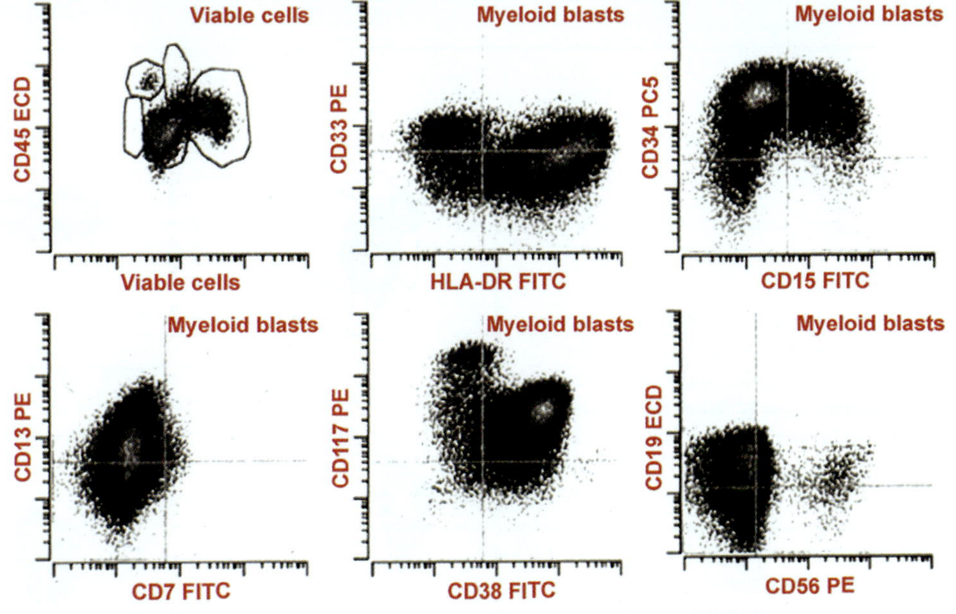

Figure 6.7 Acute myeloid leukemia with the t(8;21)(q22;q22). Note the relatively low-level expression of CD33, the aberrant coexpression of CD15 on the CD34+ blasts, and the characteristic aberrant low-level coexpression of CD19, with aberrant CD56 on a subset of myeloid blasts.

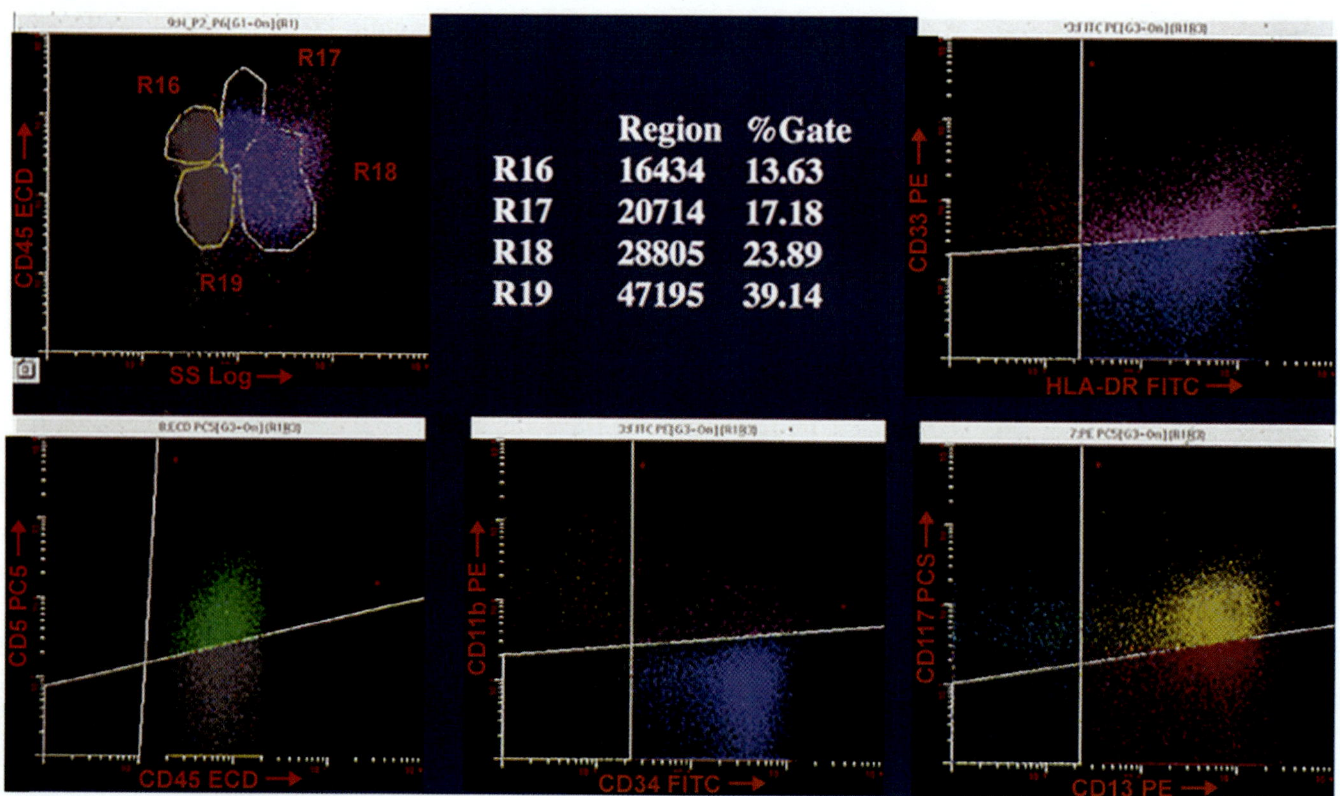

Figure 6.8 Acute myeloid leukemia with the inv(16). In addition to the markedly expanded myeloid blast population (denoted R19), note the relative prominence of both the monocytic (R17) and granulocytic (R18) populations. R16 denotes the lymphocytes. Except for the upper left histogram, all other histograms show the gated myeloid blast population. The lower left plot in the figure shows aberrant CD5 coexpression on the myeloid blasts, an occasional finding in myeloid stem-cell neoplasms.

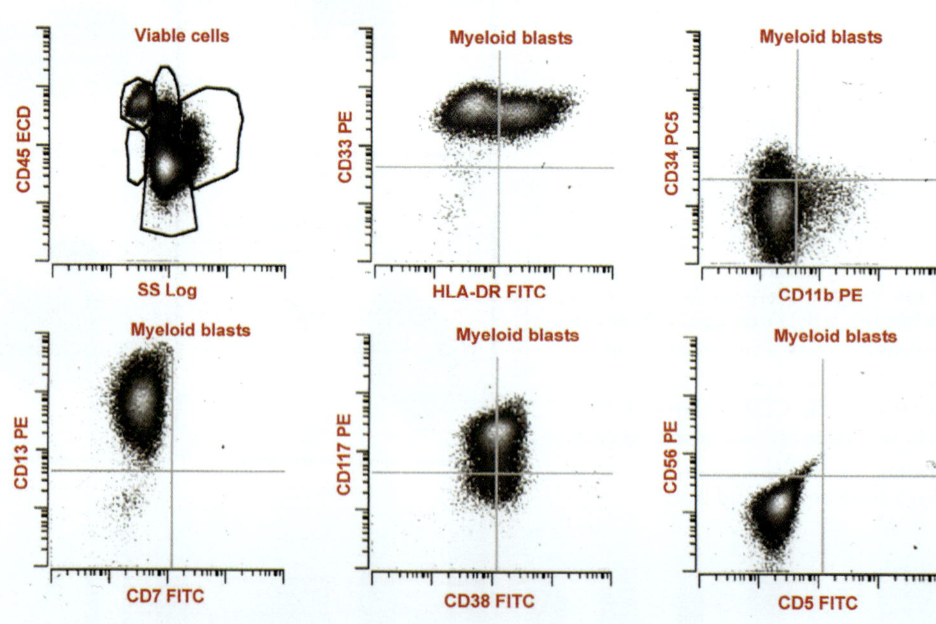

Figure 6.9 Acute myeloid leukemia with the t(15;17)(q22;q12) (acute promyelocytic leukemia). Note the characteristic loss of HLA-DR on the leukemic promyelocytes (this specimen does retain low-level HLA-DR in a subset of the leukemic cells, which is relatively unusual). In addition, note the minimal expression of CD34 with the associated expression of CD117, which is a promyelocyte-like immunophenotype.

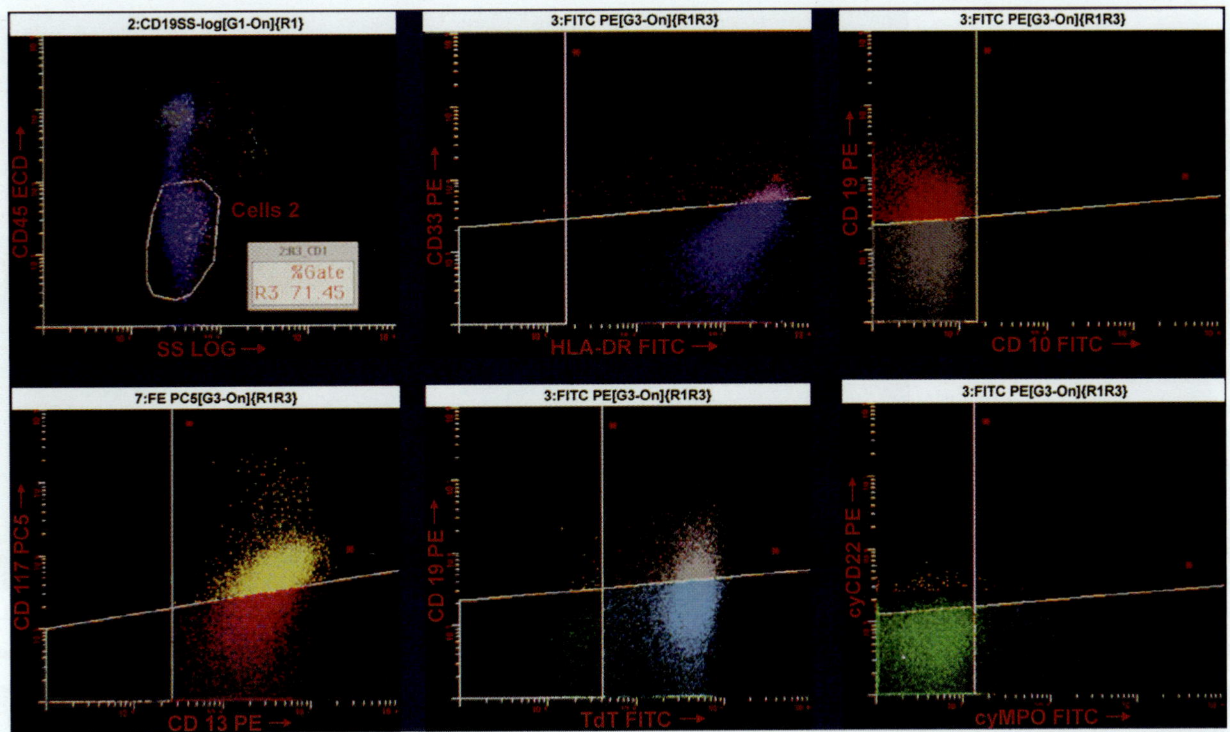

Figure 6.10   Acute biphenotypic leukemia. Note the coexpression of the B-lymphoblast–associated antigens CD19 (*upper right plot*) and TdT (*lower middle plot*), along with the myeloid-associated antigens CD117 and CD13 (*lower left plot*). Importantly, the lack of clear differentiation along either B-cell or myeloid-cell pathways, indicated by the lack of both cytoplasmic CD22 and myeloperoxidase expression in the lower right plot, leads to optimal classification as acute biphenotypic leukemia under the WHO classification system.

Figure 6.11   Paroxysmal nocturnal hemoglobinuria (PNH) involving peripheral blood. Patient tracings are shown in red and normal tracings in green. The abnormalities include loss of the GPI-linked protein CD59 on a subset of the erythrocytes (*upper right plot*), loss of CD14 on a large proportion of the monocytes (*lower middle plot*), and loss of CD66b on a large number of the neutrophils (*lower right plot*). The proportionately small size of the CD59⁻ erythrocyte population (*arrow, upper right histogram*), as compared with the abnormal leukocyte populations (*arrows, bottom right two histograms*), is presumably due to the fact that most of the affected erythrocytes are lysed in the blood shortly after release from the marrow, leaving this abnormal population relatively depleted (see also Figs. 1.59 and 1.60). (Courtesy Dr. Brent Wood.)

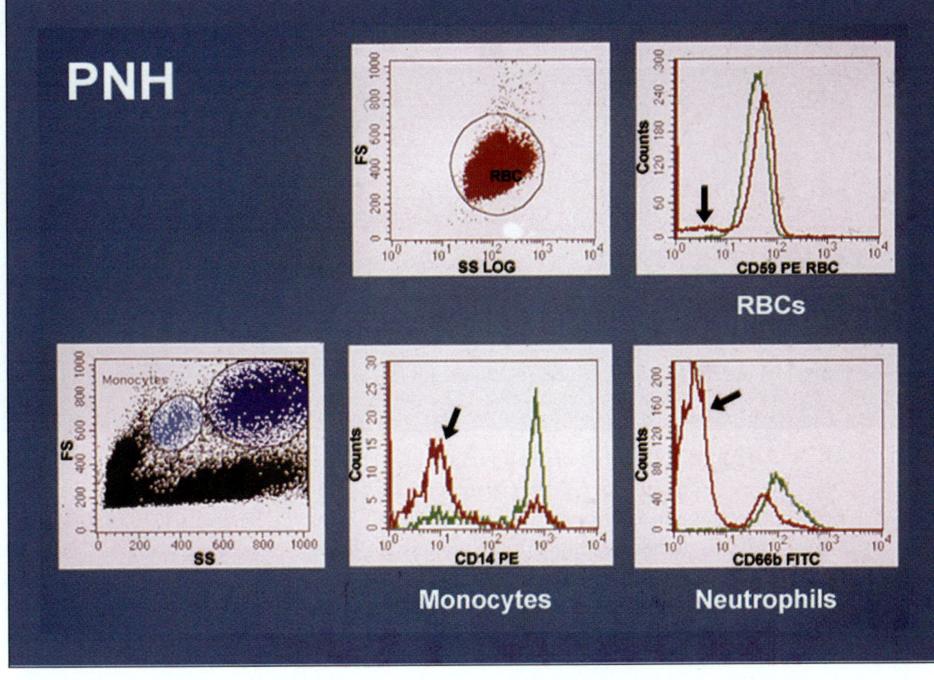

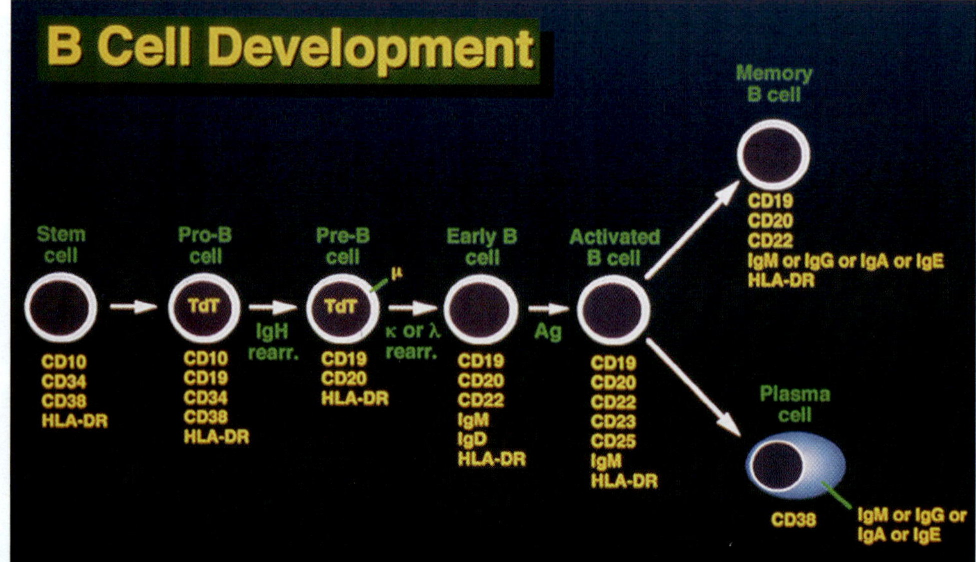

Figure 6.12 Schematic illustration of antigen expression during normal B-cell maturation. Although the germinal-center stage of B-cell development is not shown as a separate entity, it would correspond to the activated B-cell stage shown in the figure, because this stage occurs after B-cell exposure to antigen. (Courtesy Dr. Dan Sabath.)

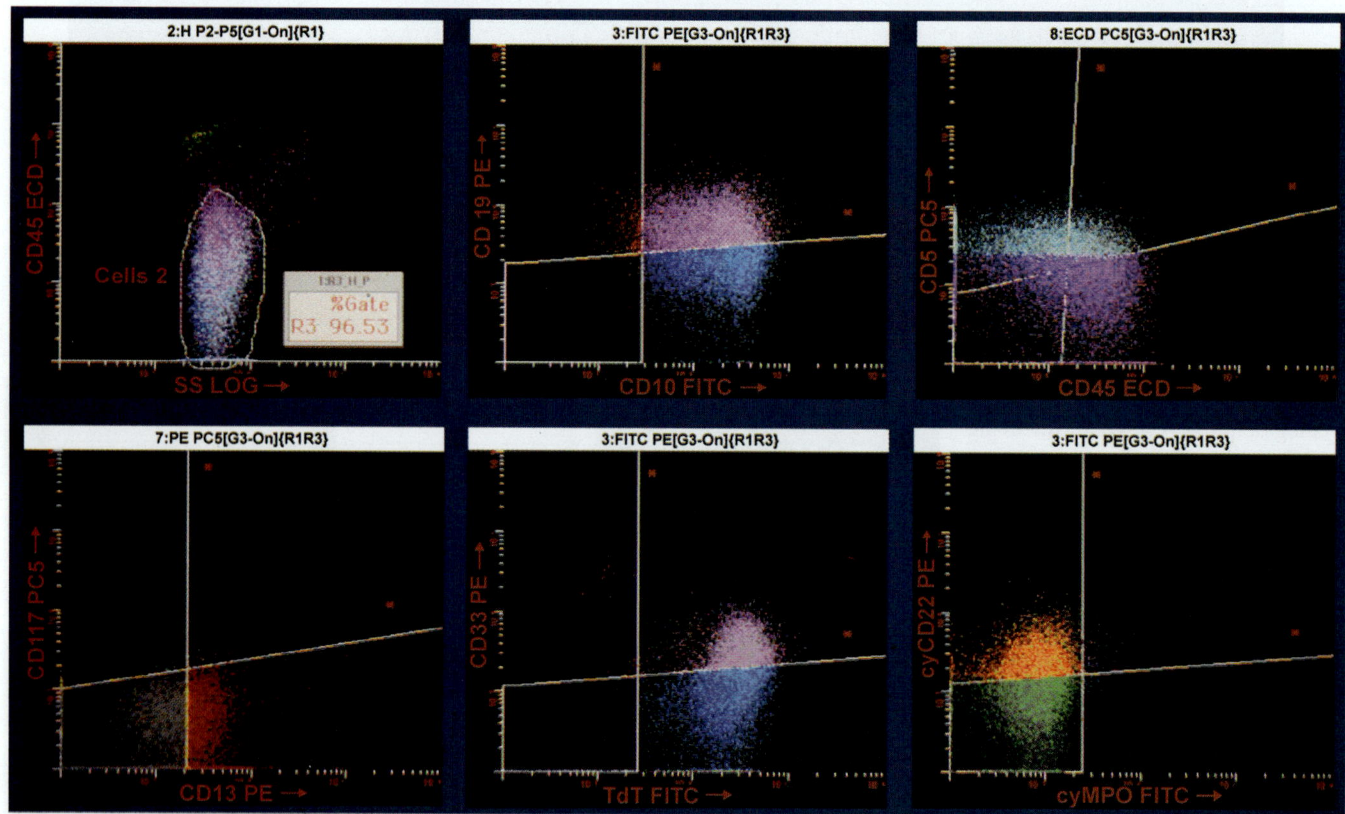

Figure 6.13 Precursor B-lymphoblastic leukemia/lymphoma. This example shows the characteristic expression of CD19, CD10 (CALLA), and TdT. Because the case also showed aberrant low-level expression of the myeloid-associated antigens CD13 and CD33, and the T-cell–associated antigen CD5, demonstration of the cytoplasmic lineage-associated antigen CD22 was used to confirm the B-lymphoid lineage of the neoplasm. This case was a Philadelphia chromosome-positive precursor B-ALL, a genetic background in which aberrant myeloid antigen expression is relatively common.

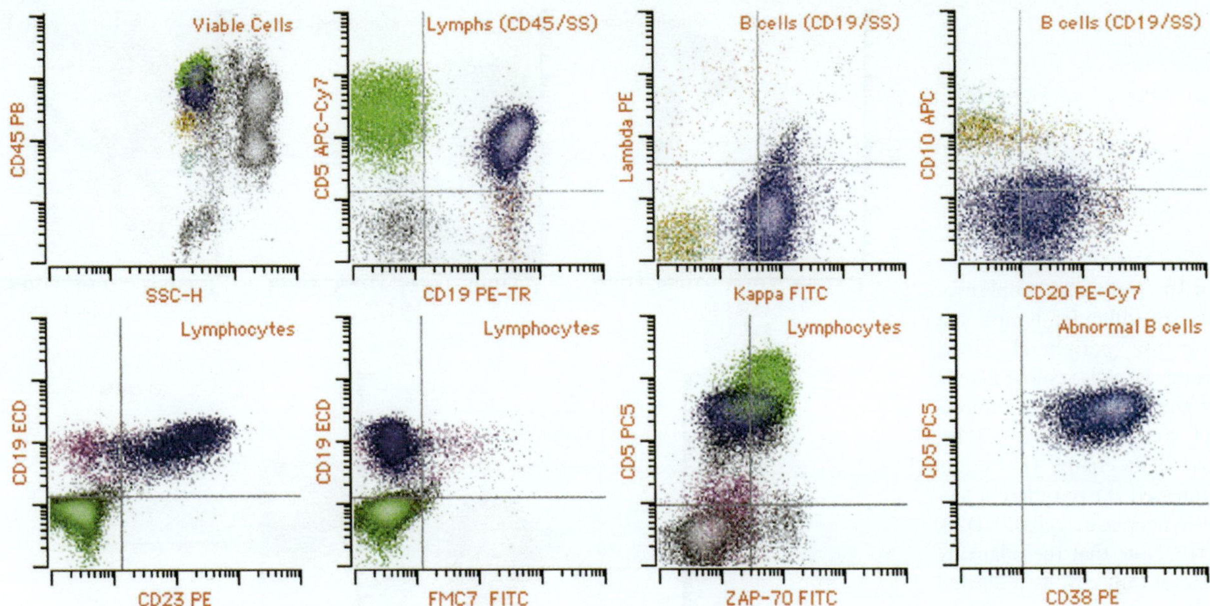

Figure 6.14 Chronic lymphocytic leukemia/small lymphocytic lymphoma. This is a typical case of CLL/SLL, (neoplastic B cells colored blue) showing the characteristic CD19, low-level surface light-chain restriction (κ in this case), low-level CD20, aberrant low-level CD5, and uniform CD23 without FMC7 on the dark blue-colored neoplastic cells. In addition, this case showed uniform expression of CD38 (*lower right plot*) and, based on the relative shift of the blue-colored B cells in relation to the green-colored T cells, was considered to be positive for ZAP-70 expression. The expression of both ZAP-70 and CD38 is an adverse prognostic indicator in CLL/SLL.

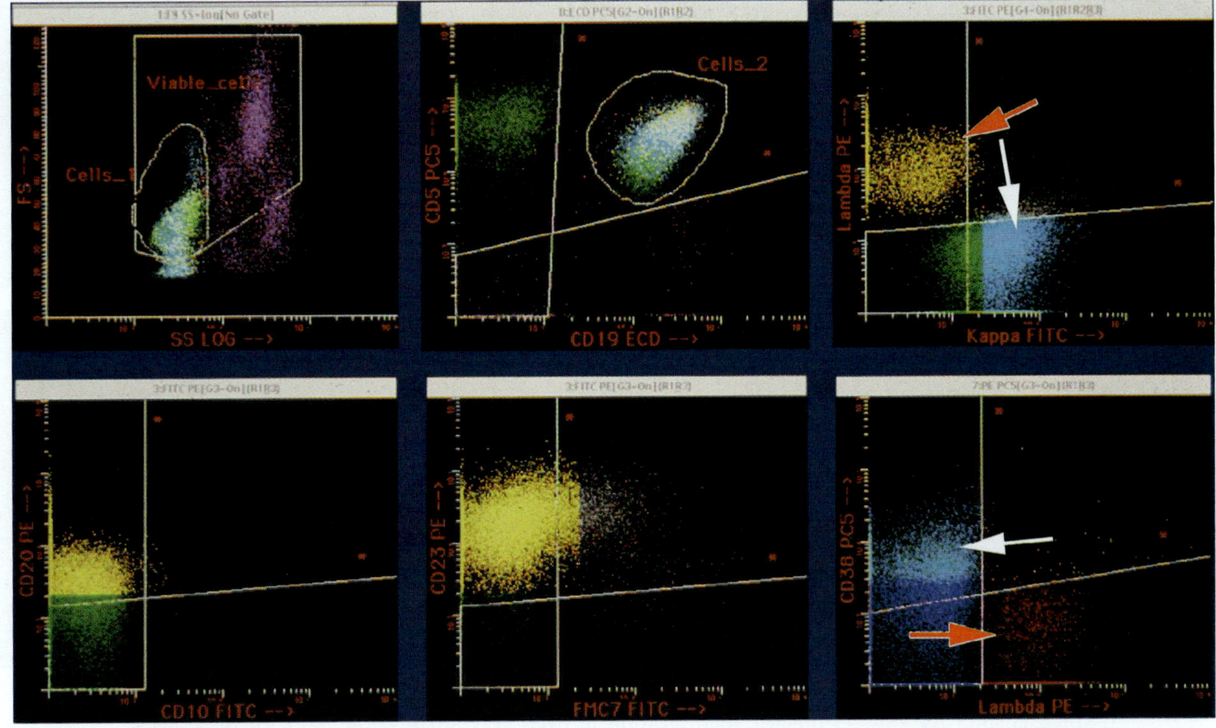

Figure 6.15 Biclonal CLL/SLL. Because CLL/SLL is such a common disease, rare patients will show the presence of two different CLL/SLL clones. In the present case, both clones showed aberrant coexpression of CD19, CD5, low-level CD20, and CD23. The predominant clone, however, was κ-restricted, (*white arrows*) whereas the minor clone was λ-restricted (*red arrows*). The lower right plot shows that the λ-restricted clone was CD38⁻ and therefore associated with a favorable prognosis, whereas the κ-restricted clone was CD38⁺ and associated with an adverse prognosis.

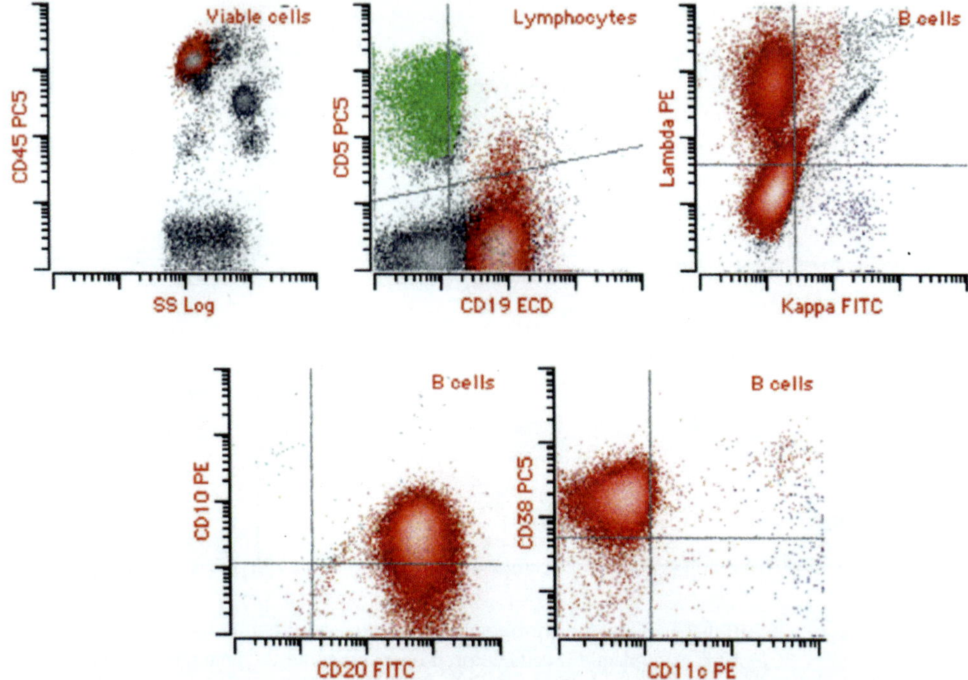

Figure 6.16 Follicular lymphoma. This case of follicular lymphoma involving the peripheral blood (neoplastic B cells colored red) showed the characteristic expression of relatively low CD19, restricted light chains (λ in this case, expressed at two different levels on the neoplastic cells), CD20, and CD10. Note that the relatively small size of the cells, as indicated by the low side scatter, would be associated with a low-grade follicular lymphoma.

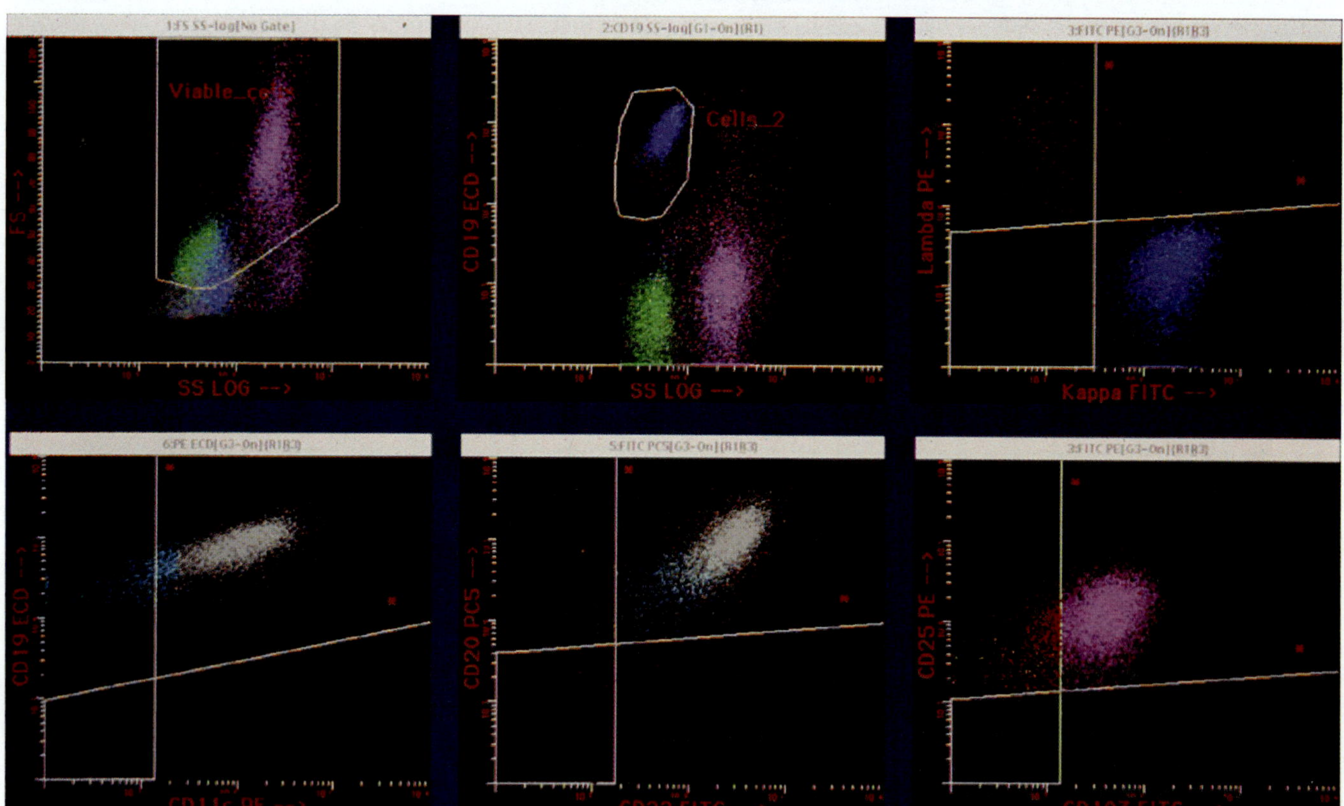

Figure 6.17 Hairy cell leukemia. Hairy cell leukemia has a very distinctive immunophenotype, which enables the flow cytometric identification of even very small populations of these cells (<0.01% in some cases). This case shows the characteristic increase in side scatter (corresponding to the increased cytoplasm in the cells) and expression of restricted surface light chains, bright CD19, CD20, CD22, and CD11c, and aberrant CD103 and CD25.

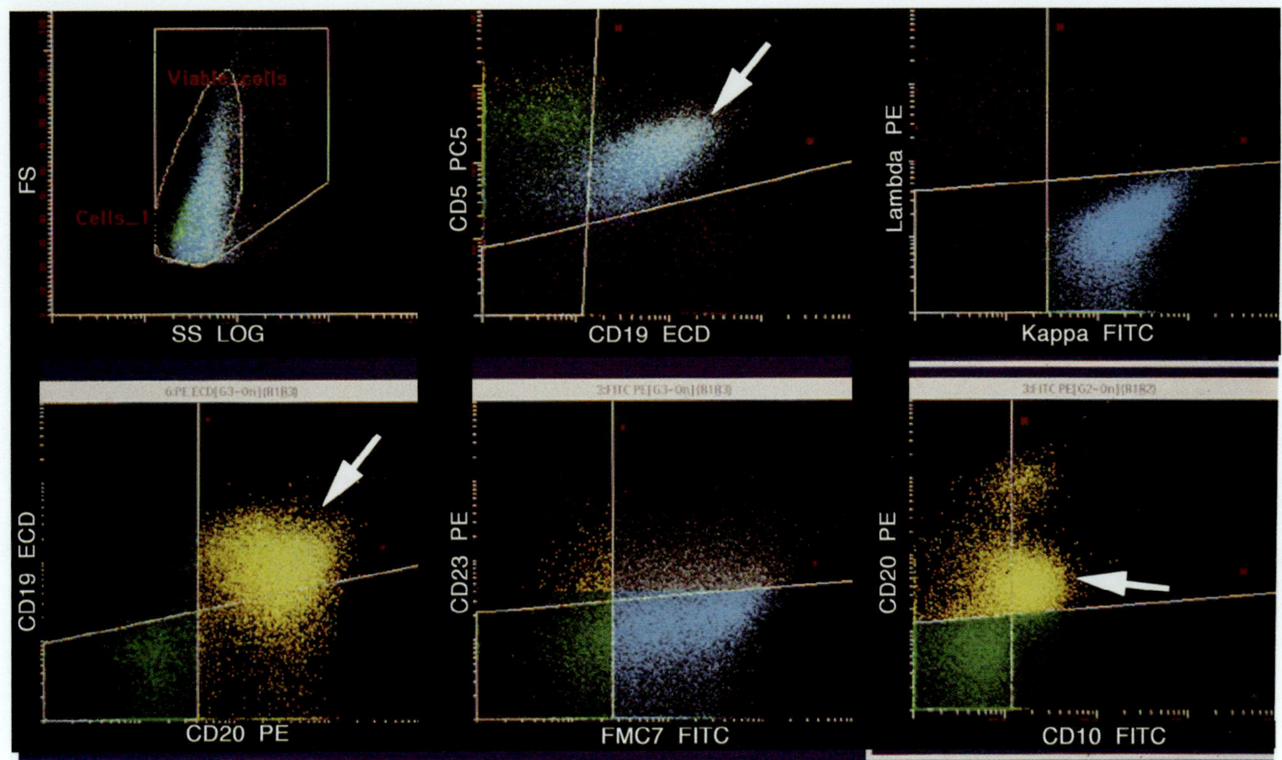

Figure 6.18 Mantle cell lymphoma. This case shows the characteristic immunophenotype of mantle cell lymphoma, including aberrant coexpression of CD5, relatively bright surface light-chain restriction and CD20 expression (compared to CLL/SLL), and expression of FMC7 without CD23 (lymphoma cells shown by *arrows*). In addition, rare cases can show low-level expression of CD10 (see *lower right plot,* from a different case).

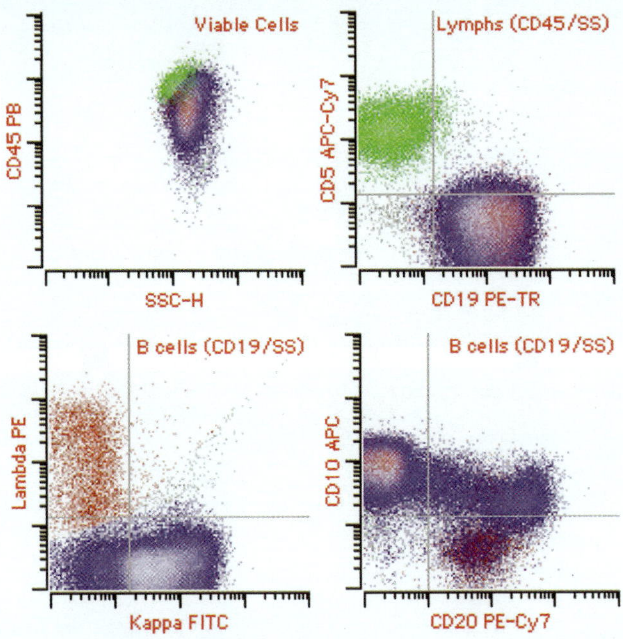

Figure 6.19 Diffuse large B-cell lymphoma (DLBCL). The immunophenotype of DLBCL can be quite varied. In this case, the neoplastic B cells (colored blue) show increased side scatter (compared with the green-colored T cells) with expression of CD19, κ-restricted light chains, CD10, and highly variable CD20, with a majority of the neoplastic cells lacking CD20.

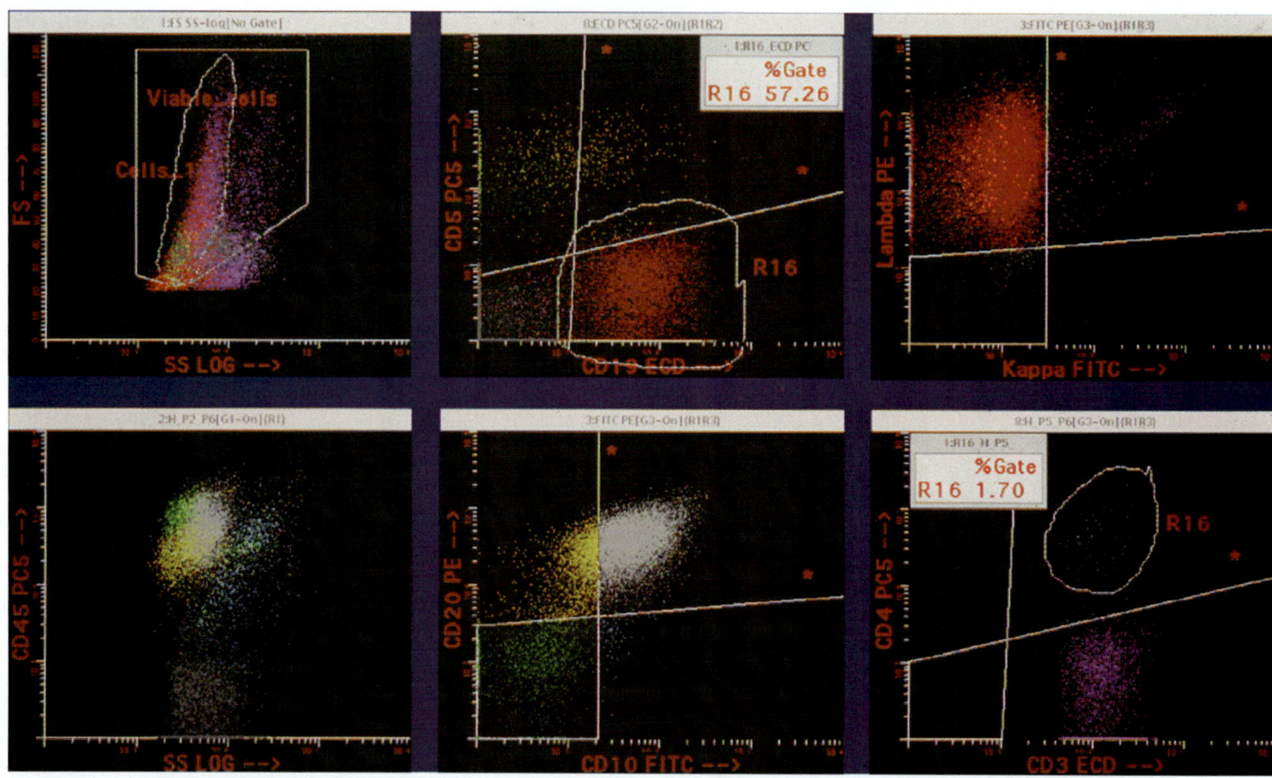

Figure 6.20 Burkitt lymphoma. This case shows the characteristic features of Burkitt lymphoma cells (*arrows*), including coexpression of CD19, CD20, and CD10, with surface light chain restriction. This case occurred in an HIV-positive male, as indicated by the virtual absence of CD4+ T cells in the lower right plot.

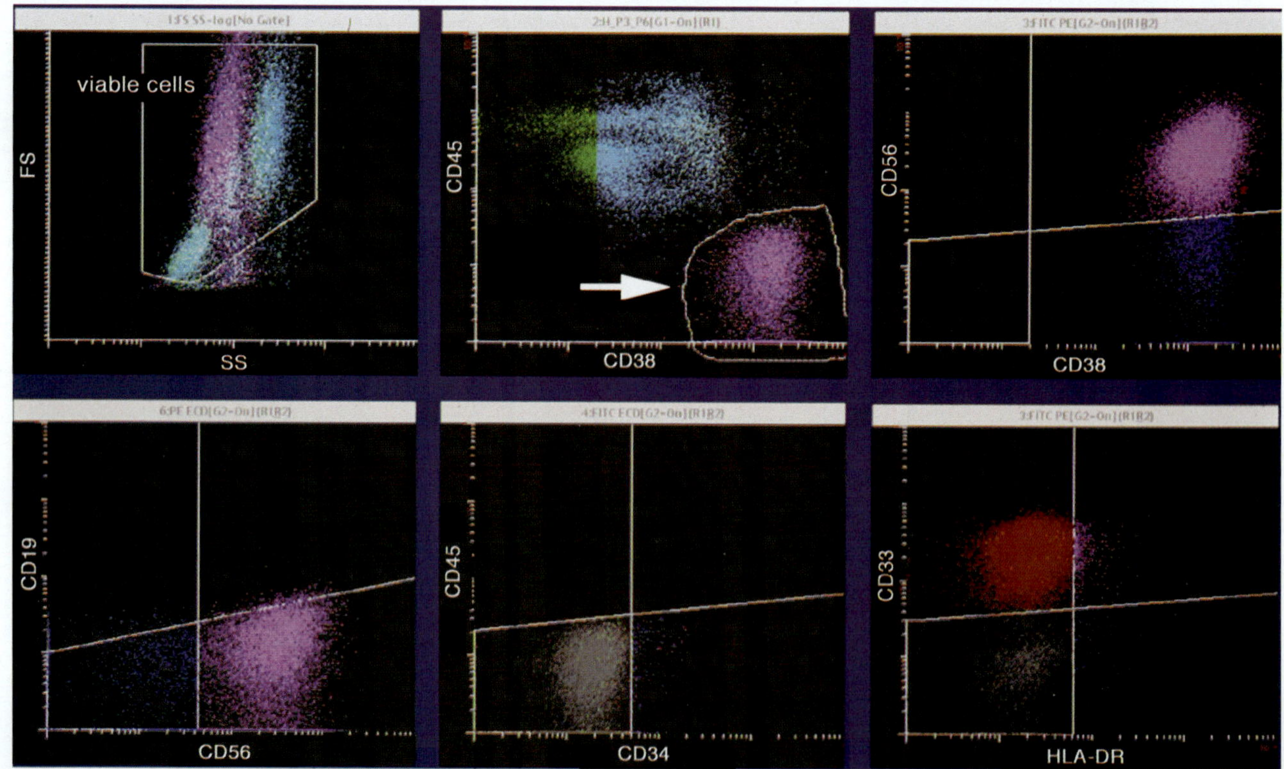

Figure 6.21 Plasma cell myeloma. This case shows the characteristic bright CD38 expression of plasma cells (*arrows*), with multiple abnormalities including loss of CD45 and CD19 and aberrant coexpression of CD56 and CD33. This case also demonstrated cytoplasmic light-chain restriction (not shown).

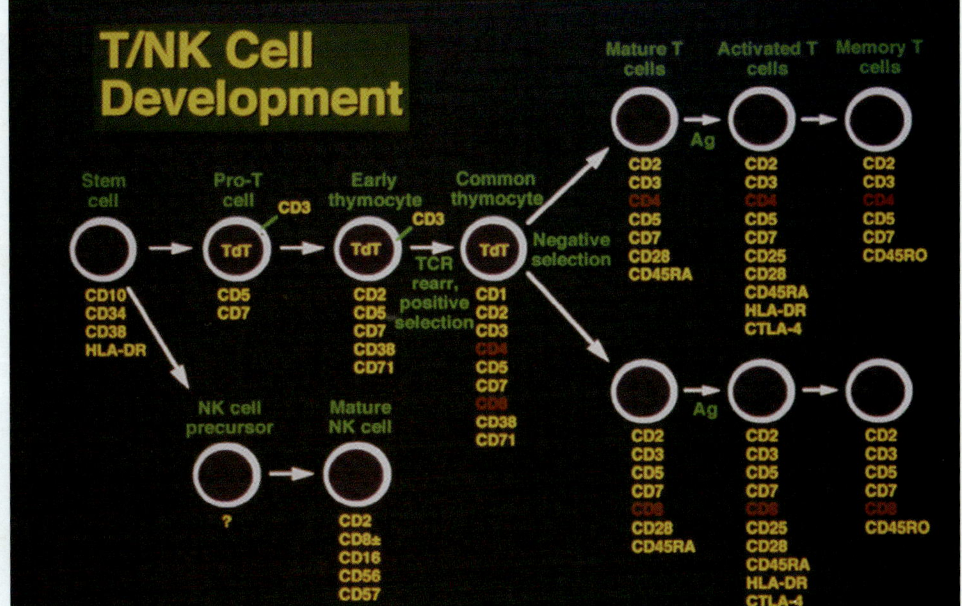

Figure 6.22 Schematic illustration of antigen expression during normal T-cell and NK-cell maturation. Note that, although the common lymphoid stem cell presumably arises in the bone marrow, most T-cell maturation occurs in the thymus. As with the B cells (Fig. 6.12), T-cell activation occurs after exposure to antigen. (Courtesy Dr. Dan Sabath.)

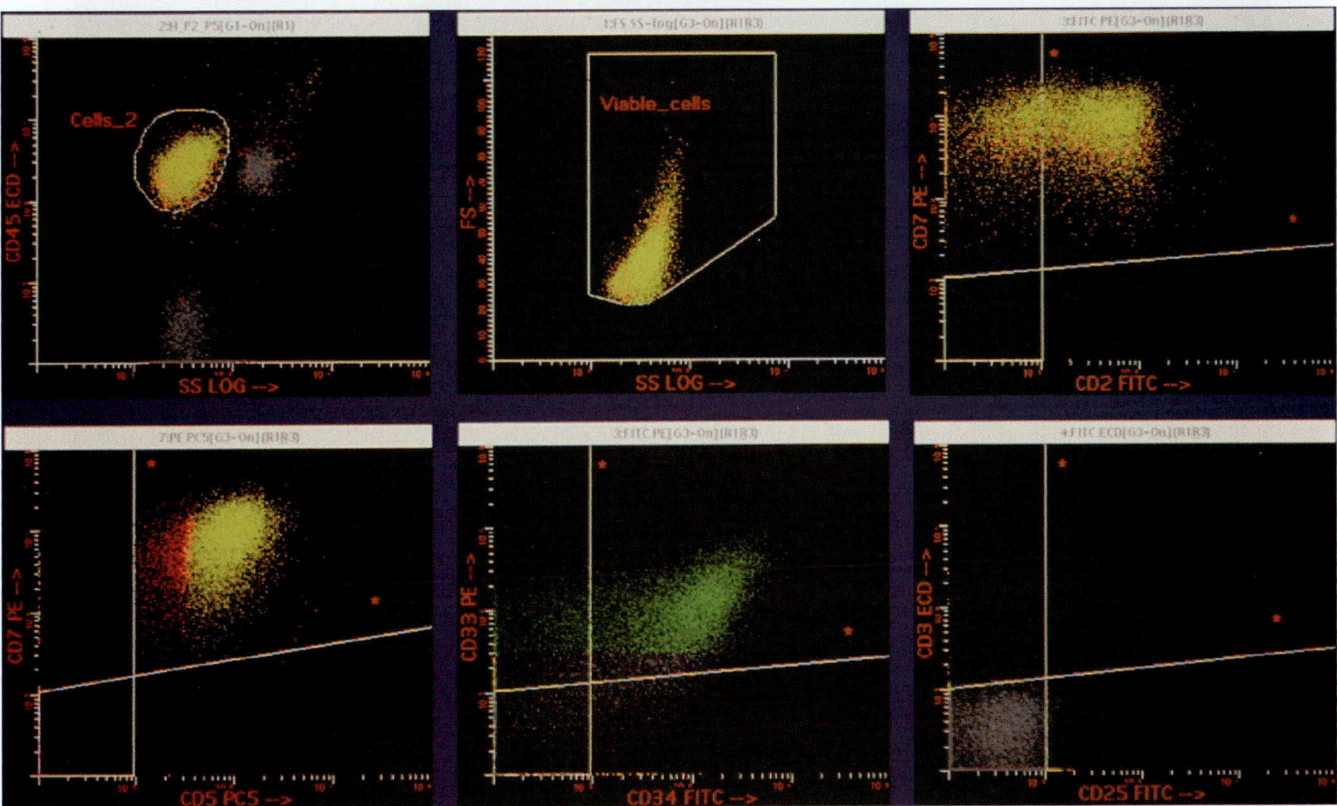

Figure 6.23 Precursor T-lymphoblastic leukemia/lymphoma of immature thymocyte stage. Precursor T-ALL can show immunophenotypic features reminiscent of any stage during early T-cell development. This case has an immature thymocyte immunophenotype, with expression of CD2, CD5, CD7, and CD34, but without CD3, CD4, or CD8. Aberrant coexpression of the myeloid-associated antigen CD33 is present in this case, as shown in the lower middle plot. TdT was also expressed (not shown).

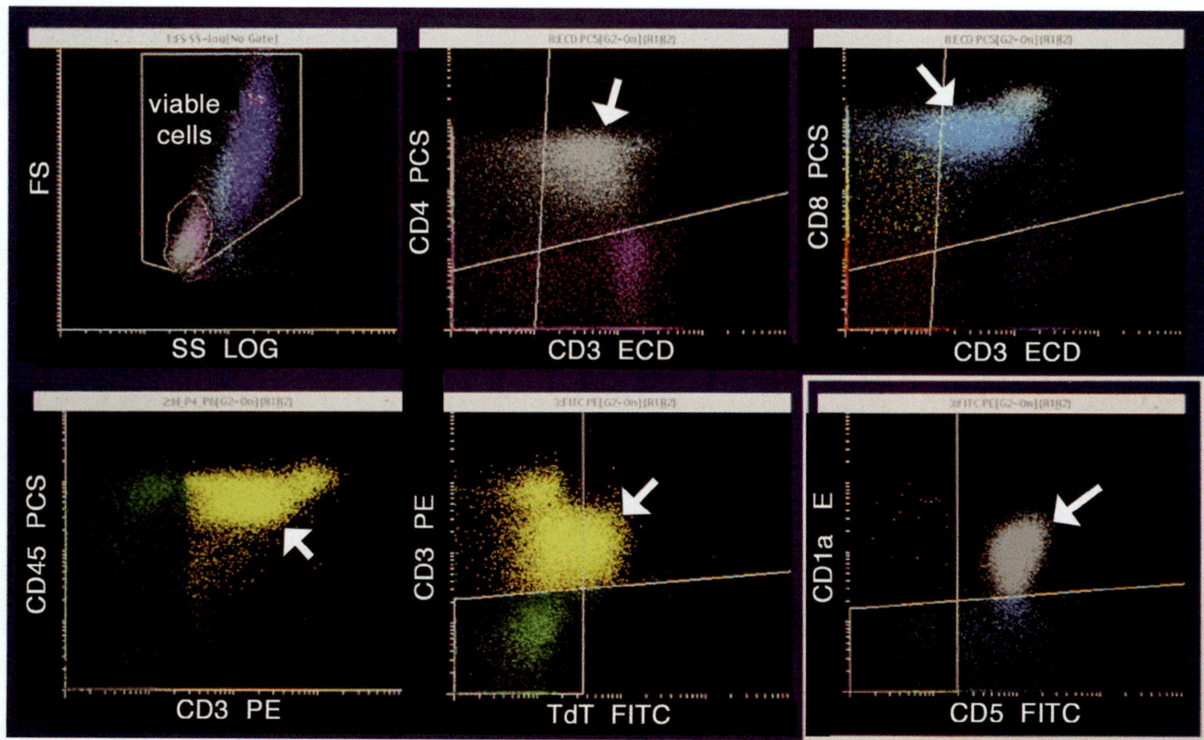

Figure 6.24 Precursor T-lymphoblastic leukemia/lymphoma of common thymocyte stage. In contrast to Figure 6.23, the present case shows coexpression of low-level CD3, CD4, CD8 and TdT, as well as CD1a, common thymocyte immunophenotype. As indicated in the lower left plot, the level of CD45 expression in precursor T-ALL is often close to that of a mature T-cell, in contrast to precursor B-ALL, in which the level of CD45 is often quite low (Fig. 6.13).

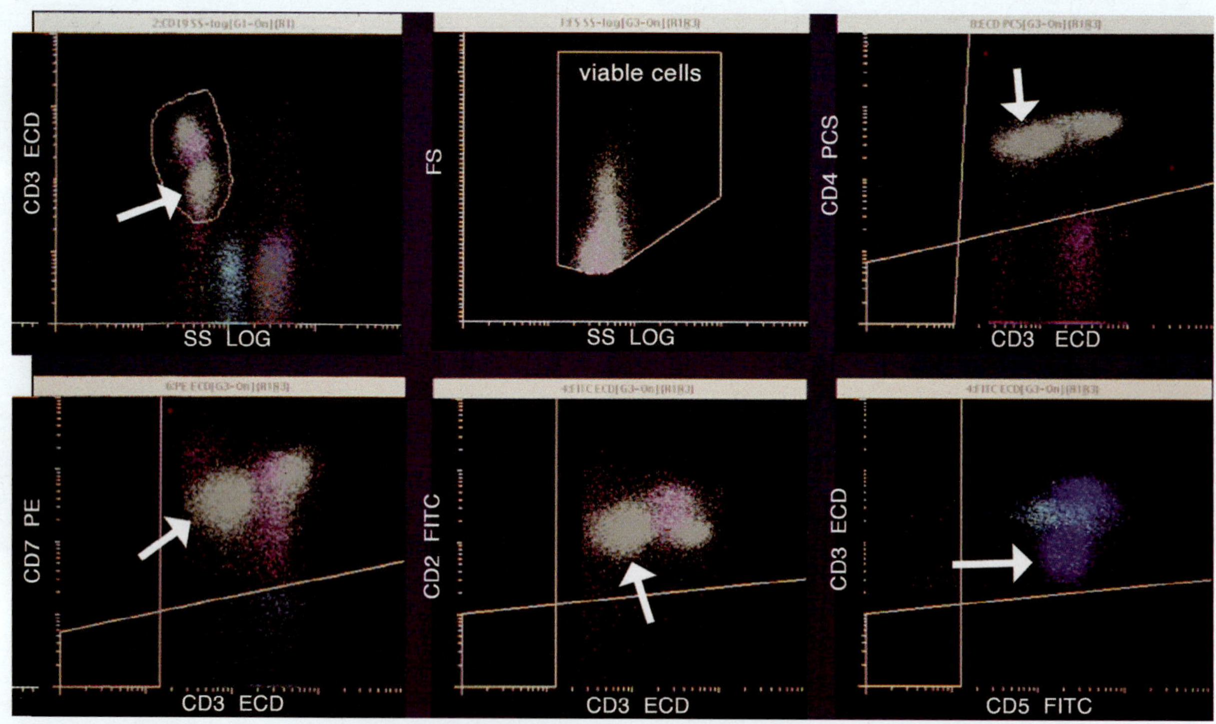

Figure 6.25 T-cell prolymphocytic leukemia (T-PLL). Note the relatively distinctive T-cell subpopulation showing decreased CD3, with relatively normal levels of CD4, CD2, CD7, and CD5. Unlike this case, up to 20% of T-PLLs show aberrant coexpression of CD4 and CD8.

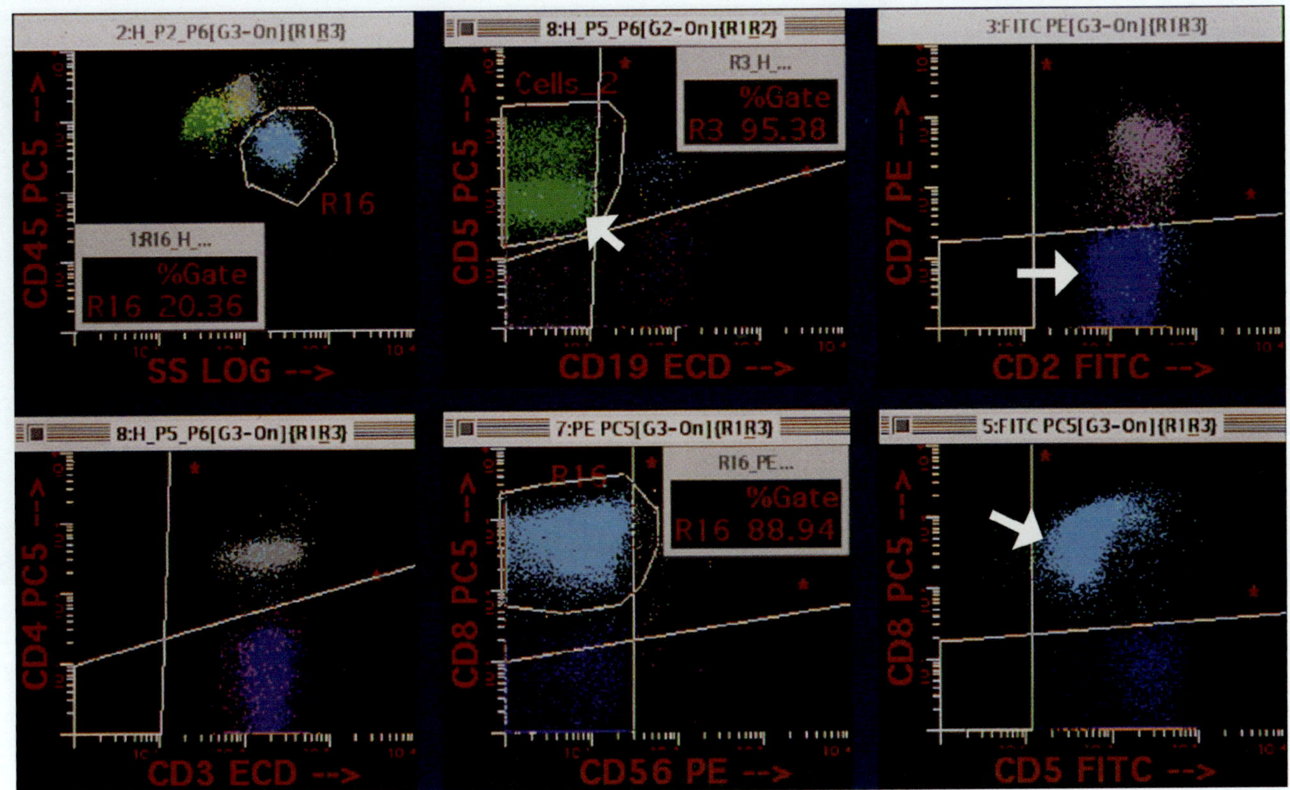

Figure 6.26 T-cell large granular lymphocytic leukemia (T-LGL). This case shows most of the common immunophenotypic features of T-LGL leukemia. The histogram in the upper left shows neutropenia (only 20% neutrophils in the R16 gate among the leukocytes), a characteristic of this disorder. In addition, this case demonstrates mild loss of CD5 and complete absence of CD7 (*arrows*), the two most common antigens showing aberrant loss on the neoplastic CD8$^+$ T cells in this disorder. Finally, there is a marked excess of CD8$^+$ over CD4$^+$ T cells.

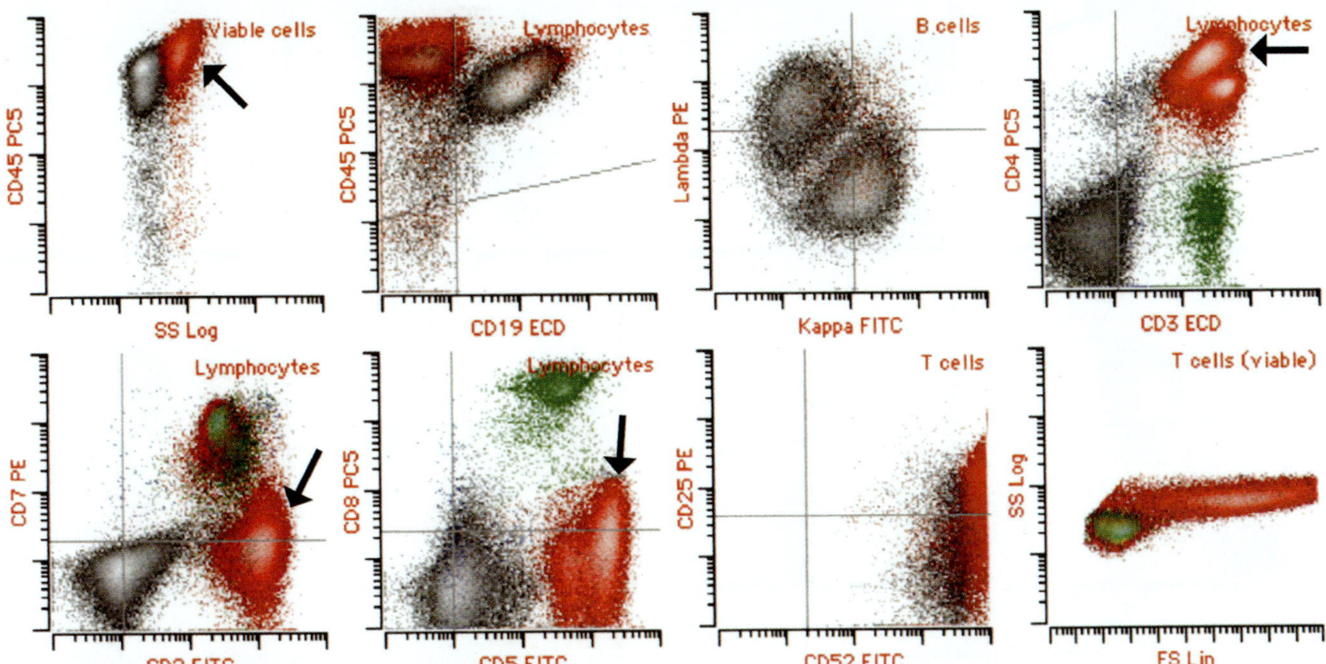

Figure 6.27 Mycosis fungoides or Sézary syndrome. This case illustrates lymph node involvement by a transformed case of MF/SS. Note the increased size (FS) of the red-colored neoplastic cells (*right lower histogram*); the increased CD4, CD5, and CD45; the aberrant loss of CD7 (*arrows*); and the relatively normal level of CD2. Like most mature T-cell neoplasms, this case strongly expressed CD52.

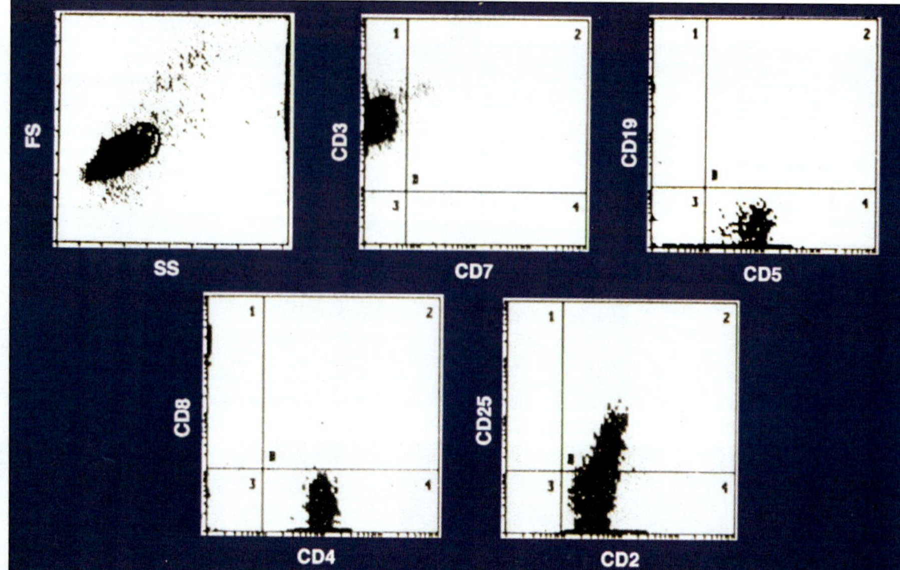

Figure 6.28   Adult T-cell leukemia/lymphoma (ATLL). This case shows a typical immunophenotype of ATLL, including coexpression of CD2, CD3, CD4, and CD5, with aberrant loss of CD7 and variable expression of CD25.

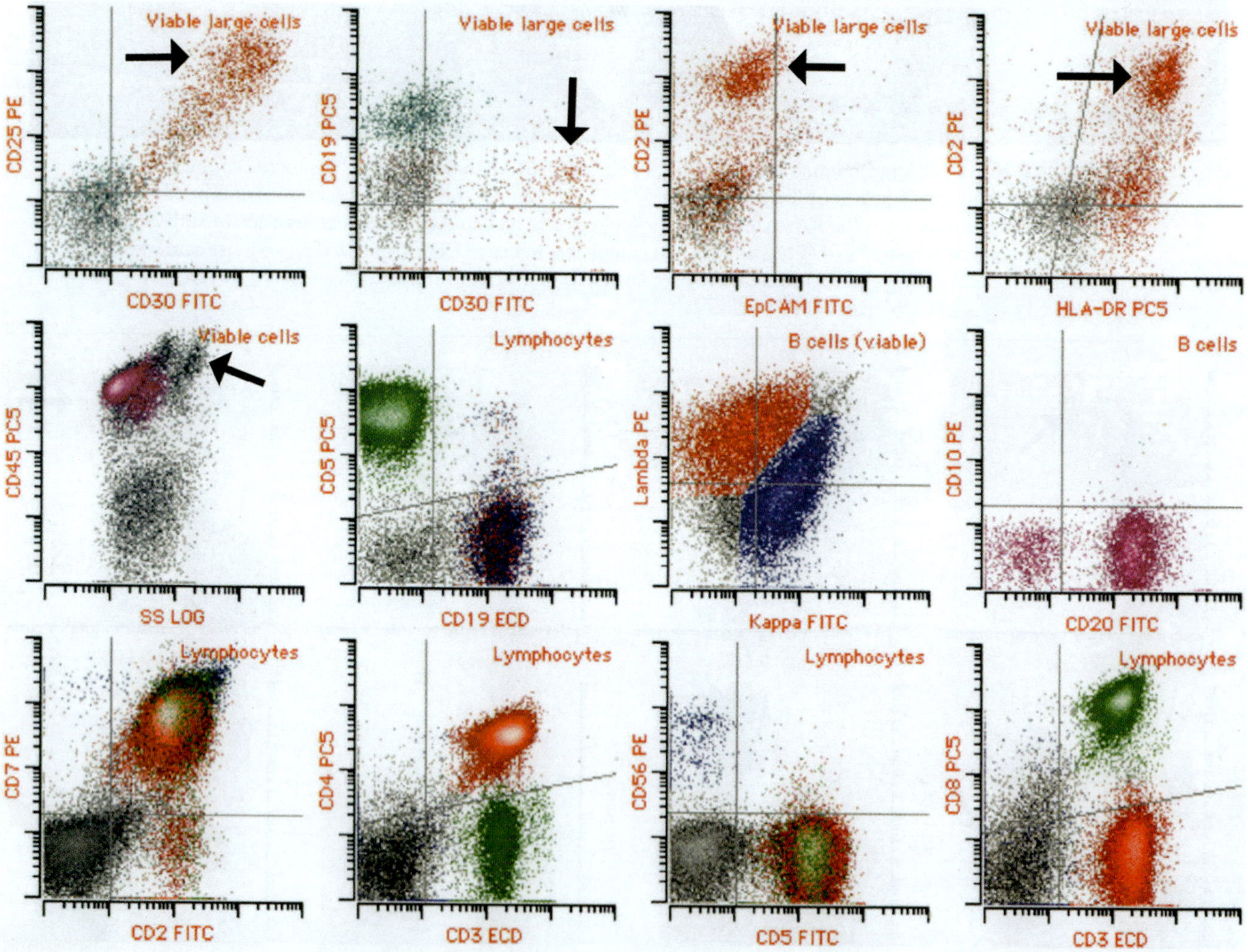

Figure 6.29   Anaplastic large-cell lymphoma, T-cell type (ALCL). This case, in which the lymph node was only partially involved by ALCL, shows a predominant population of normal B cells and T cells (*lower two rows of plots*). However, gating on the bright CD45⁺ cells with relatively high side scatter (*arrow, left middle histogram*) identified a population of very large cells coexpressing bright CD30, CD25, CD2, and HLA-DR, without the B-cell antigen CD19 or the carcinoma-associated antigen EpCAM (*arrows, top row of histograms*). This is a typical immunophenotype for anaplastic large-cell lymphoma. This lymphoma expressed ALK protein by immunohistochemistry (not shown).

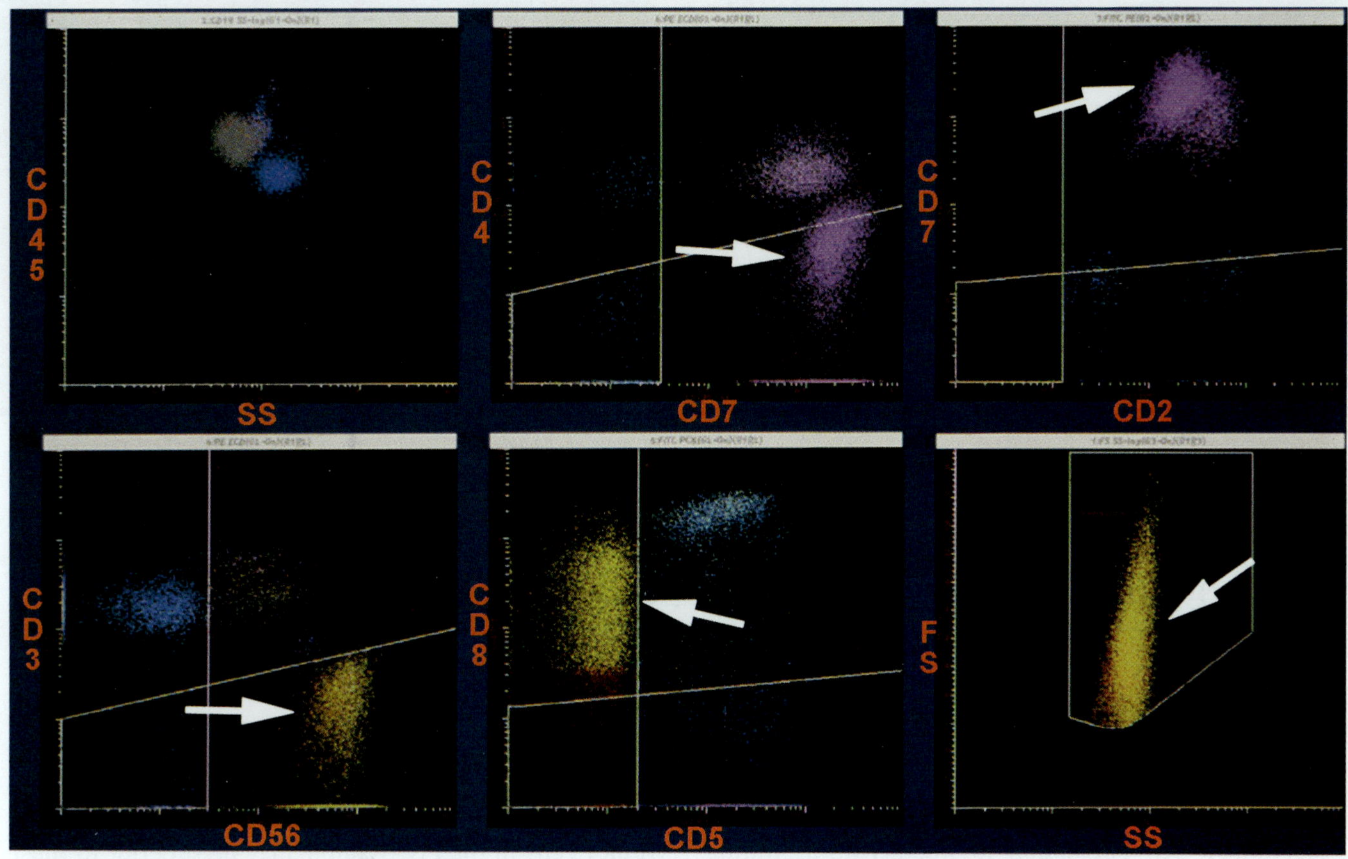

Figure 6.30   Aggressive NK-cell leukemia. This case illustrates expression of CD2, bright CD7, and uniform CD8 and CD56, without surface CD3, a typical NK-cell immunophenotype. The increased forward scatter of these cells, however, suggests a significantly greater size than normal NK cells, a finding confirmed by the large-cell morphology seen on a peripheral blood smear.

Cytology and Laser Scanning Cytometry

William R. Geddie, MD, FRCPC

THE ROLE OF CYTOLOGY IN DIAGNOSING LYMPHOPROLIFERATIVE AND OTHER HEMATOLOGIC DISORDERS

Hematolymphoid cells can be seen in every type of exfoliative cytology specimen and commonly constitute the predominant cell population in fine-needle aspiration biopsy samples obtained from a variety of organs. Such samples must be recognized as lymphoid and correctly stratified into reactive and neoplastic categories. The examination of specimens using classical cytologic methods, usually involving the Papanicolaou stain and monolayer preparations of various types, serves this triage role well and, in some settings, these techniques suffice for diagnosis. In this paradigm confirmation and subtyping of hematolymphoid malignancies, are deferred to the histologic examination of subsequent excisional or core biopsy material.

The utility of fine-needle aspiration biopsy of lymph nodes as a diagnostic modality has been questioned and remains controversial. But the same tools that are available for the study of the bone marrow (Romanowsky Giemsa-type stains, cell surface marker and molecular studies, cytogenetics and interphase fluorescence in situ hybridization [FISH]) can also be applied to evaluating cytologic specimens and often may permit specific diagnoses.

For a variety of reasons most young patients who are to be treated with curative intent have an excisional biopsy sample taken at some point. Cytology specimens may, however, be the best cellular material available for diagnosis. In some cases, excisional biopsy material is necrotic, fibrous, crushed, or badly fixed, and a repeat biopsy is not possible or cannot be justified to the patient. In other cases, such as primary effusion lymphoma, a cytology specimen may be the only diagnostic

material available. In such instances, the ability to maximize the diagnostic yield from the cytology samples is extremely important. For the same reason fine-needle aspiration (FNA) should be performed in conjunction with core biopsy samples. FNA produces, on average, more tumor cells, in a cell suspension suitable for flow cytometry or other ancillary tests, than are obtained by an average core biopsy. Furthermore, the condition of the tumor cells in the FNA sample may be superior to those in the core.

Even when an excisional nodal biopsy is planned, preoperative FNA of the involved lymph node or other lesion is extremely valuable for the following reasons:

- FNA can be performed at several sites, and the best site for excisional biopsy chosen.
- The diagnosis of a lymphoproliferative disorder can be made and staging investigations initiated.
- Material can be harvested for ancillary tests, thus shortening the workup of the subsequent surgical biopsy specimen.
- The findings may obviate the need for an excisional biopsy.

Based on the findings of the cytologic examination, a decision not to perform an excisional biopsy may be made for the following reasons:

- Limited further information would be gained (and the risk benefit ratio to the patient is unacceptably high).
- Clinical urgency mandates immediate treatment.
- Observation only is indicated (as with indolent lymphoma).
- It would be useful to preserve the lesion as a marker of response to treatment.
- The cytology specimen confirms recurrence of a disease already diagnosed.
- Biopsy is surgically difficult or impossible.

A cytology sample alone, whether exfoliative or FNA, may be sufficient for treatment of a lymphoproliferative disorder when the following conditions are met:

- The diagnosis has been based on a good specimen that has been well prepared, allowing for confirmation of the morphologic findings in many fields.
- Pathognomonic morphologic findings, immunophenotype, FISH (fluorescence in-situ hybridization), molecular studies, or histochemical stains can confirm the diagnostic impression.
- The adjuvant techniques themselves are of good quality, with appropriate controls.
- Proliferation studies have been performed.
- Clinicopathologic and radiologic correlation has taken place.

In some diseases (such as small lymphocytic lymphoma), these conditions may easily be met. In others, such as Hodgkin lymphoma, they may be met with difficulty. In some disorders in which diagnosis relies primarily on architectural patterns (such as Castleman disease), diagnosis by cytologic means may be impossible. A diagnosis will be possible only if the handling of the material optimizes the assessment of morphology and permits all necessary ancillary investigations.

LASER SCANNING CYTOMETRY AS AN ANCILLARY TECHNIQUE IN CYTOLOGIC DIAGNOSIS OF LYMPHOMA

Some lesions aspirate easily and yield more than enough cells for morphologic assessment, flow cytometry, and other ancillary tests. However the need to preserve material for additional studies makes it highly desirable to utilize an immunophenotyping method that requires less than the one million or more cells typically used in flow cytometry for a full B-cell and T-cell panel.

In slide-based cytometry, labeled cells on a glass surface are interrogated as they are moved past a laser by a precisely controlled stage. Emitted fluorescence is collected by photomultiplier tubes in a manner exactly analogous to flow cytometry. Commercially available instruments exsist (CompuCyte®) for which analytic methods have been developed. In the immunophenotyping methods described by Clatch (ref), a standardized cell suspension is introduced into the potential space between two pieces of glass separated by a "spacer manifold" with adhesive on both surfaces of the top panel (top panel, Fig. 7.5).

After the cell suspension is introduced into this space, the cells sediment by gravity and adhere through electrostatic forces caused by sialic acid residues on the cells. A pre-diluted three- or four-antibody mixture containing 1.5 µL of each primary antibody then replaces the supernatant fluid. After reacting with these cells for 20 minutes in the dark, the unbound antibody is washed by introducing saline at one end of the well and absorbing it with blotting paper at the other end.

When the resulting slide is examined using the laser scanning cytometer, a "contour" is placed around each cell by the instrument software (middle panel, Fig. 7.5). A variety of parameters, including forward scatter signal and multispectral fluorescence within the set contour, are recorded and can be used to create conventional histograms. The XY coordinates of each contoured event on the slide are also "remembered" as part of the list mode file so that cells making up populations can be relocalized and examined morphologically before or after staining. Although the morphology of the cells has usually suffered as a result of several incubations, different cell types can be recognized well enough to confirm gating strategies (lower panel, Fig. 7.5).

Diagram 7.1

Sample Processing
FNA Sample
"Dry aspirate"
Hemodiluted sample or fluid
Divide material into 3 direct smears
Use one drop for direct smear or prepare air dried cytospin
Make cell suspension in PBS
Air dried smear
Wet alcohol fixed smear
Air dried smear
Diff-Quik
MGG
Papanicolou stain
Rapid assessment
Nonhematolymphoid (e.g., metastatic carcinoma)
- Repeat for preparation of cell block or cytospin slides
Hematolymphoid
Purulent material microorganisms (bacteria, fungi) "Negative" staining of mycobacteria Granulomas
Normal or hyperplastic
Abnormal
Repeat for culture
Repeat aspiration for cell suspension for surface marker studies, FISH, molecular
- (for fluids do cell count and start studies)
- check cellularity to ensure adequacy before leaving patient

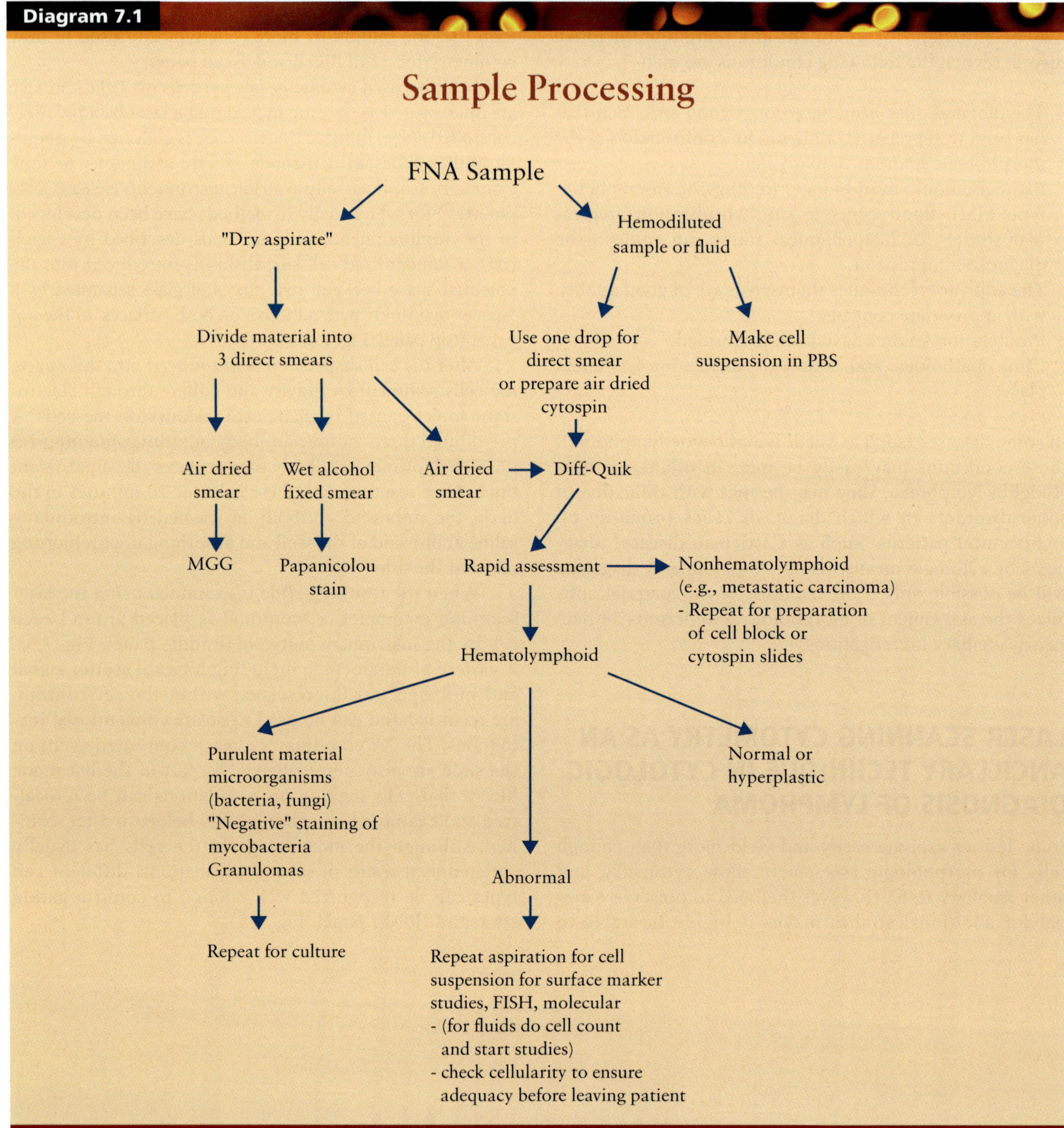

Diagram 7.2

Diagnostic Pathway

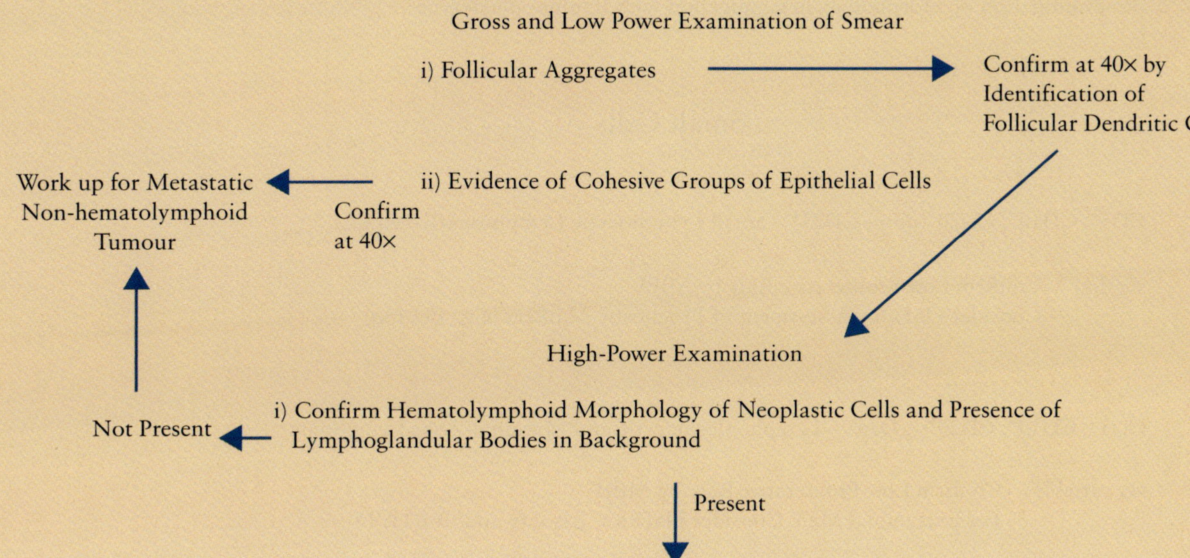

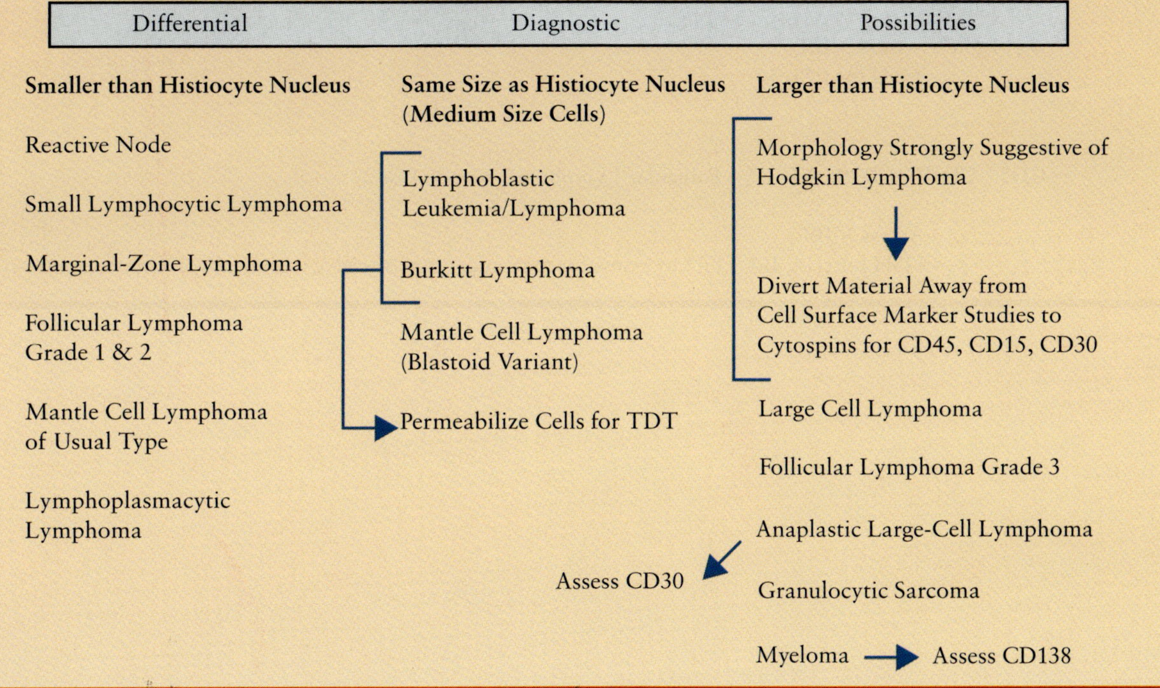

Diagram 7.3

Diagnostic Pathway: Small Cells

-Re-examination of Morphology in conjunction with Immunophenotype

Small Cells

$CD5^+$, $CD10^-$, $CD20^+$(dim), $CD23^+$ - Small Lymphocytic Lymphoma/B-cell CLL

sIg dim   - Confirm Low Proliferative Rate by MIBI
      - Consider FISH for Assessment of Prognostic Markers (e.g., del 13q)

$CD5^-$, $CD10^-$, $CD20^+$ $CD23^-$ - Lymphoplasmacytic and Marginal-Zone Lymphoma

sIg variable   - Confirm Low Proliferative Rate by MIB1
      - For Extranodal MZL Consider FISH for Trisomy and/or t(11; 18)

$CD5^+$, $CD10^-$, $CD20^+$(bright), $CD23^-$ - Mantle Cell (Classic Type)

sIg bright - Assess MIBI
      - FISH for t(11; 14)

$CD5^-$, $CD10^+$, $CD20^+$, $CD23^{\pm}$ - Follicular Lymphoma (Grade 1 or 2)

      - Assess MIBI
      - FISH for t(14; 18) [FISH to assess for rearrangement of cMyc if clinically in transformation]

Diagram 7.4

Diagnostic Pathway: Medium Cells

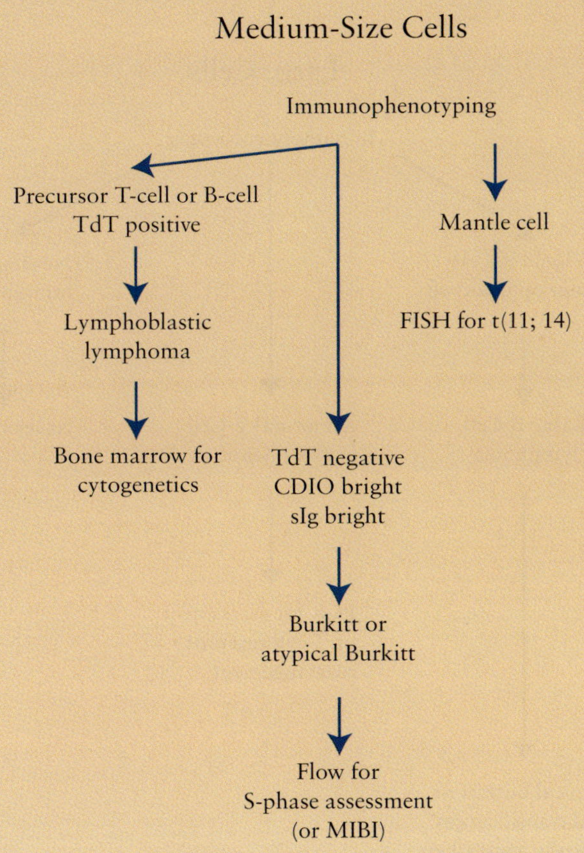

Medium-Size Cells

Immunophenotyping

Precursor T-cell or B-cell
TdT positive

Mantle cell

Lymphoblastic
lymphoma

FISH for t(11; 14)

Bone marrow for
cytogenetics

TdT negative
CDIO bright
sIg bright

Burkitt or
atypical Burkitt

Flow for
S-phase assessment
(or MIBI)

Diagram 7.5

Diagnostic Pathway: Large Cells
Large Cells
Immunophenotyping
Clonal B-Cell immunophenotype
No diagnostic immunophenotype
Large B-Cell lymphoma
Abnormal T-Cell or NK phenotype
Excisonal biopsy
PCR for assessment of T-cell receptor rearrangement
Atypical Burkitt or "dual translocation" (clinically aggressive)
FISH for t(14;18) and cMyc

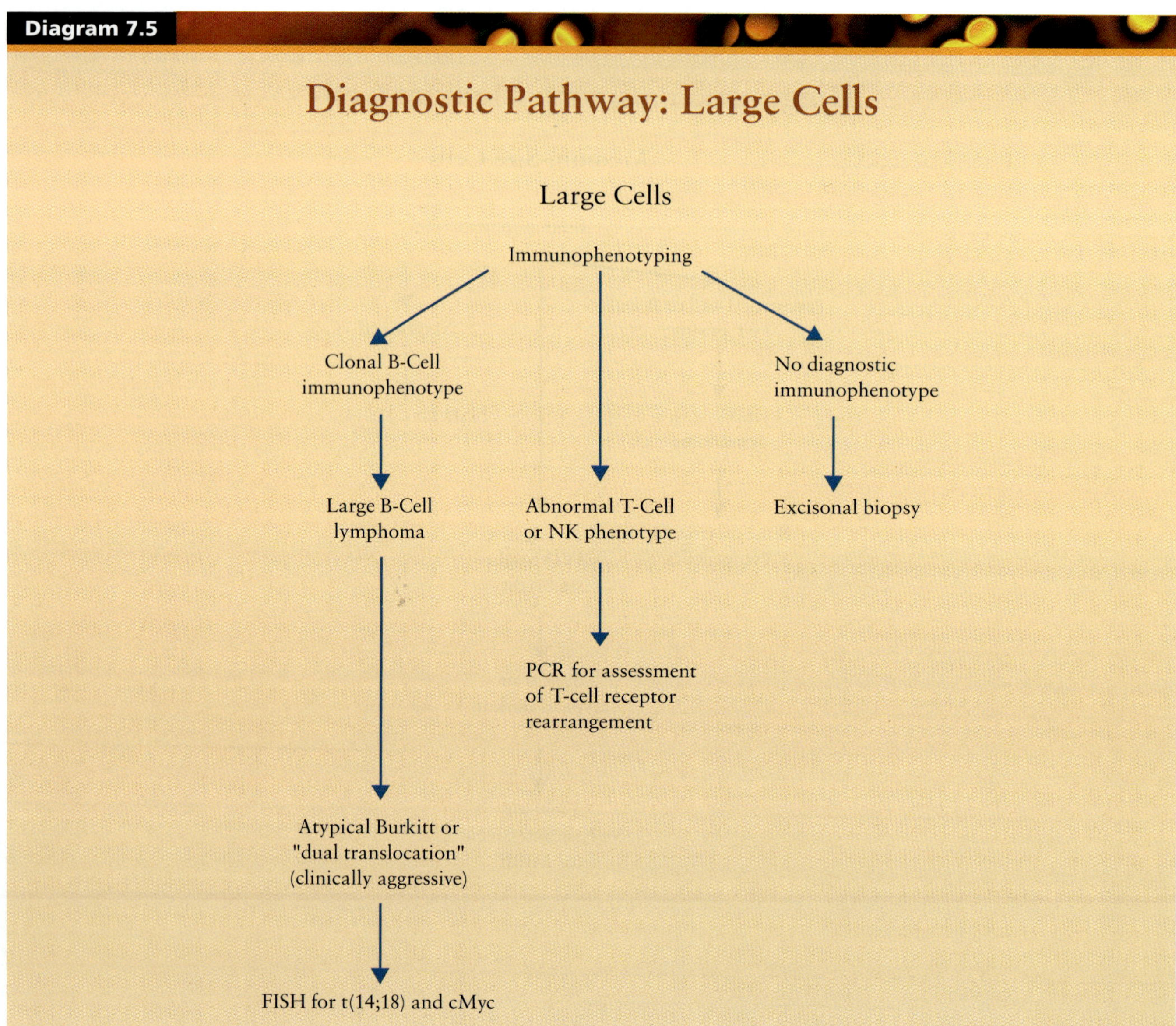

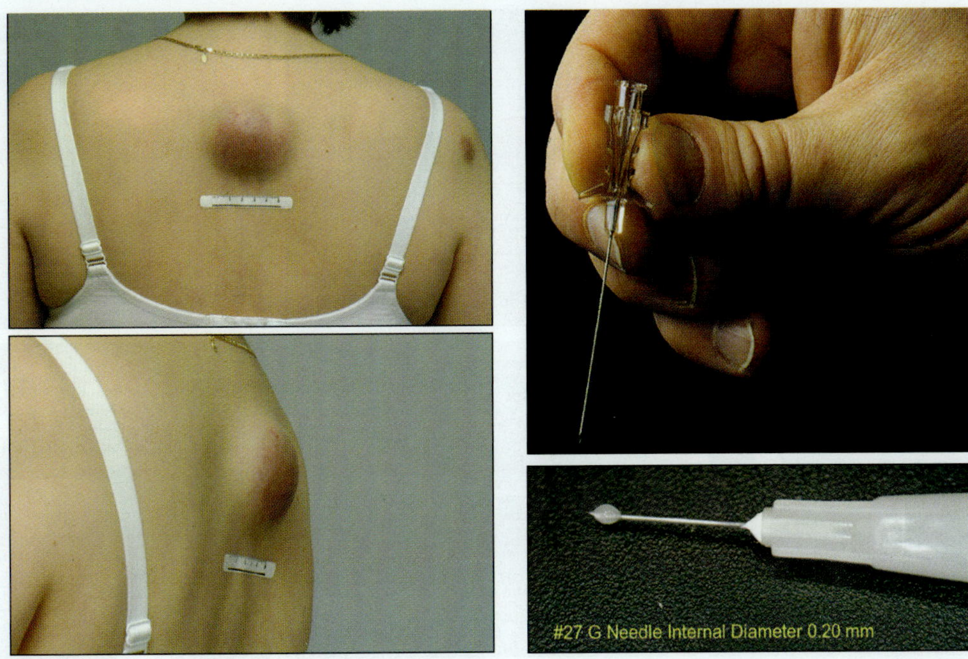

Figure 7.1   Technique of FNA biopsy. In addition to lymph nodes, a variety of other subcutaneous lesions, such as the cutaneous lymphoma illustrated here, are amenable to sampling by fine-needle biopsy. Many cytology textbooks emphasize the use of a syringe, sometimes manipulated with a syringe holder such as the Cameco. However many lesions, in particular smaller lesions such as the deposits seen on this patient's right shoulder, are more easily sampled with a needle alone, using the so-called *Zajdela* or pipette technique. The lesion is fixed with one hand (the left, for a right-handed operator), and the needle held by the operating hand is introduced through the skin and into the subcutaneous lesion. The change in density between skin, subcutaneous fat and lesional tissue is easily appreciated. With the needle in the lesion, 10 to 20 short strokes or *reciprocations* are made, taking care to remain within the boundaries of the lesion. The cellular material obtained by the cutting action of the beveled end of the needle rises by capillary action within the needle, which should be removed if blood or cellular material is observed within the hub.

Using this method, a drop of cellular material containing thousands to millions of cells can be obtained even with a needle as small as 27G (*right lower panel*). (Zajdela, de Maublanc MT, Schlienger P, Hage C. Cytologic diagnosis of periorbital tumores using fine-needle sampling without aspiration. *Diagn Cytopathol* 1986;2:17–20.)

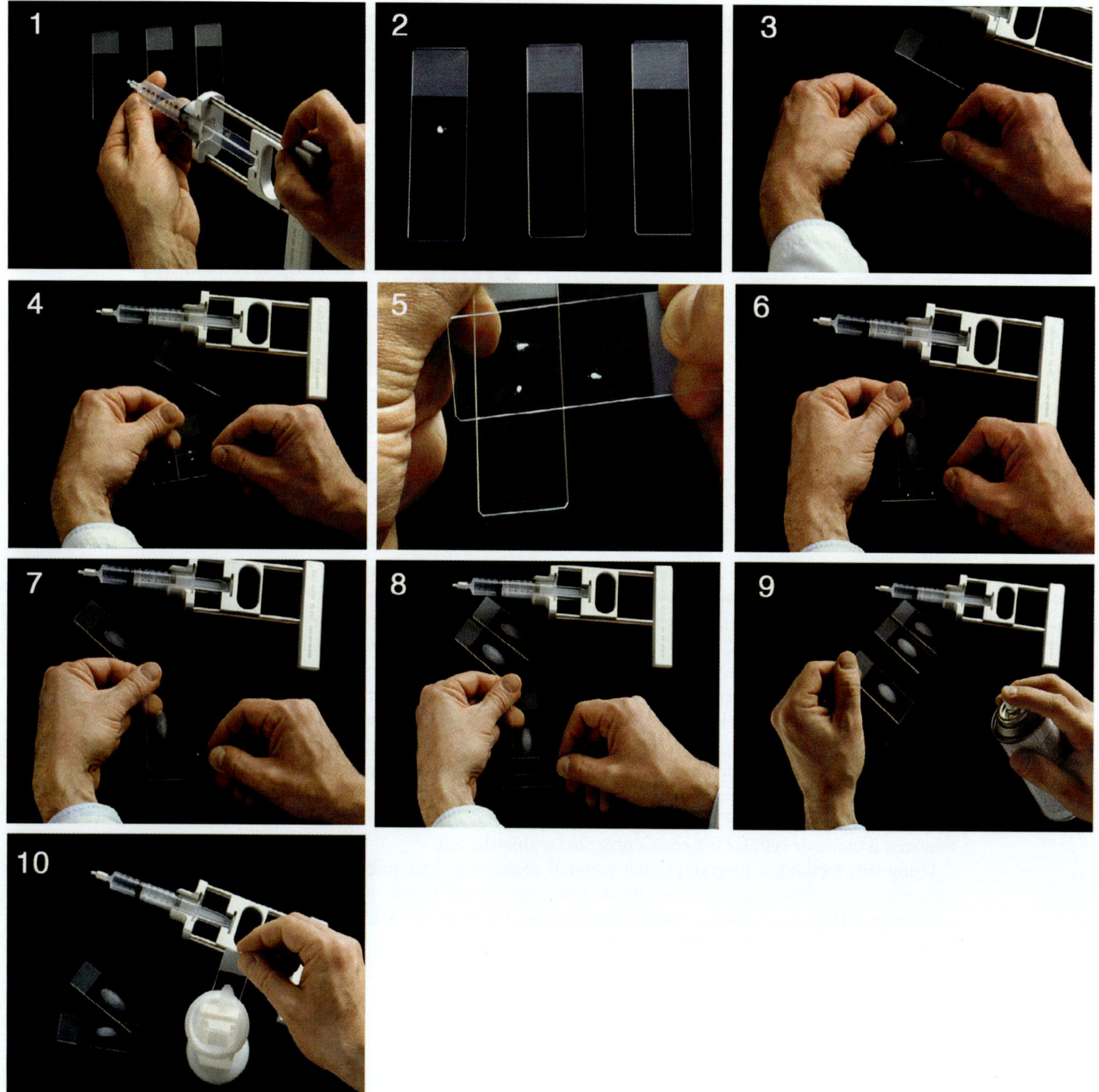

Figure 7.2 Smear preparation technique. The Cameco syringe holder may be very useful in manipulating the material obtained by fine-needle sampling. The needle used for the biopsy is attached to a syringe already filled with air. With the bevel of the needle down and just above the slide near the frosted end, the cellular material in the needle is expelled gently in one place. A right-handed operator holds this receiving slide by the upper left-hand corner and, with his right hand places the edge of a clean slide about 1 cm away from the cellular material. He gently lowers it onto the drop of material to pick up some (about one-third) of the sample. The slide is then moved to the left and the process repeated. The slide in the operator's right hand is then flipped over (note that, in picture no. 5, the two drops of cellular material now appear on the top of the slide in the aspirator's right hand). This slide is now lowered gently on top of the original drop of material. The material spreads by capillary action. The smearing slide is kept absolutely parallel to the bottom slide and drawn without pressure down the length of the slide. If this maneuver is performed correctly, almost no cellular material will remain on the smearing slide. The smearing slide in the aspirator's right hand is now flipped over again and the smearing process is repeated using the two drops of cellular material picked up from the original drop, which are now applied to two other clean slides. Usually the first two smears are allowed to air-dry for Romanowsky Giemsa-type stains, and the last smear is fixed while still wet, using either alcoholic spray fixative or by dropping the slide into a Coplin jar. (Löwhagen's technique.) (Stanley MW, Lowhagen T. *Fine Needle Aspiration of Palpable Masses.* Stoneham, MA: Butterworth-Heinemann, 1993:23–41.)

PATTERNS IN UNSTAINED ASPIRATES

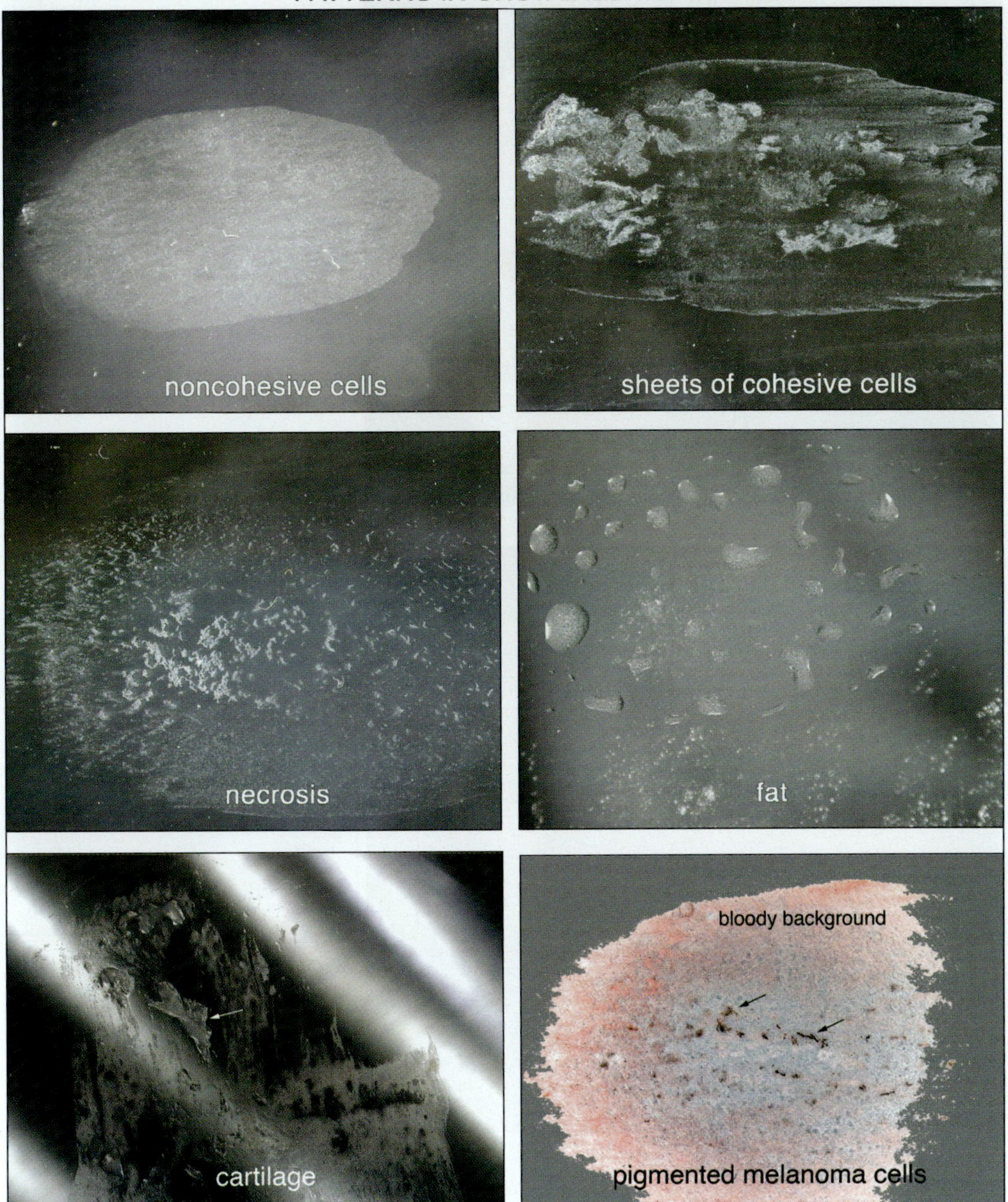

Figure 7.3   Patterns in unstained aspirate smears. Cellular material of different types can be appreciated immediately after smear preparation. A pure lymphoid aspirate, usually referred to as a "dry" aspirate, gives a smooth or slightly granular smear indicative of evenly applied noncohesive cells. Cohesive cells, usually epithelial, are seen as aggregates on the unstained smear, whereas necrosis gives a flocculent, ropy, or greasy "sebum-like" smear. Fat is recognized as individual droplets of oily material. In aspirates of melanoma, melanin pigment sometimes makes the smear gray or black (*arrows*). Cartilage, difficult to spread out, can be seen as flecks of white, almost glassy, material (*arrow*). Purer blood gives an evenly disbursed, shiny appearance, as long as the sample has been smeared immediately to avoid clotting.

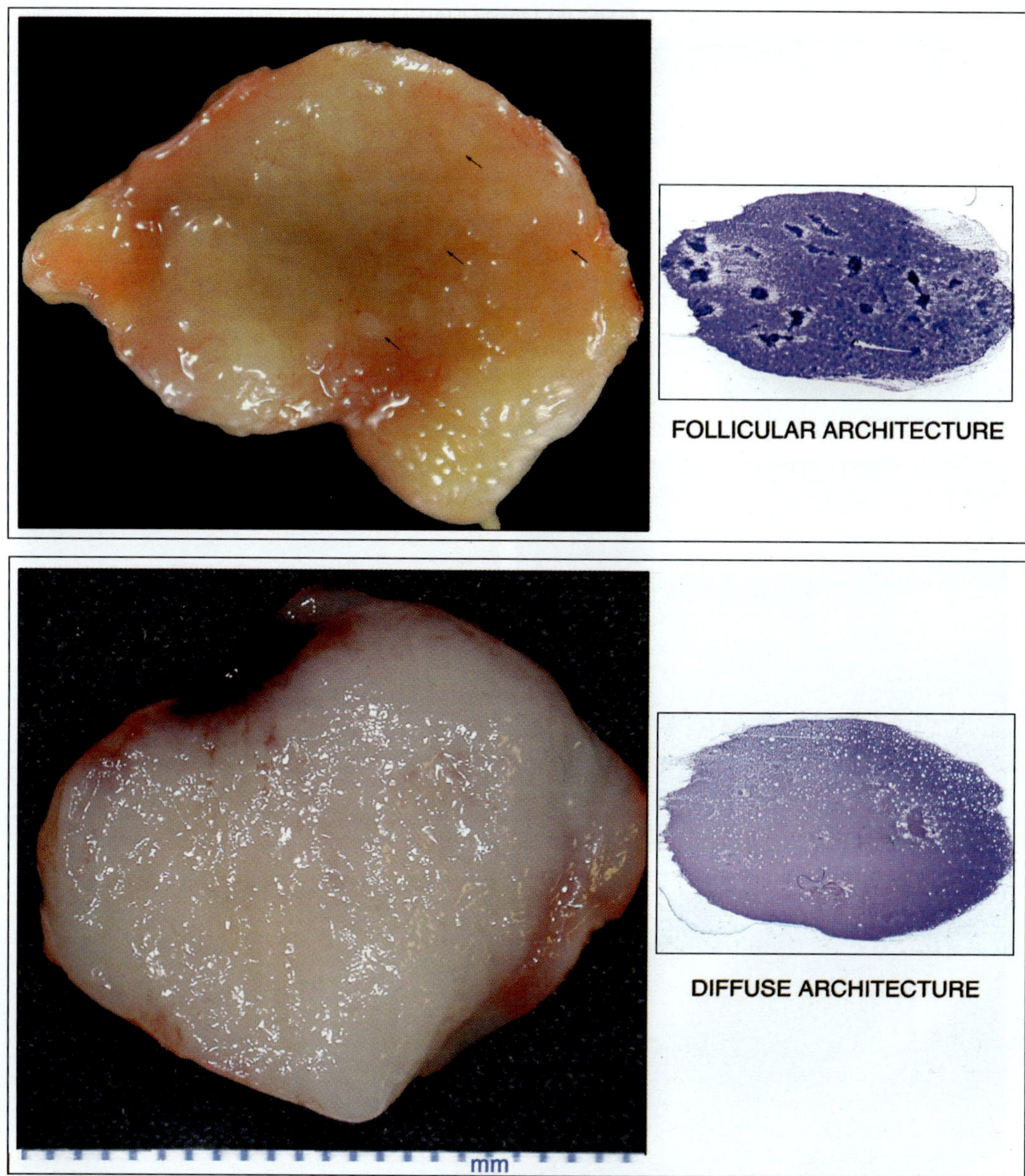

Figure 7.4   Gross recognition of lymph node architecture. Lymphoid follicles or germinal centers less than 1 mm in size can be recognized on gross inspection of excised lymph nodes (*arrows, upper left panel*). These structures can be aspirated in their entirety by 27G needles having an internal diameter of 0.2 mm. These intact follicular aggregates are seen easily as small round dots on the stained smear (*upper right panel*). When a diffuse lymphoid infiltrate is aspirated, the resulting smear does not show any evidence of aggregated cells (*lower panels*).

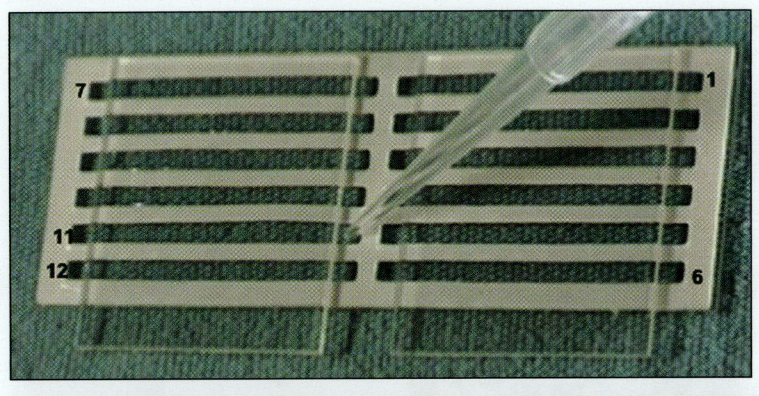

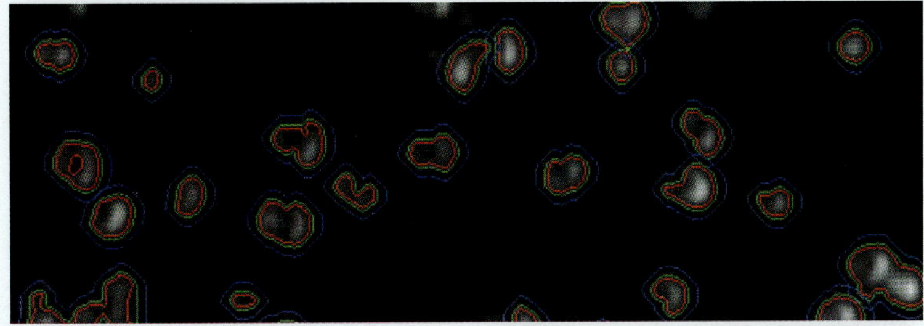

Metastatic Seminoma – Relocalization of unstained cells

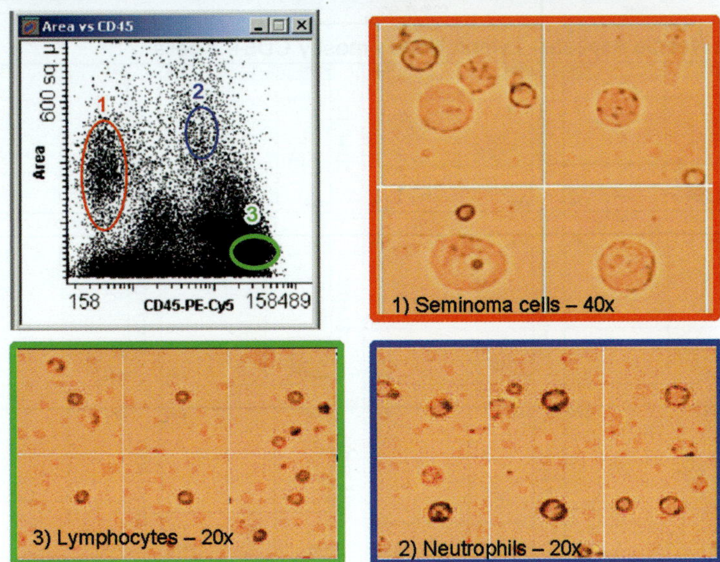

Figure 7.5   *Top panel:* This is a typical example of a "Clatch" slide used on the laser scanning cytometer. In the immunophenotyping methods described by Clatch, a standardized cell suspension is introduced into the potential space between two pieces of glass separated by a spacer manifold with adhesive on both surfaces. Each scattergram corresponds to one of the 12 areas or lanes on the slide. *Middle panel:* Laser scanning cytometer contouring. *Bottom panel:* Initial gating occurs in a cell size (laser scatter) vs. CD45 histogram based on all of the cells on the slide. Populations of interest can be relocalized for morphologic assessment. The images are based on forward laser scatter in these unstained cells. (Clatch R. Immunophenotyping of Hematological malignancies by laser scanning cytometry. In: Darzynkiewicz Z, Crissman HA, Robinson JP, eds. *Methods in Cell Biology*, Vol 64. 3rd ed. San Diego: Academic Press, 2001:213–342.)

Infectious Mononucleosis

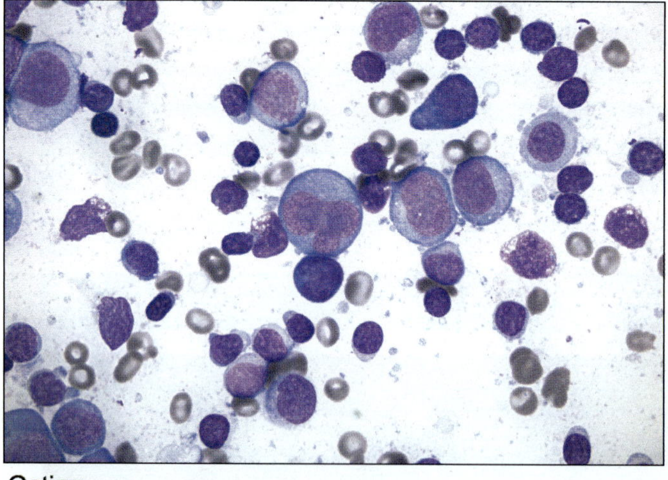

Gating

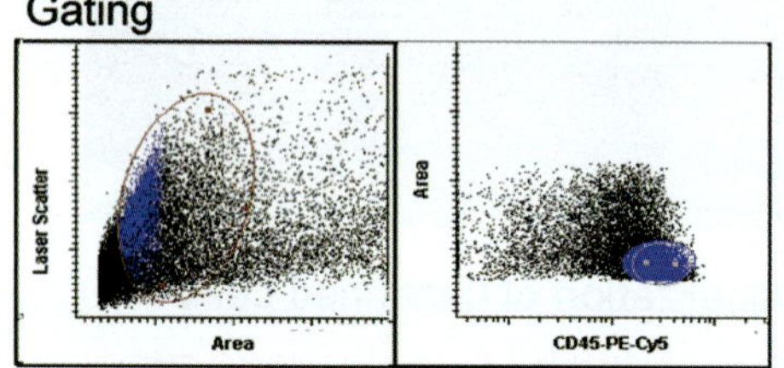

Fine Needle Aspirate - Lymph Node - **mostly CD8+ T cells**

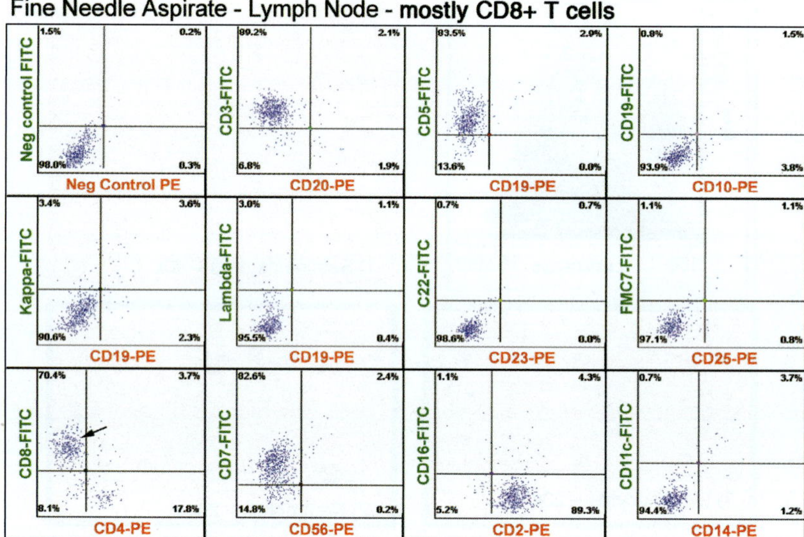

Figure 7.6 Acute viral lymphadenopathy with immunoblastic reaction (infectious mononucleosis). In viral lymphadenopathies, of which infectious mononucleosis is the prototype, numerous smudge cells and necrotic cells are seen in the background of a highly cellular smear dominated by atypical lymphocytes. Many cells with eccentric deep blue cytoplasm are present. Immunoblasts, frequently binucleate and, showing huge inclusion-like nucleoli, may mimic Reed-Sternberg cells. Mitoses are frequently numerous and the MIB1 fraction, if assessed, is very high. Immunophenotyping usually shows a T-cell predominance with inverted CD4:CD8 ratio (*arrow*). It can be difficult to find a "clean" gate because of the large number of necrotic cells.

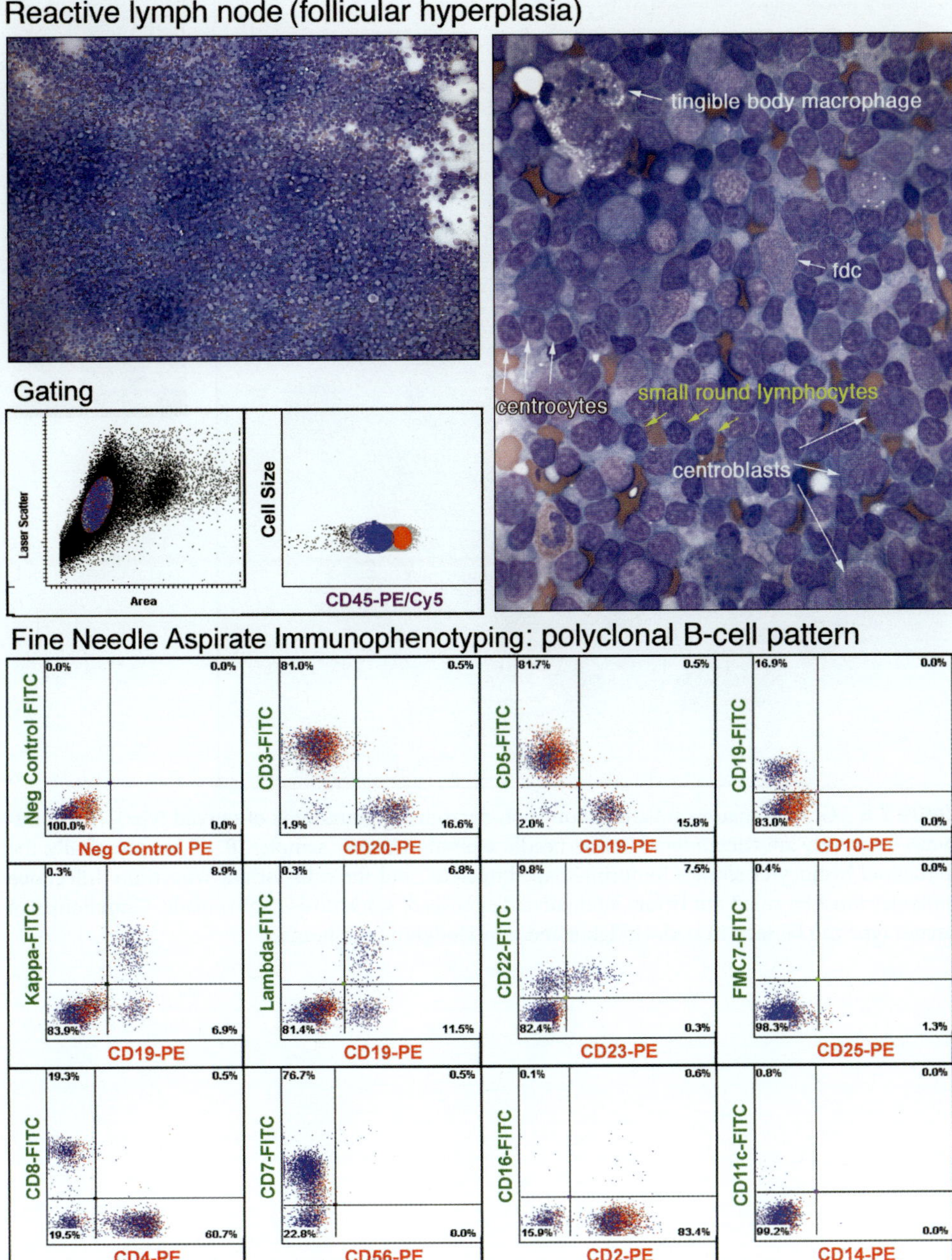

Figure 7.7   Reactive lymph node (follicular hyperplasia). In the morphologic assessment of aspirates from a hyperplastic node, intact germinal centers containing follicular dendritic cells and tingible-body macrophages can be recognized in the context of a highly heterogeneous population. The latter include small and transformed lymphocytes (centrocytes and centroblasts) and usually some plasmacytoid cells. Immunophenotypic analysis will show variable proportions of T cells and B cells. T cells are appropriately subdivided into T-helper and T-suppressor subsets (no evidence of subset restriction), and there is no evidence of antigen loss or aberrant antigen expression. The B cells are polytypic, κ-positive cells are predominant, and no significant number of B cells failing to express surface antigen can be found.

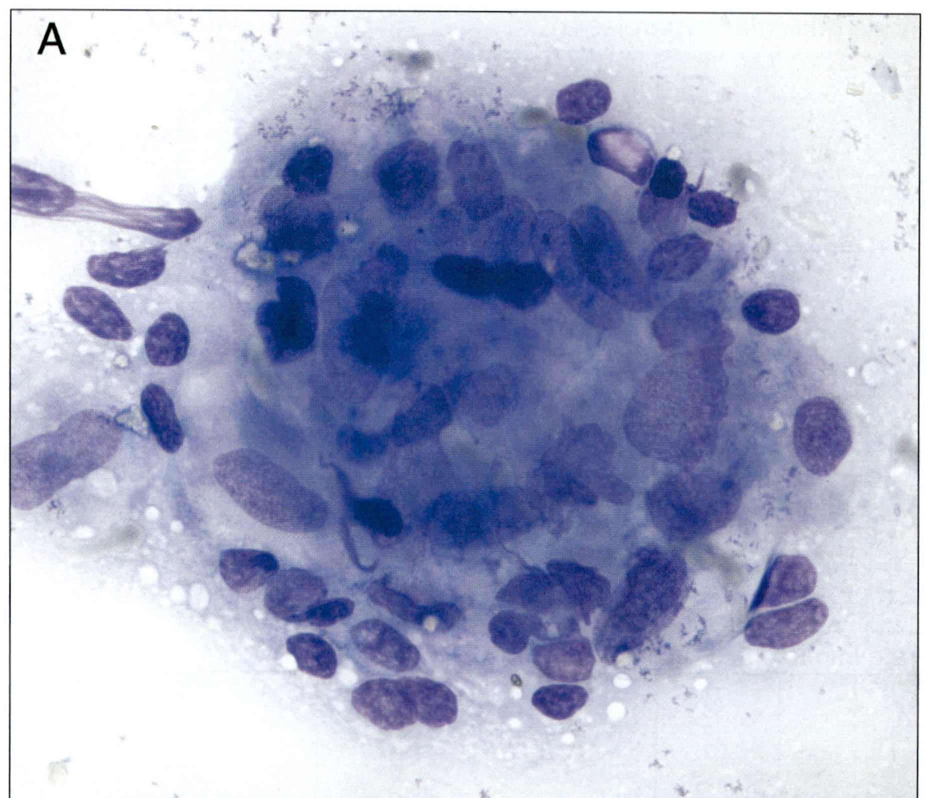
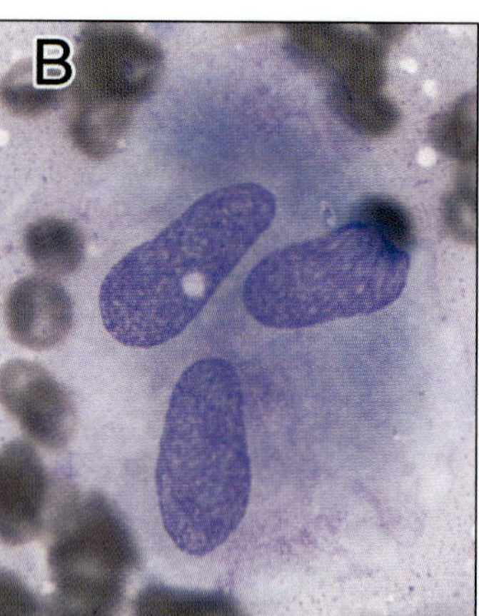

Figure 7.8   Granulomatous inflammation (non-necrotizing granuloma of sarcoid type). **A.** Granulomas frequently are encountered in fine-needle aspiration biopsy samples. **B.** Characteristically, the epithelioid histiocytes show a footprint-shaped nucleus, and the cells form a syncytium. Infectious etiologies must be ruled out before a tentative diagnosis of sarcoidosis can be made. Granulomas of sarcoid type can be seen in both Hodgkin and non-Hodgkin lymphoma.

Chronic lymphocytic leukemia (CLL)/Small lymphocytic leukemia (SLL)

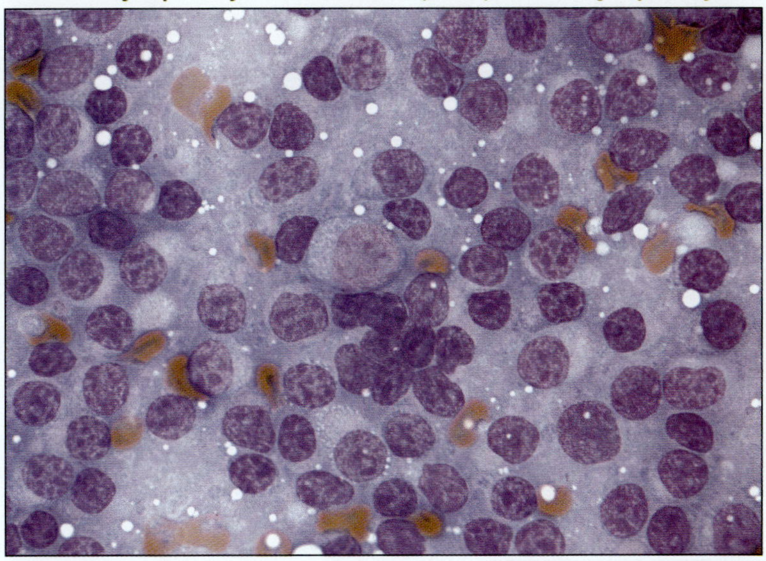

Gating

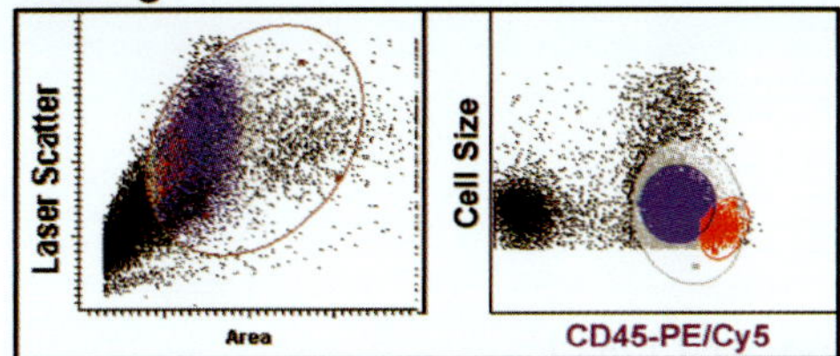

Fine Needle Aspirate Immunophenotyping: kappa restricted CD5+/CD23+ B cells

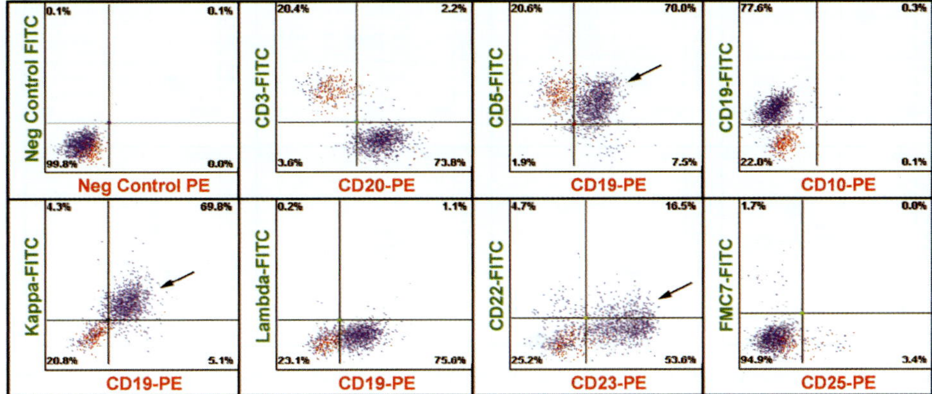

Figure 7.9   Small lymphocytic lymphoma with or without B-cell chronic lymphocytic leukemia. Aspirates of lymph nodes involved by small lymphocytic lymphoma, or enlarged in patients with known B-cell chronic lymphocytic leukemia, are frequently encountered. Often a rapid increase in lymph node size prompts concern about possible transformation. Pseudo-follicles or proliferation centers may be evident on low-power examination of a smear, which is otherwise dominated by small lymphoid cells slightly larger than normal lymphocytes, with round nuclei and clumped chromatin. Plasmacytoid cells often are observed. Prolymphocytes and para-immunoblasts (the large cell in the center of this photomicrograph) are always found. Immunophenotyping shows the typical pattern of dim CD20, absent FMC7, dim sIg with light chain restriction and coexpression of CD5 and CD19 (*arrows*). *Note*: The initial gating of the "cell size versus CD45" laser scanning cytometry histogram has colored the brighter CD45$^+$ and smaller cells red. These cells are T cells.

Prolymphocytic transformation in CLL

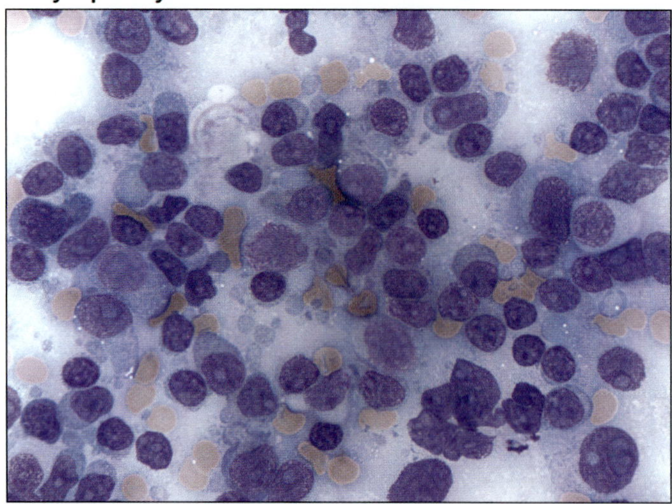

Gating

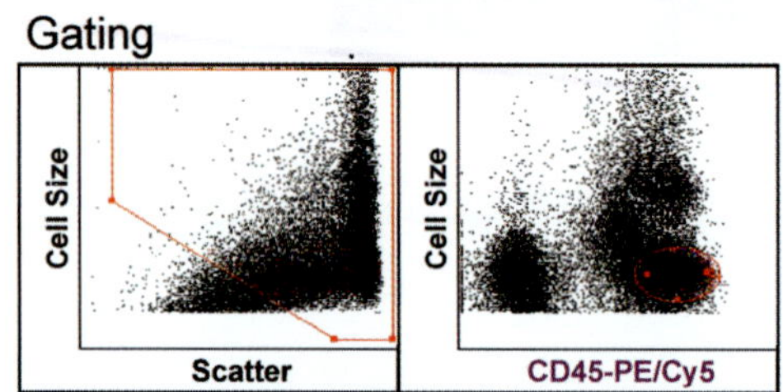

Lymph Node Aspirate Immunophenotyping - CLL/PLL

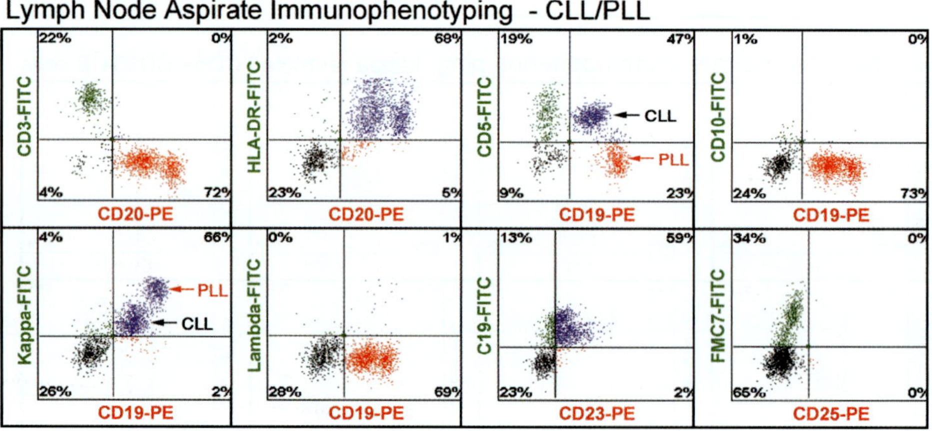

Figure 7.10   Prolymphocytic transformation in chronic lymphocytic leukemia. *Top panel:* Numerous prolymphocytes with medium-sized nuclei, dispersed chromatin, and small nucleoli are noted, as well as para-immunoblasts. Immunophenotyping by laser scanning cytometry shows two distinct populations of brightness in the CD20$^+$ and CD19$^+$ neoplastic B cells. Typical CLL cells are dimly CD20$^+$ and CD19$^+$, dimly sIg$^+$ with κ–light-chain restriction, and coexpress CD5 and CD23. They are FMC7$^-$. Prolymphocytes are brighter for CD20, CD19, and sIg, and they have lost CD5 and CD23. They are FMC7$^+$. *Note:* In these histograms the quadrants, rather than populations, have been colored.

Follicular lymphoma

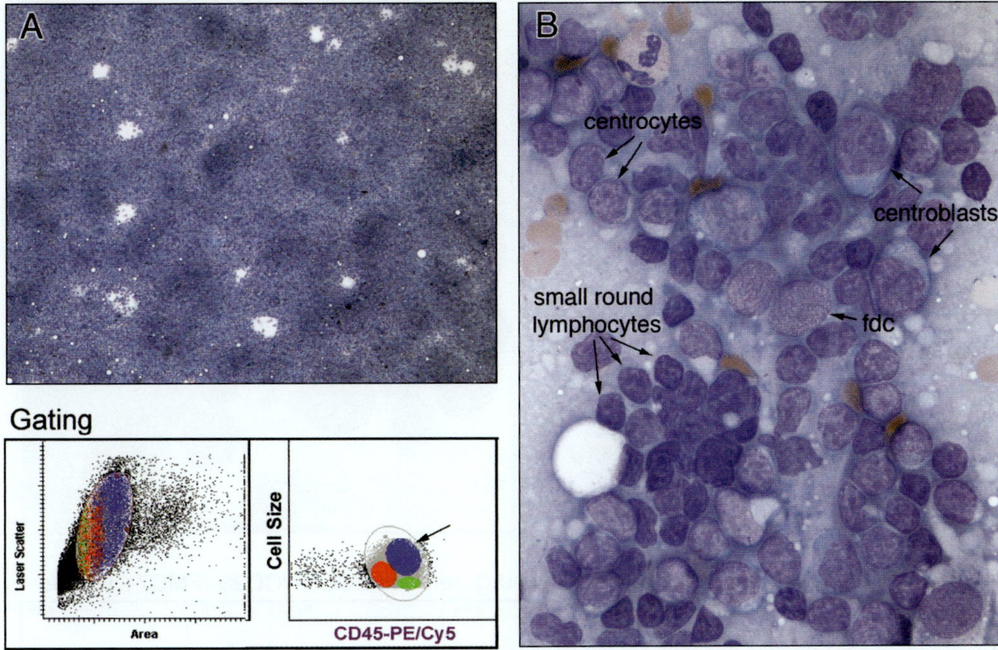

Fine Needle Aspirate Immunophenotyping: lambda CD10+ B cells

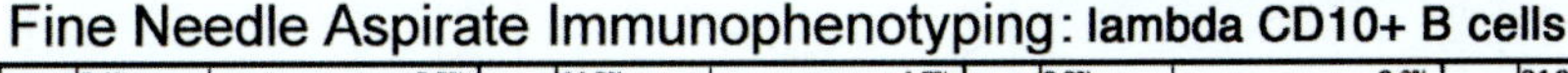

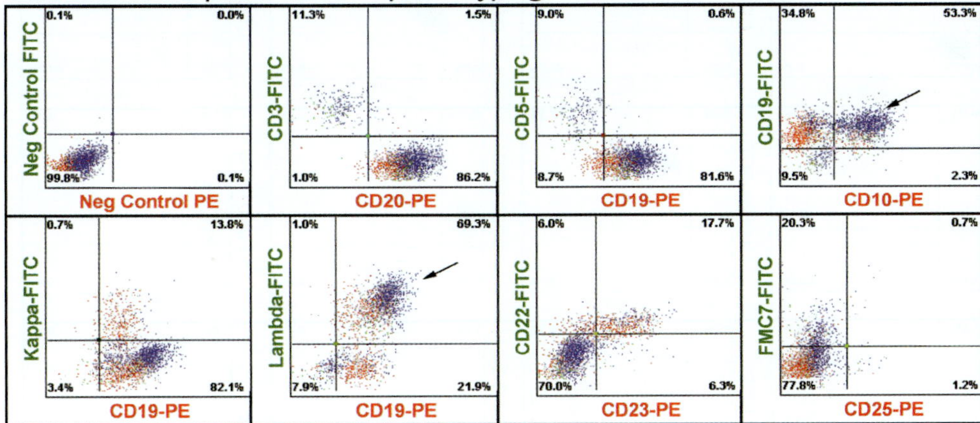

Figure 7.11 Follicular lymphoma. Statistically, follicular lymphoma is the most frequently encountered lymphoproliferative disorder in fine-needle aspiration cytology. In a smear prepared by the method shown, follicular aggregates are usually visible at low power. The follicular dendritic cell (FDC) meshwork binding these follicles together is evident at high-power examination. FDCs, frequently seen as "kissing" nuclei, are characterized by a finely reticulated chromatin and small central nucleoli. Within the follicular aggregates small round lymphocytes, centrocytes characterized by clumped chromatin without nucleoli, and centroblasts characterized by more open chromatin and one or more peripherally placed nucleoli are also present. Immunophenotypic analysis typically shows a B-cell predominance, but the clonally restricted population may be partially obscured by polytypic B cells, depending on the extent of lymph node involvement. The clonally restricted B cells are typically CD10[+](*arrows*) and often express CD23. FISH for t(14;18) may be useful in equivocal cases. The MIB1 fraction is typically lower than 25%. The proportion of centroblasts within the follicular aggregates corresponds roughly to the grading system of Mann and Berard.

Mantle cell lymphoma (blastoid variant)

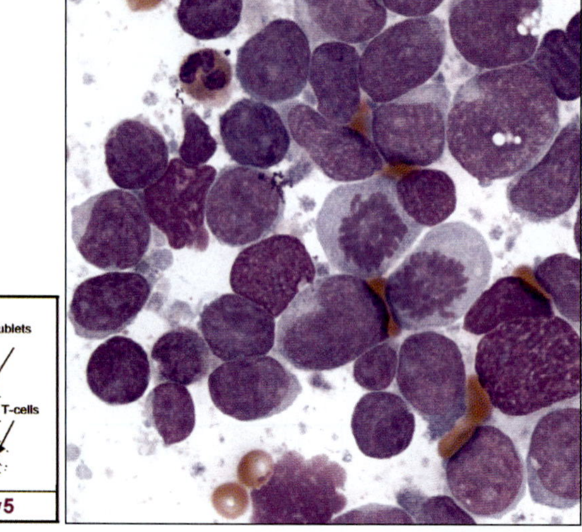

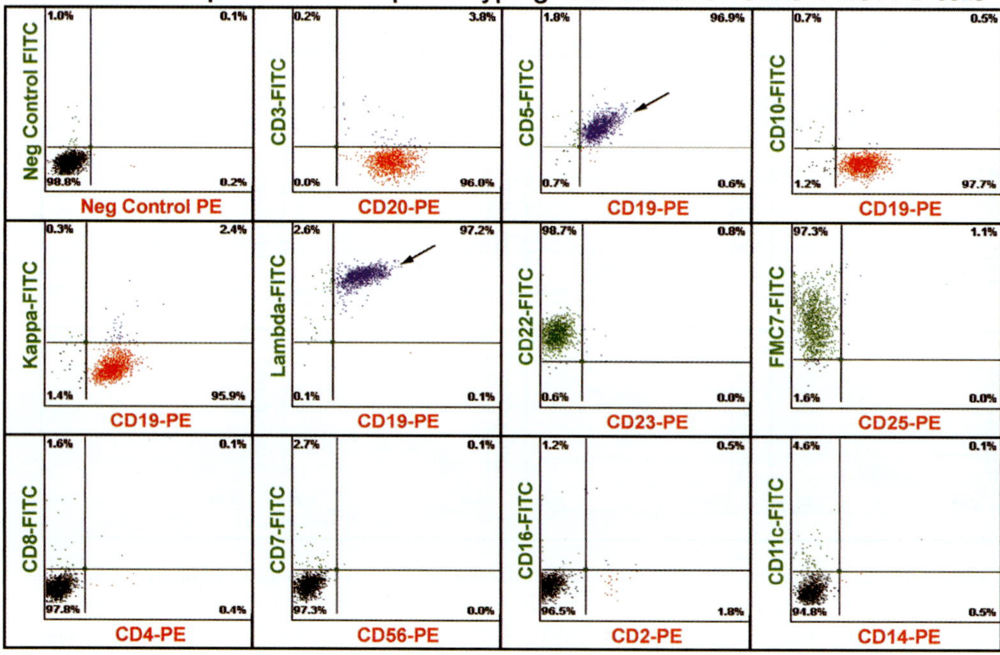

Figure 7.12 Mantle cell lymphoma. The morphology of mantle-cell lymphoma is highly variable, although the immunophenotype is quite constant. In this example, as is typical, the cells are brightly CD20[+] and FMC7[+] and very brightly sIg[+] (λ–light-chain restricted), and they show the usual coexpression of CD5 (*arrows*) and lack of expression of CD10. The cytomorphology in this case is that of the "blastoid" variant. The cells were tetraploid, and all showed the t(11;14). More typically, a highly monotonous population of slightly enlarged and irregular lymphocytes, interrupted only by occasional histiocytes, is seen on the smear. The MIB1 proliferation fraction may be highly variable in mantle-cell lymphoma. In this example, the immunophenotyping histograms show the convention of "colored quadrants."

Marginal cell lymphoma

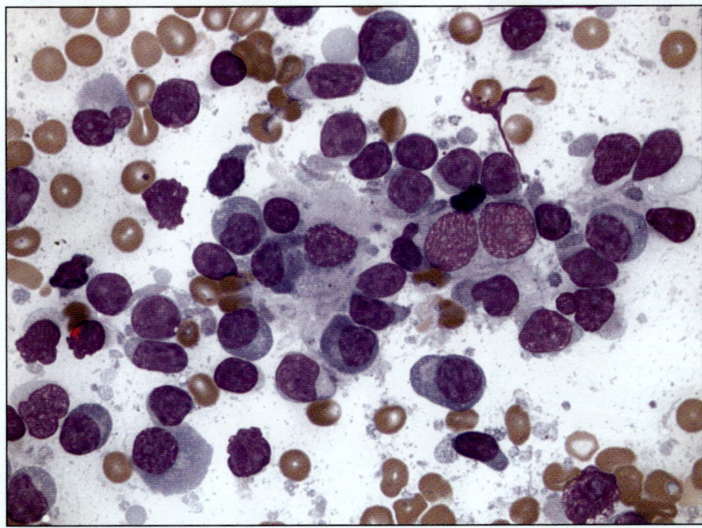

Gating

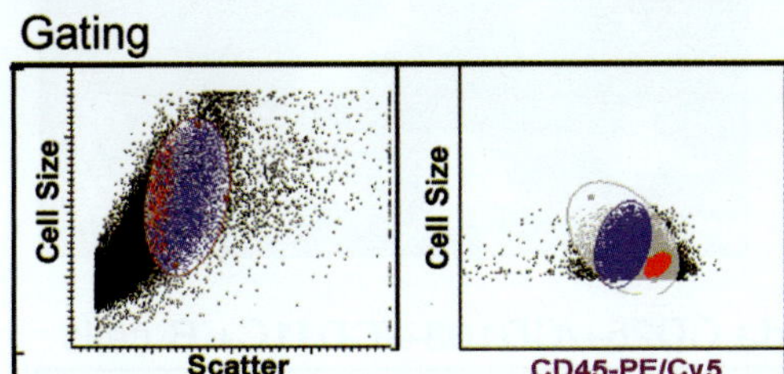

Fine Needle Aspirate Immunophenotyping: kappa CD23-/FMC7- B cells

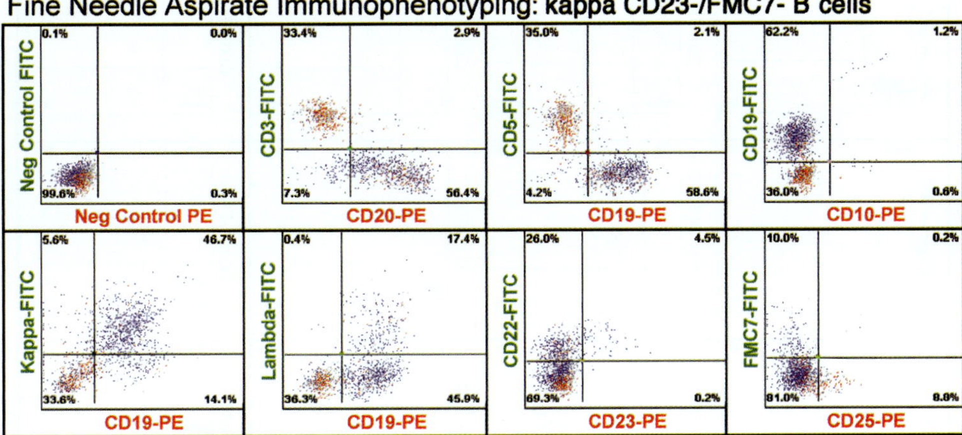

Figure 7.13 Marginal zone lymphoma. Because the immunophenotype is *null* or nonspecific, and the t(11;18) is often not present, it is difficult to make a definitive diagnosis of nodal marginal zone lymphoma from fine-needle aspiration. This example shows the typical lack of CD5 and CD10 in the clonally restricted B-cell population. Usually, some remnants of follicular architecture are evident in the smear, and high-power examination shows plasma cells and plasmacytoid cells. Monocytoid B cells are less evident in Romanowsky Giemsa stain preparations than in paraffin sections.

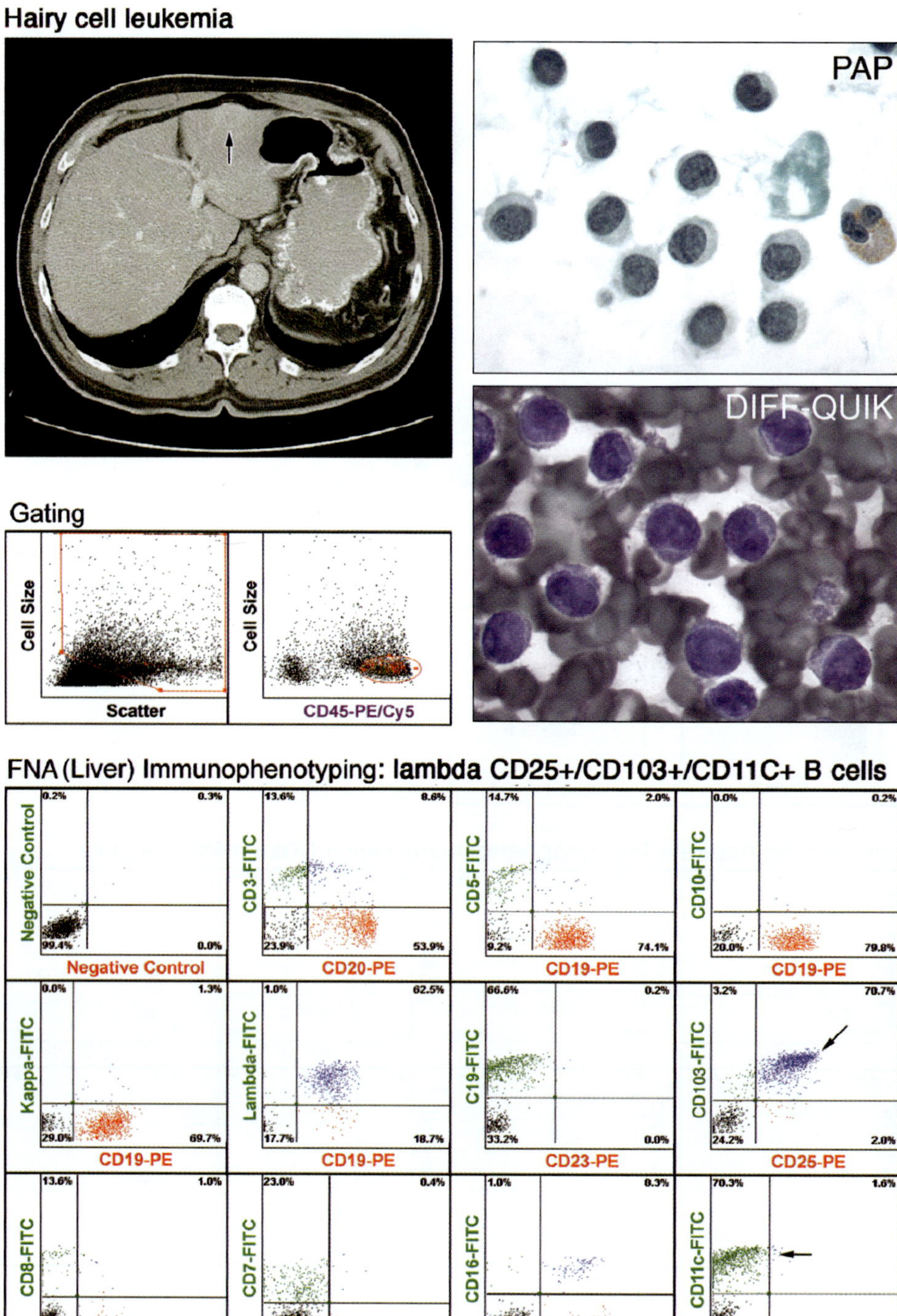

Figure 7.14   Hairy cell leukemia (HCL). Axial CT shows a liver mass in a patient with a history of hairy cell leukemia believed to be in hematologic remission. It was thought unlikely that this represented organ involvement by HCL. Fine-needle aspiration of the liver nodule showed a population of monotonous cells with slightly indented or reniform nuclei. Air-dried and Diff-Quik-stained cells revealed variable numbers of fine cytoplasmic protrusions. The immunophenotyping in this case shows an artifact due to poor regulation of the photomultiplier tube collecting signal from FITC. In each case, saturation has occurred, making CD20, FMC7 and CD11c appear less bright than would be expected from HCL. Nonetheless, the immunophenotype, brightly CD20$^+$, dimly sIg$^+$ with λ–light-chain restriction, coexpression of CD25 and FMC7, and expression of CD11c is characteristic (*arrows*).

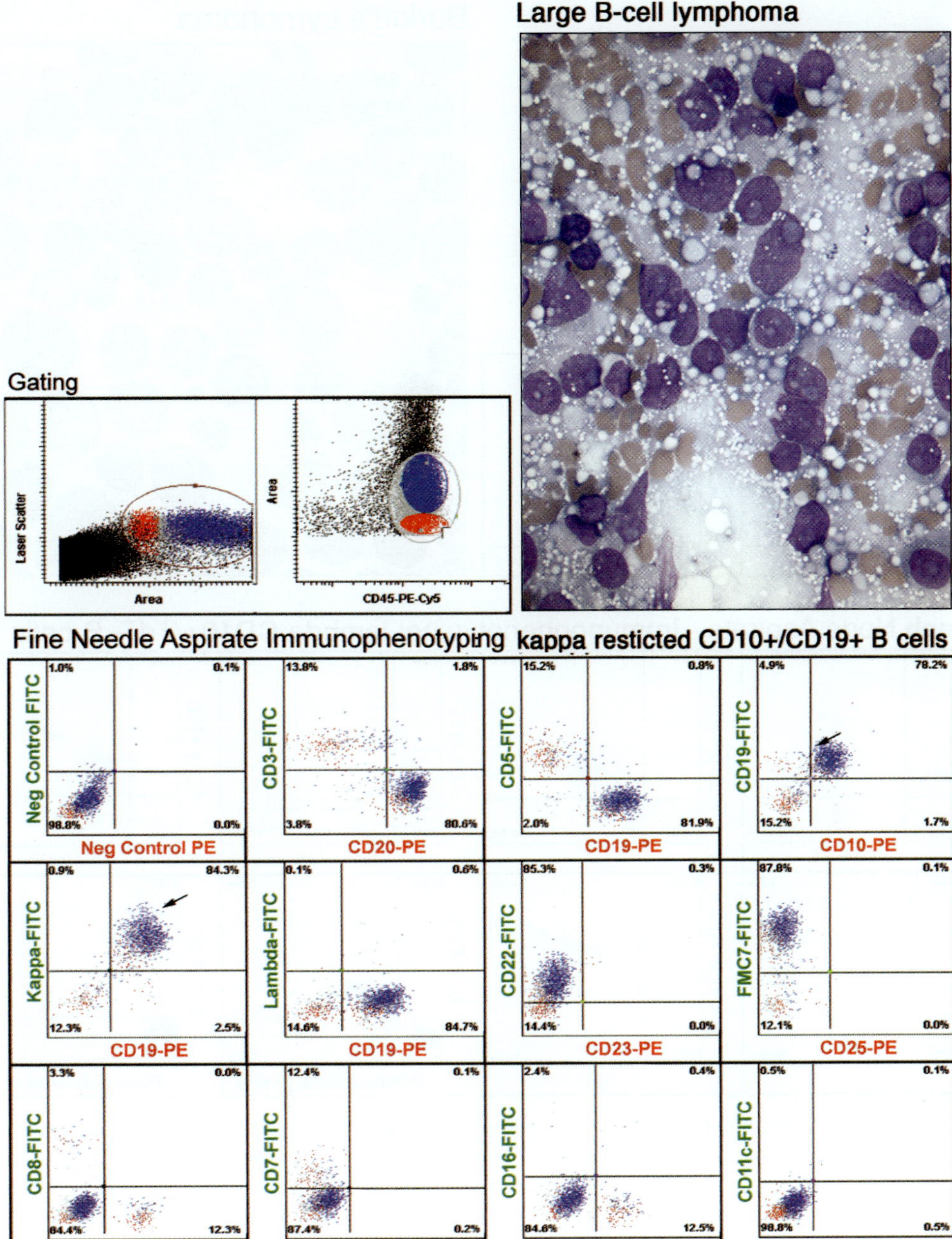

Figure 7.15 Large B-cell lymphoma. Large B-cell lymphoma represents the second most frequently encountered lymphoproliferative disorder in cytology. The morphology is extremely heterogeneous, united only by the finding of significant numbers of morphologically abnormal large cells with prominent nucleoli. Immunophenotyping usually shows expression of surface immunoglobulin with light-chain restriction but, in some cases, the cells fail to express surface immunoglobulin. A significant percentage of cases show expression of CD10 (*arrows*), in some cases raising the possibility of Burkitt or atypical Burkitt lymphoma as a differential diagnosis. Note that in the gating histogram in this case the neoplastic population is significantly larger than the non-neoplastic T cells. In most cases of follicular lymphoma grade 3, intact follicular aggregates are present in the smear. Aspiration cytology, however, cannot reliably distinguish between diffuse large B-cell lymphoma and follicular lymphoma grade 3 in all cases.

Burkitt's Lymphoma

Gating

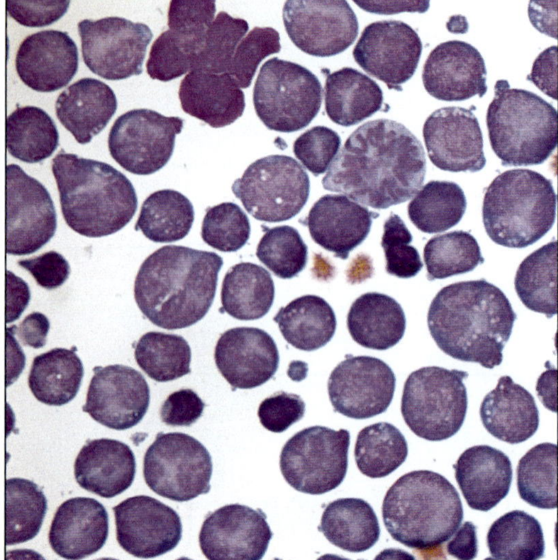

Lymph Node Aspirate - Immunophenotyping: lambda CD10+/TdT- B cells

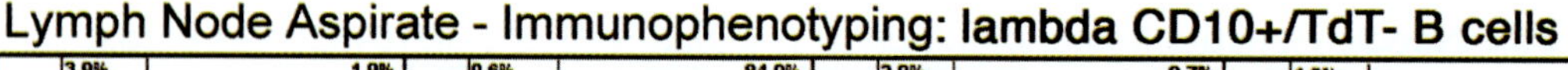

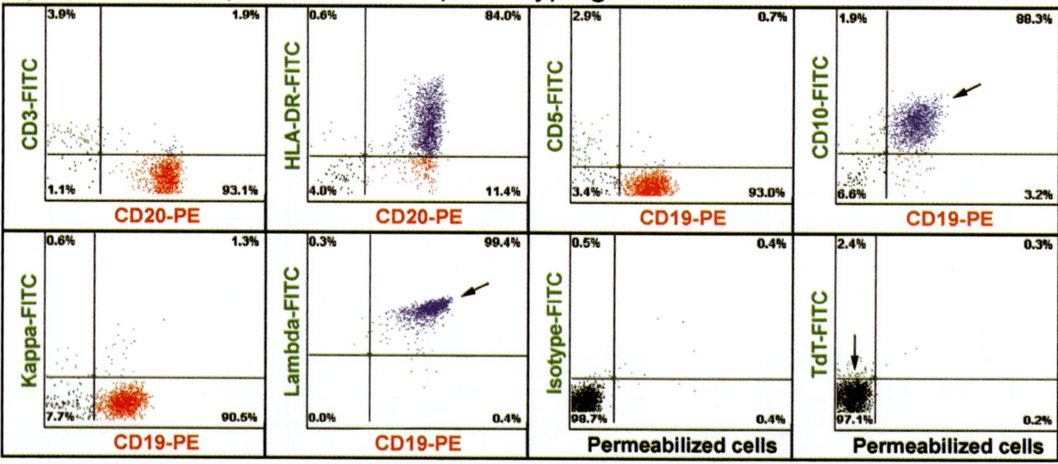

Figure 7.16 Burkitt and Burkitt-like (atypical Burkitt) lymphoma. Aspirates from Burkitt or Burkitt-like lymphoma are usually highly cellular, but may contain large amounts of apoptotic debris and necrotic cells. The diagnosis is suggested by the typical medium-sized blasts with a narrow rim of deep blue cytoplasm containing variable numbers of vacuoles. The typical brightly CD20+, HLA DR+, CD10+, and brightly sIg+ immunophenotype is illustrated (*arrows*). Immunophenotyping by laser scanning cytometry using Clatch's method provides the opportunity of permeabilizing cells already *in situ* on the slide, reapplying antibody and looking for evidence of cytoplasmic antigens such as TdT (colored quadrants).

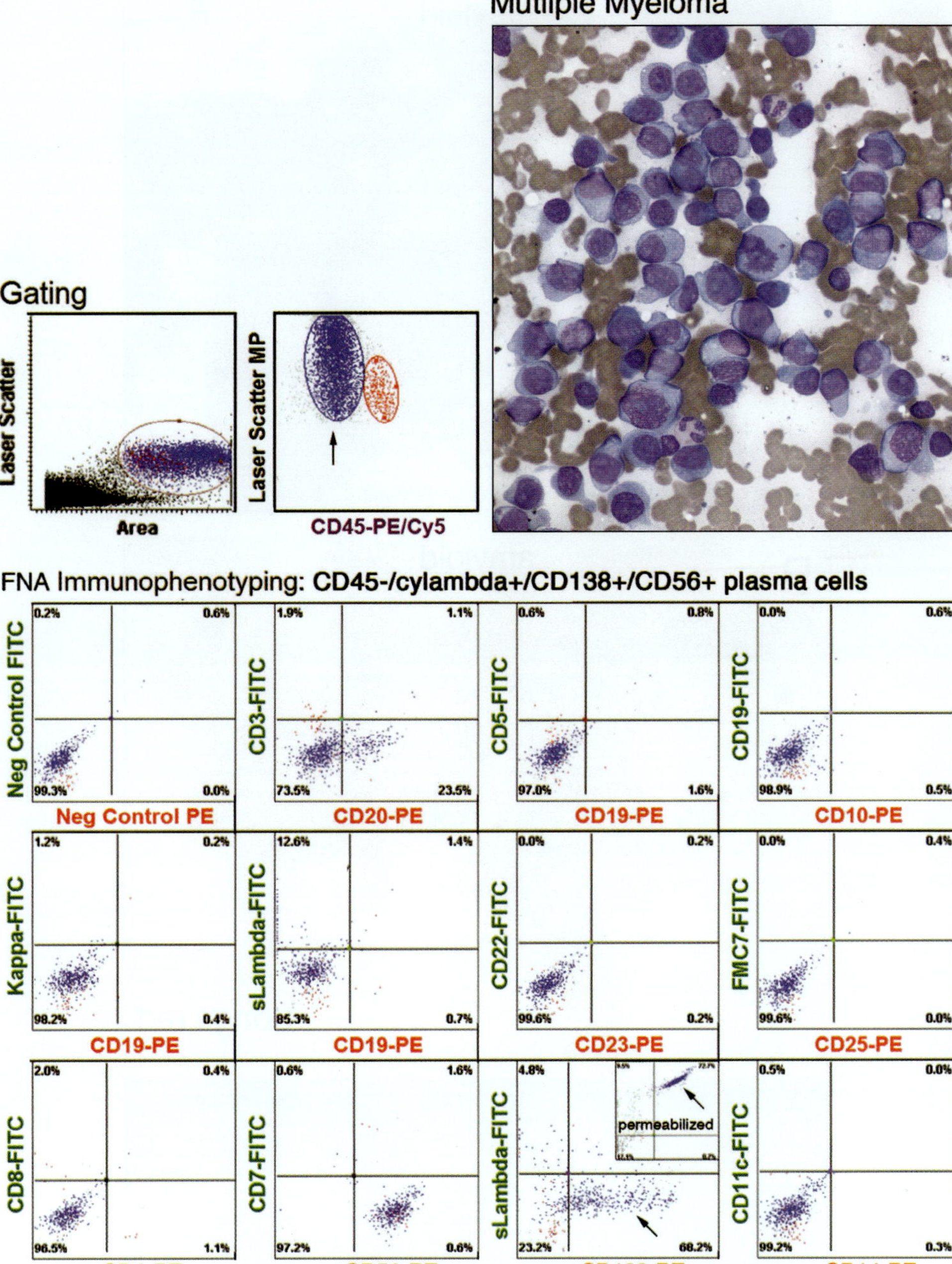

Figure 7.17   Plasma cell myeloma (plasmacytoma). Plasmacytomas frequently are aspirated in patients with known myeloma and occasionally are the first specimen obtained on presentation. When all the cells demonstrate typical plasma cell morphology, immunohistochemical demonstration of light-chain restricted strong cytoplasmic immunoglobulin, and positivity for CD138 is usually sufficient for confirmation of the diagnosis. Immunophenotyping may be useful when less well-differentiated populations are present or a majority of the cells have "plasmablastic" morphology, as in this case. Laser scanning cytometry shows a dominant population of CD45-dim or negative cells, which fail to express surface immunoglobulin, but in which strong cytoplasmic immunoglobulin can be demonstrated after permeabilization and restaining of the cells (*arrows*).

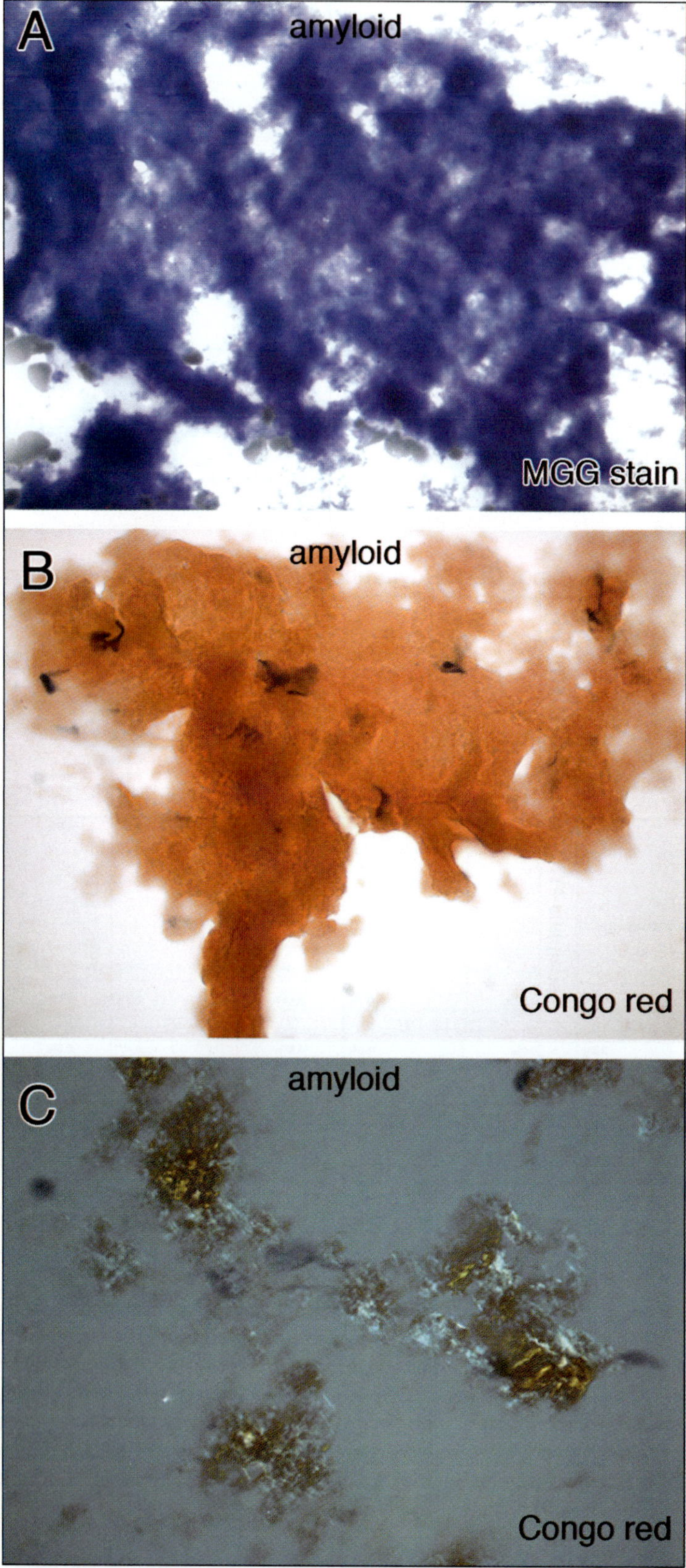

Figure 7.18 Amyloidosis. Rarely, amyloid may be aspirated from lymph nodes or other subcutaneous masses, as in this patient with plasma-cell myeloma. In air-dried and Romanowsky Giemsa-stained material, the pattern superficially resembles necrosis, but no outlines of cells are visible. Congo-red staining and polarized light microscopy confirm the diagnosis.

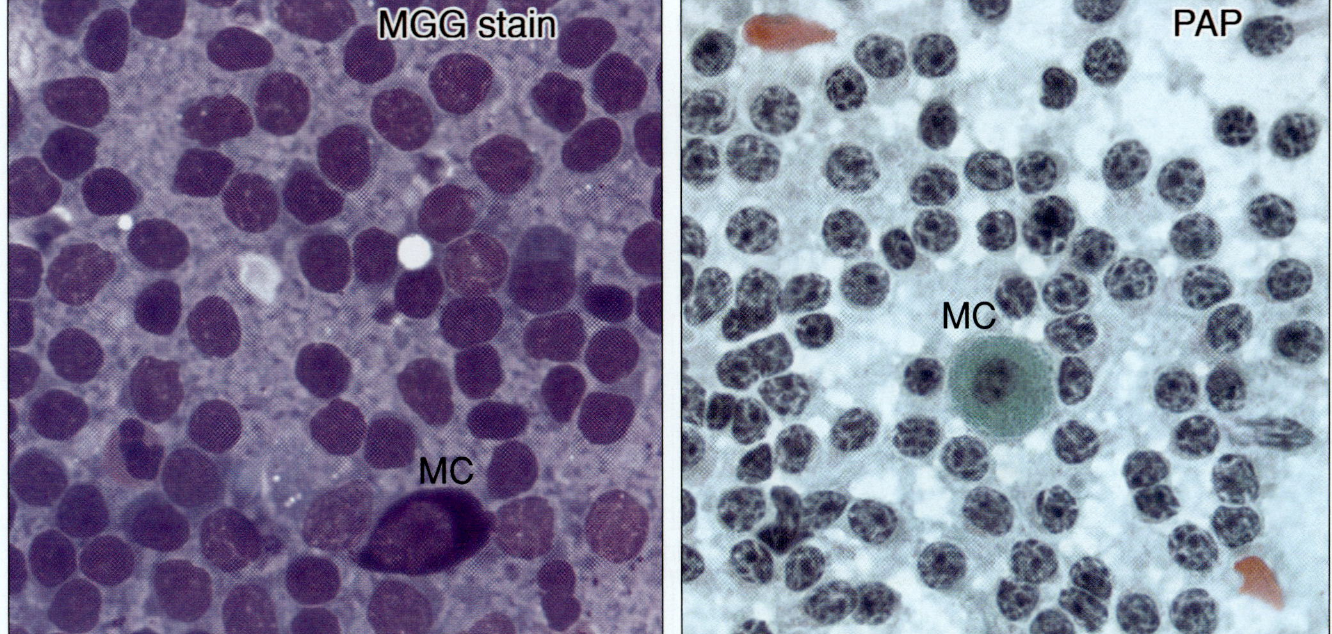

Figure 7.19 Lymphoplasmacytic lymphoma in patient with Waldenström macroglobulinemia. In this case, the May-Grunwald-Giemsa-stained smears show extremely heavy background staining due to the high levels of IgM (*left panel*). The characteristic clock-face nuclear morphology is better seen in the Papanicolaou-stained slide (*right panel*). Without clinical and other laboratory findings, FNA biopsy samples of lymphoplasmacytic lymphoma cannot be differentiated from marginal-zone lymphoma. Many cases of lymphoplasmacytic lymphoma do contain significant numbers of mast cells (MC).

Reactive T cells in CSF

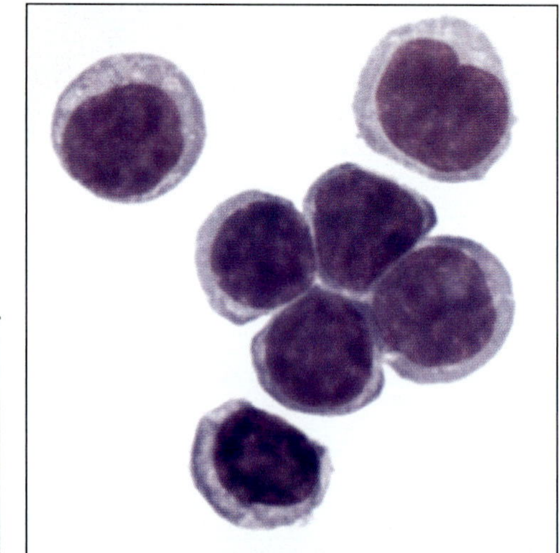

Gating

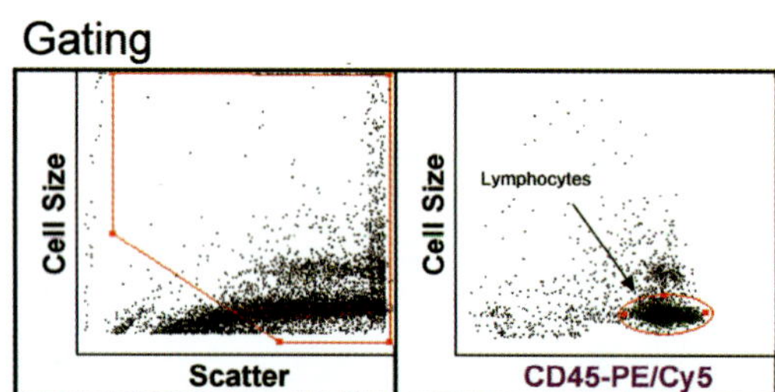

Cerebrospinal Fluid Immunophenotyping: normal T-cell pattern

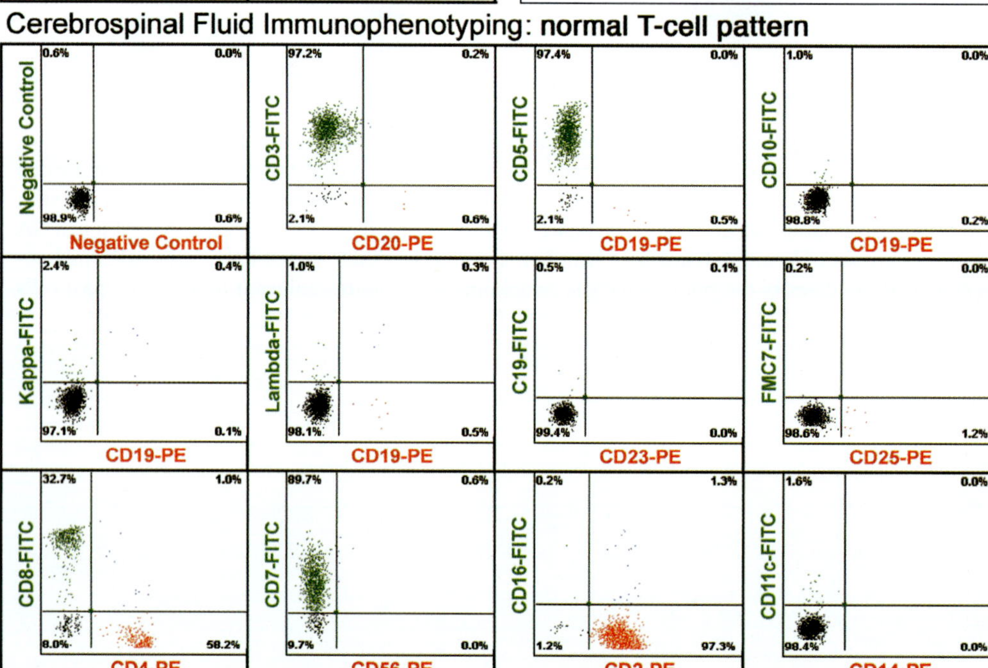

Figure 7.20 Reactive lymphoid population in cerebrospinal fluid (CSF). The low total cell number in small aliquots of CSF may make immunophenotypic analysis difficult. In patients with a history of lymphoma or imaging findings suspicious for leptomeningeal disease, a full panel of T-cell, B-cell, NK, and myeloid antigens may be desired. As in the case illustrated here, the morphologic findings may appear to be those of reactive lymphocytes, but some cells can show nuclear irregularity that can cause diagnostic ambiguity. Cytospin preparations are notorious for exaggerating nuclear lobulations or indentations. Laser scanning cytometry can provide assessment of a full panel of antigens using as few as 50,000 to 60,000 cells, as seen in this example of CSF lymphocytosis caused by pseudotumor cerebri (colored quadrants).

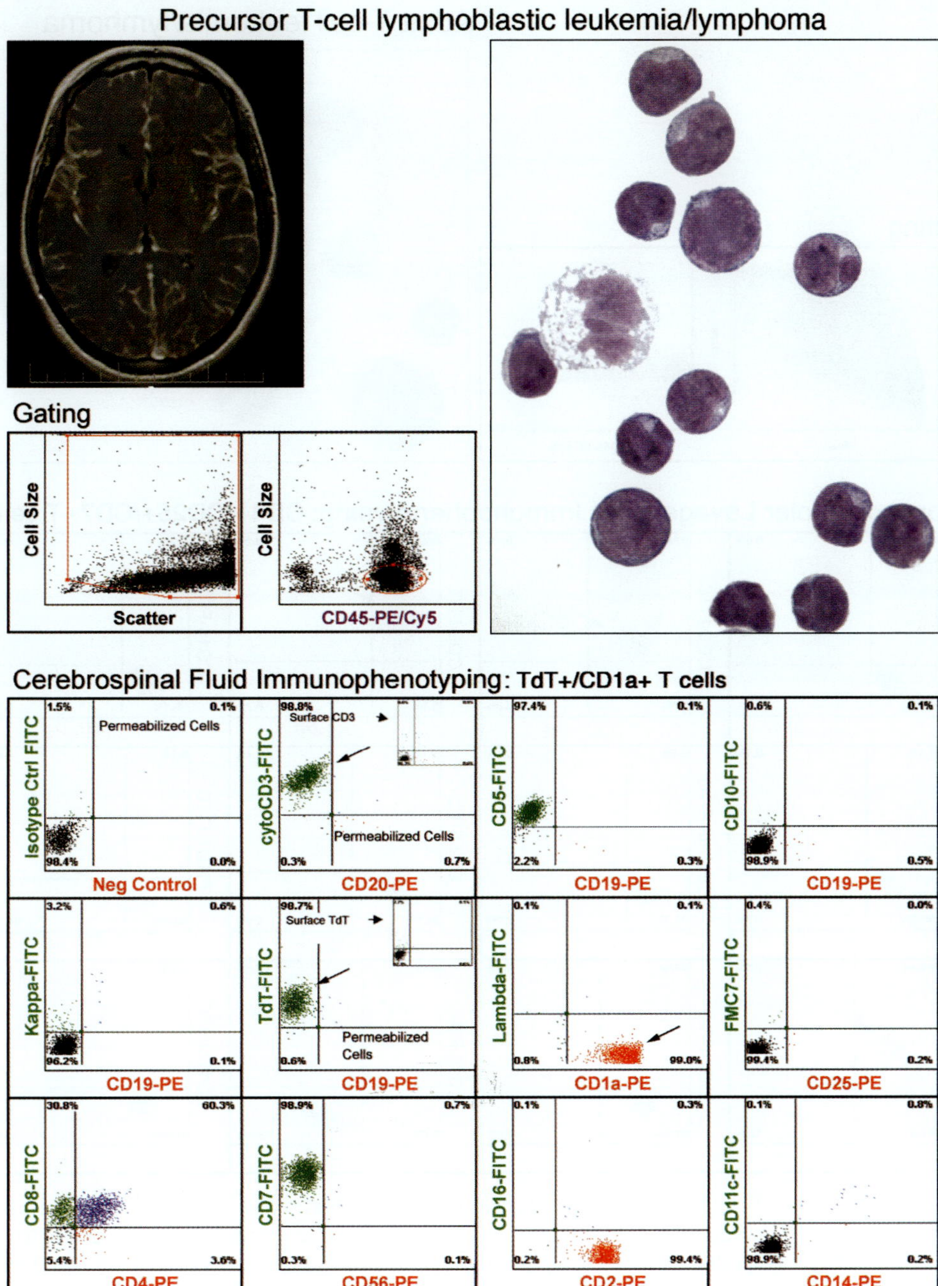

Figure 7.21 Precursor T-cell lymphoblastic leukemia lymphoma (T-ALL). In this patient with treated T-ALL, leptomeningeal enhancement suggested CNS relapse. About 60,000 cells were available for assessment. The blasts seen morphologically are confirmed as T-ALL by the absence of surface CD3 with uniform cytoplasmic CD3, co-expression CD4 and CD8 positivity for CDIa, and presence of TdT (*arrows*). Cytoplasmic antigens were demonstrated by permeabilizing and restaining cells found negative in the initial analysis, shown in insets (colored quadrants).

Adult T-cell leukemia/lymhoma

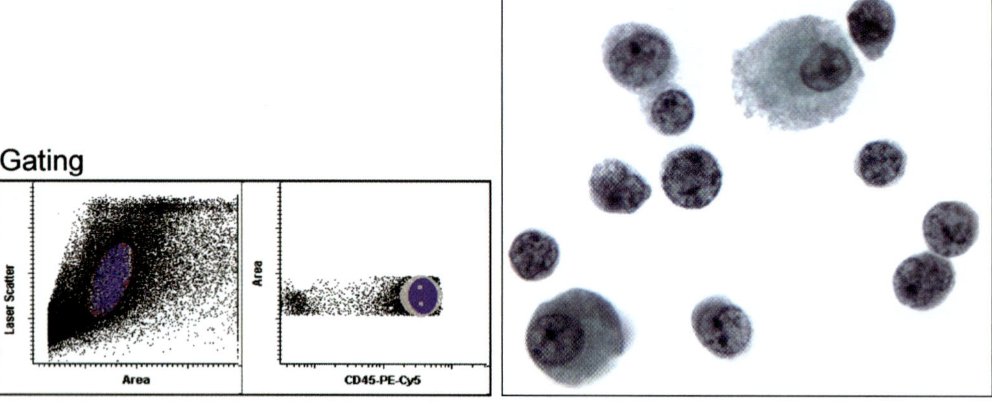

Bronchoalveolar Lavage Fluid Immunophenotyping: CD4+/CD25+/CD7- T cells

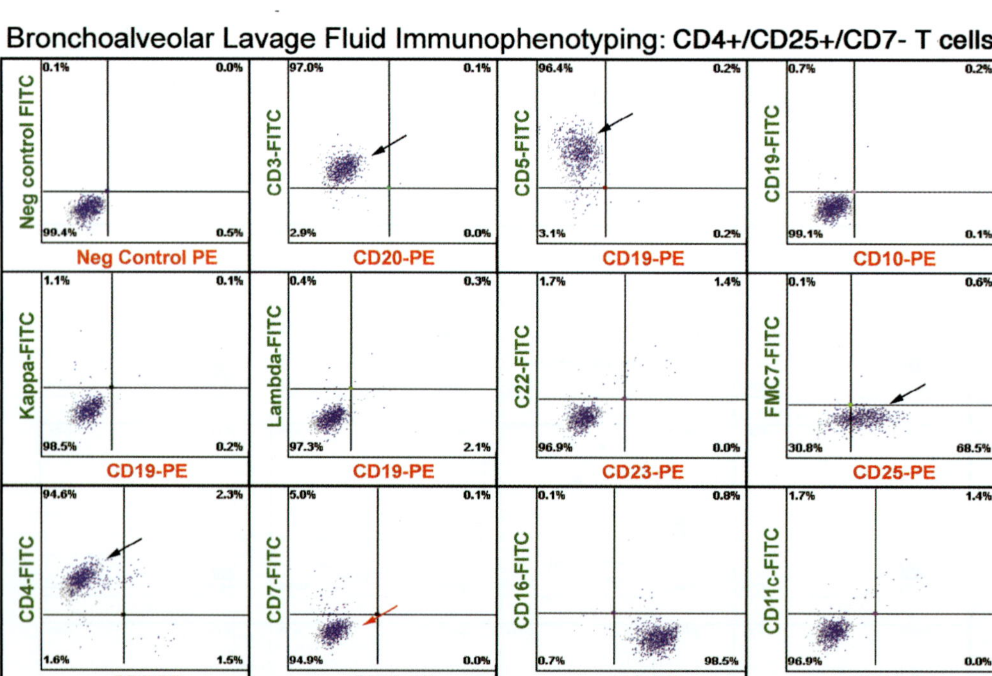

Figure 7.22   Adult T-cell leukemia/lymphoma (ATLL) in bronchoalveolar lavage fluid. This patient with a history of "smoldering" ATLL underwent bronchoalveolar lavage to investigate pulmonary infiltrates. Morphologically abnormal lymphocytes were found in Papanicolaou-stained Thin-Prep slides. Laser scanning cytometric immunophenotyping shows that these cells demonstrate an abnormal T-cell phenotype, with complete loss of CD7, subset restriction (CD4), and expression of CD25 (*arrows*), confirming parenchymal infiltration by ATLL.

Thymoma

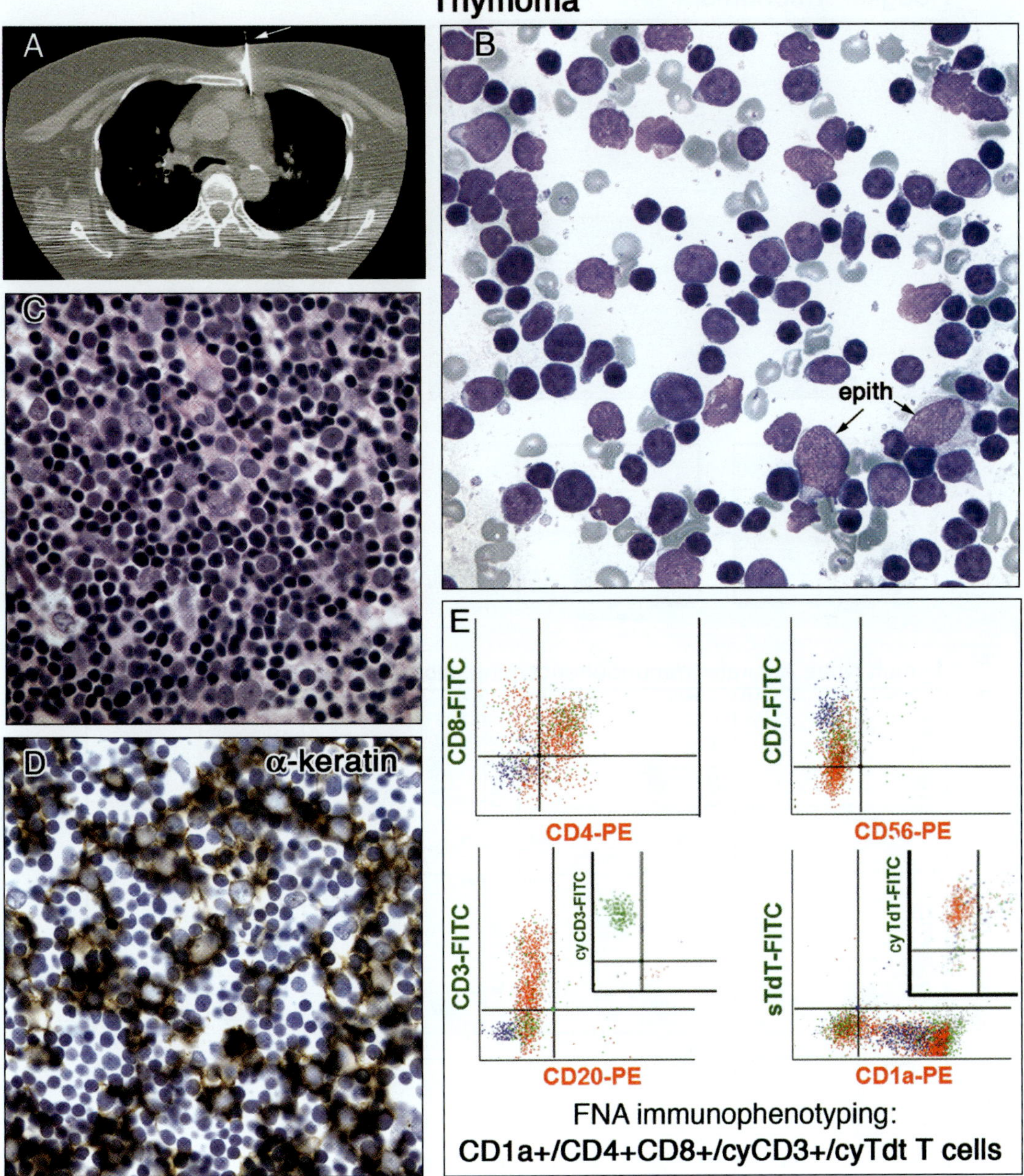

Figure 7.23 Thymoma. The imaging differential diagnosis of an anterior mediastinal mass may include both thymoma and lymphoblastic lymphoma. Panel A shows an axial computed tomography (CT) scan of the thorax and highlights a needle placed through the chest wall into an anterior mediastinal mass. Thymic epithelial cells ("epith" in *panel B*) may be difficult to appreciate in the cytology smears. Sections taken from the cell block reveal dual populations of small lymphoid cells and larger epithelioid cells. Immunohistochemistry (*panel D*) displays the keratin-positive epithelial cells. Scanning cytometry (*panel E*) in this case showed an initial gating histogram in which there were three populations of brightness for CD45. The CD45-dim cells have been colored blue, the intermediate population green, and the CD45-bright cells red. The CD45-dim and intermediate cells (blue and green) are negative for surface CD3, and were dimly positive for CD5, and positive for CD10. The CD45-bright cells (*red*) show a "smear" pattern of variable expression of sCD3 from negative to bright and demonstrated a bimodal pattern of expression of CD5 (dim and moderate), and were negative for CD10. Note the inset in the top right-hand corner of the CD3 versus CD20 histogram, illustrating strong expression of cytoplasmic CD3 in all cells. The CD45-dim cells (*blue*) are double negative for CD4/CD8, and the CD45-intermediate cells (*green*) are double positive, as are the majority of the CD45-bright (*red*) cells. The blue population is bright for CD7 and intermediate for CD1a, whereas the red population again shows a "smear" of positivity for CD7. Note that all the cells are TDT$^+$ after fixation and permeabilization. These findings illustrate the full maturation sequence of T cells, typical of thymocytes as found in thymoma.

Hodgkin lymphoma

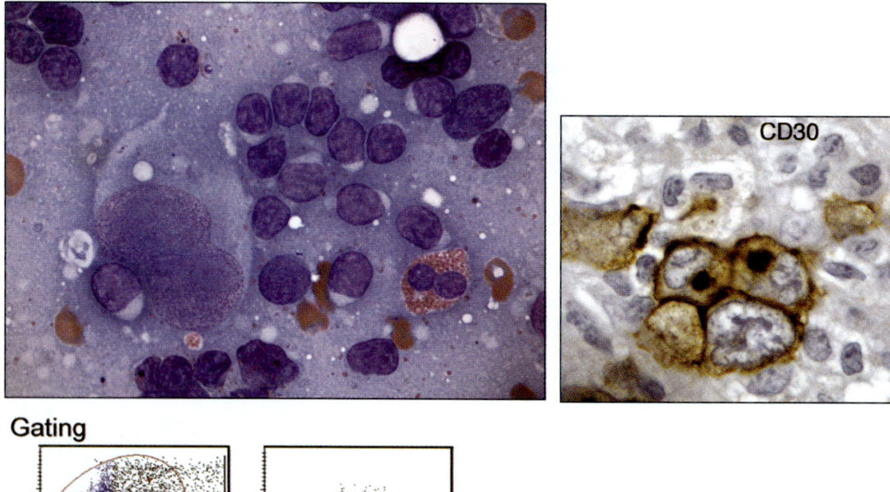

Gating

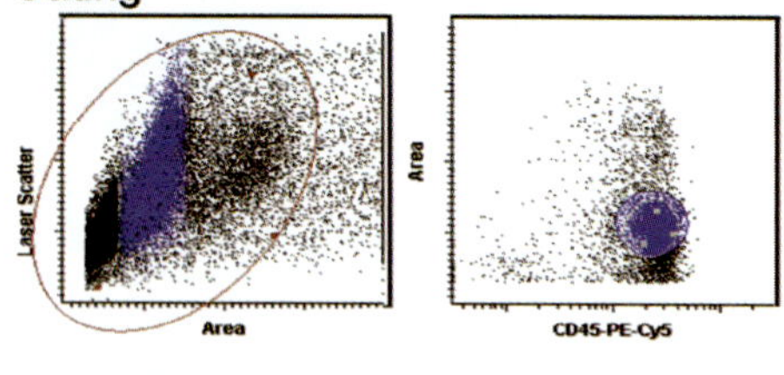

Lymph Node Aspirate Immunophenotyping: mostly CD4+ T cells

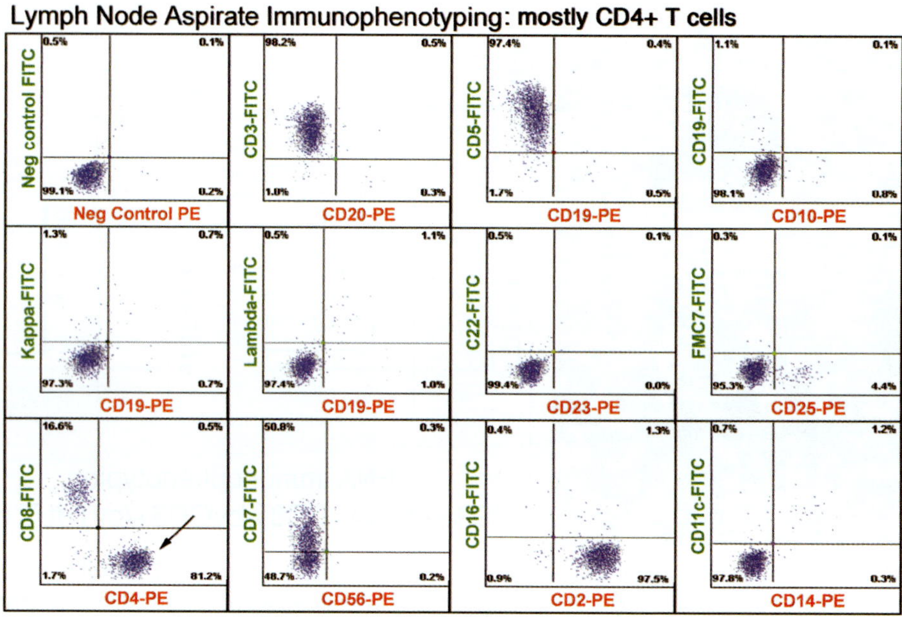

Figure 7.24 Classical Hodgkin lymphoma. Aspirates from Hodgkin lymphoma usually show a characteristic pattern of large pleomorphic cells set against a background of morphologically normal small lymphocytes and variable numbers of granulocytes. Hodgkin cells (mononuclear RS cells) and classical Reed-Sternberg cells are characterized by extremely fragile, pale cytoplasm, and bare nuclear forms are common. In May-Grunwald-Giemsa-stained preparations, the huge inclusion-like nucleoli are usually pale-blue structures against a finely reticulated purple nucleus. In some cases, the diagnostic immunophenotype of classical Hodgkin lymphoma (CD45$^-$, CD15$^+$, CD30$^+$) can be confirmed in cell block material (as illustrated here) or in cytospin preparations. Because of the fragility of the cytoplasm, staining in cytospin preparations is often inadequate or ambiguous. Cell surface marker immunophenotyping using any modality is usually not useful. If performed, a dominant population of T cells with normal immunophenotype showing a strong predominance of CD4 T-helper cells is found (*arrow*).

Chloroma (acute monocytic leukemia)

Gating and Compensation

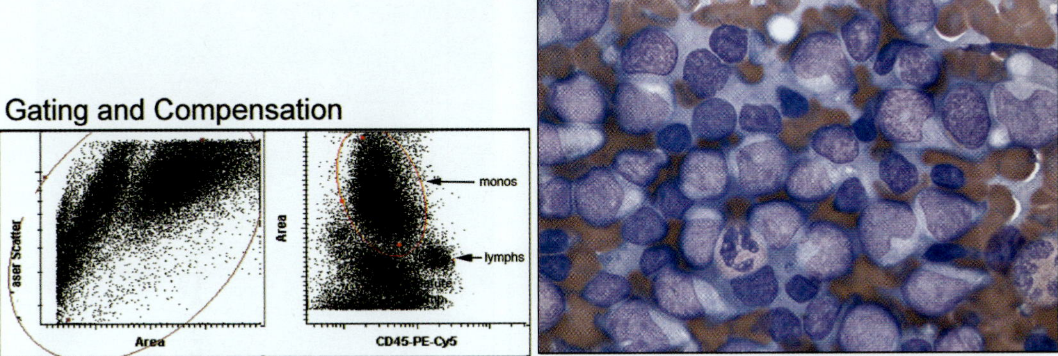

Fine Needle Aspirate Immunophenotyping: CD11C+/CD14+/CD4+ monocytic precursors

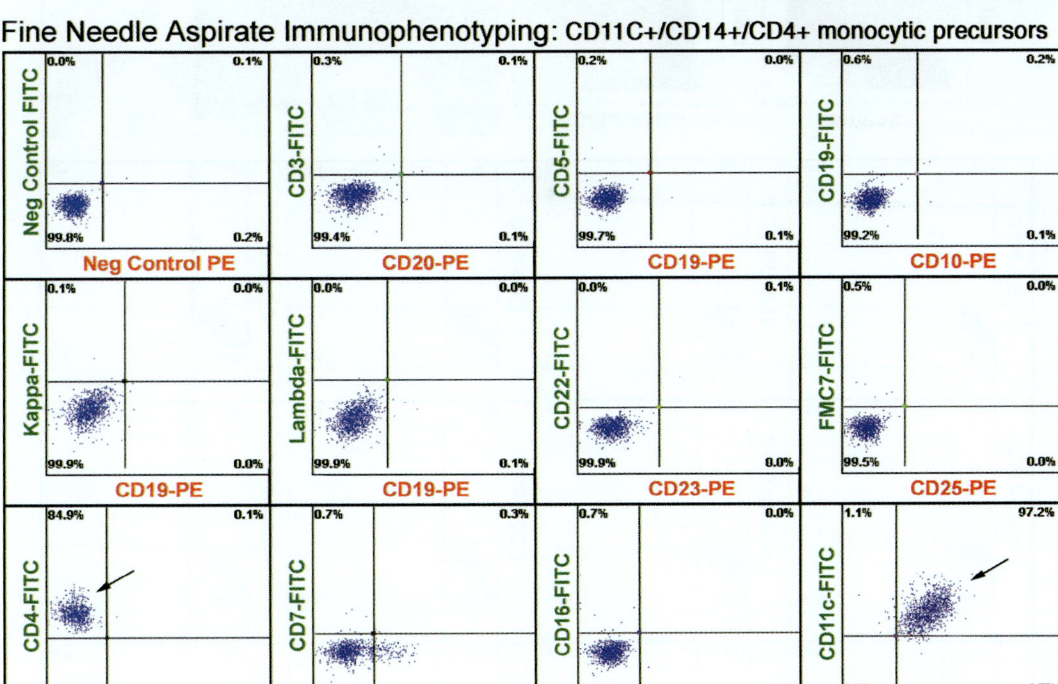

Figure 7.25 Chloroma (granulocytic sarcoma of lymph node) in acute monoblastic leukemia. This patient was referred to an ear, nose, and throat (ENT) surgeon for cervical lymphadenopathy. Fine-needle aspiration of cervical nodes showed large blast-like cells with histiocytic or monocytic features. Immunophenotyping showed that these cells were dimly positive for CD45 and positive only for CD4, CD11c, and CD14, in the usual lymphoid panel used for lymph node assessment (*arrows*). Examination of peripheral blood and bone marrow confirmed acute monoblastic leukemia.

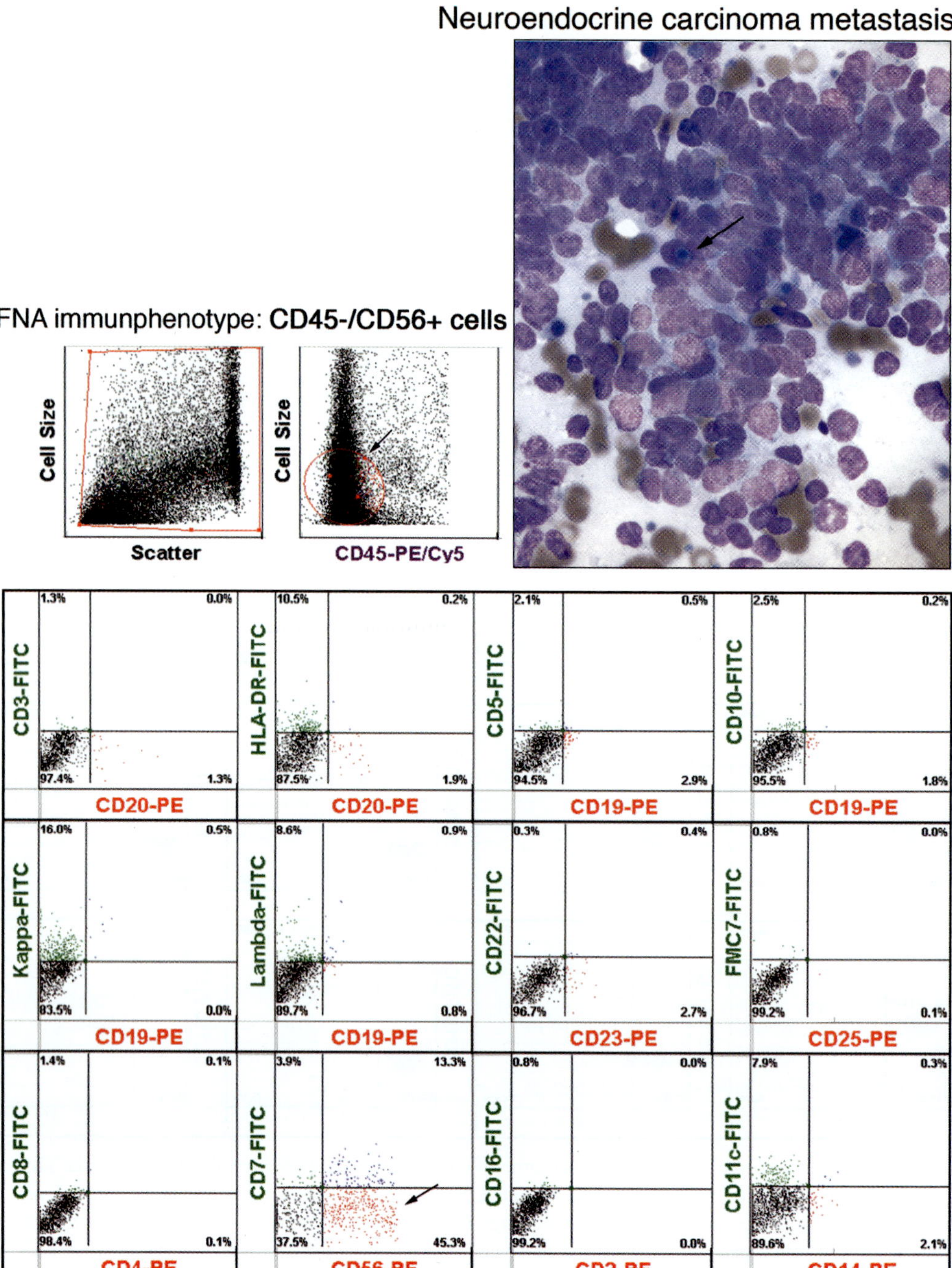

Figure 7.26 Metastatic small-cell anaplastic carcinoma. Lymph nodes involved by poorly differentiated neuroendocrine neoplasms occasionally may be misclassified as malignant lymphoma. The diagnosis usually is clarified by the absence of lymphoglandular bodies in the background of a smear and the finding of occasional cohesive groups of cells displaying nuclear molding. Another useful finding illustrated here is the presence of the so-called "blue bodies." These structures usually represent the punctate accumulation of cytokeratin filaments within the cytoplasm of these neuroendocrine-type cells. Subjected to cell surface marker immunophenotyping, the cells are CD45$^-$ and are usually negative for all lymphoid markers except CD56 (*arrow*).

Approach to the Microscopic Evaluation of Blood and Bone Marrow

Douglas C. Tkachuk, MD, FRCPC, and Jan V. Hirschmann, MD

EXAMINATION OF THE PERIPHERAL BLOOD

Slide Preparation and Staining

Preparations for examining peripheral blood can employ either cover slips or slides. With the former, a drop of blood is placed on a cover slip and a second one is set over the first. Sliding the two apart creates smears on both, which can then be stained and mounted on slides. For preparations using slides, a drop of blood is put near the end of one slide, and a second slide (the spreader) is placed at a 30- to 45-degree angle medial to the blood. The spreader is pulled back into the blood, allowing it to extend along the slide's edge. The spreader is then rapidly pushed forward to produce the smear. Machines also can prepare blood films, either using a similar spreading procedure or by spinning a slide with a drop of blood on it, using centrifugal force to spread the blood across the glass.

The dyes used for blood smears contain a mixture of eosin and methylene blue that Romanowsky, a Russian protozoologist, first employed in 1890 to see malaria parasites. Subsequent modifications are May-Grünwald-Giemsa and Wright stains, the former commonly used in Europe, the latter in North America. Both contain eosin and methylene azures, which are derivatives of methylene blue. Eosin is acidic and gives a red to orange color to the alkaline components of cells, such as hemoglobin and the granules of eosinophils, which contain an alkaline spermine derivative. The alkaline methylene azures give a blue to bluish-purple color to the acidic cellular elements, including the nucleic acids (DNA, RNA), nucleoproteins, and the granules of basophils, which contain the acid heparin.

Slide Examination

Properly stained slides are usually pink. Bluish discoloration can arise from too thick a smear, an overly lengthy staining time, or excessively alkaline buffer in the dyes. The slide also may be blue because the blood contains excessive amounts of plasma proteins in such diseases as multiple myeloma.

Microscopic examination should begin at low power ($\times$10 or $\times$20 objective) to determine the adequacy of staining; to detect abnormalities in cell number, type, or aggregation; and to find the optimal area to examine platelets, red cells, granulocytes, and lymphoid cells. For red cells, the best location occurs where the erythrocytes are in a single layer, close to one another, but not overlapping. White cells often are seen best in the thicker portions of the slide. A view at higher power ($\times$40 to $\times$50 objective) allows an assessment of cell size and number and a closer examination of the individual elements. Oil immersion lenses ($\times$50 and $\times$100) provide greater magnification to see finer objects, such as cytoplasmic granules, cellular inclusions, and chromatin patterns in the nucleus.

EXAMINATION OF THE BONE MARROW ASPIRATE SMEAR AND THE CLOT SECTION

Slide Preparation and Staining

The technique used to prepare slides from bone marrow aspirates is similar to that used for making blood films and should result in well-separated spicules of marrow at one end of the slide (see Fig. 8.15). Care should be taken to ensure that bone marrow spicules are present in the drop of marrow fluid applied to the slide. Another method, the "pull" technique, is used to prepare crush (or squash) preparations that result in marrow spicules being concentrated in the central area of the slide. This facilitates accurate differential marrow cell counts and the appreciation of megakaryocyte numbers. After spreading, the aspirate smears are allowed to air dry; this is followed by fixation in methanol and then staining, either manually or automatically using a dipping-style slide stainer, with May-Grünwald-Giemsa or Wright stains.

The three most common histochemical stains used to evaluate aspirates in the hematology lab are Prussian blue (Perl) for iron stores and the myeloperoxidase (MPO) and nonspecific esterases (α-naphthyl butyrate or acetate) to evaluate the myeloid and monocytic lineages, respectively. Occasionally, other histochemical stains can be performed on aspirates including Sudan black as an alternative to MPO, toluidine blue to accentuate the metachromatic staining properties of granules in mast cells and basophils, and periodic acid-Schiff (PAS) to assess immature erythroid and T-cell precursors. On occasion, particularly when neither flow cytometry nor biopsy sections are available, selective immunohistochemistry or immunofluorescence panels can be performed on aspirate smears. Immunostains performed on aspirate smears, particularly for cell surface markers, often are difficult to interpret due to excessive nonspecific background staining. In addition, interphase fluorescent in-situ hybridization (FISH) for diagnostic chromosomal abnormalities, polymerase chain reaction (PCR) for assaying clonal B- and T-cell populations, and reverse transcriptase PCR (RTPCR) for detecting oncogenic fusion transcripts can be performed on aspirate smears for both diagnostic and minimal residual disease detection.

Slide Examination

Aspirate smears are first evaluated at low magnification using a 5× or 10× objective lens to ensure the sample contains spicules and is representative of the marrow cavity. Examination should be directed to areas near spicules containing intact marrow cells devoid of cytoplasmic stripping and excessive air-drying artifact (see Fig. 8.16). Abnormal cellular aggregates (e.g., clumps of metastatic cancer cells), and numbers of megakaryocytes are also best appreciated at low power (see Fig. 8.17). In normal aspirates, segmented granulocytes should be the predominant cell type seen at medium power (×20 to ×40) and an attempt to approximate the relative ratio of myeloid to erythroid cells (the M:E ratio) should be assessed at this magnification. Abnormal granulocytic and mononuclear patterns are best appreciated during low- to medium-power examinations of aspirates (see Figs. 8.21 and 8.22). At higher magnifications, using either high dry (60×) or oil immersion (100×) objective lenses, each of the major three hematopoietic lineages (megakaryocytes, myeloid, and erythroid) should be examined cytologically. Plasma cells, lymphocytes, and abnormal cells, including blasts, other immature precursors, and non-hematolymphoid cells, should be enumerated.

Clotted bone marrow left over from aspirate smears can be fixed in formalin with or without mercury chloride (B5) and further processed (embedded in paraffin and stained with hematoxylin and eosin [H&E]) on an automated tissue processor. These "clot sections" can be valuable complements to aspirate smears from which cellularity and the relative cytologic composition of the bone marrow cavity can be readily evaluated (see Figs. 8.46 and 8.47). If necessary, immunohistochemical studies also can be performed on clot sections. In certain situations, such as the frequent marrow sampling required as part of treatment-monitoring protocols in certain hematologic diseases (e.g., acute leukemia and chronic myelogenous leukemia [CML]), clot sections suffice as alternatives to biopsies.

EXAMINATION OF THE BONE MARROW BIOPSY AND THE TOUCH PREP

Slide Preparation and Staining

Apart from a decalcification step, bone marrow core biopsies are prepared as are most other surgical biopsy specimens, using an automated tissue processor. The latter includes formalin fixation, paraffin embedding, and cutting 3- to 5-micron sections for H&E staining on glass slides. Special stains routinely used for interpreting the biopsy are Gomori's silver stain for reticulin, trichrome stain for collagen, and various immunohistochemical panels used to determine lineage-specific antigen expression on cells.

Slide Examination

A systematic approach should be employed in the morphologic interpretation of all hematopoietic tissues, and the core biopsy is no exception. At low power, the length of biopsy specimen should be recorded, and any distortion of overall cellular architecture (e.g., metastases, necrosis, fibrosis, granulomas, lymphoid nodules) or abnormalities in the bony trabeculae noted. At medium magnification, the relative ratio of myeloid to erythroid cells is best appreciated, as well as megakaryocyte numbers. Myeloid maturation is assessed at high power by comparing the relative number of cells with round nuclei (blasts, promyelocytes, and myelocytes) to those with segmented nuclei (metamyelocytes, bands, and neutrophils). Maturation in the erythroid line is estimated by comparing the proportion of larger erythroid cells with open chromatin and distinctly round, smooth nuclear contours (immature precursors) to the smaller forms with closed nuclei (mature precursors). Small mature lymphocytes are slightly larger than mature erythroids, have closed chromatin patterns, and typically display slightly irregular nuclear contours.

Bone marrow touch preps (imprints) should be made routinely from core biopsy specimens. Using forceps, the fresh core biopsy is gently pressed three or four times against a glass slide, allowed to air dry, and then fixed and stained similarly to blood and aspirate smears. Touch preps are sometimes useful as a "quick look" alternative to the biopsy that can, especially if aspirates do not contain marrow (*dry tap*), give clues to the identity of the prominent cell type in marrow specimens (see Figs. 8.48 and 8.49).

Table 8.1

Hematology reference values in normal adults

Test	Men		Women	
	Conventional Units	SI	Conventional Units	SI
Hemoglobin	14.0–17.4 g/dL	140–175 g/L	12.3–15.3 g/dL	123–153 g/L
Hematocrit (volume of packed red cells)	41.5–50.4	0.415–0.504	36–45	0.36–0.45
Red cell count	$4.5–5.9 \times 10^6/\mu L$	$4.5–5.9 \times 10^{12}/L$	$4.5–5.1 \times 10^6/\mu L$	$4.5–5.1 \times 10^{12}/L$
White cell count	$4.4–11.3 \times 10^3/\mu L$	$4.4–11.3 \times 10^9/L$	$4.4–11.3 \times 10^6/\mu L$	$4.4–11.3 \times 10^9/L$
Mean corpuscular volume (fl)	80–96	80–96	80–96	80–96
Mean corpuscular hemoglobin (pg)	27.5–33.2	27.5–33.2	27.5–33.2	27.5–33.2
Mean corpuscular hemoglobin concentration	33.4–35.5 g/dL	334–355 g/L	33.4–35.5 g/dL	334–355 g/L
Platelet count	$150–450 \times 10^3/\mu L$	$150–450 \times 10^9/L$	$150–450 \times 10^3/\mu L$	$150–450 \times 10^9/L$
Reticulocyte count	0.5%–2.5%	0.005–0.025	0.5%–2.5%	0.005–0.025
Reticulocyte count	$22,500–147,500/mm^3$	$22.5–147.5 \times 10^9/L$	$22,500–147,500/mm^3$	$22.5–147.5 \times 10^9/L$
Sedimentation rate (Westergren) <50 yrs. of age (mm/h)	0–15	0–15	0–20	0–20

SI, Systéme International d'Unites.
Adapted with permission from *Wintrobe's Clinical Hematology*, 11th Edition, page 2697.

Table 8.2

Red blood cell values at various ages: Mean and lower limit of normal (−2 SD)

Age	Hemoglobin (g/dL) Mean	−2 SD	Hematocrit (%) Mean	−2 SD	Red Cell Count (1,012/L) Mean	−2 SD	Mean Corpuscular Volume (fl) Mean	−2 SD	Mean Corpuscular Hemoglobin (pg) Mean	−2 SD	Mean Corpuscular Hemoglobin Concentration (g/dL) Mean	−2 SD
Birth (cord blood)	16.5	13.5	51	42	4.7	3.9	108	98	34	31	33	30
1 to 3 days (capillary)	18.5	14.5	56	45	5.3	4.0	108	95	34	31	33	29
1 wk	17.5	13.5	54	42	5.1	3.9	107	88	34	28	33	28
2 wk	16.5	12.5	51	39	4.9	3.6	105	86	34	28	33	28
1 mo	14.0	10.0	43	31	4.2	3.0	104	85	34	28	33	29
2 mo	11.5	9.0	35	28	3.8	2.7	96	77	30	26	33	29
3 to 6 mo	11.5	9.5	35	29	3.8	3.1	91	74	30	25	33	30
0.5 to 2.0 yr	12.0	0.5	36	33	4.5	3.7	78	70	27	23	33	30
2 to 6 yr	12.5	11.5	37	34	4.6	3.9	81	75	27	24	34	31
6 to 12 yr	13.5	11.5	40	35	4.6	4.0	86	77	29	25	34	31
12 to 18 yr												
Female	14.0	12.0	41	36	4.6	4.1	90	78	30	25	34	31
Male	14.5	13.0	43	37	4.9	4.5	88	78	30	25	34	31
18 to 49 yr												
Female	14.0	12.0	41	36	4.6	4.0	90	80	30	26	34	31
Male	15.5	13.5	47	41	5.2	4.5	90	80	30	26	34	31

SD, standard deviation.

These data were compiled from several sources. Emphasis is on recent studies using electronic counters and on the selection of populations that are likely to exclude individuals with iron deficiency. The mean ±2 SD can be expected to include 95% of the observations in a normal population. From Dallman PR. In: Rudolph A, ed. *Pediatrics,* 16th ed. New York: Appleton-Century-Crofts, 1977; and Lubin BH. Reference values in infancy and childhood. In: Nathan DG, Oski FA, eds. *Hematology of infancy and childhood,* 4th ed. Philadelphia: WB Saunders, 1993 (22). Reprinted with permission from *Wintrobe's Clinical Hematology,* 11th Edition, page 2701.

Table 8.3

Differential counts from bone marrow aspirates from 12 healthy men

	Mean (%)	Observed Range (%)	95% Confidence Limits (%)
Neutrophilic series (total)	53.6	49.2–65.0	33.6–73.6
Myeloblasts	0.9	0.2–1.5	0.1–1.7
Promyelocytes	3.3	2.1–4.1	1.9–4.7
Myelocytes	12.7	8.2–15.7	8.5–16.9
Metamyelocytes	15.9	9.6–24.6	7.1–24.7
Band	12.4	9.5–15.3	9.4–15.4
Segmented	7.4	6.0–12.0	3.8–11.0
Eosinophilic series (total)	3.1	1.2–5.3	1.1–5.2
Myelocytes	0.8	0.2–1.3	0.2–1.4
Metamyelocytes	1.2	0.4–2.2	0.2–2.2
Band	0.9	0.2–2.4	0–2.7
Segmented	0.5	0–1.3	0–1.1
Basophilic and mast cells	0.1	0–0.2	—
Erythrocytic series (total)	25.6	18.4–33.8	15.0–36.2
Pronormoblasts	0.6	0.2–1.3	0.1–1.1
Basophilic	1.4	0.5–2.4	0.4–2.4
Polychromatophilic	21.6	17.9–29.2	13.1–30.1
Orthochromatic	2.0	0.4–4.6	0.3–3.7
Lymphocytes	16.2	11.1–23.2	8.6–23.8
Plasma cells	1.3	0.4–3.9	0–3.5
Monocytes	0.3	0–0.8	0–0.6
Megakaryocytes	0.1	0–0.4	—
Reticulum cells	0.3	0–0.9	0–0.8
Myeloid to erythrocyte (M:E) ratio	2.3	1.5–3.3	1.1–3.5

Reprinted with permission from *Wintrobe's Clinical Hematology*, 11th Edition, page 2701.

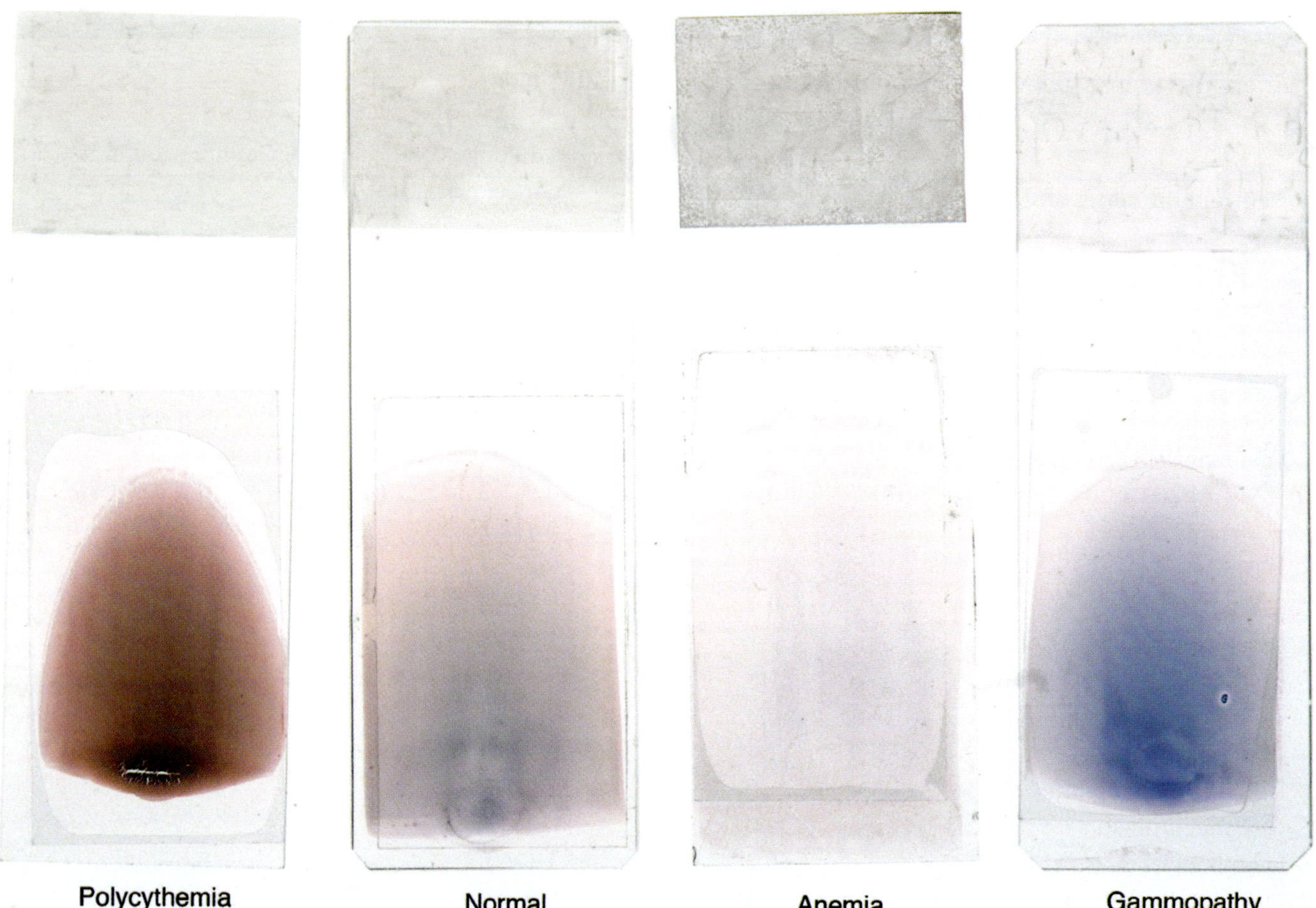

Figure 8.1. Macroscopic appearance of blood films. The color of blood smears can reflect severe underlying abnormalities in hematocrit and the presence of abnormal circulating immunoglobins. The smear on the left, from a patient with polycythemia vera and a hemoglobin of 20 g/dL, appears noticeably darker than the normal (hemoglobin = 14 g/dL) and pale anemic sample (hemoglobin = 7). The blood film on the right, from a case of myeloma, is blue because circulating monoclonal immunoglobins take up the basophilic stains used in blood smears.

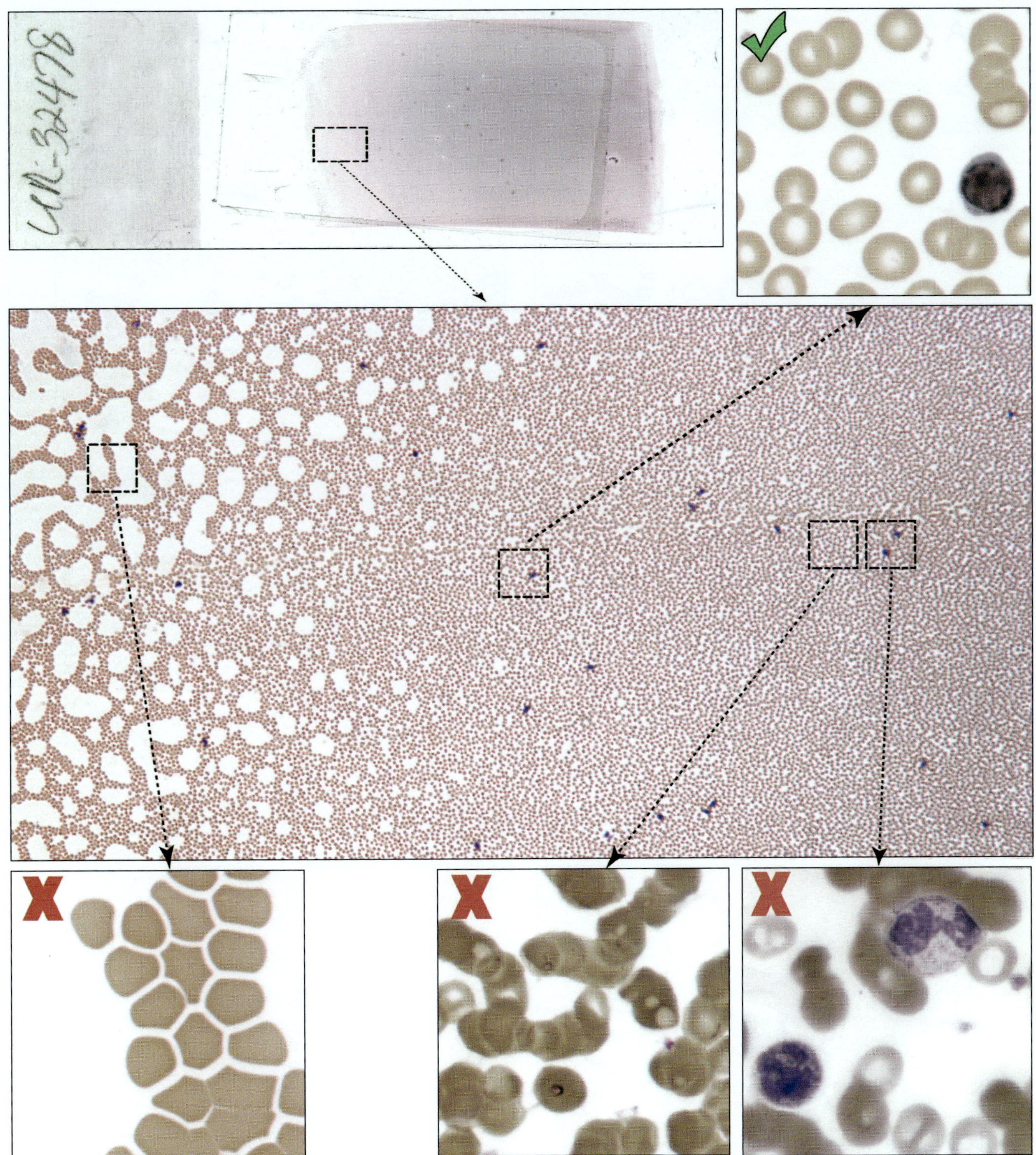

Figure 8.2. Microscopic approach to blood films. Selecting the correct area to examine is essential in properly assessing blood films. Regions where red blood cells are well-spaced and almost touch each other are optimal for examining erythrocytes (*right upper panel*). Erythrocytes, when examined too closely to the edge of the slide, appear misshapen and falsely hyperchromic (*left lower panel*), whereas those too distant often appear shrunken and aggregated (*right lower panels*).

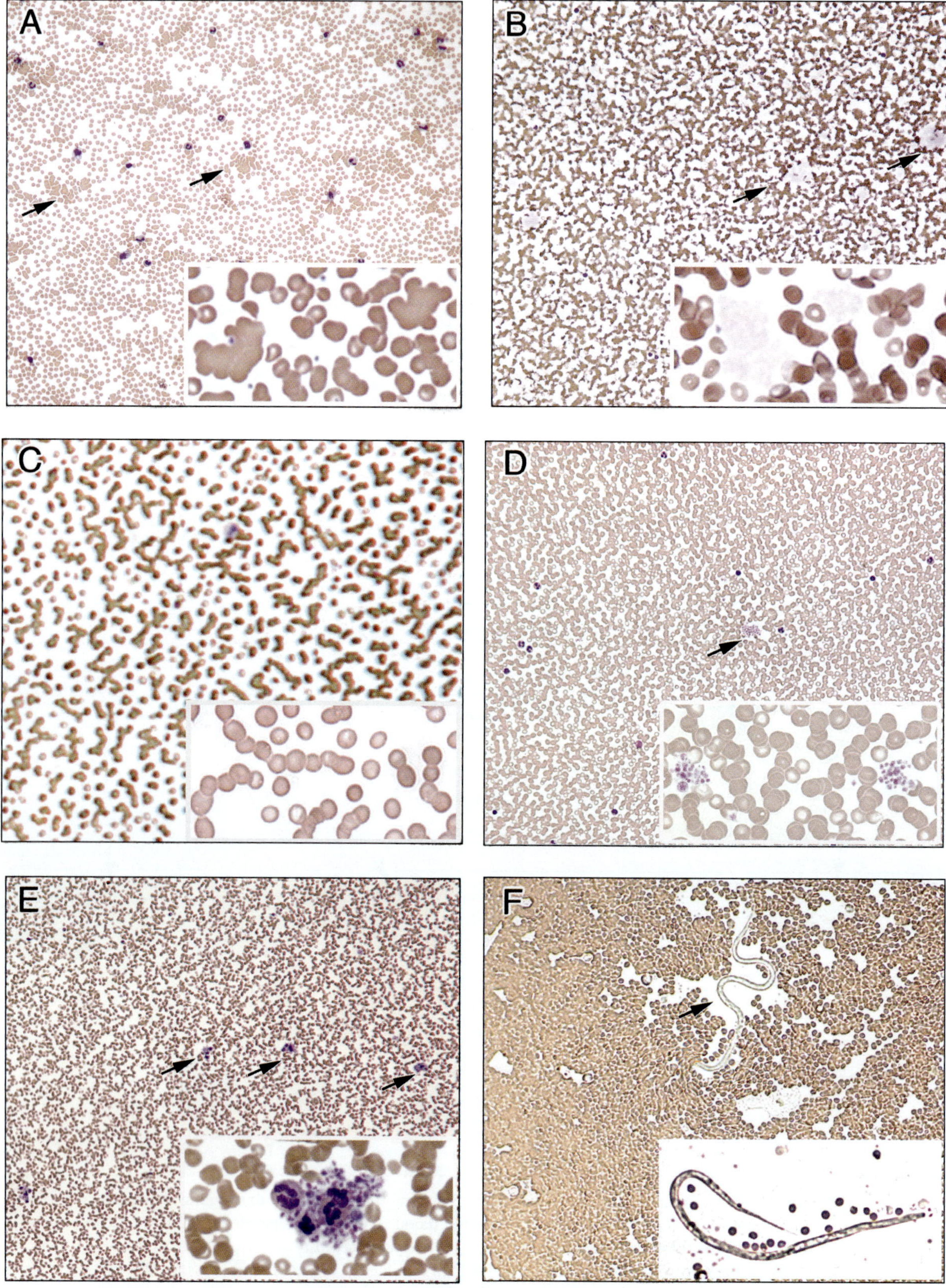

Figure 8.3.   Examining blood films at low magnification. Abnormal aggregates, precipitated proteins, and parasites are best seen by examining large areas of the smear at low-power magnification. Shown here are RBC aggregation from cold agglutinins (**A**), precipitates of cryoglobulins (**B**), rouleaux formation from serum monoclonal gammopathy (**C**), platelet aggregation (**D**), platelet and leukocyte aggregates (**E**), and infection of the blood with microfilaria (**F**).

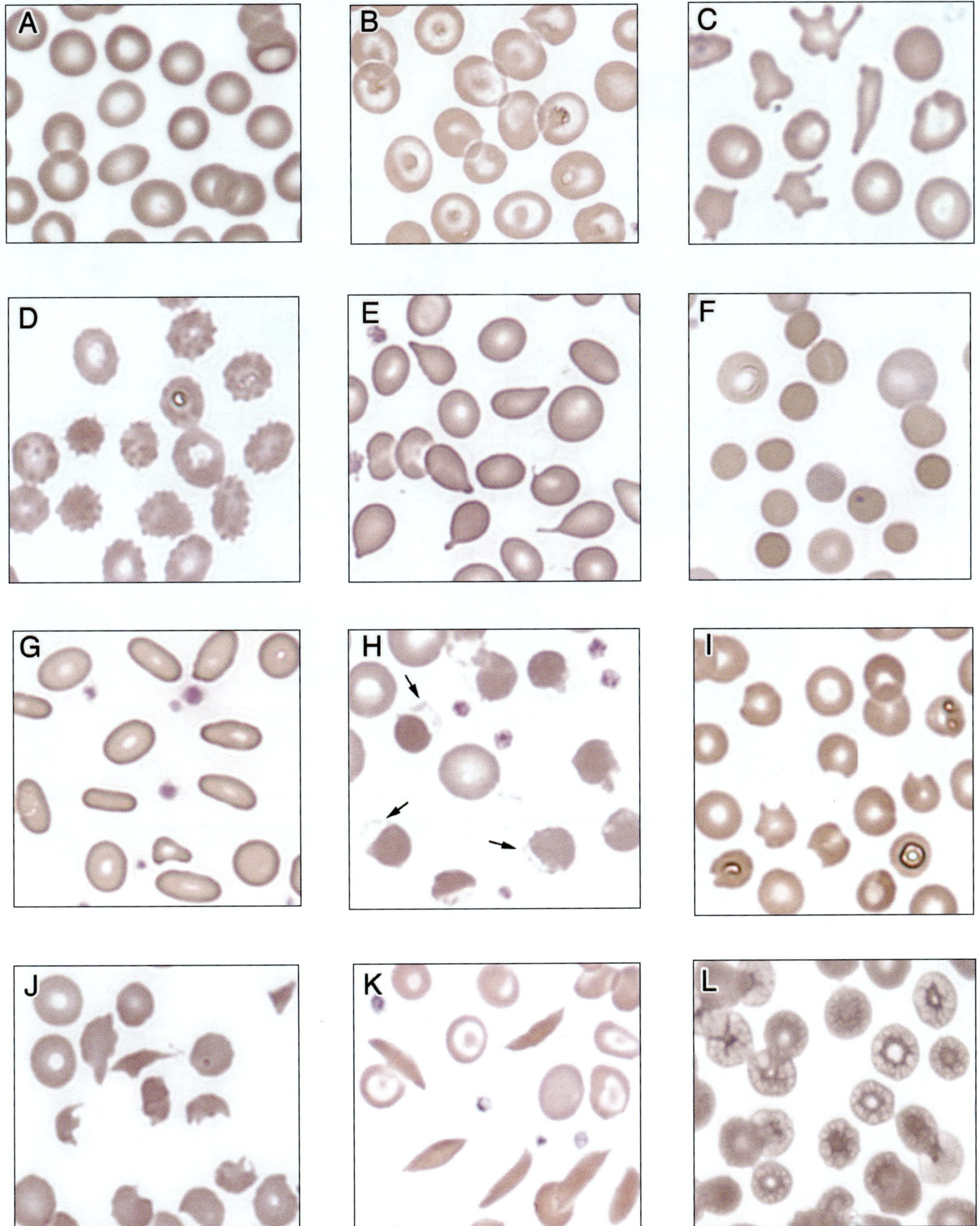

Figure 8.4. Red blood cell morphology: Abnormally shaped forms (poikilocytes). Normal red blood cells (**A**) and various abnormal forms are shown, including: targets (**B**), spur cells (acanthocytes) (**C**), burr cells (echinocytes) (**D**), teardrops (dacrocytes) (**E**), spherocytes (**F**), ovalocytes (**G**), blister cells (*arrows*, **H**), bite cells (**I**), schistocytes (**J**), sickle cells (**K**), and erythrocytes displaying dehydration artifact (**L**).

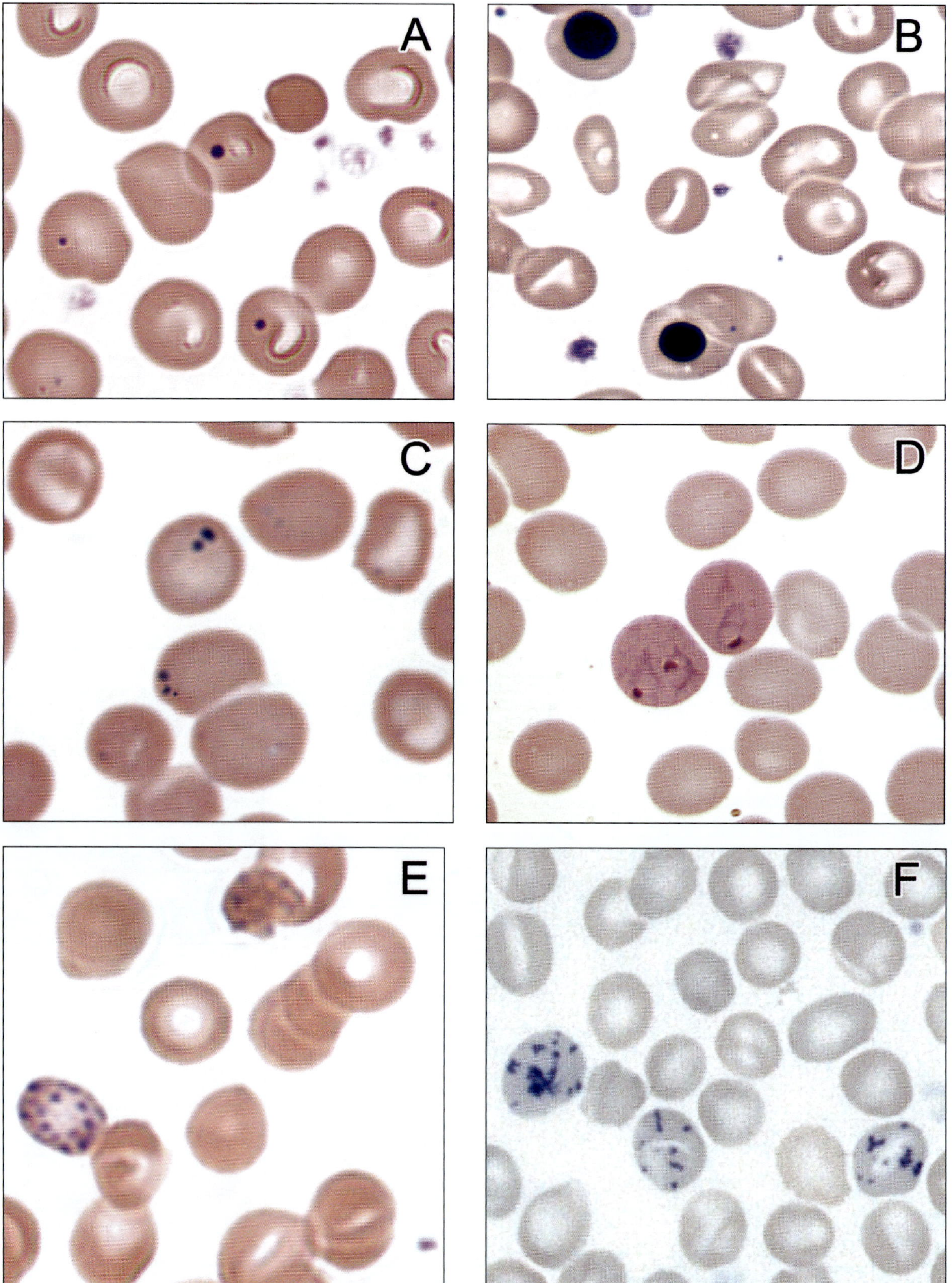

Figure 8.5. Red blood cell morphology: Abnormal inclusions. Howell-Jolly bodies (**A**), nucleated red blood cell precursors (**B**), Pappenheimer bodies (**C**), trophozoites of *Plasmodium vivax* (**D**), coarse basophilic stippling in a case of lead poisoning (**E**), and crystal violet supravital stain demonstrating Heinz-body inclusions in a patient who has undergone a splenectomy (**F**).

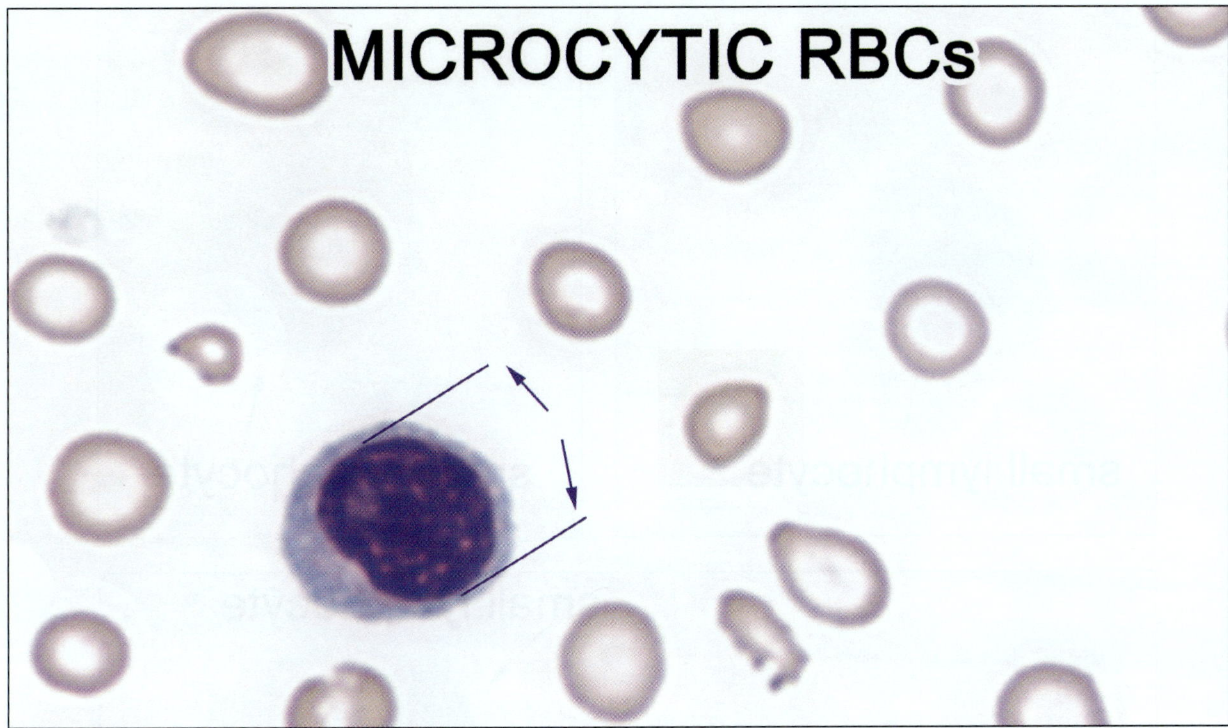

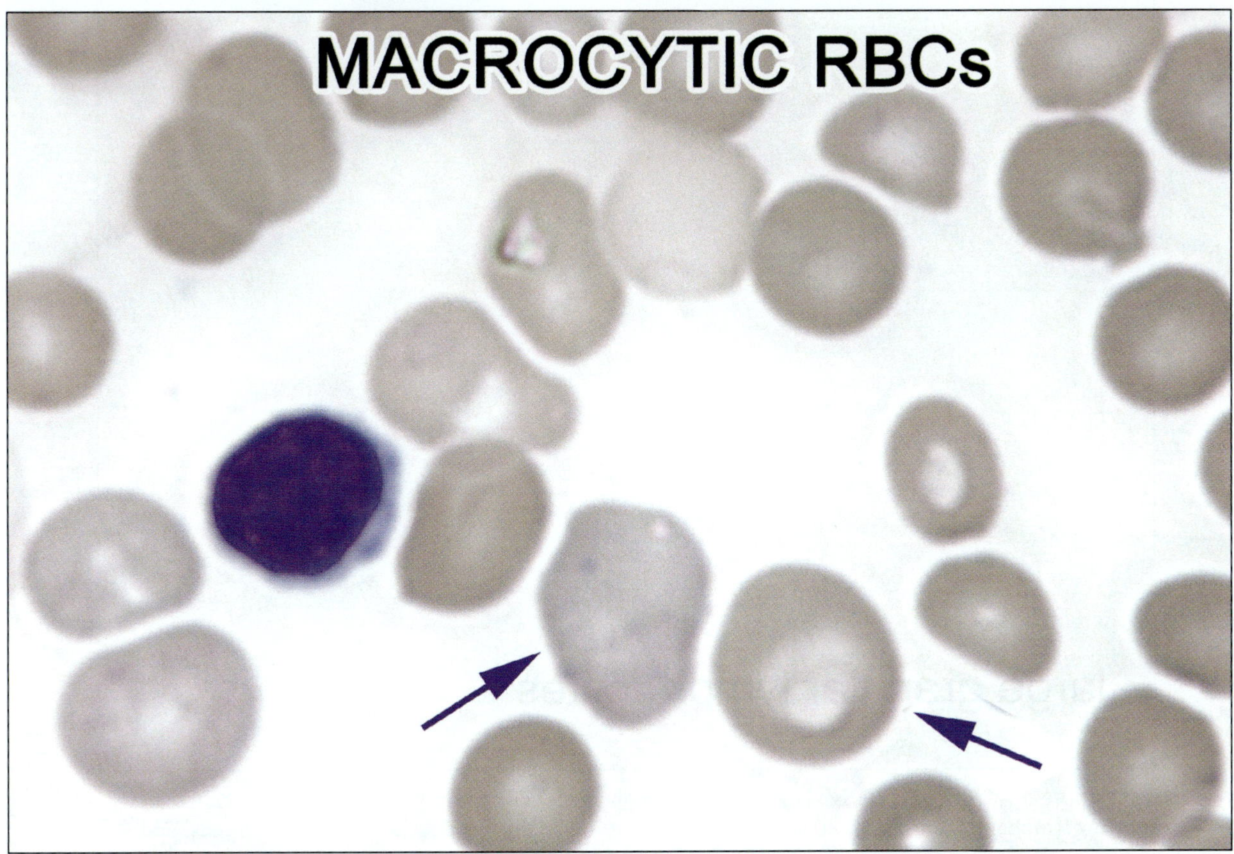

Figure 8.6. Red blood cell mporphology: Size. Red blood cell size is best measured by automated hematology analyzers, but severe size differences can be estimated by comparing the diameters of red cells to those of lymphocyte nuclei. Normal erythrocytes are approximately the same size as the nuclei of small lymphocytes. The top panel shows numerous microcytic red cells that are significantly smaller than the diameter of the lymphocyte nuclei. The bottom panel demonstrates two macrocytic red cells, the one on the left a polychromatophilic RBC (*arrows*).

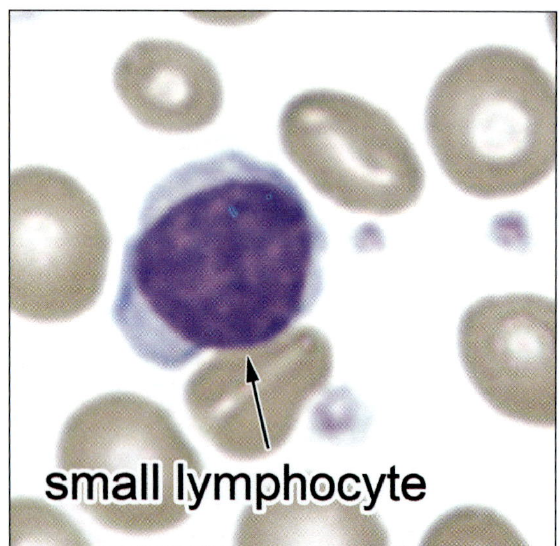

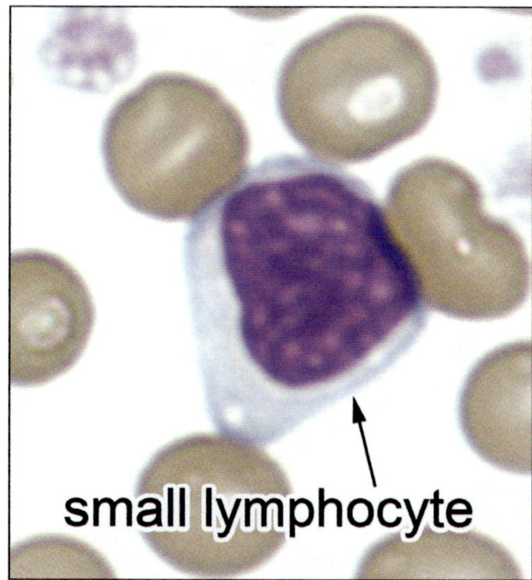

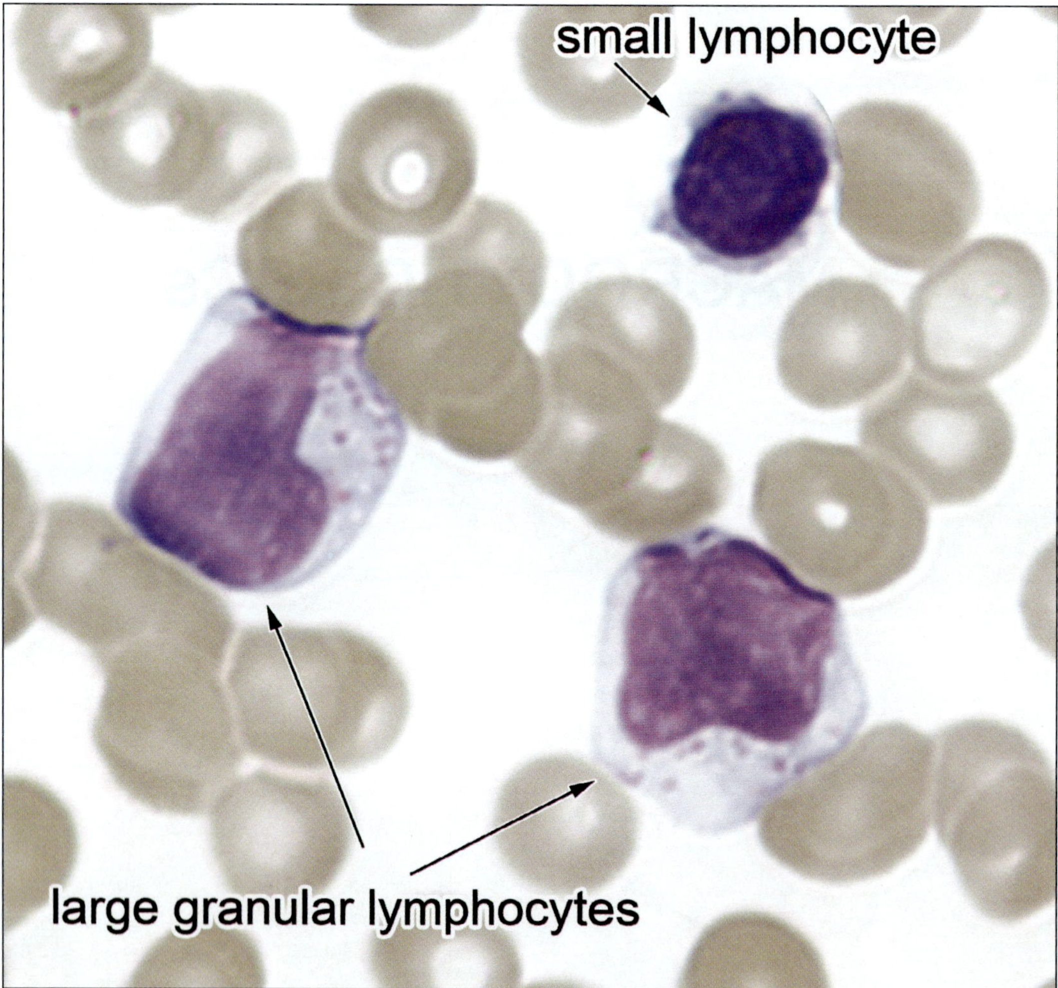

Figure 8.7.   Lymphocyte and large granular lymphocyte (LGL) morphology. Normal small circulating lymphocytes are usually 10 to 15 microns in size (slightly bigger than normal red blood cells) and typically have high nuclear:cytoplasmic (N:C) ratios, with scant amounts of slightly basophilic staining cytoplasm. Lymphocyte nuclei are usually smoothly contoured with a mature (or "closed") chromatin pattern and absent nucleoli. The appearance of large granular lymphocytes (LGLs) is somewhat more variable, but they generally have moderate N:C ratios and neutral-staining cytoplasm that often contains purplish granules. The chromatin of LGLs is often slightly more "open" than that of small lymphocytes.

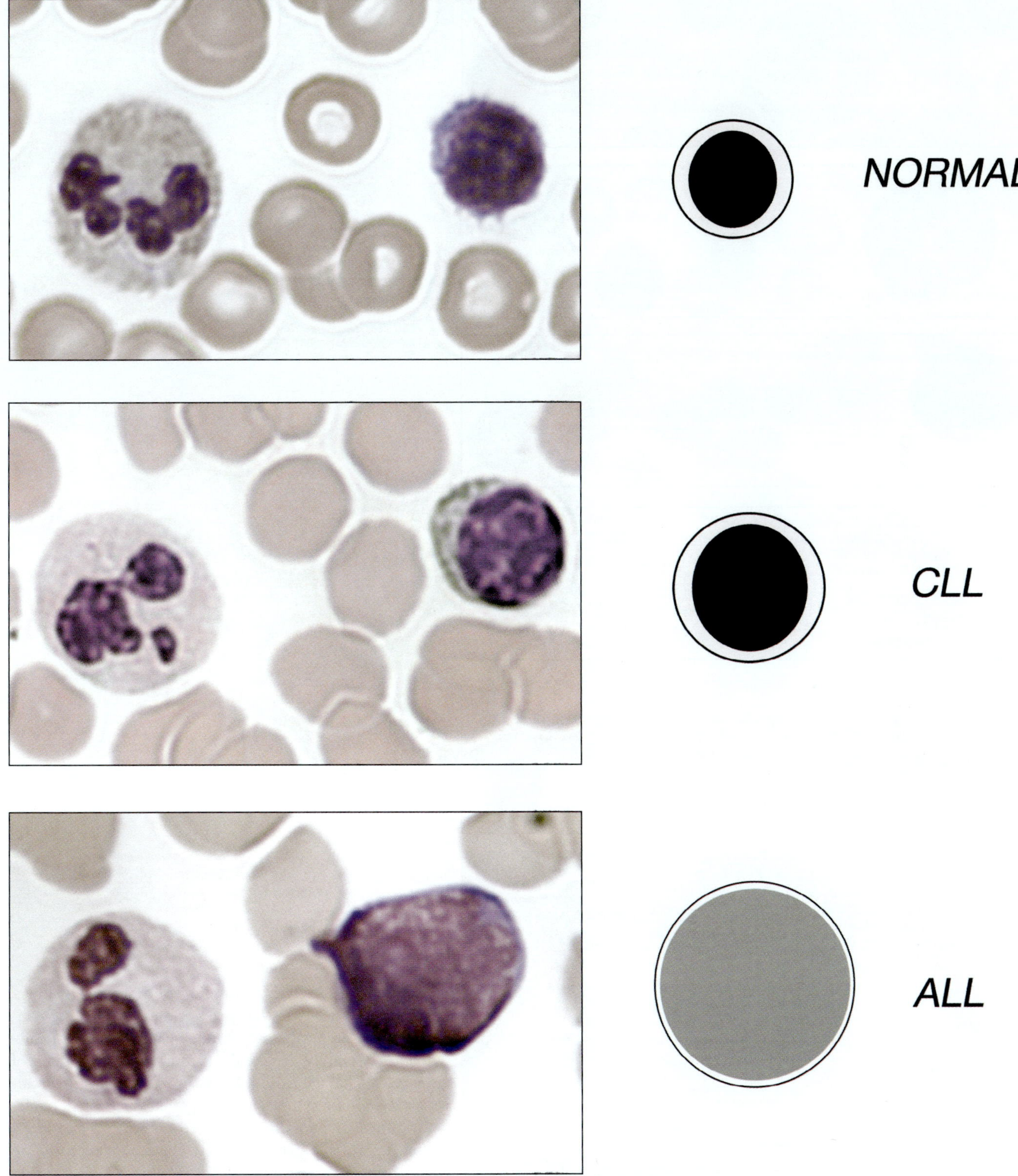

Figure 8.8. Morphology of the small neoplastic lymphoid disorders: Chronic lymphocytic leukemia (CLL) and acute lymphoid leukemia (ALL). Two common neoplastic conditions featuring small, neoplastic lymphoid cells are CLL and ALL (*middle* and *bottom panels*, respectively). The designation "ALL" includes both precursor B- and T- lymphoblastic leukemia. CLL cells are variable in appearance and typically look very much like slightly larger versions of normal small lymphocytes. CLL cells can display clumped or "soccer ball" chromatin. The L1 type of lymphoblast shown here usually has a high nuclear:cytoplasmic (N:C) ratio with an immature or "open" chromatin.

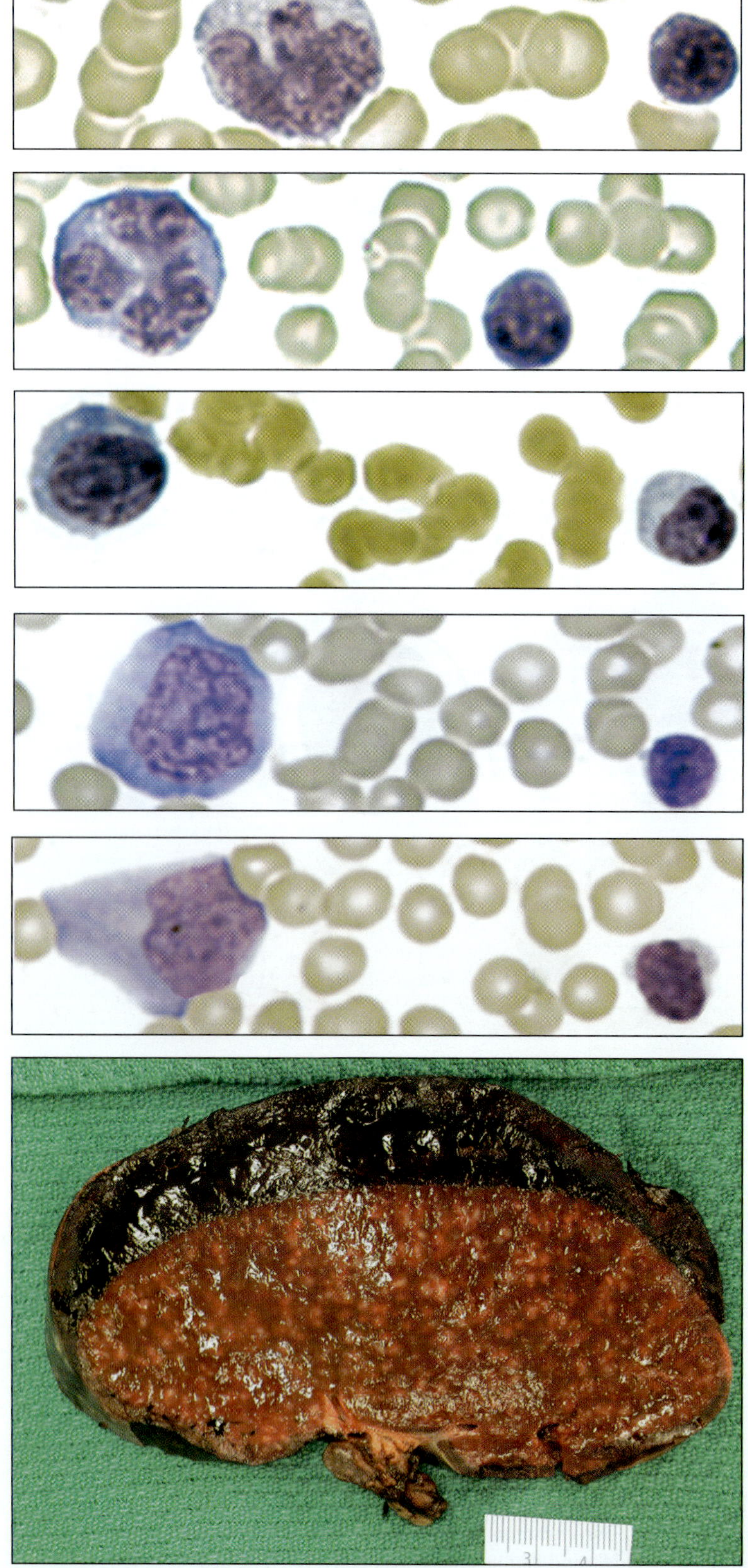

Figure 8.9. "Atypical" lymphocyte morphology, infectious mononucleosis. When referring to circulating lymphocytes, "atypical" is a confusing term that generally denotes benignity, despite the pleomorphic appearance of the cells. Characteristic features include large size, abundant basophilic cytoplasm that is often vacuolated, nucleoli, diffuse or partially condensed chromatin, and large, often irregularly shaped nuclei. The top five panels are from different cases of infectious mononucleosis showing the variable appearance of the atypical lymphocytes seen with this particular disease. For comparison, normal lymphocytes are shown on the right side of each panel.

SMALL CELL NEOPLASTIC LYMPHOID DISORDERS

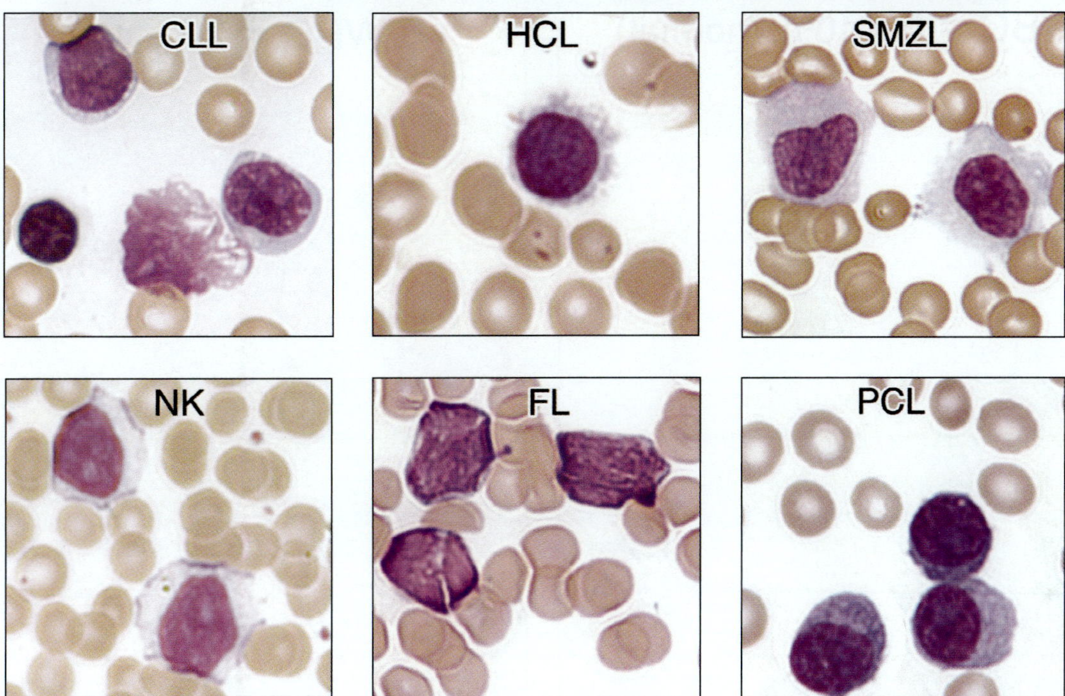

LARGE CELL NEOPLASTIC LYMPHOID DISORDERS

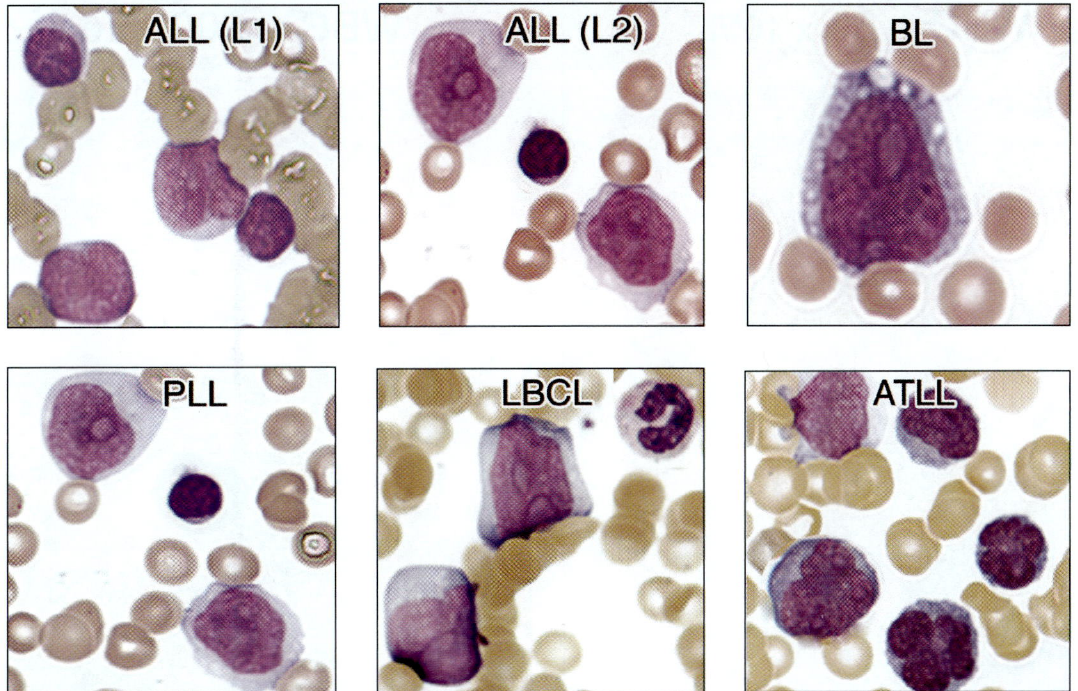

Figure 8.10. Small and large neoplastic lymphoid disorders. Peripheral blood smears from various lymphoproliferative disorders that feature primarily small and large cells are shown in the top and bottom panel sets, respectively: CLL, chronic lymphocytic leukemia/lymphoma; HCL, hairy cell leukemia; SMZL, splenic marginal zone lymphoma; NK, NK leukemia; FL, peripheralized follicular lymphoma; PCL, plasma cell leukemia; ALL(L1), acute lymphoblastic leukemia with L1 type blasts; ALL(L2), acute lymphoblastic leukemia with L2 type blasts; BL, Burkitt lymphoma/leukemia with L3 type blasts; PLL, prolymphocytic leukemia; LBCL, peripheralized large B-cell lymphoma; and ATLL, adult T-cell lymphoma/leukemia.

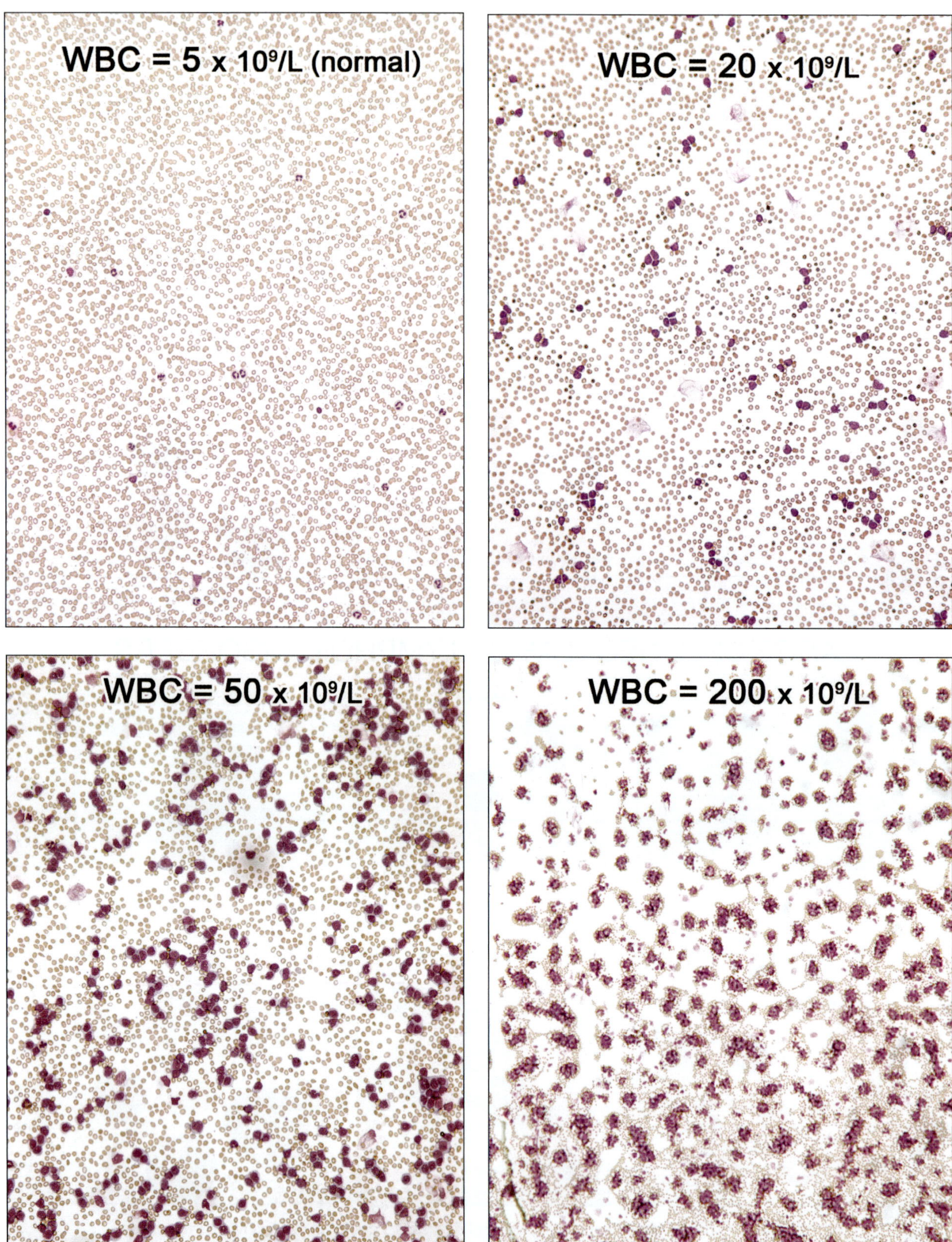

Figure 8.11. Leukocyte morphology: Low-power morphology. Leukocytes are best counted by automated hematology analyzers, but an approximate estimate of white cell numbers (the "leukocrit") can be done during examination at low magnification by comparing the ratio of white cells to erythrocytes (normal is approximately 1 to 500).

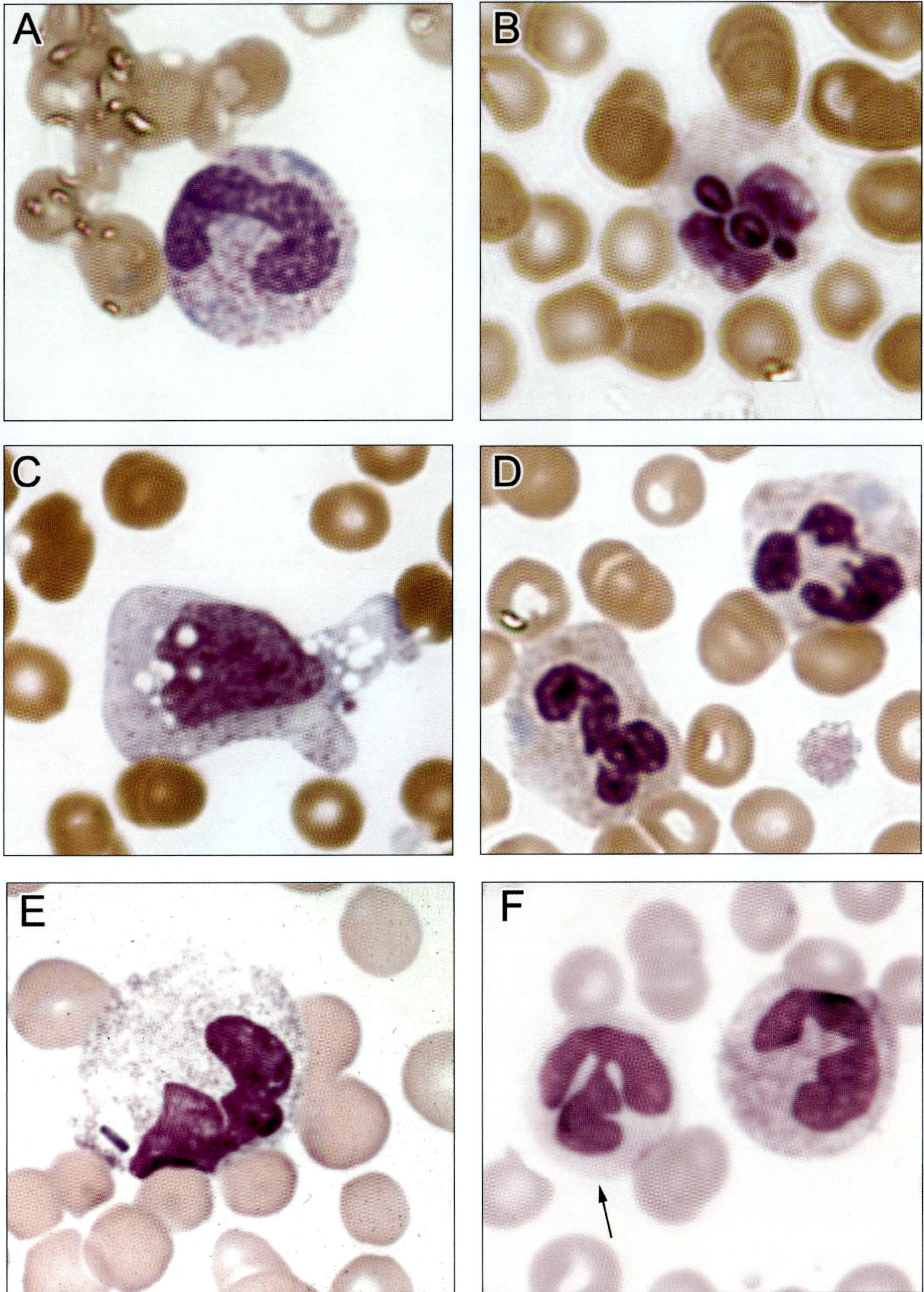

Figure 8.12.   Granulocyte morphology: Cytoplasmic features. **A:** Band showing "toxic changes," including increased cytoplasmic granulation and numerous bluish Döhle bodies. **B:** Circulating band ingesting a budding-yeast (*Candida albicans*). **C:** Monocyte showing "toxic changes," including cytoplasmic granulation and vacuolization. **D:** May-Hegglin anomaly with large Döhle-like inclusions and giant platelets. **E:** Neutrophil ingesting bacteria in a case of sepsis from *Clostridium perfringens*. (Courtesy Dr. I. Quirt.) **F:** A dysplastic hypogranular neutrophil lacking cytoplasmic granulation (*arrow*) and a normal neutrophil.

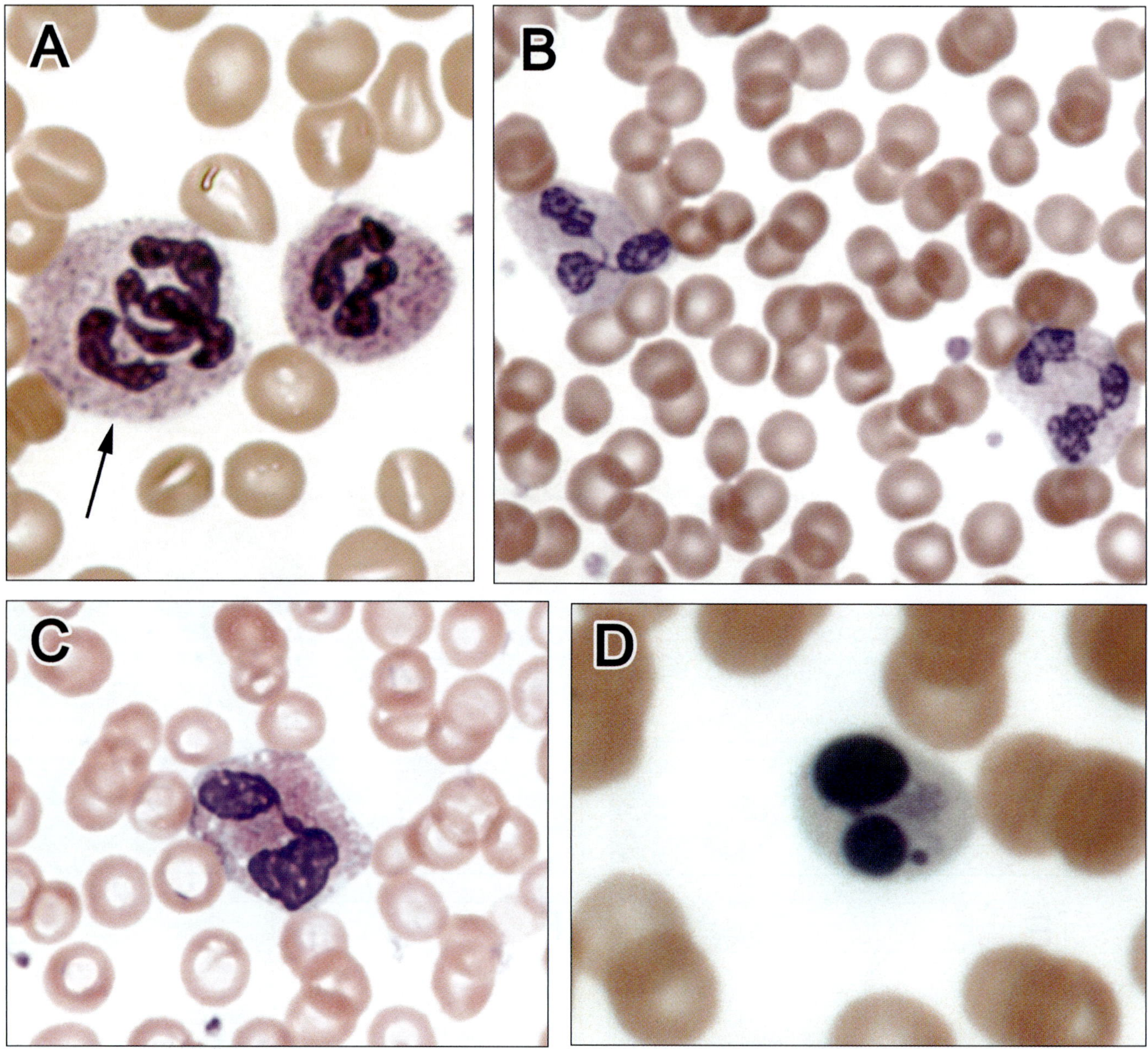

Figure 8.13.   Granulocyte morphology: Nuclear features. **A:** Giant hypersegmented neutrophil (*arrow*) from a case of vitamin B$_{12}$ deficiency. **B:** Hypersegmented neutrophils from antifolate chemotherapy. **C:** Dysplastic neutrophil (pseudopelgeroid cell) in case of myelodysplastic syndrome. This neutrophil, which has two lobes connected by a thin filament, resembles the neutrophils in the hereditary abnormality called Pelger-Huet anomaly. **D:** Degenerating neutrophil.

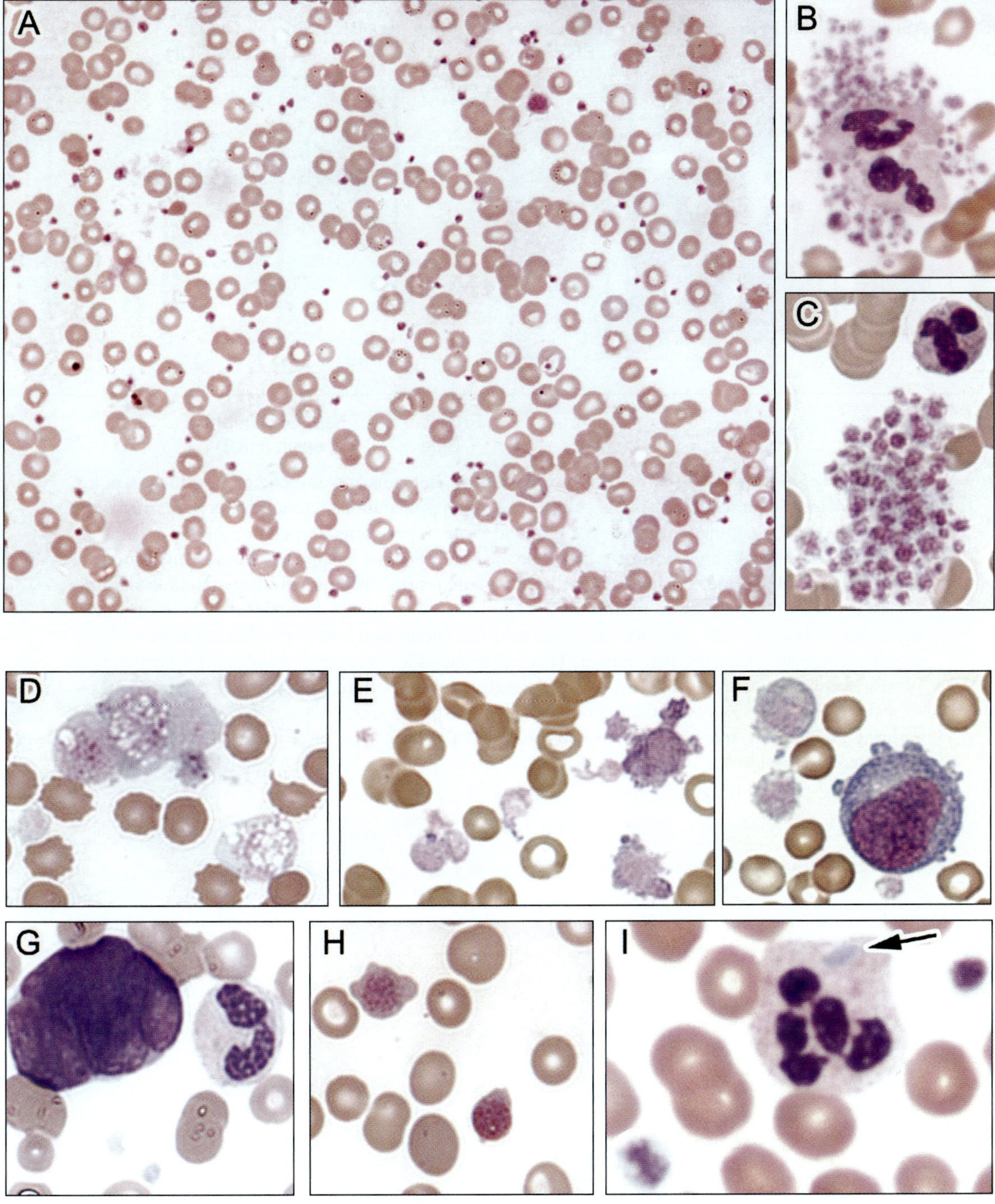

Figure 8.14.   Platelet abnormalities. **A** through **C**, Thrombocythemia and thrombocytopenia. **A:** Increased numbers of platelets in a case of essential thrombocythemia with a platelet count of 500 × 10^9/L (normal range is between 150 and 400 × 10^9/L). Platelet numbers are best measured using automated hematology analyzers, but estimates can be made microscopically by assuming that 7 to 20 platelets per oil immersion field represent a normal platelet count. **B and C:** Platelet satellitism and aggregation, respectively, from EDTA exposure in blood collection tubes. This phenomenon often leads to falsely low measurements of platelet numbers by automated hematology analyzers and can be avoided by using heparin or citrate as anticoagulants in collection tubes. **D** through **I:** Abnormal platelet morphology. **D:** Giant platelets in primary myelofibrosis, cellular phase. **E:** Bizarre platelets in essential thrombocythemia. **F:** Giant platelets and a megakaryoblast in acute megakaryoblastic leukemia. **G:** Stripped megakaryocytic nucleus. **H:** Bernard-Soulier syndrome. This congenital bleeding disorder is characterized by thrombocytopenia and large platelets. (Courtesy Dr. M. Abdelhaleem.) **I:** May-Hegglin anomaly. Large Döhle-like inclusions (*arrow*) and giant platelets are illustrated here (see also Fig. 8.12).

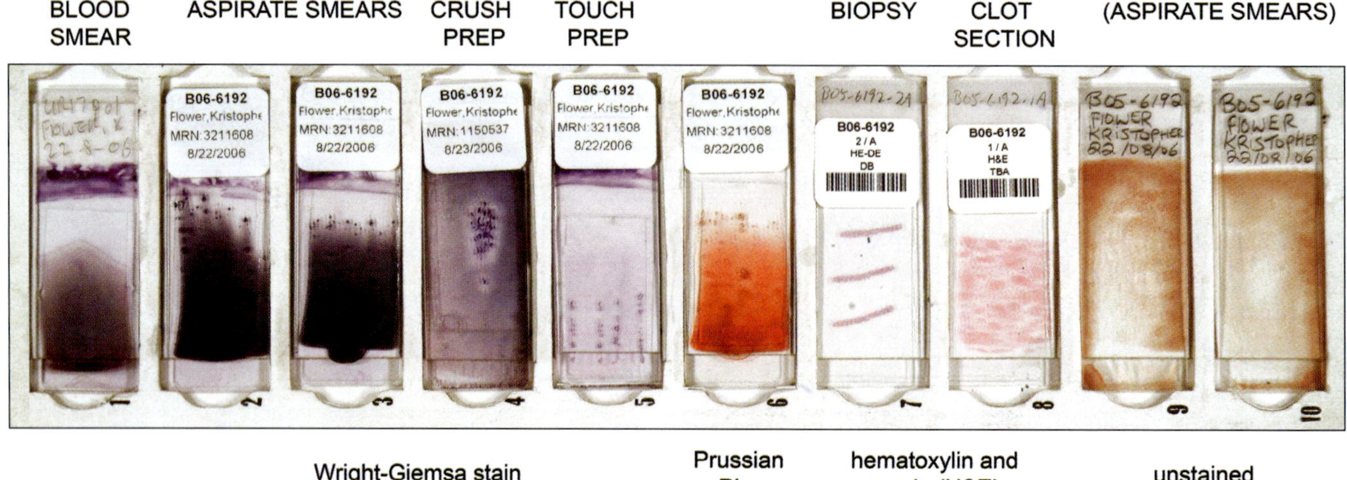

Figure 8.15.   Bone marrow staining and special studies. Bone marrow samples are routinely sent for Wright-Giemsa staining of the aspirate smears and touch preparations ("touch preps"); hematoxylin and eosin (H&E) staining is used for the clot and biopsy specimens. Depending on the indication for the marrow sampling, specimens also can be sent for flow cytometry, fluorescence-in situ-hybridization (FISH), molecular assays, and cytogenetic testing. Additionally, Prussian blue staining for iron studies, reticulin stains, immunohistochemistry, various histochemical stains (e.g., esterase, myeloperoxidase), special stains for fungi and acid-fast bacilli, and bacterial cultures can be ordered as appropriate for each particular patient. This figure shows a typical tray of slides for interpretation of a bone marrow sample (*from left to right*): Peripheral blood film, two marrow aspirate smears ("push" technique), a crush preparation of marrow aspirate smear ("pull" technique), touch or imprint preparation, marrow aspirate smear stained for iron, core biopsy, clot section, and two unstained aspirate smears.

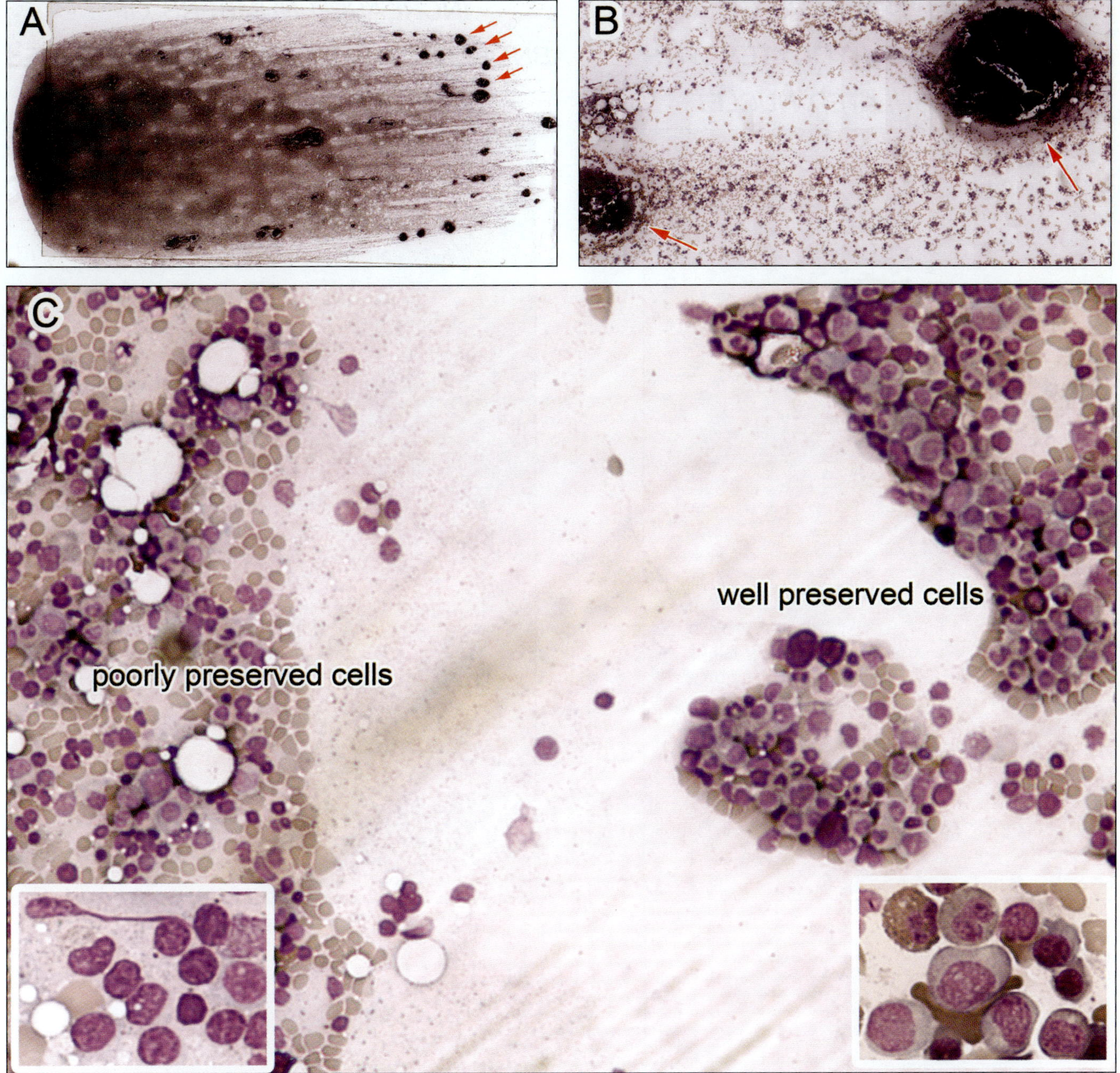

Figure 8.16. Microscopic approach to aspirate smears. A through C: Selecting the correct area to examine is essential in assessing marrow smears properly. The best regions are near particles (*arrows*) containing well-preserved clusters of cells that represent the actual cellular content of the marrow cavity. Areas of the aspirate where marrow cells are well-spaced and almost touch each other are optimal (*right side of lower panel*). One should avoid trying to evaluate areas where the cells are stripped of cytoplasm and/or display excessive air-dry artifact (*left side of lower panel*).

NORMAL NUMBERS OF NORMAL MEGAKARYOCYTES WITH MULTILOBULATED NUCLEI

INCREASED NUMBERS OF ABNORMALLY SMALL MEGAKARYOCYTES WITH UNILOBULATED NUCLEI

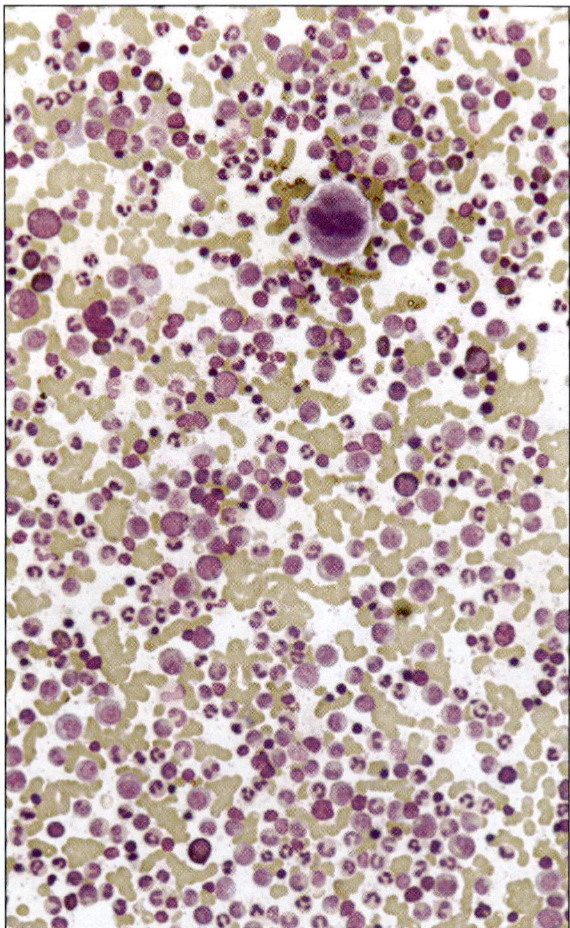

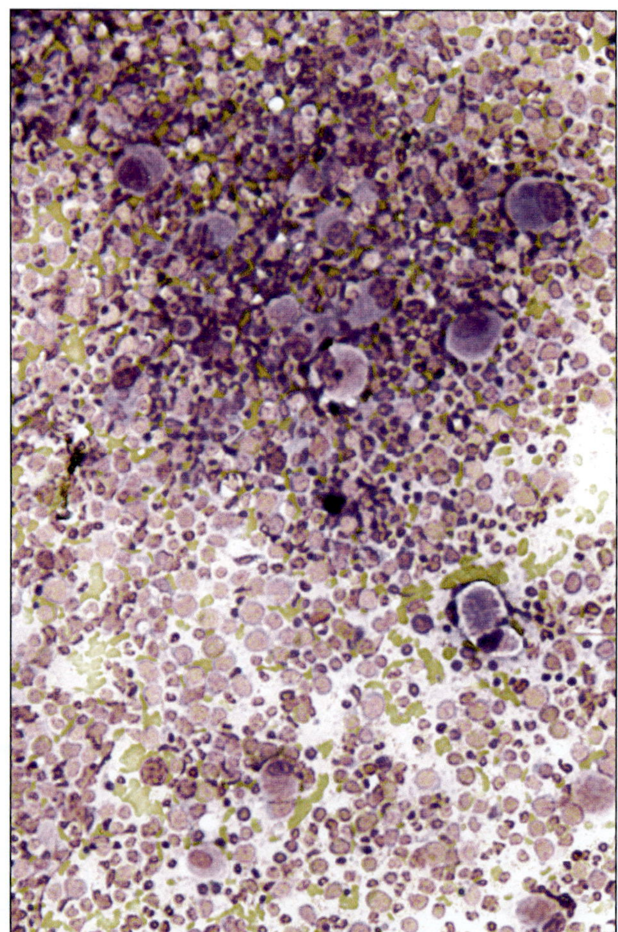

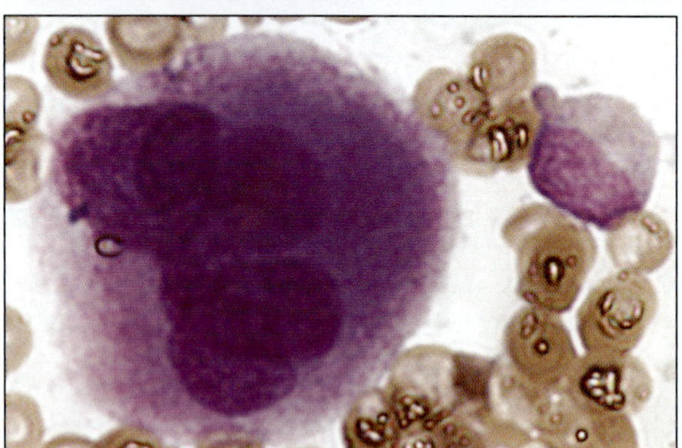

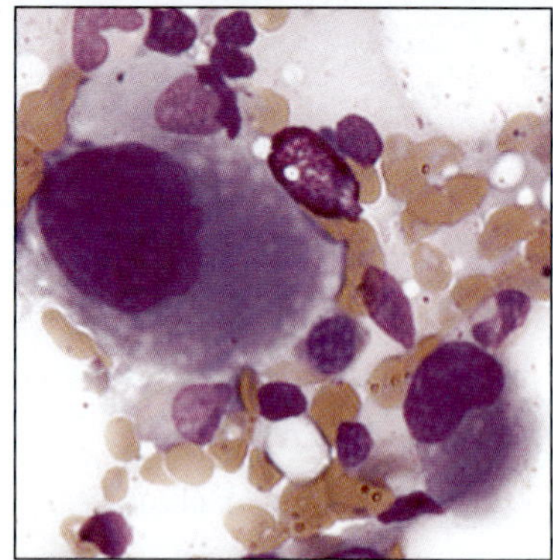

Figure 8.17.   Assessing megakaryocytes in the aspirate smear. Megakaryocytes are relatively rare in normal bone marrow specimens, representing approximately 1% of all nucleated cells. To assess megakaryocytes adequately, careful examination at low magnification is necessary. Megakaryocytes are the largest cells in the marrow (at least twice as large as a promyelocyte) and typically have polyploid nuclei.

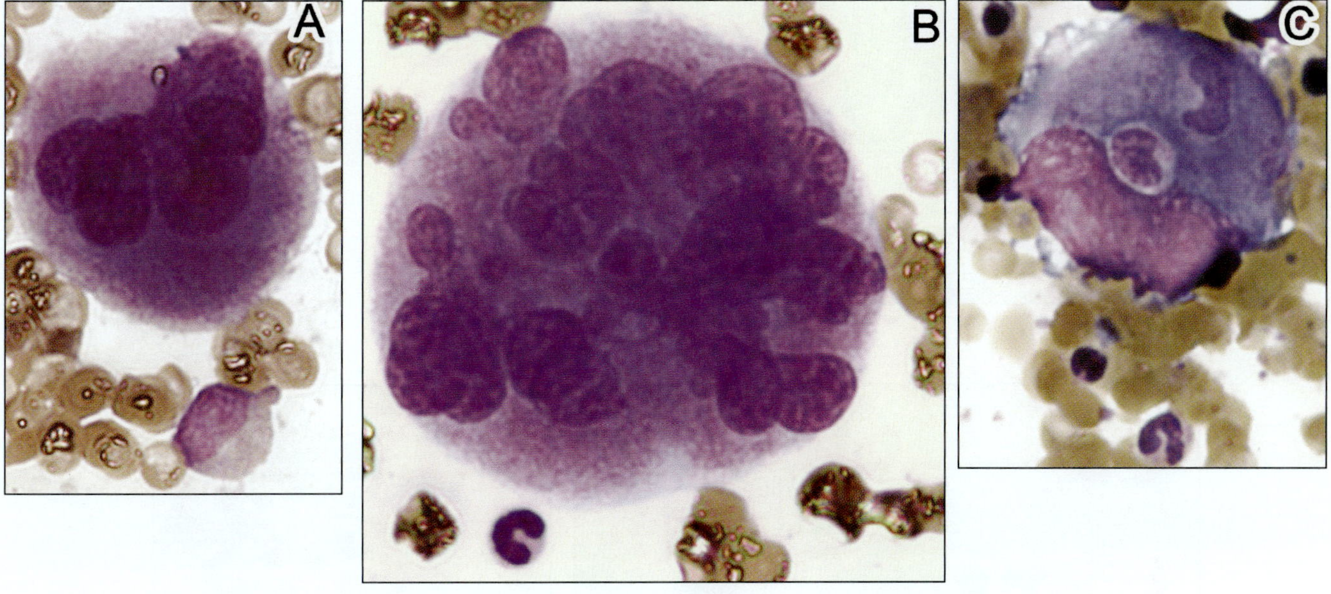

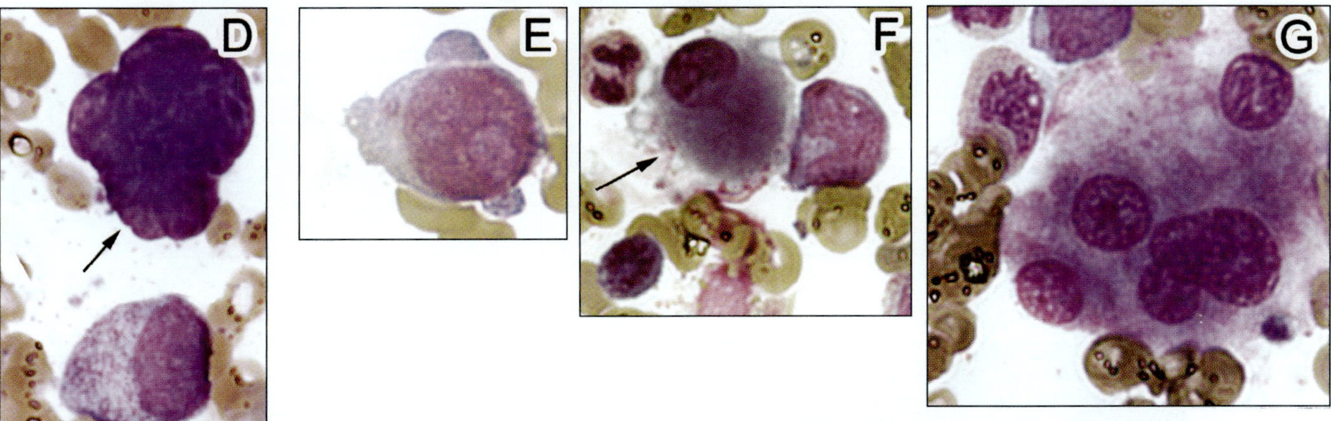

Figure 8.18. Morphology of the megakaryocyte. A through D: Variations of normal megakaryocytes. A normal megakaryocyte with multiple contiguous nuclear lobes (A), a "mature" megakaryocyte from a case of essential thrombocythemia with prominent nuclear lobulations (B), an example of emperipolesis (the presence of an intact cell within a megakaryocyte) (C), and a stripped megakaryocyte nucleus (*arrow*, D). E through G: Dysplastic megakaryocytes. A megakaryoblast (E), a micromegakaryocyte with a unilobular nucleus (F), and a megakaryocyte with separated nuclear lobulations (G).

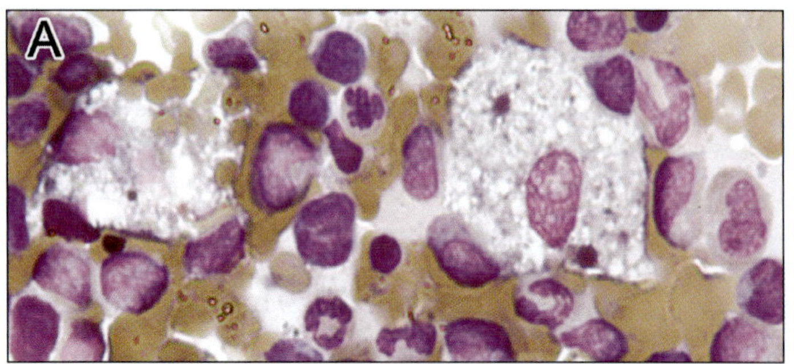

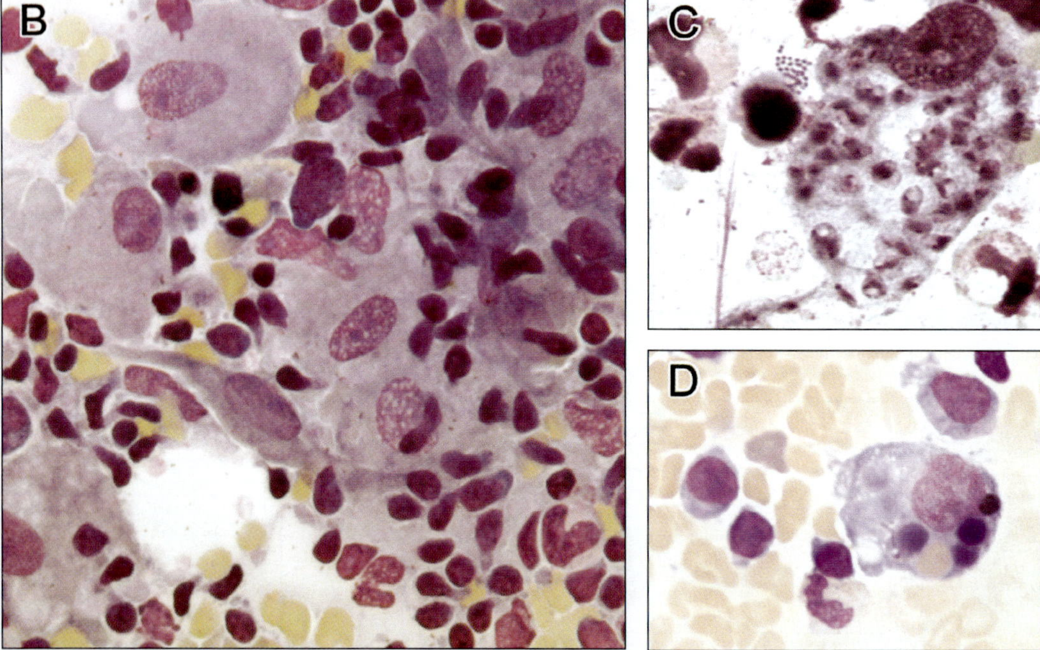

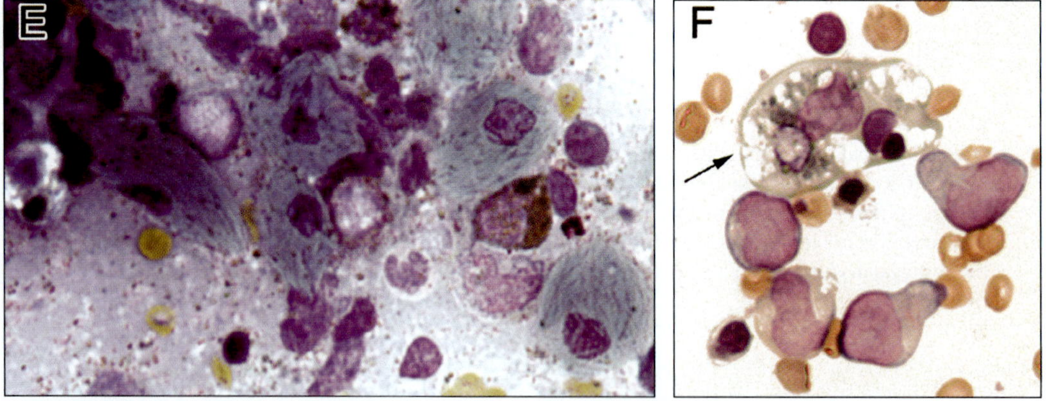

Figure 8.19. Histiocytes in the aspirate smears. **A:** An occasional histiocyte with tingible (stained) bodies is not an unusual finding in the aspirate smear. Often the engulfed material can be shown with appropriate stains to represent siderotic granules in patients with excess iron stores. **B** and **C:** Infectious-related histiocytosis. Granulomatous inflammation with clusters bon histiocytes admixed with lymphocytes in a case of tuberculosis (**B**), amastigotes in a marrow histiocyte from a case of visceral leishmaniasis (**C**), and a fatal case of Epstein-Barr virus–associated hemophagocytic syndrome (**D**). **E** and **F:** Marrow histiocytosis associated with hematopoietic malignancies. Sea-blue histiocytes of chronic myelogenous leukemia (**E**) and hemophagocytosis (*arrow*) associated with a case of T-cell lymphoproliferative disorder involving the bone marrow (**F**).

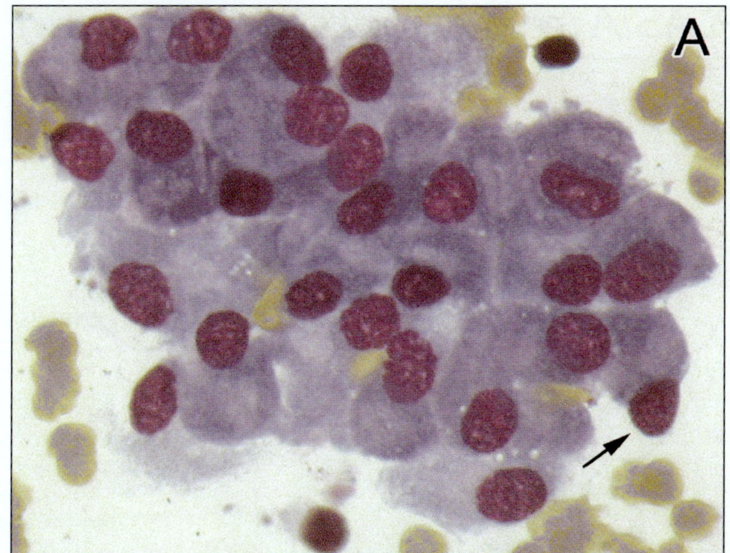
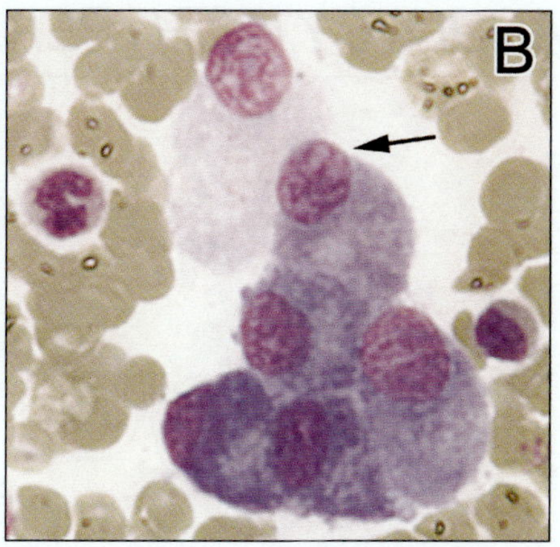
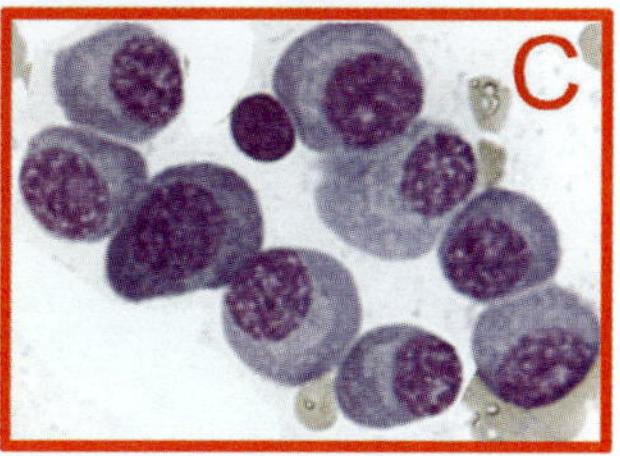
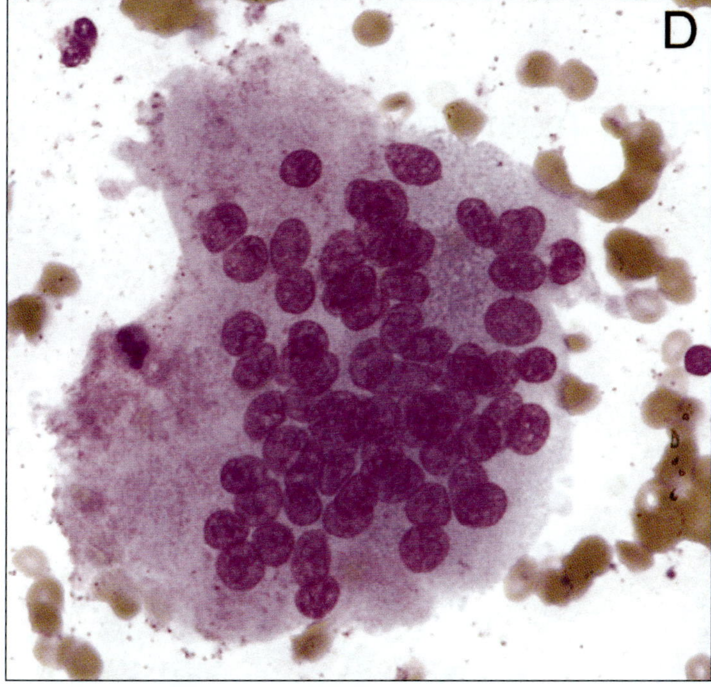
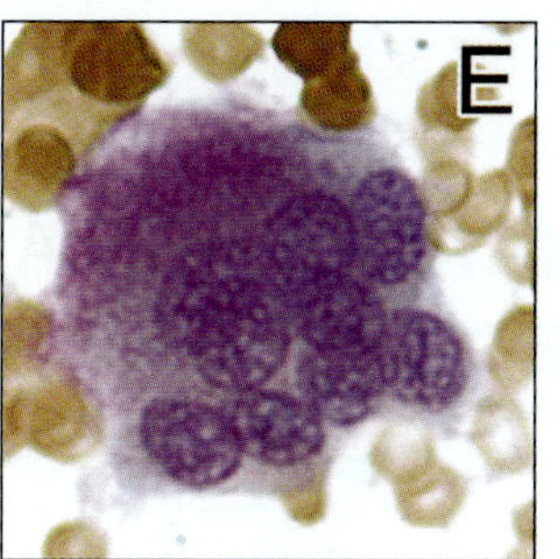
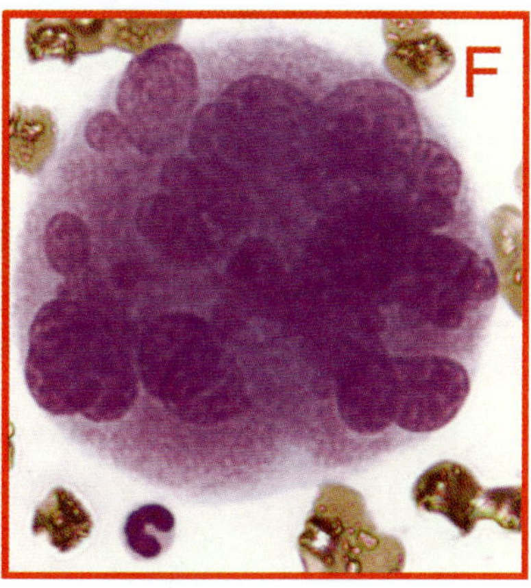

Figure 8.20. Bone cells in aspirate smears. **A** and **B**: Clusters of osteoblasts with the characteristic extruding or "pouting" nuclei (*arrows*). **C**: Plasma cells, shown here for comparison, are smaller than osteoblasts and do not have extruding nuclei. **D** and **E**: Osteoclasts with numerous well-separated and uniformly sized nuclei resembling "pennies on a plate." (Courtesy Dr. J. Lazarchick.) **F**: Megakaryocytes, one shown here for comparison, have variably sized nuclei with contiguous lobulations.

GRANULOCYTIC HYPERPLASIA (POST CYTOKINE ADMINISTRATION)

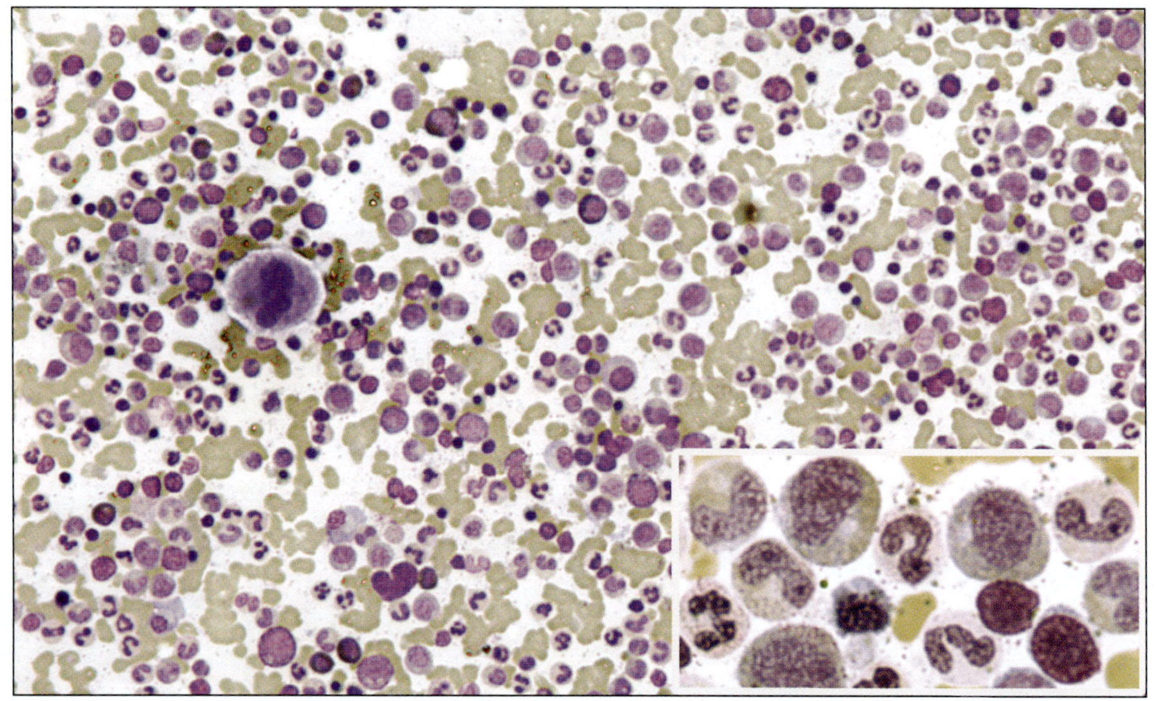

MATURATION ARREST (POST VIRAL INFECTION)

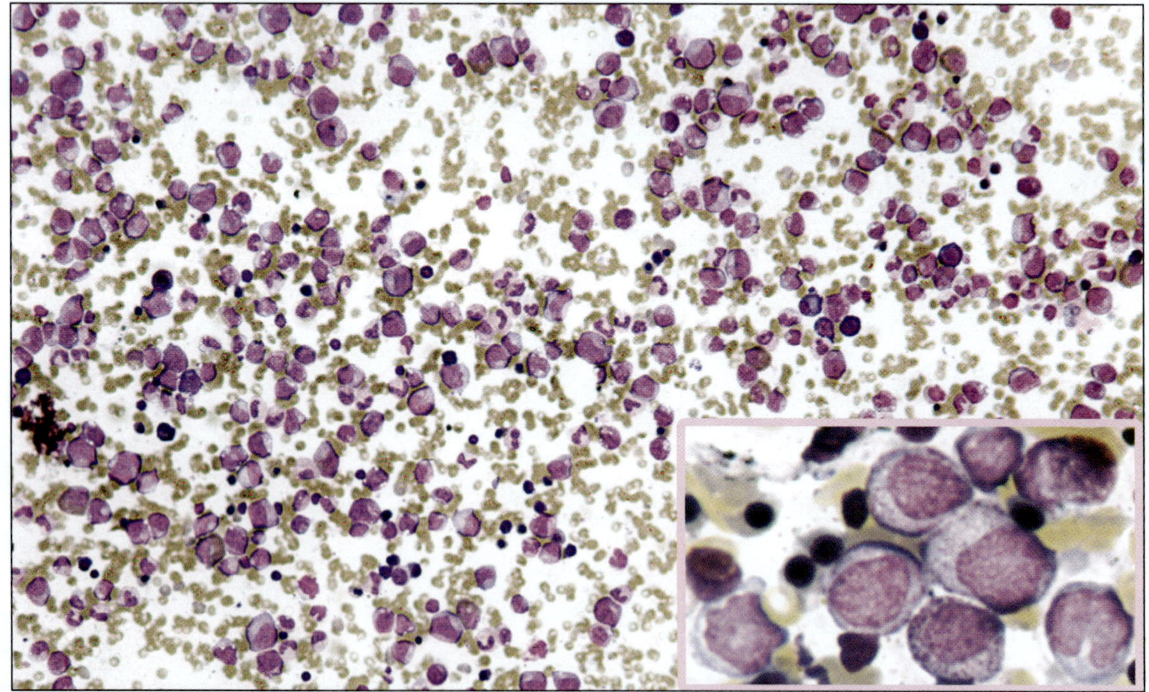

Figure 8.21.   "Granulocytic pattern" in aspirate smear. Diverse etiologies may give similar morphologic findings, and clinical correlation often is necessary to elucidate the proper pathologic diagnosis. Both aspirates show predominant numbers of immature granulocytic precursors.

MARROW INVOLVED BY LYMPHOMA (CLL)

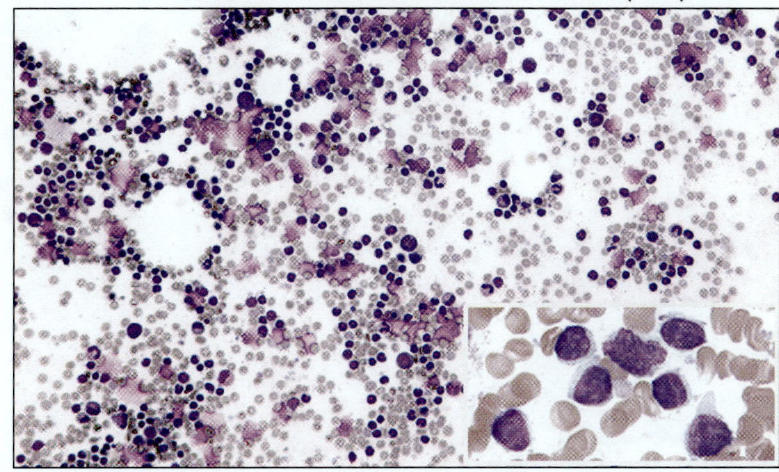

ACUTE LEUKEMIA (AML)

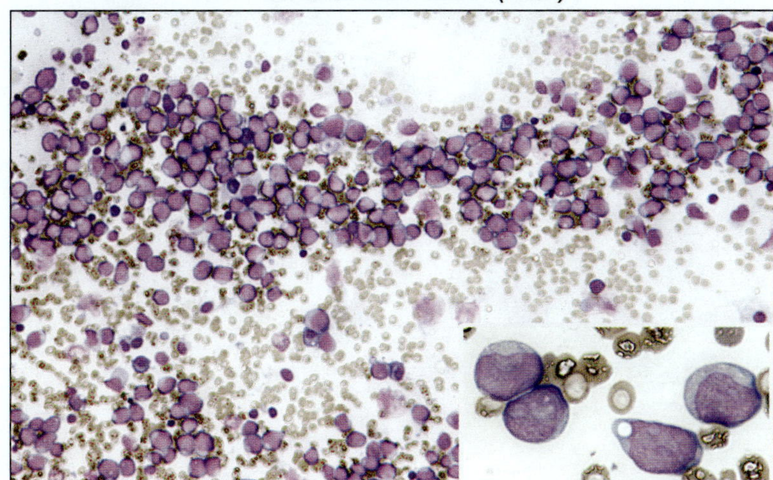

ERYTHROID HYPERPLASIA (THALASSEMIA)

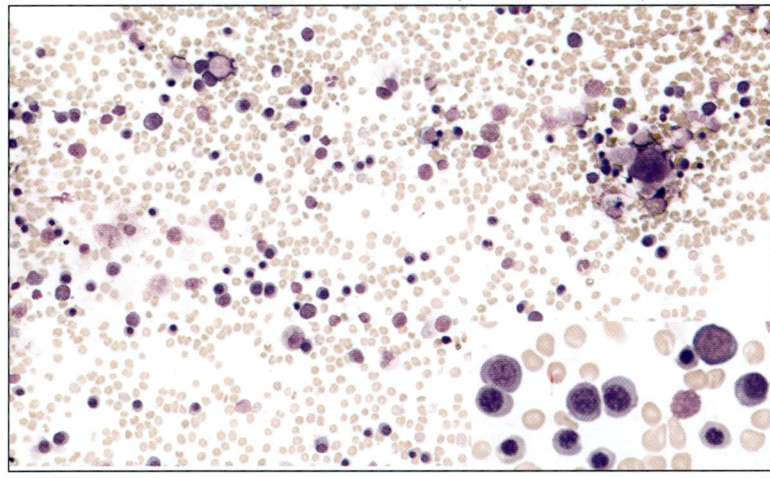

Figure 8.22. "Mononuclear pattern" in aspirate smear. The most common cells in the marrow are segmented granulocytic precursors and, at low-power magnification, these should predominate. The top two panels demonstrate a mononuclear pattern composed mostly of a monotonous cell population (mature lymphoid and primitive hematopoietic, *upper and middle panels, respectively*) that is best appreciated at low magnification. The lower panel consists mainly of a heterogeneous population of mononuclear cells, in this particular case, of mature erythroid origin.

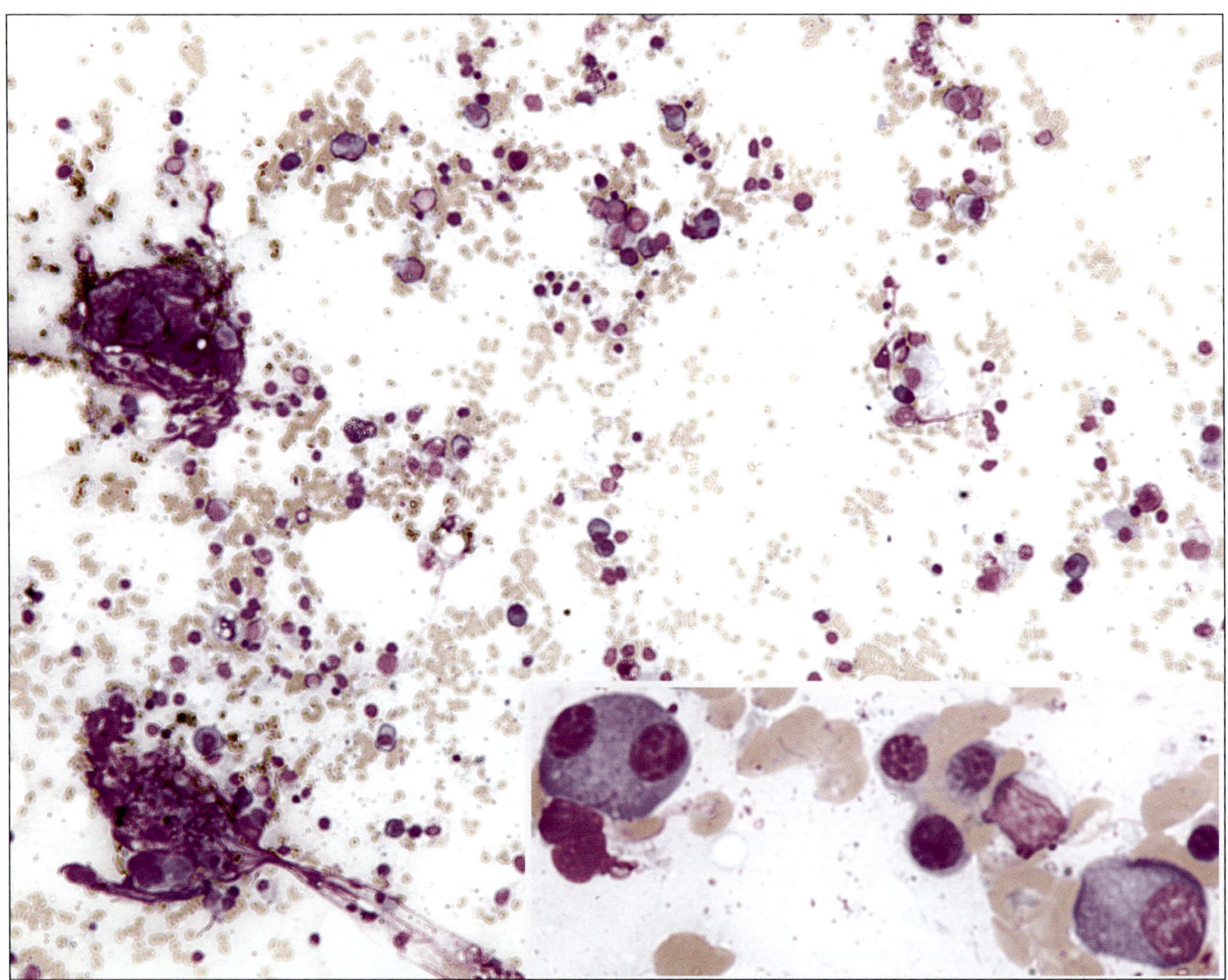

Figure 8.23. Aplastic aspirate. When viewing supposedly aplastic aspirate smears it is important to evaluate whether the sample is representative. The presence of marrow particles and some evidence of hematopoiesis ensure the aspirates are from the marrow cavity and not merely peripheral blood. Plasma cells and lymphocytes often appear disproportionately increased in aplastic smears from diverse etiologies, and the examiner should be cautious in diagnosing myeloma or lymphoprolifera-tive disorders in this setting.

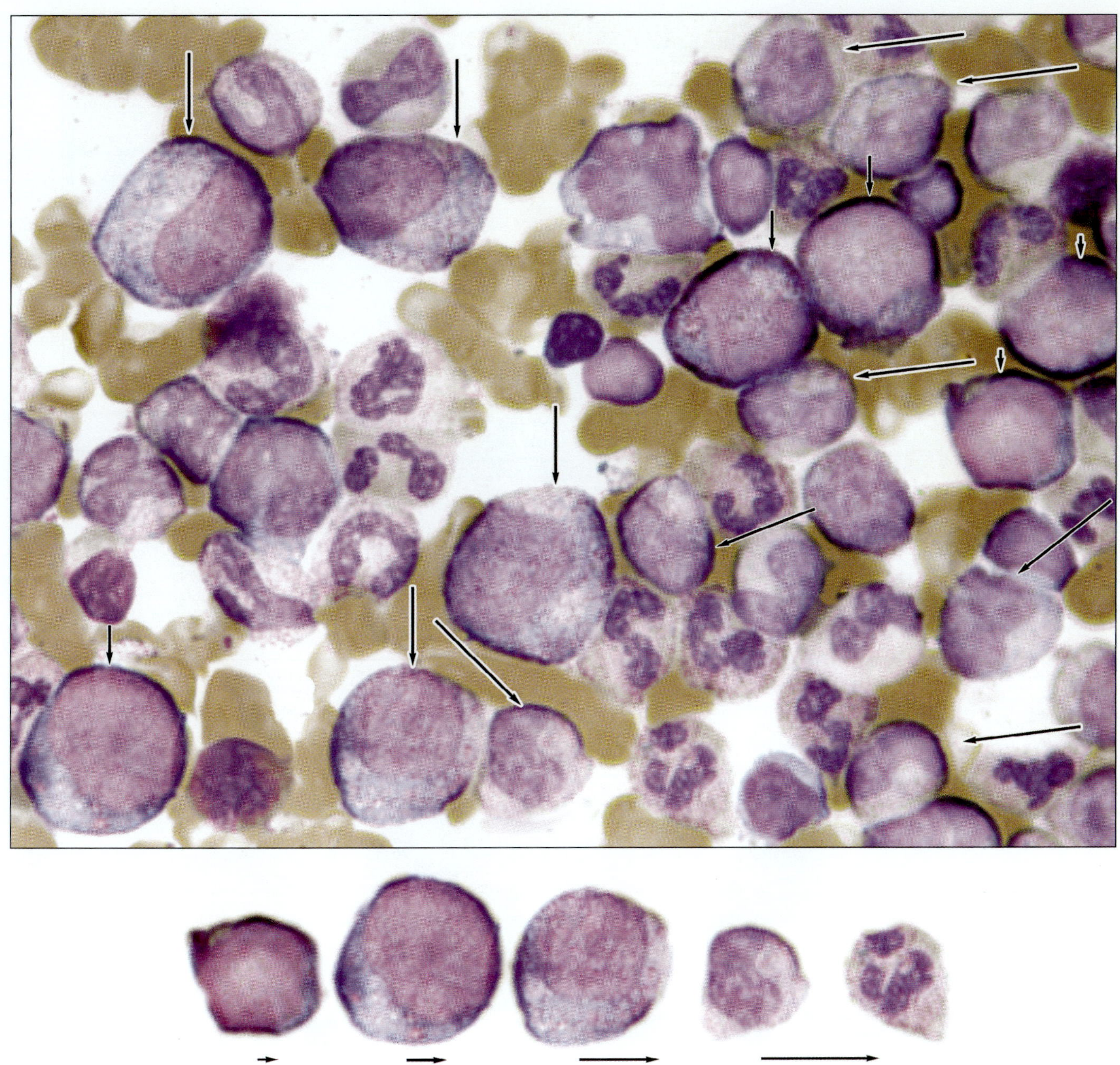

Figure 8.24. Morphology of granulocytic precursors in marrow. In this composite figure, the spectrum of immature to mature myeloid precursors is designated by a series of lengthening arrows.

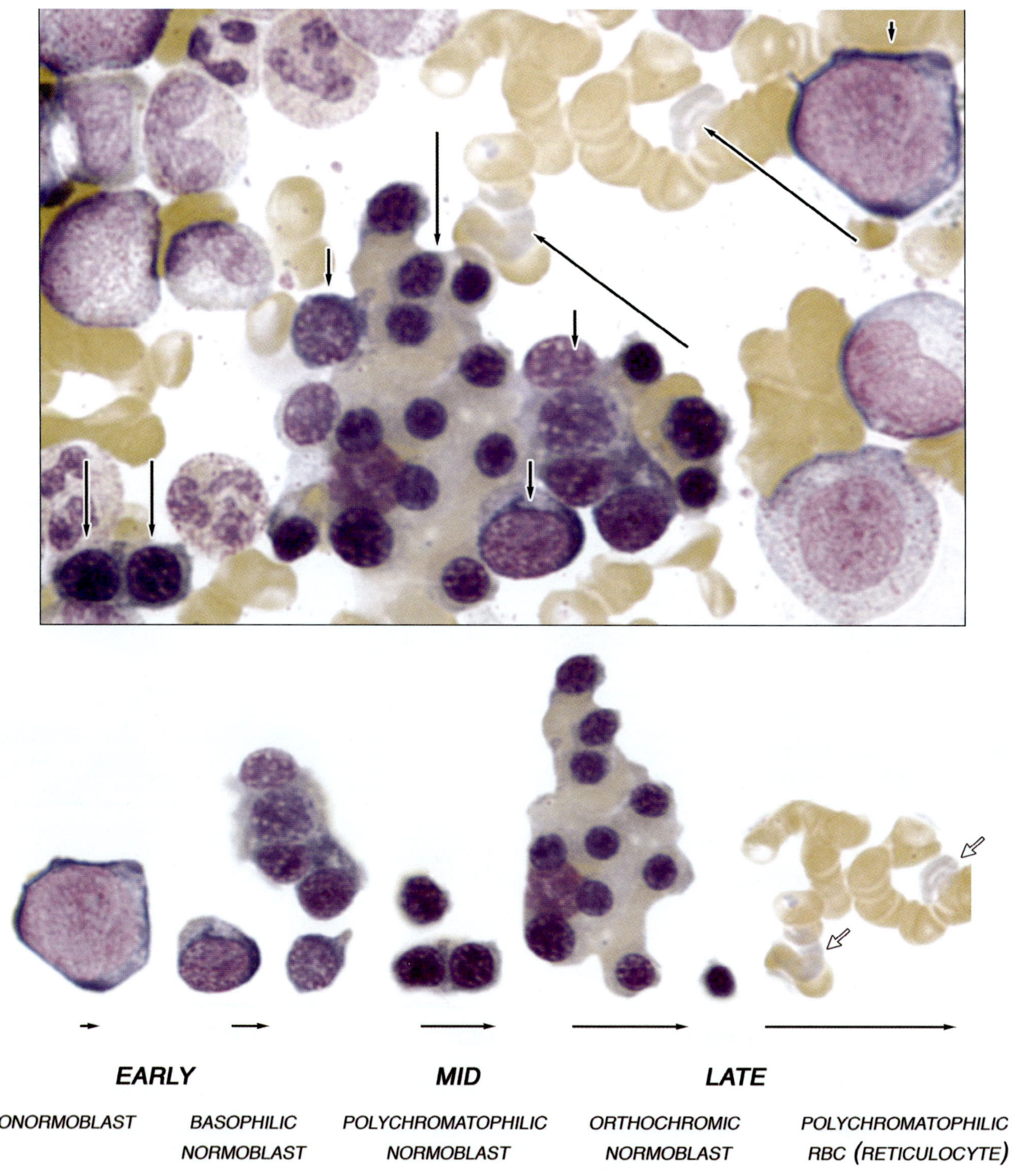

Figure 8.25.   Morphology of erythroid precursors in marrow. In this composite figure, the spectrum of immature to mature erythroid precursors is designated by a series of lengthening arrows.

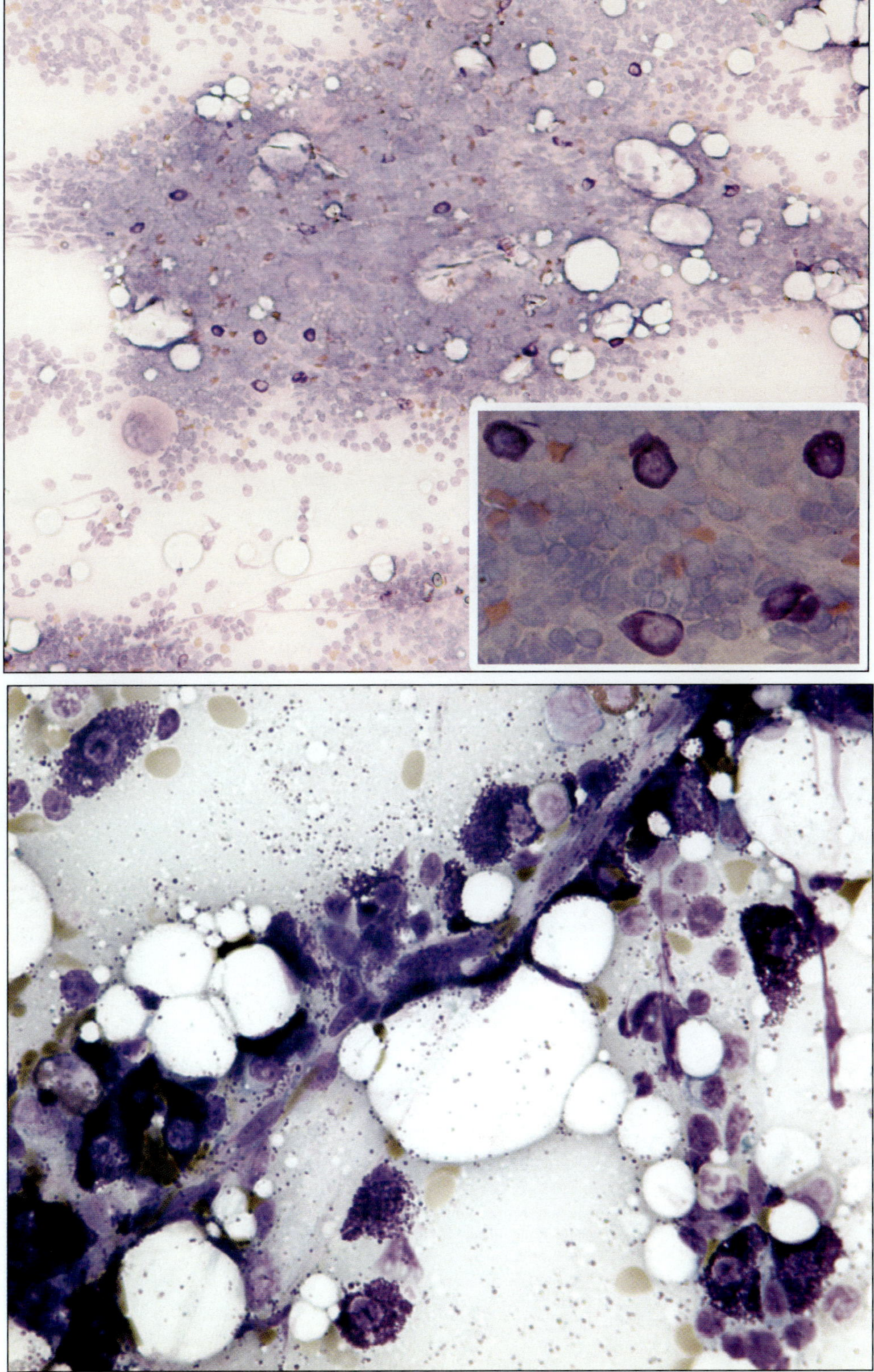

Figure 8.26.　Mast cells. Normally, mast cells constitute less than 1% of all the nucleated marrow cells. They often are enmeshed in the stroma of marrow particles, making them difficult to appreciate in standard aspirate preparations. The top panel is a smear stained with toluidine blue that shows normal numbers of mast cells in this rather large marrow particle. They display metachromatic staining, in which the color of the cell components is different from that of the dye used. The bottom panel, from a case of systemic mastocytosis, illustrates a Wright-Giemsa–stained aspirate demonstrating numerous heavily granulated mast cells.

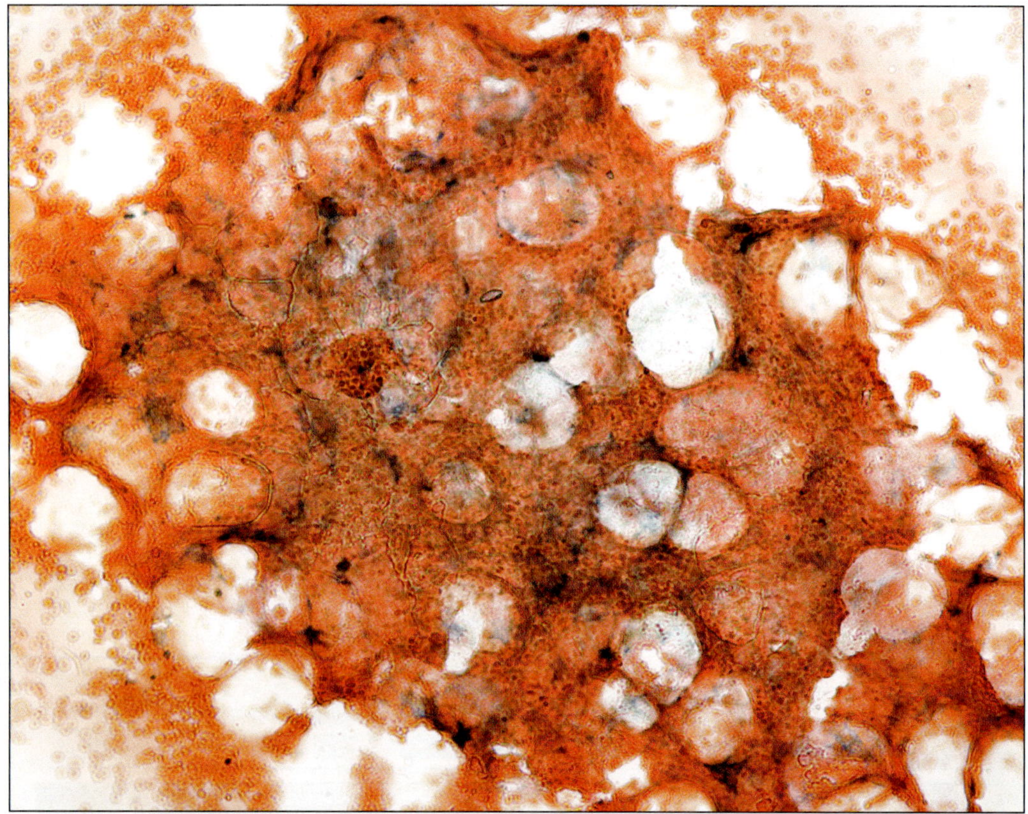

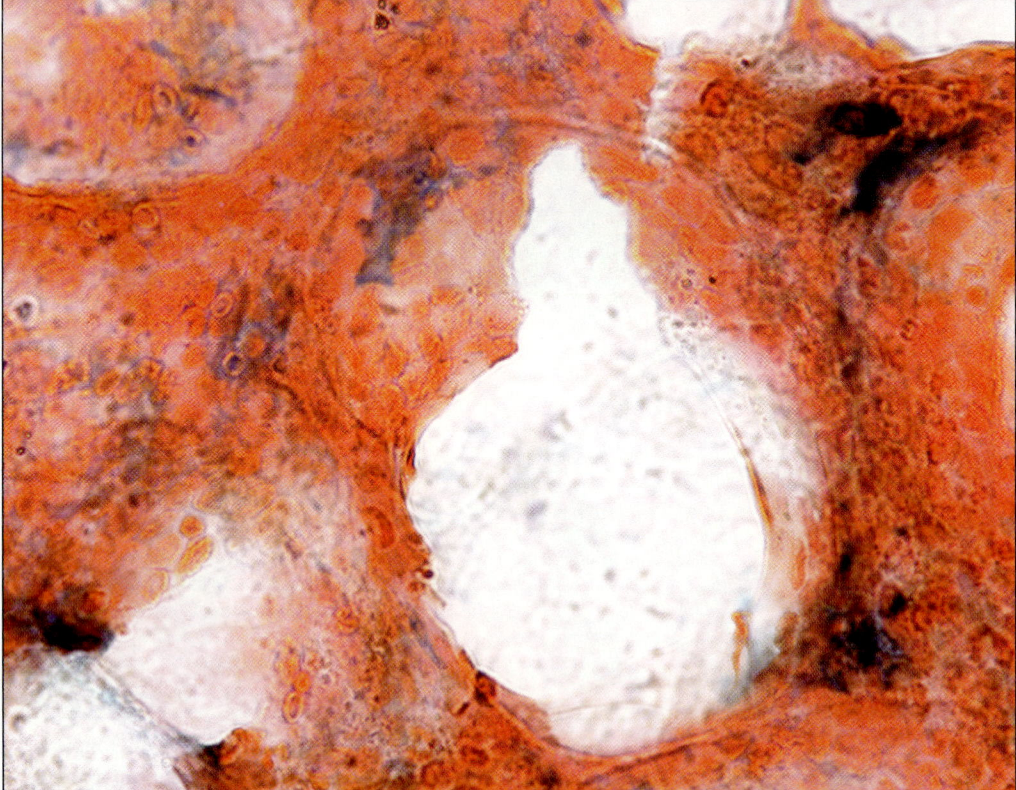

Figure 8.27.   Prussian blue iron stains. Staining the bone marrow for iron is the gold standard for assessing body iron stores. Individual histiocytes scattered throughout the aspirate smear show the normal pattern of fine granular blue staining for iron (see also Fig. 1.9).

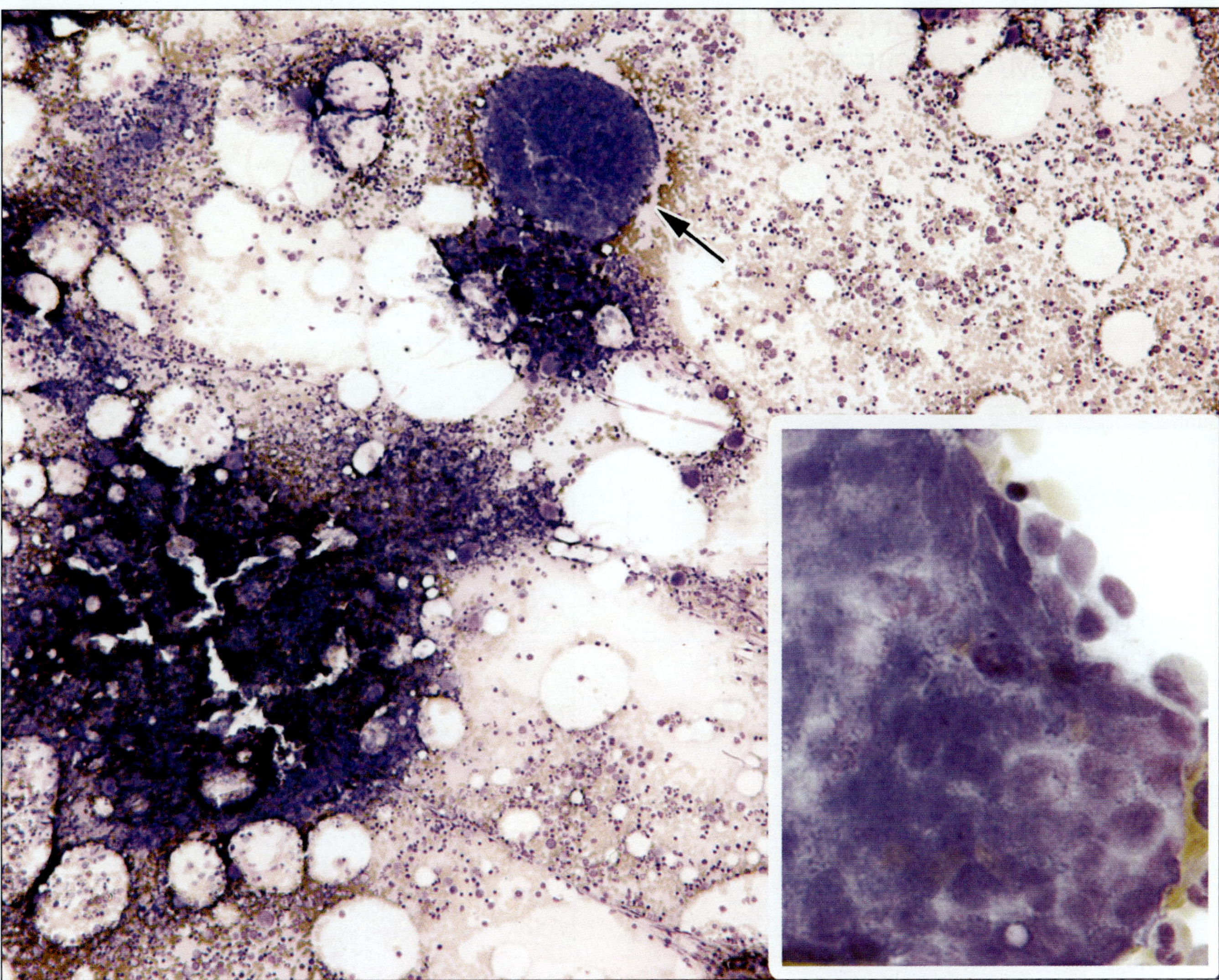

Figure 8.28.   Metastatic breast carcinoma. This aspirate smear shows a large, thick cohesive cluster of malignant cells with smooth borders. Examination at higher power reveals poorly preserved, large collections of highly atypical cells. This cluster was the only evidence of metastatic malignancy in all six aspirate smears evaluated in this particular case.

LOOSE AGGREGRATE OF HEMATOPOIETIC CELLS

COHESIVE CLUSTER OF CARCINOMA

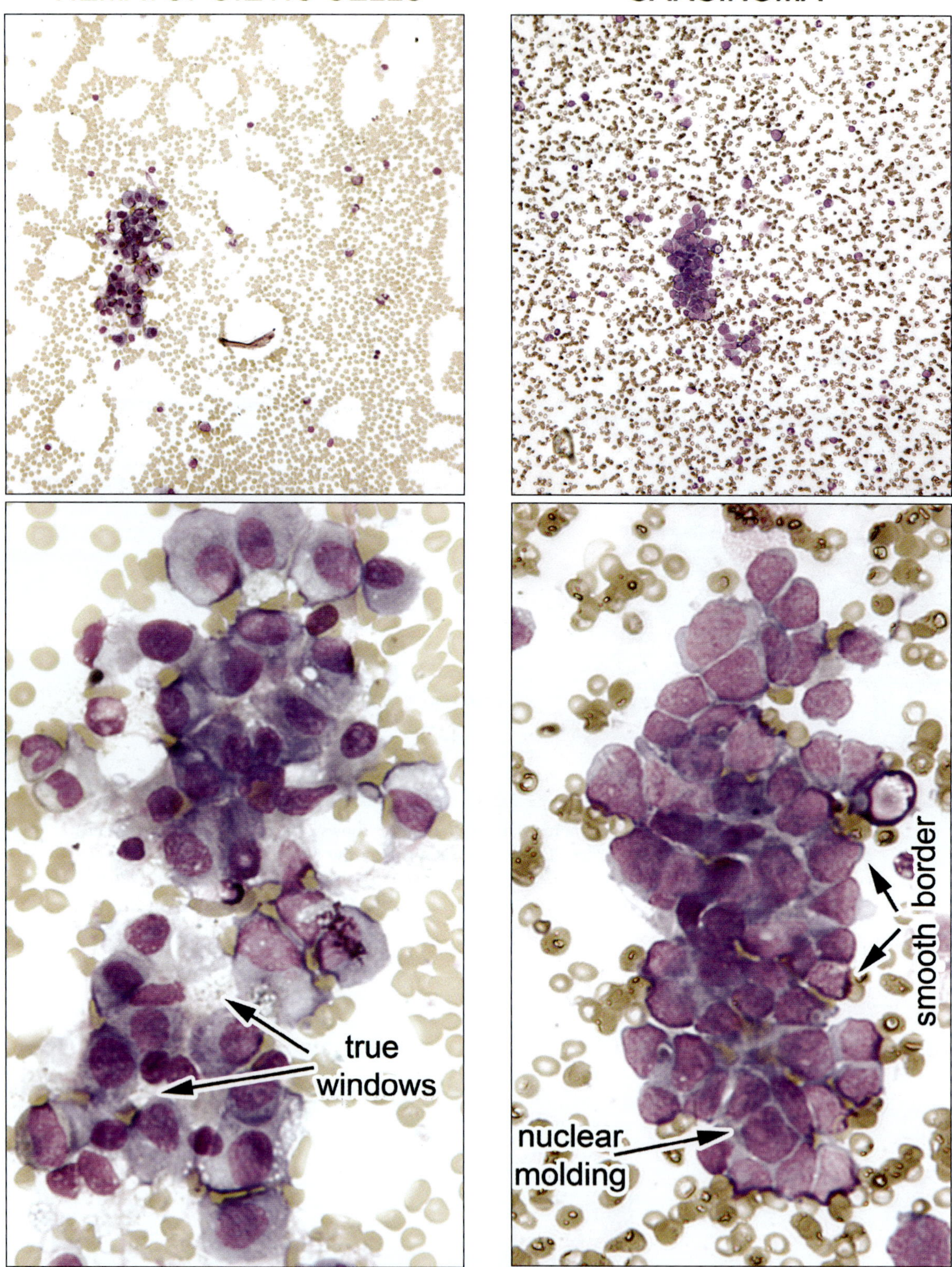

Figure 8.29.   Hematopoietic verses nonhematopoietic cells in aspirate smear. Tight clusters of degenerating large cells in aspirate smears strongly suggest marrow involvement by extrinsic neoplasms that are neither lymphoid nor hematopoietic in origin. Morphologic differences between collections of hematopoietic cells and cohesive clumps of nonhematopoietic cancer cells are illustrated here, with examples of acute monocytic leukemia and metastatic small cell carcinoma of the lung (*left* and *right panels*, respectively).

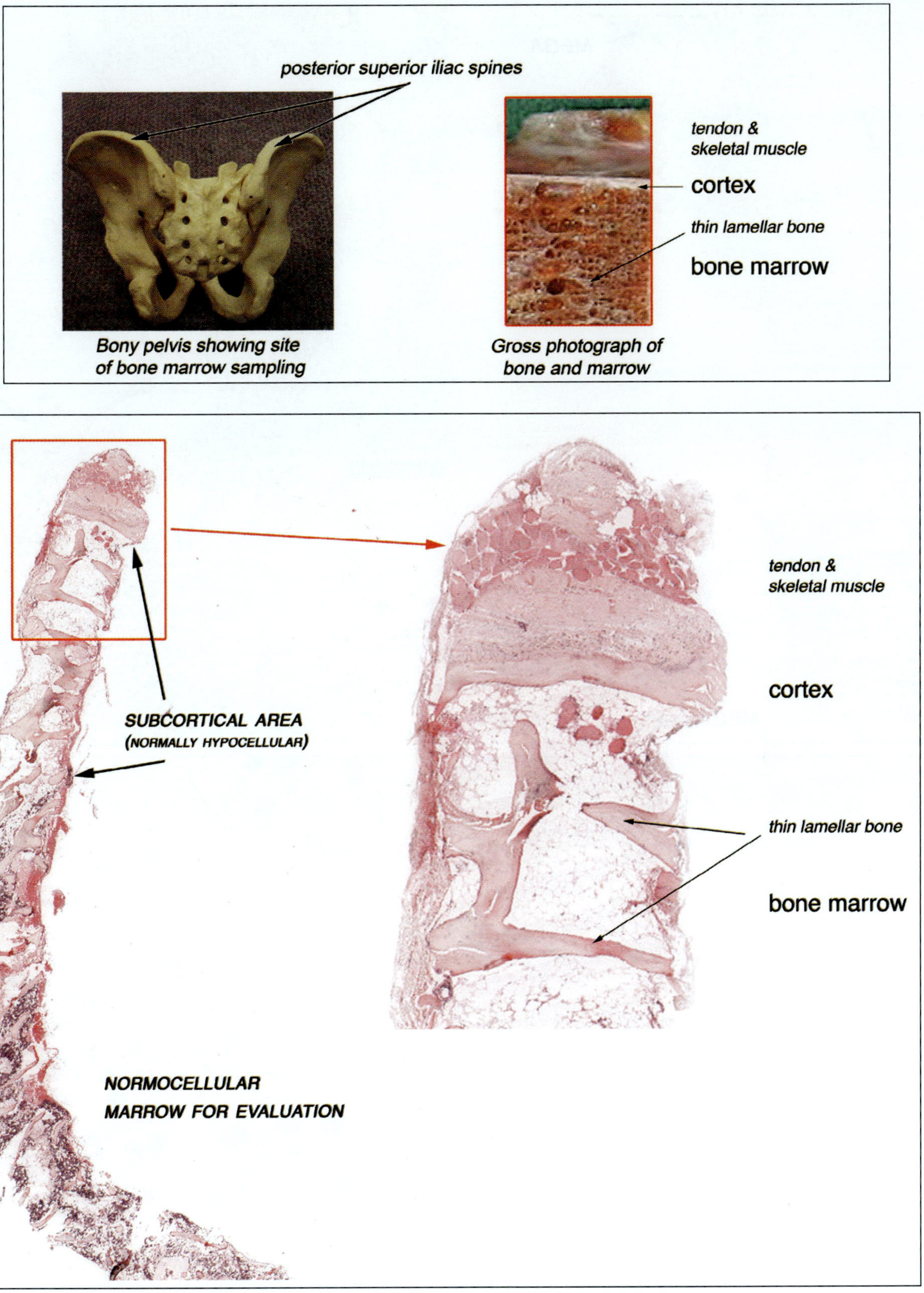

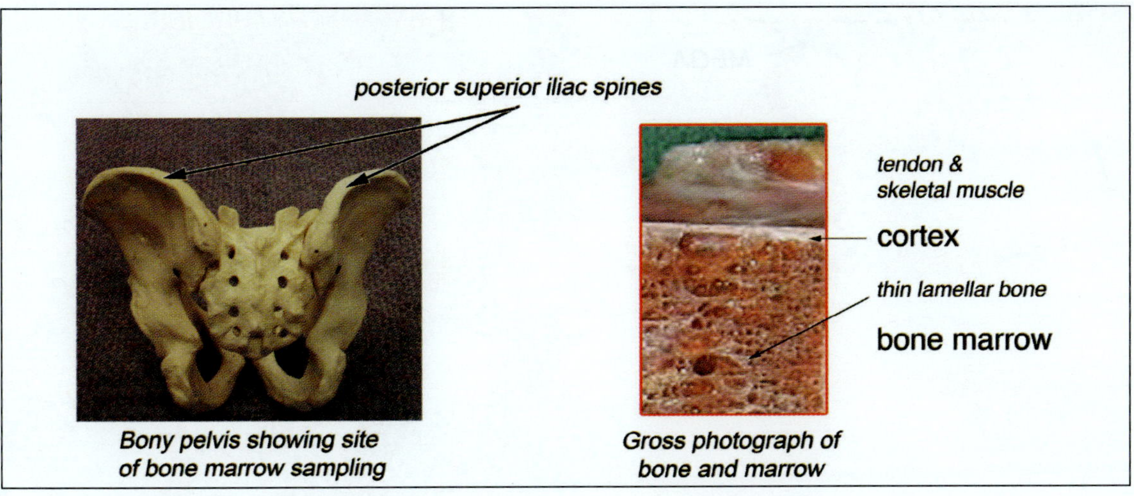

Figure 8.30.   Anatomy of the bone marrow. This composite figure shows the relationships between the skeletal anatomy of the bone marrow biopsy site and the microscopic features of biopsy interpretation.

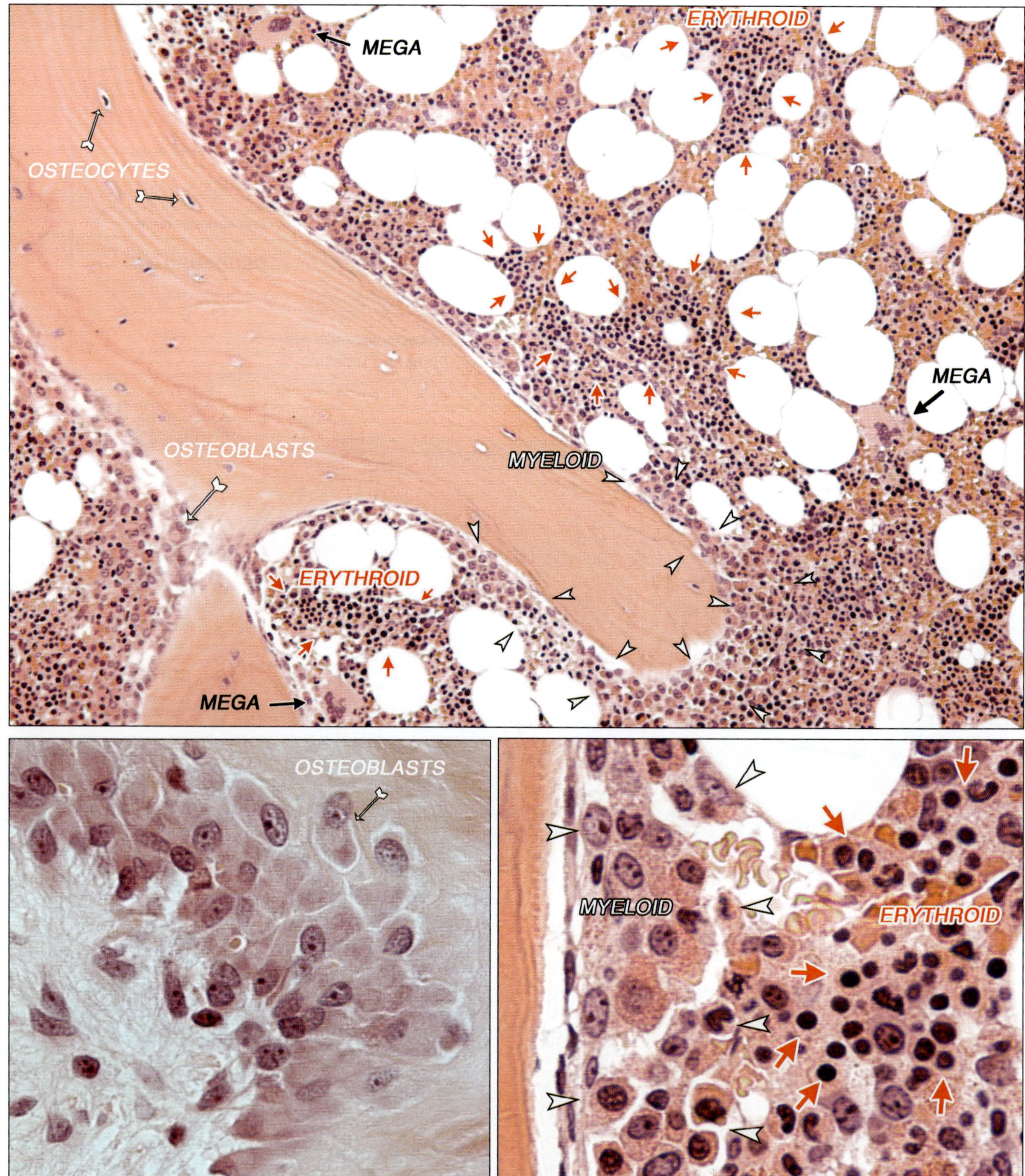

Figure 8.31. Microanatomy of the bone marrow biopsy. The three major hematopoietic lineages of the marrow—megakaryocytic (MEGA, *black arrows*), myeloid (*white arrows*), and erythroid (*red arrows*)—all tend to cluster together and are recognizable in biopsy specimens. The myeloid series tend to collect near bony trabeculae and perivascular spaces.

MILD INCREASE IN MEGAKARYOCYTES

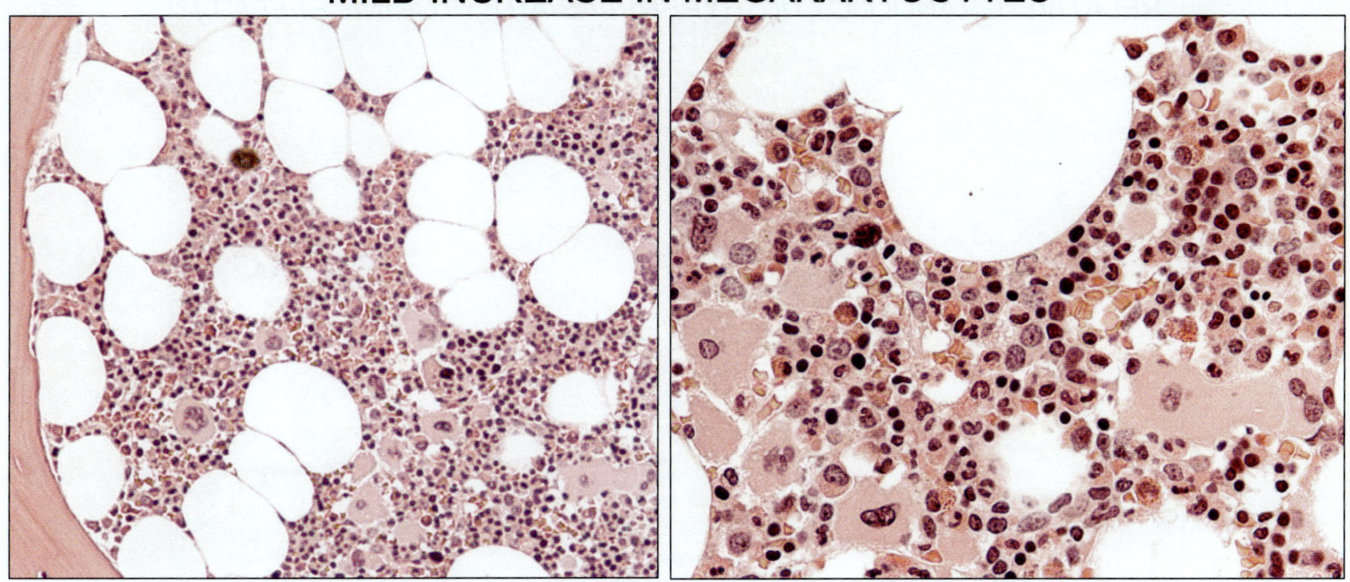

SEVERE INCREASE IN MEGAKARYOCYTES

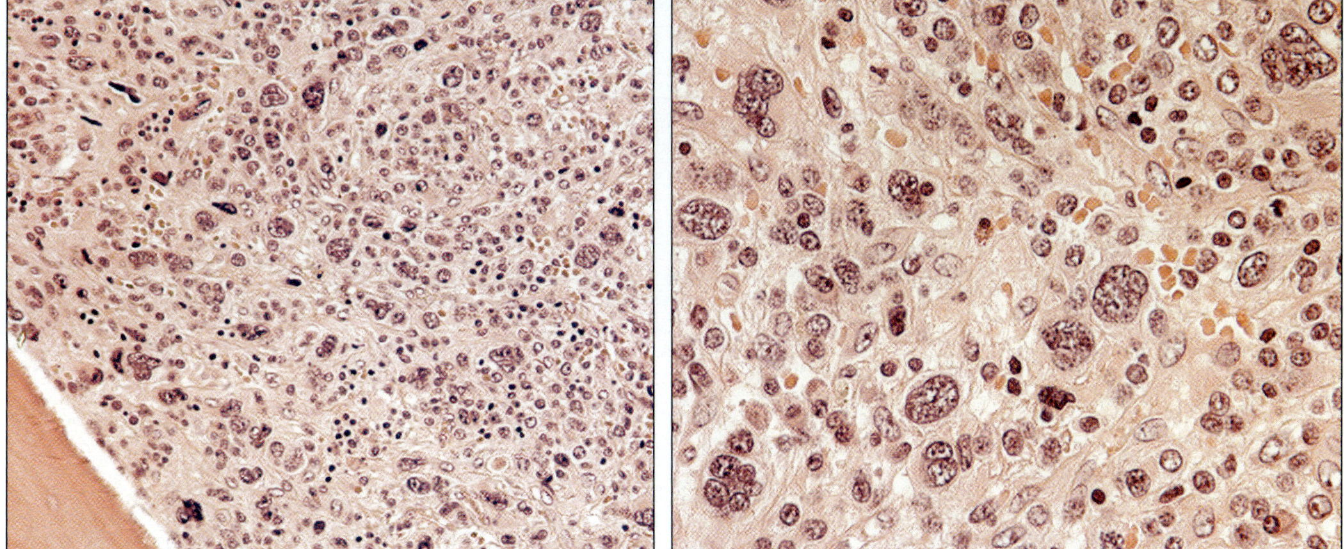

Figure 8.32.   Megakaryocytes. Increases in megakaryocyte can be best appreciated using low and medium magnification of the core biopsy. Architectural distortion (swirling and lining up of individual marrow cells) consistent with significant marrow fibrosis is present in the bottom panels.

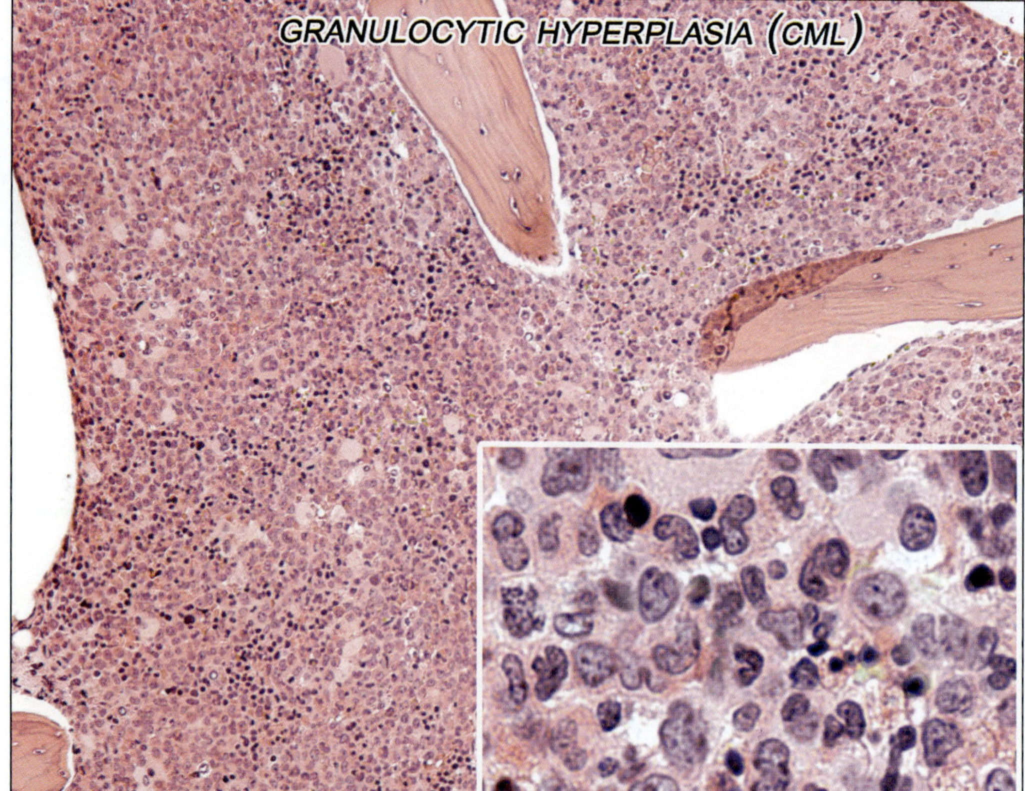

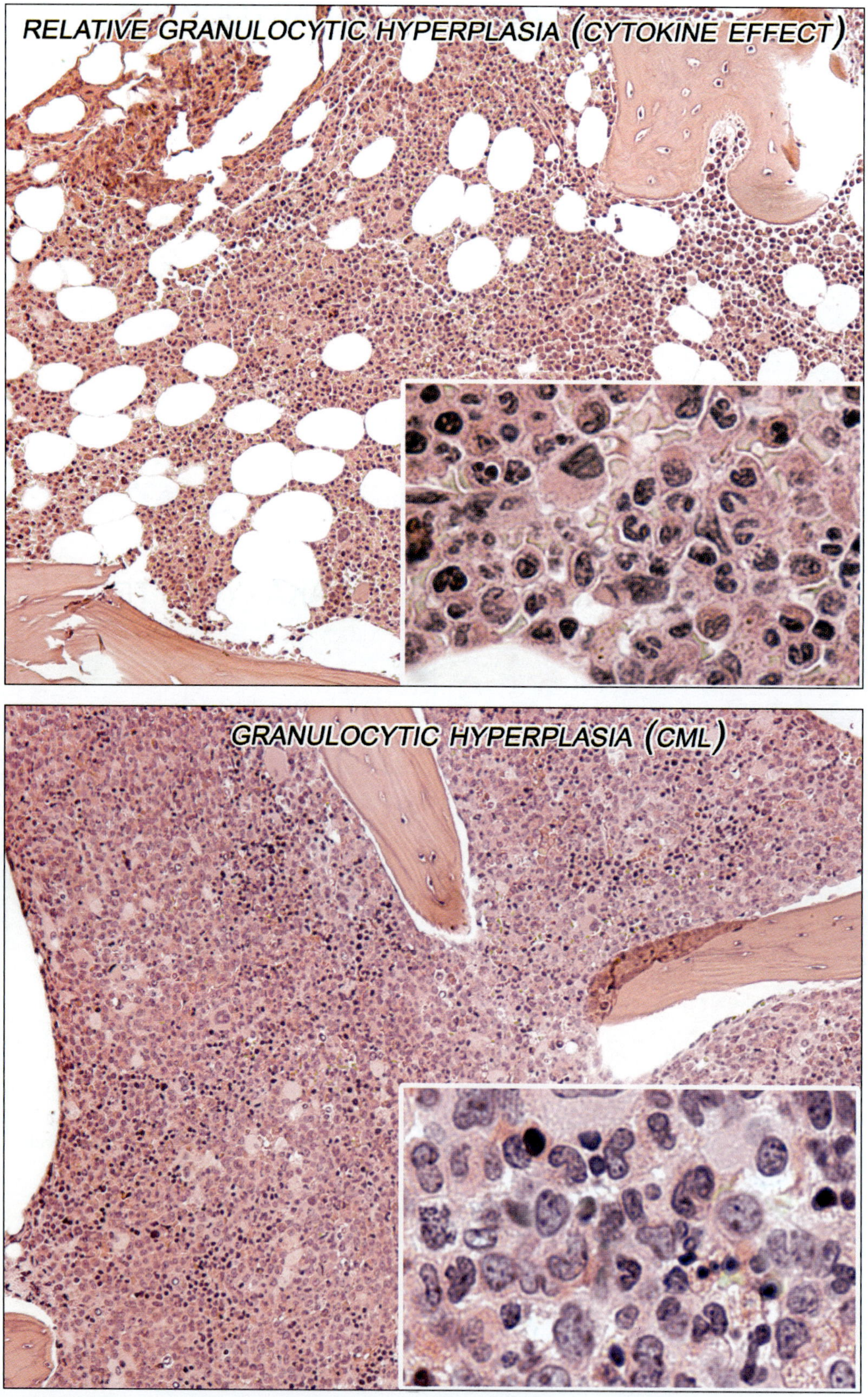

Figure 8.33. "Granulocytic pattern" in biopsy. Relative and absolute increases in granulocytic precursors are readily seen in the top and lower figures, respectively.

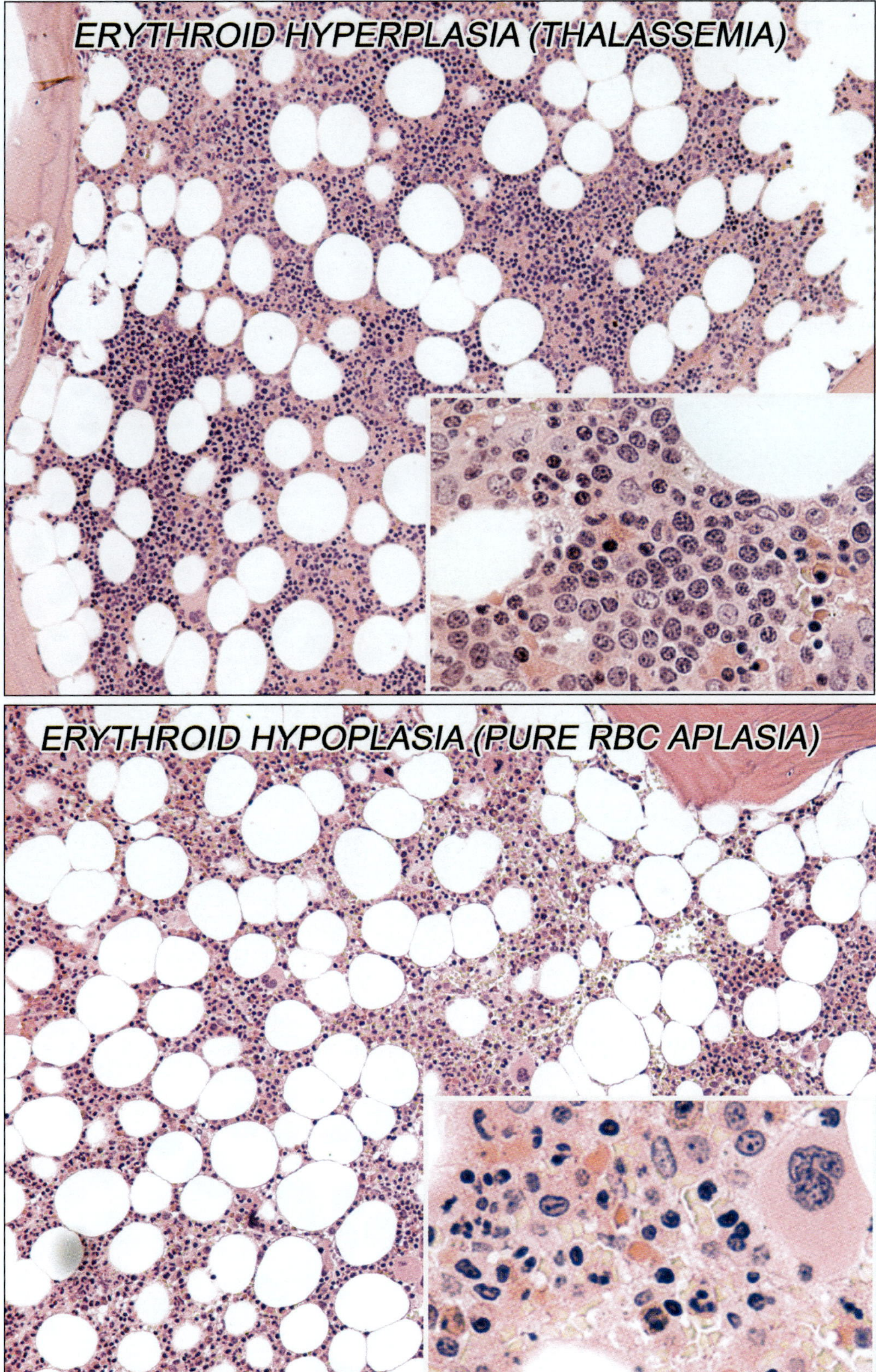

Figure 8.34. Erythropoiesis in biopsy. An absolute increase in erythroid precursors that results in a "mononuclear pattern" is shown in the top panel. The bottom panel shows a severe decrease in erythroid precursors giving the biopsy a "granulocytic" appearance. Increased and decreased erythropoiesis is apparent in these two biopsy specimens.

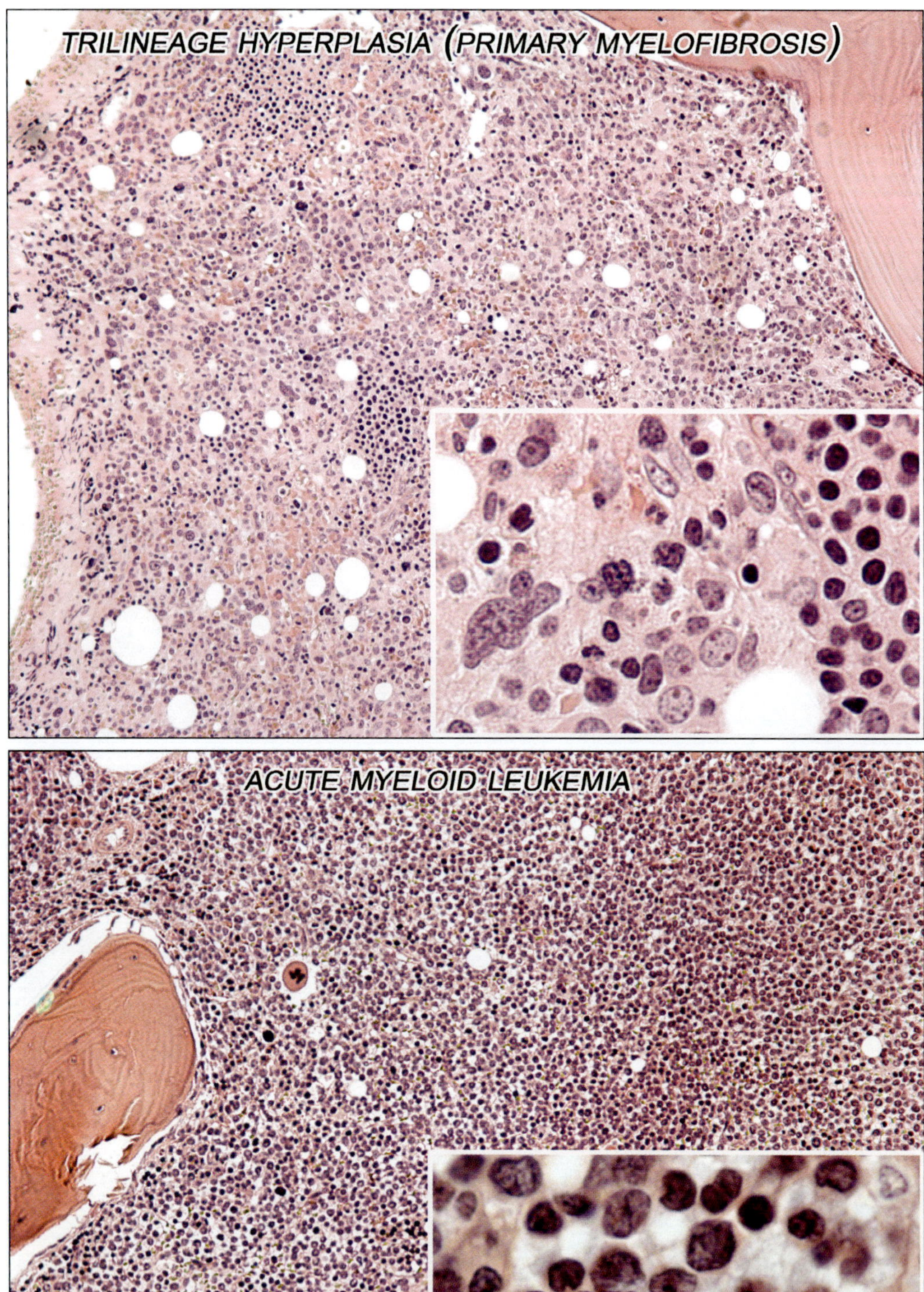

Figure 8.35. Hyperplastic patterns in biopsy. Two hyperplastic marrow specimens are illustrated here. One contains a heterogeneous mixture of mature hematopoietic precursors typical of the myeloproliferative syndromes (*top panel*). The bottom panel shows the expansion of a homogenous population of immature hematopoietic cells characteristic of acute leukemia.

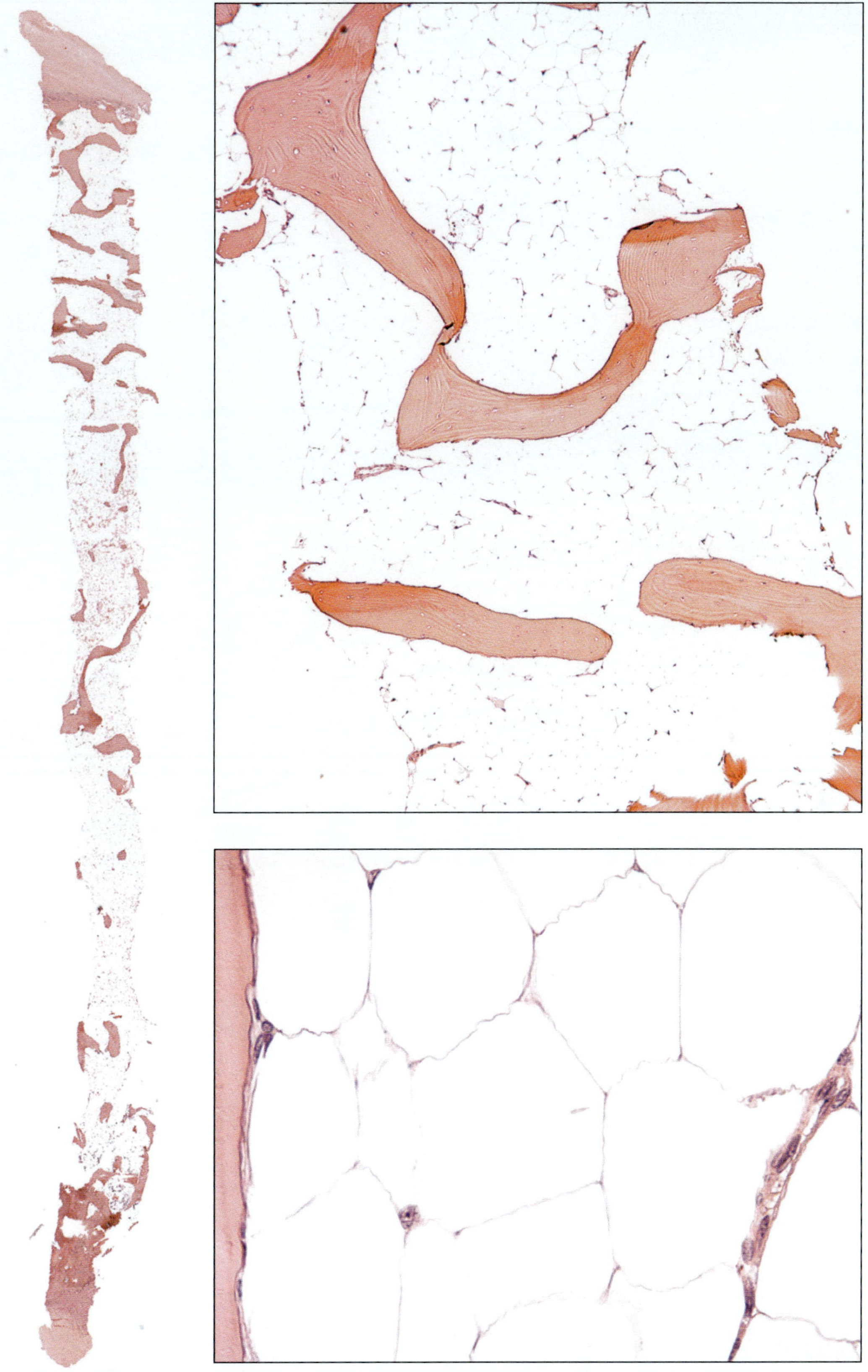

Figure 8.36. Hypoplastic patterns in biopsy. This biopsy from a case of aplastic anemia shows profound hypocellularity and virtually no evidence of hematopoiesis. The differential diagnosis of a bone marrow biopsy almost devoid of hematopoiesis includes congenital and idiopathic causes of aplastic anemia, hypocellular myelodysplastic syndromes, and paroxysmal nocturnal hemoglobinuria. Plasma cells and mast cells often appear disproportionally increased in hypoplastic specimens.

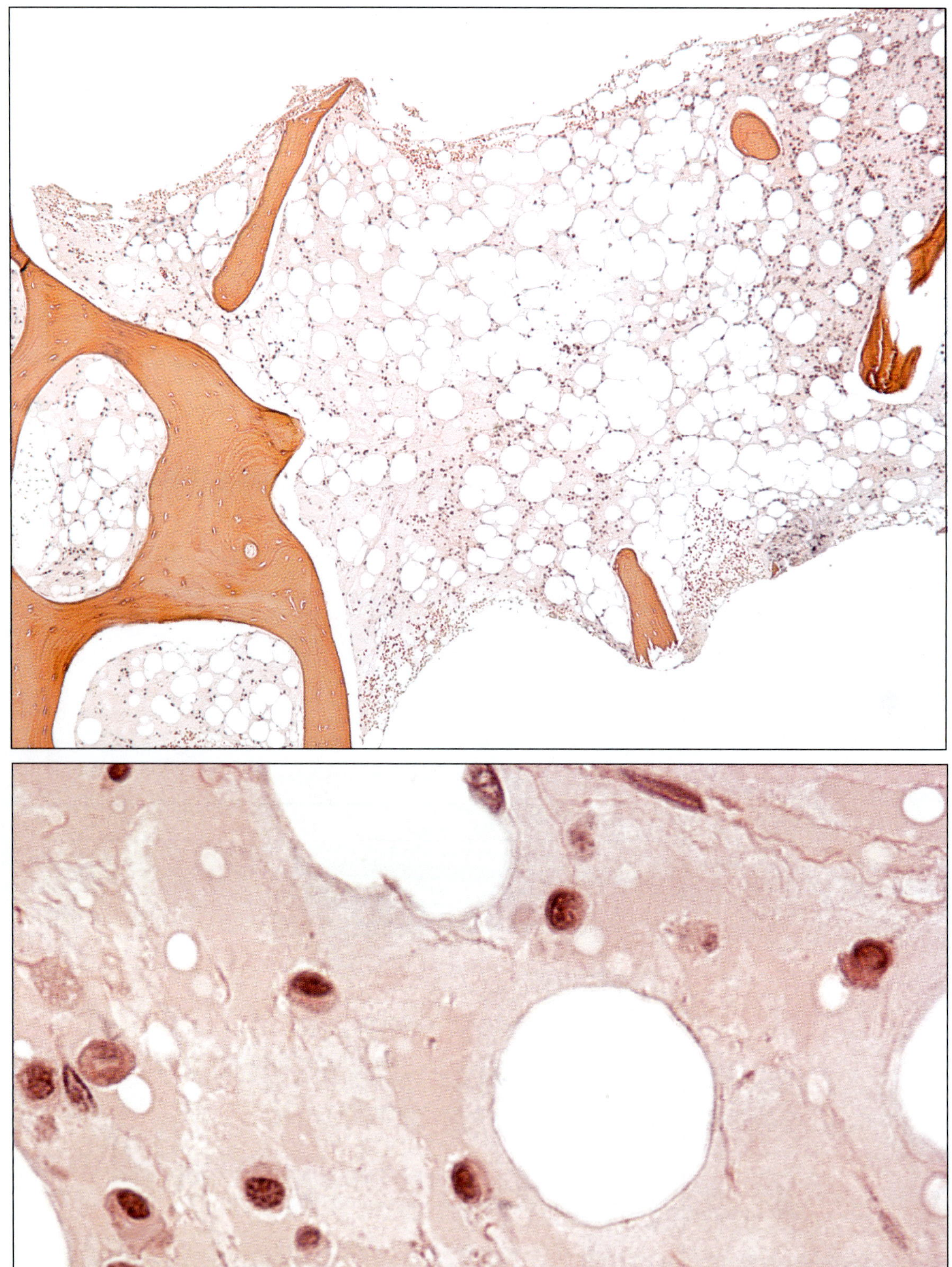

Figure 8.37.   Serous atrophy. In this condition, an amorphous gelatinous ground substance replaces fat and hematopoietic cells. Causes include chronic systemic dysfunctions, such as HIV and malnutrition.

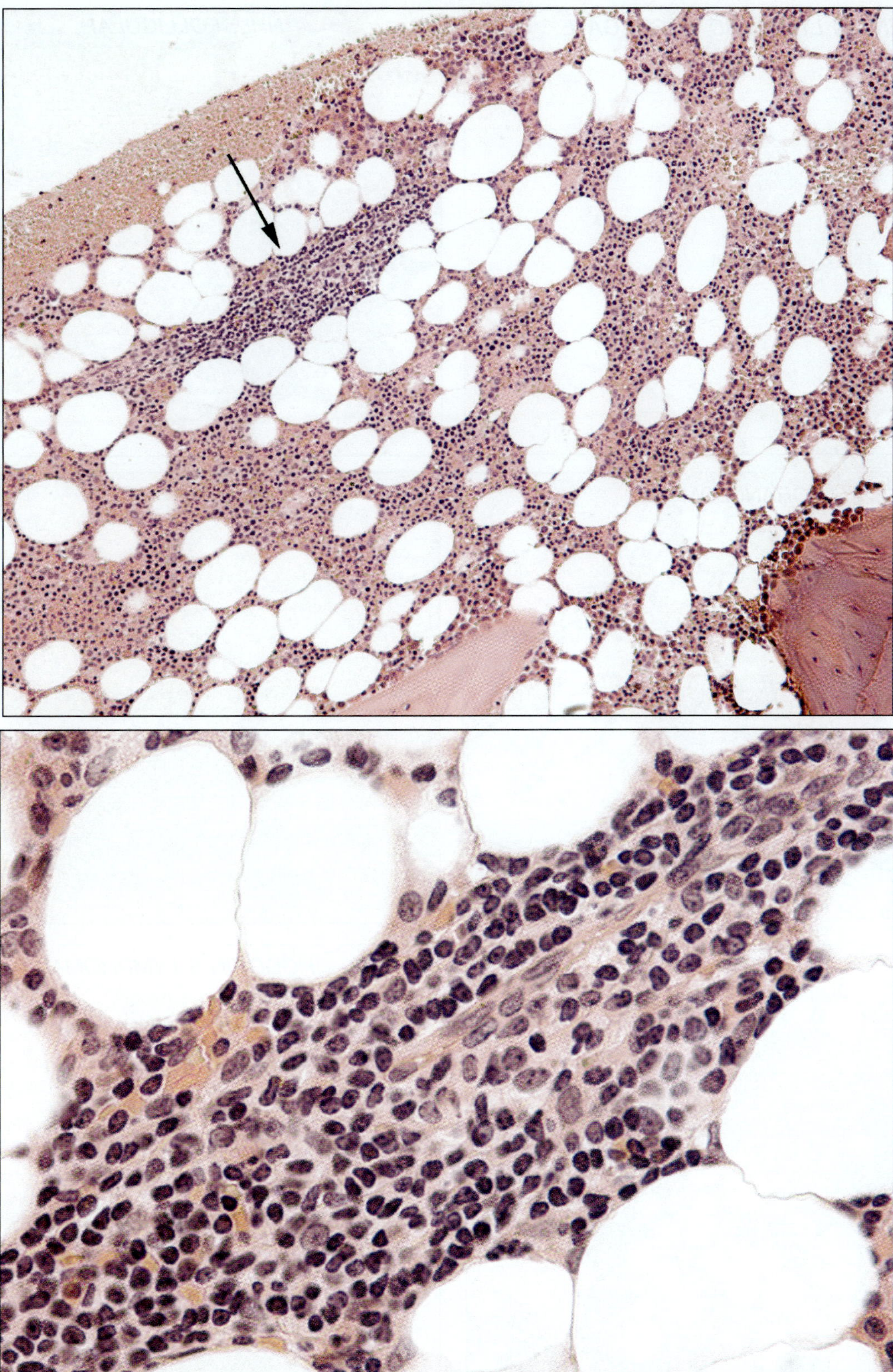

Figure 8.38. Lymphoid aggregates of the bone marrow. Benign lymphoid nodules of the bone marrow increase with age and are more frequent in women and patients with autoimmune diseases. Benign nodules usually consist mostly of small mature lymphocytes with smooth nuclear contours that are well-demarcated, small in size, and few in number. Other benign features include perivascular location and lack of significant CD10+ cells. This is an example of a small perivascular lymphoid nodule (*arrow*).

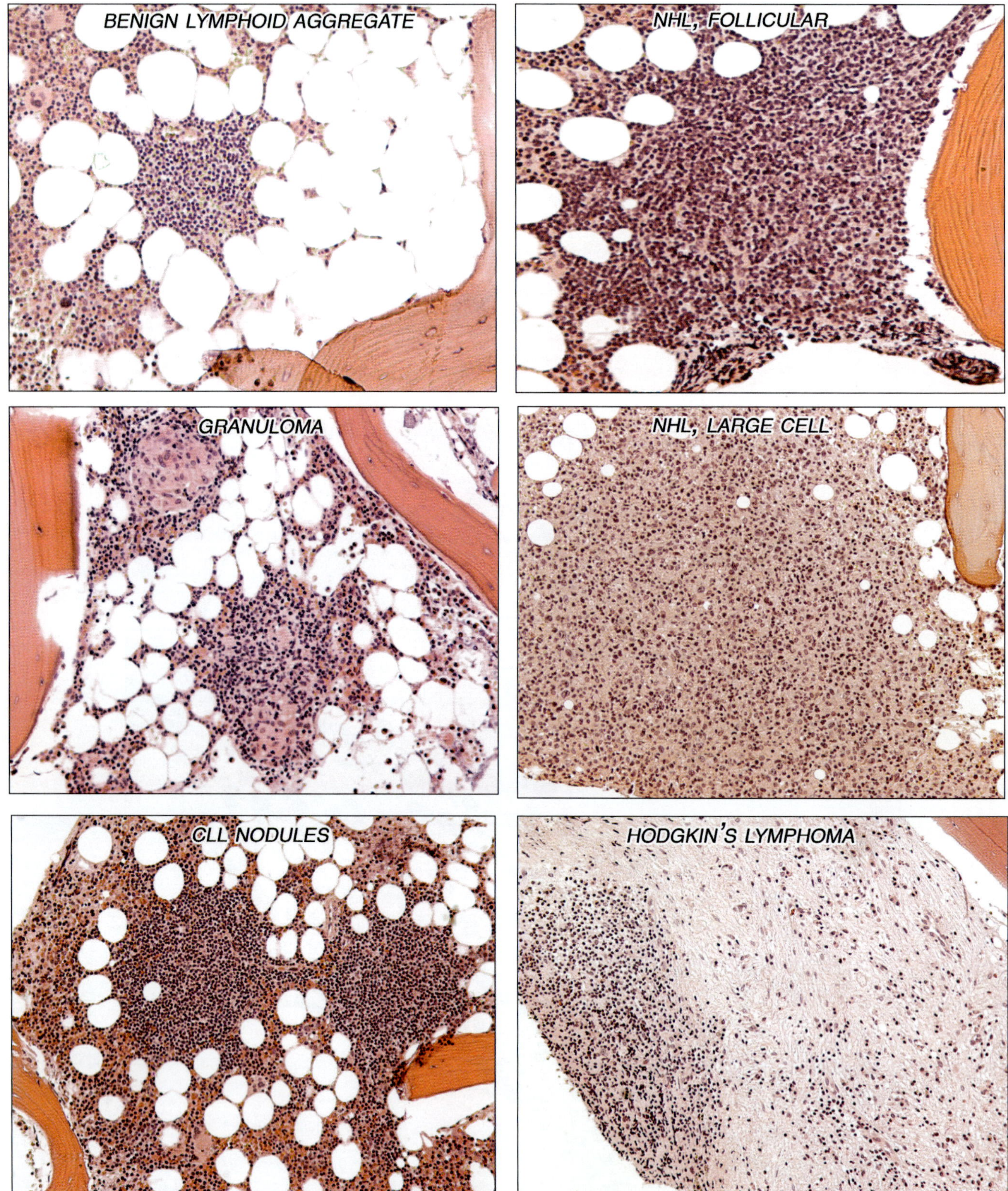

Figure 8.39. Benign and malignant lymphoid nodules. These biopsies show a benign lymphoid nodule, two incidental granulomas, nodular involvement of the marrow by chronic lymphocytic leukemia (CLL), follicular lymphoma, diffuse large B-cell lymphoma, and Hodgkin lymphoma.

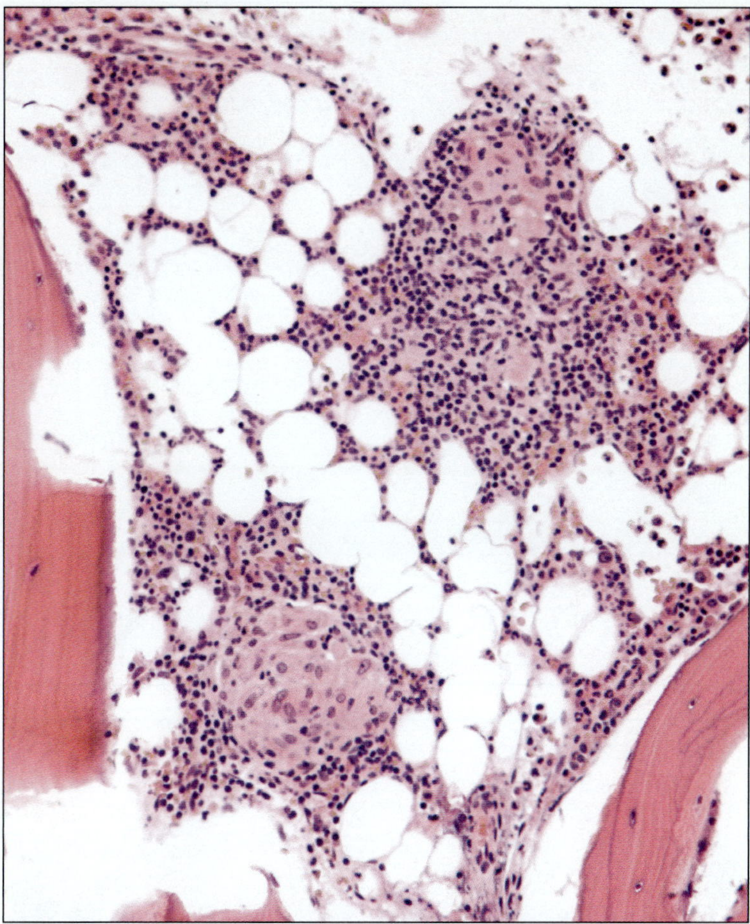

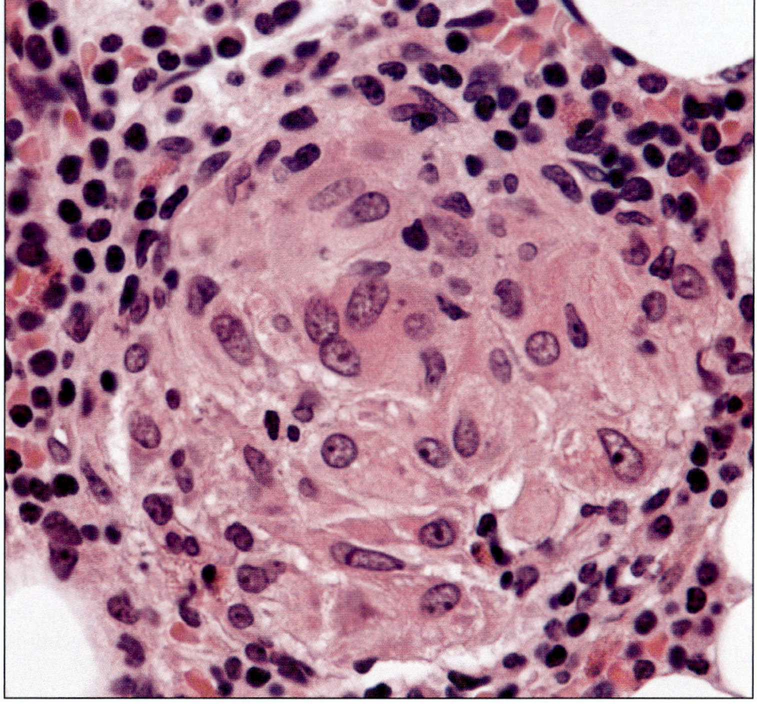

Figure 8.40. Bone marrow granulomas. This biopsy shows two discrete noncaseating granulomas from a patient with sarcoidosis. Other causes of bone marrow granulomas include lymphoid and nonlymphoid malignancies, infectious diseases, drugs, foreign bodies, and connective tissue diseases.

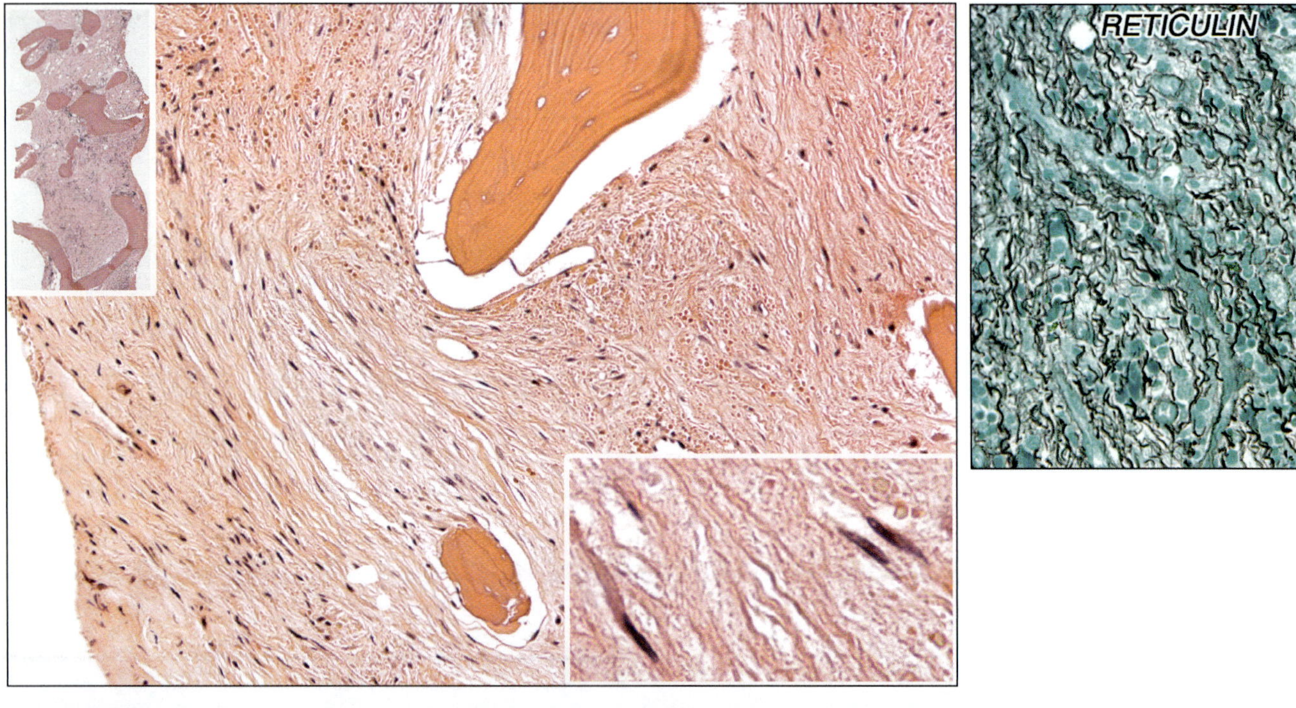

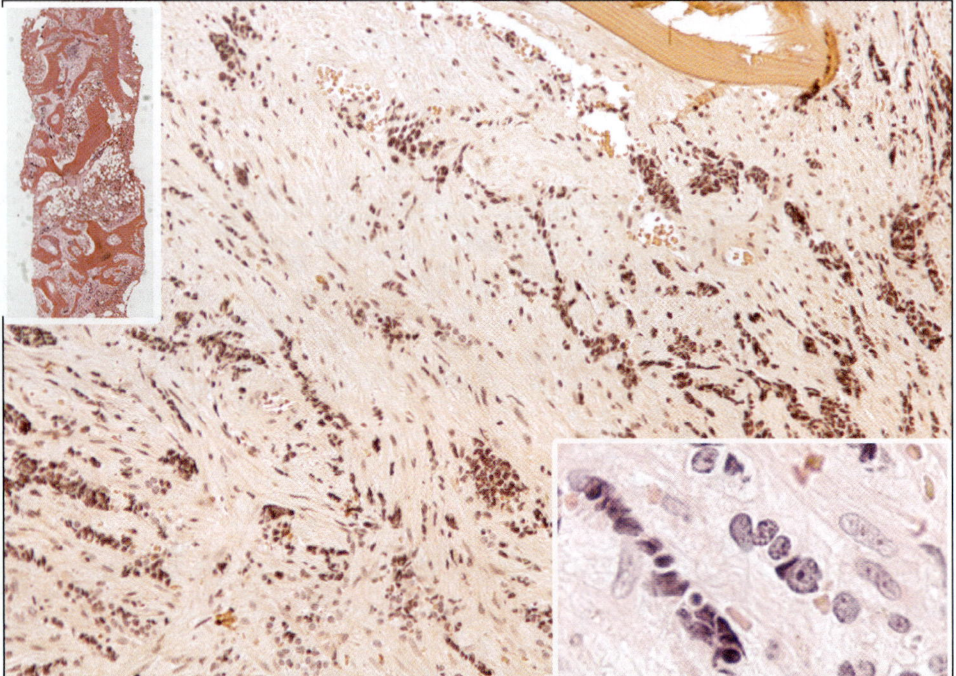

Figure 8.41.   Bone marrow fibrosis. Two cases of severe marrow fibrosis are shown here. The top panels are from a case of primary myelofibrosis with spindle-shaped fibroblasts and collagen replacing the entire marrow cavity. Reticulin stains on the right side show an increase in thickened fibers that encircle individual marrow cells. The bottom panel is a case of secondary marrow fibrosis from metastatic breast carcinoma. Note the malignant cells lining up in rows ("Indian filing") and the swirling patterns between the strands of collagenous fibrosis.

BONY TRABECULAE PATTERNS IN BIOPSY

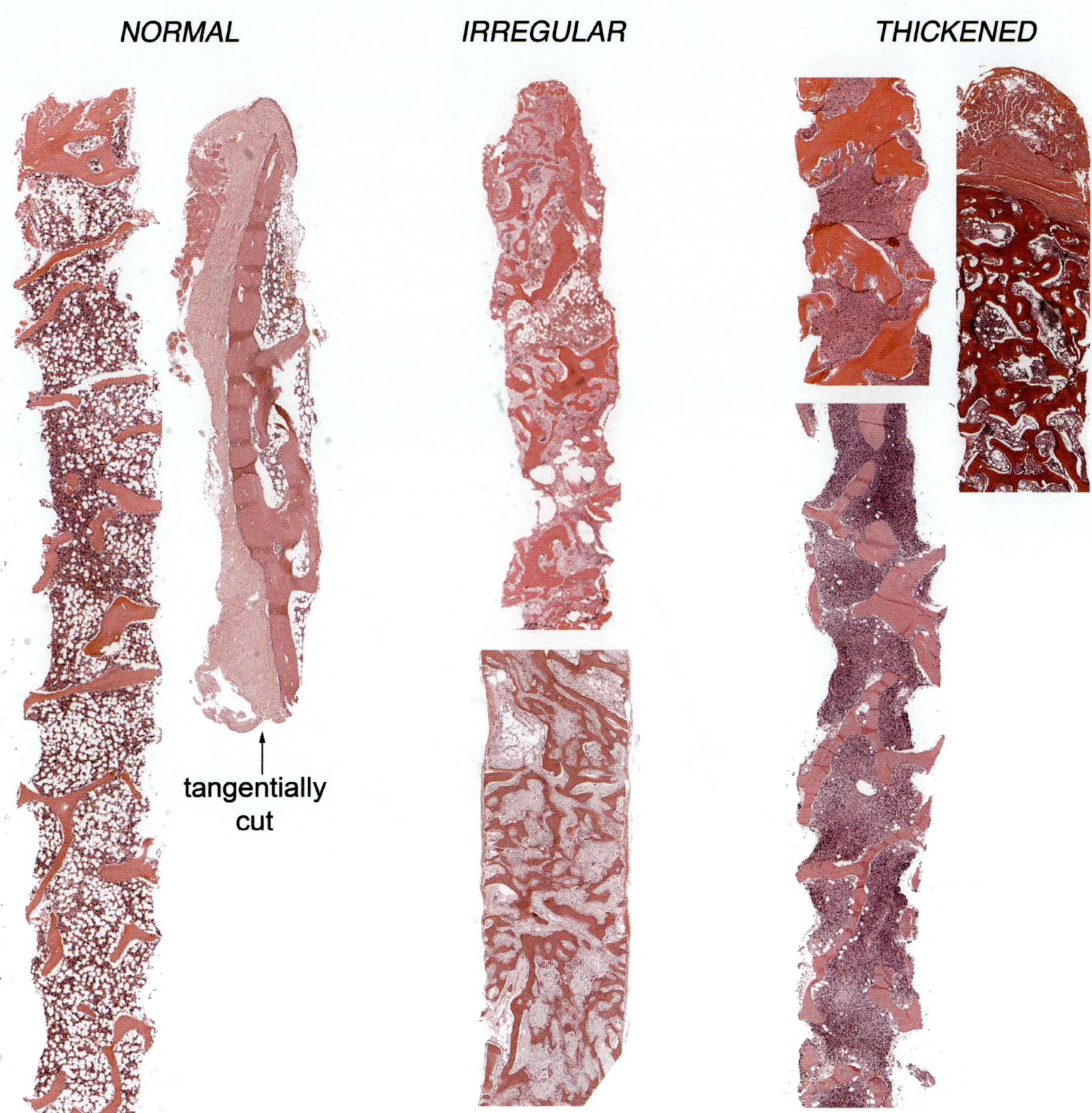

Figure 8.42. Bony trabeculae patterns in biopsy. Aside from the thickened area immediately subjacent to the cortex, normal bone marrow biopsies (shown here on the *left*) consist of numerous, thin, bony trabeculae. Various conditions that cause increased bone resorption and formation are associated with irregular and thickened bony trabeculae and include primary and secondary bone disease (renal disease), primary and metastatic bone tumors, non-neoplastic disorders of bone, fracture (and previous biopsy) site repair, infections, circulatory disorders, osteoporosis, osteomalacia, and metabolic disorders (e.g., hyperparathyroidism). The normal biopsy shown here illustrates the thickened paracortical bone that is exaggerated in the tangentially cut specimen. The middle biopsy beneath the irregular pattern label is from a patient with chronic renal disease and secondary hyperparathyroidism; the biopsies on the tright are all cases of primary myelofibrosis.

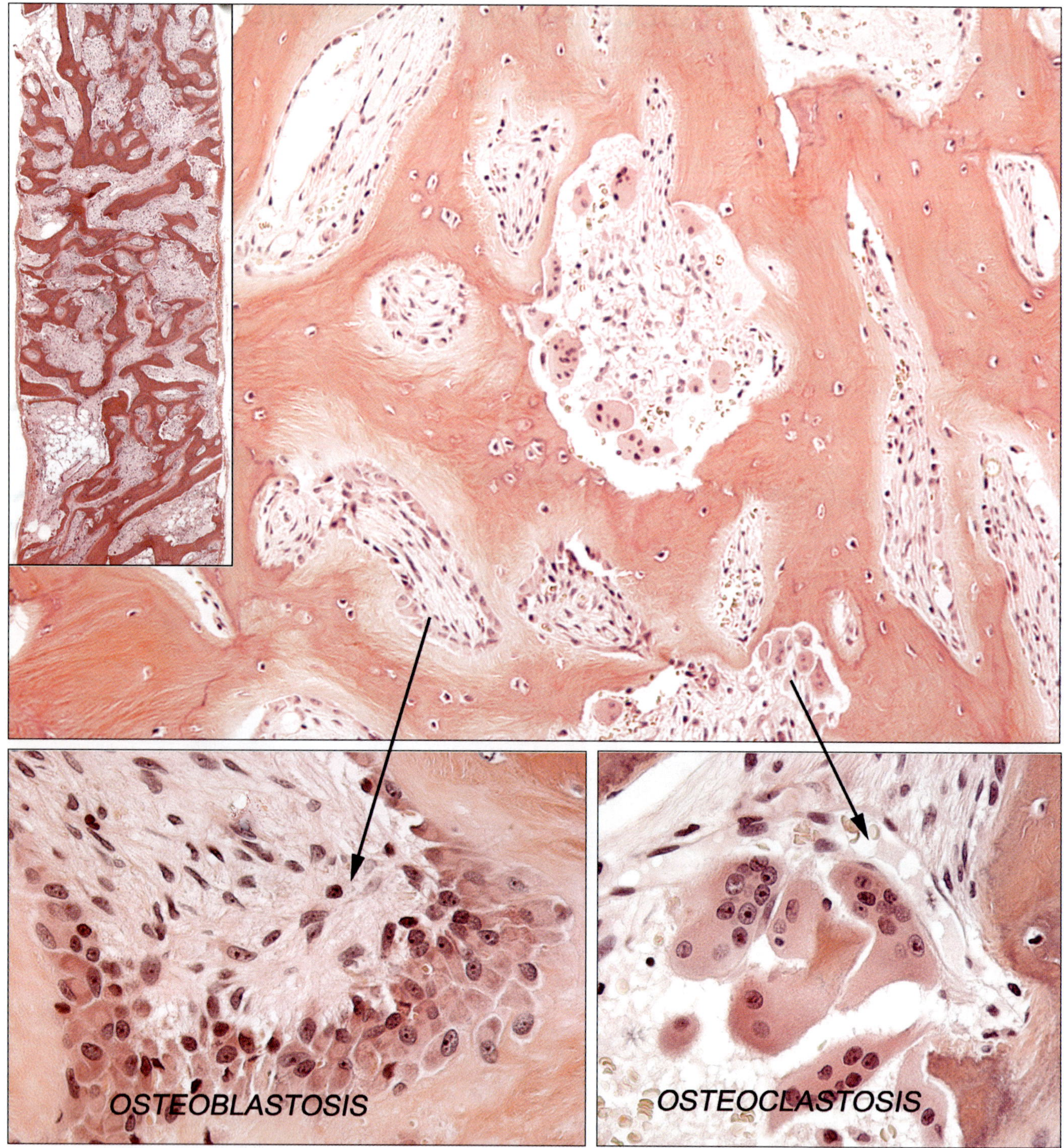

Figure 8.43.   Renal osteodystrophy. This biopsy shows thickened and thinned, irregular bony trabeculae with osteoclastosis, osteoblastosis, and evidence of abnormally increased bone turnover.

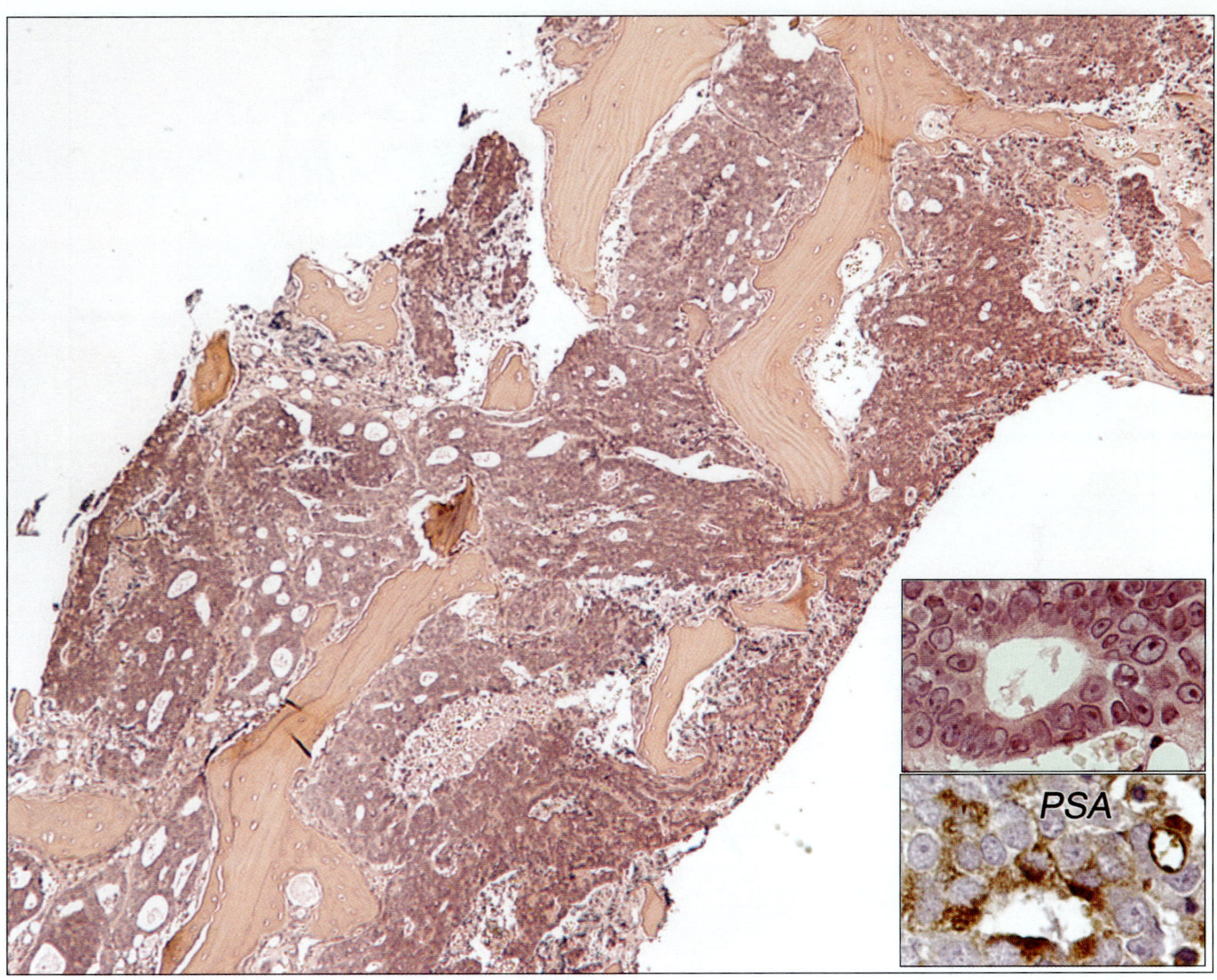

Figure 8.44. Metastatic adenocarcinoma. Malignant gland-forming cells replace the marrow in this case of metastatic prostate adenocarcinoma. Immunostains for prostate-specific antigen (PSA) were positive. Metastatic carcinoma in bone marrow typically forms cohesive rests of cells distributed in a sinusoidal pattern of involvement that may be associated with necrosis.

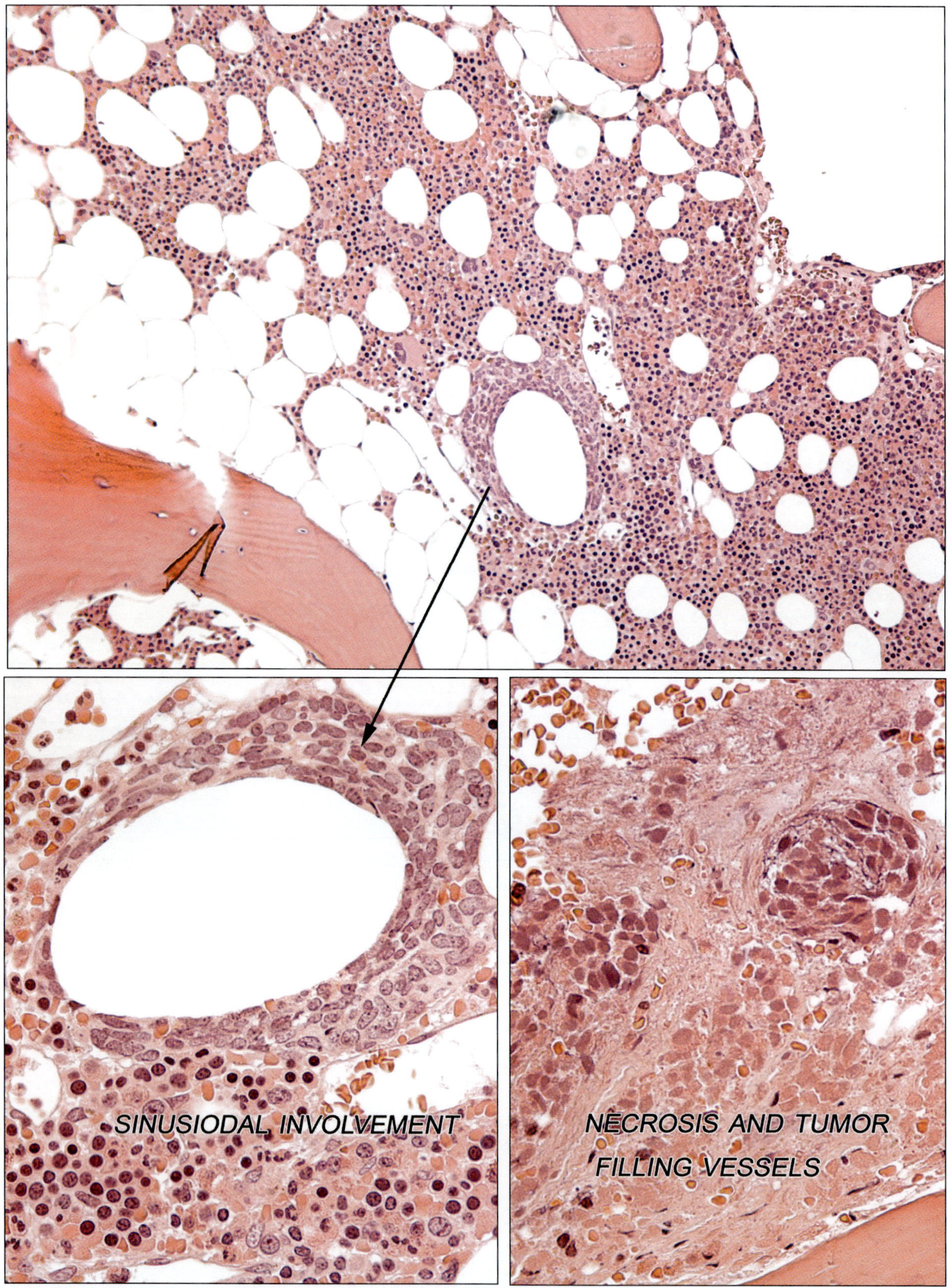

Figure 8.45. Bone marrow necrosis. Vessels and sinuses are involved by necrotic tumor metastases in this case of metastatic breast carcinoma.

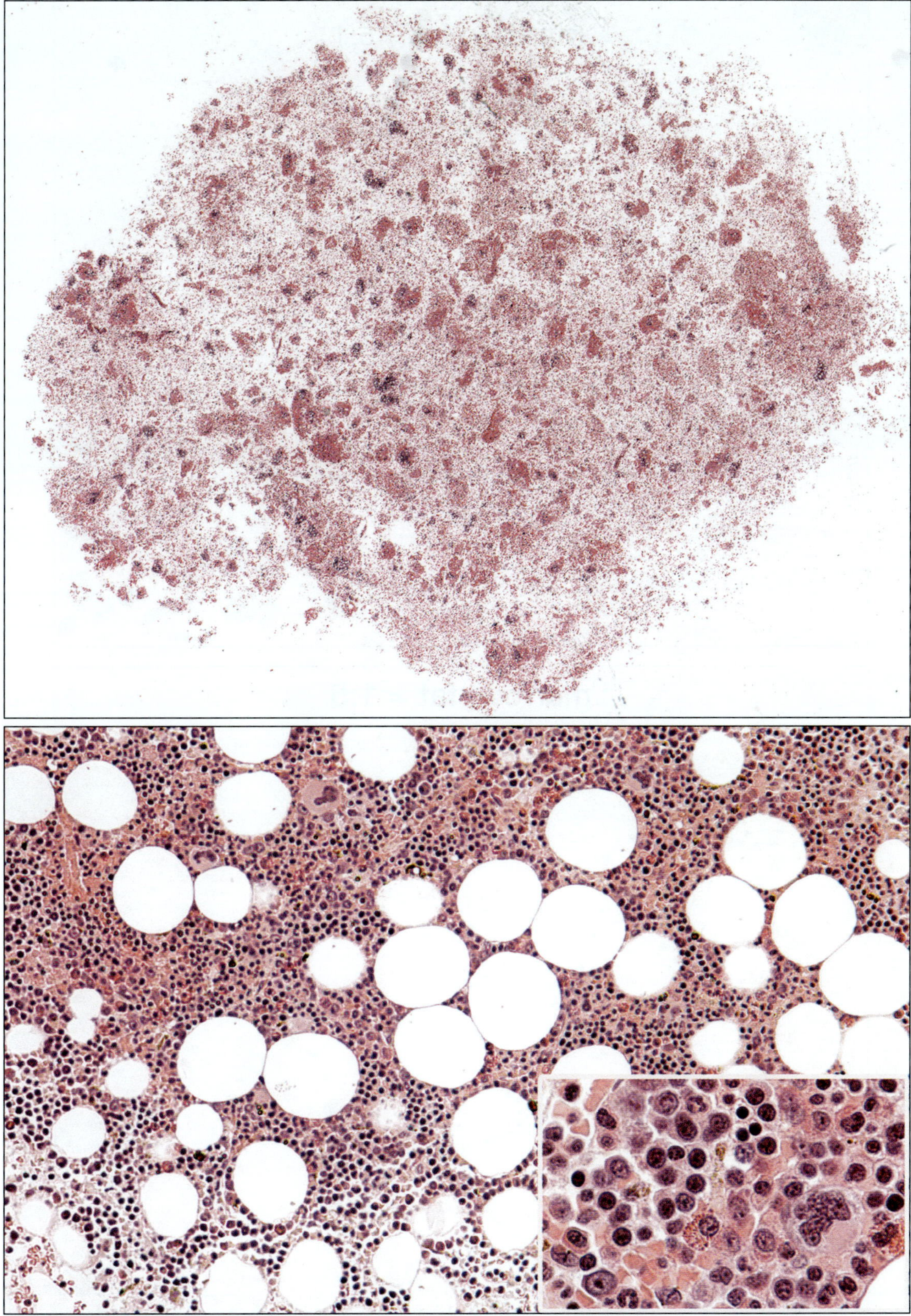

Figure 8.46 Clot section. The clot section, much like the biopsy, allows one to assess cellularity, composition, and to some degree, architectural features of the bone marrow. Additionally, immuno-histochemical stains can be used on clot sections to further elucidate the lineage of cells. This clot section shows the typical findings in a middle aged adult with a marrow:fat ratio of approximately 1.1 that shows mixed trilineage hematopoiesis.

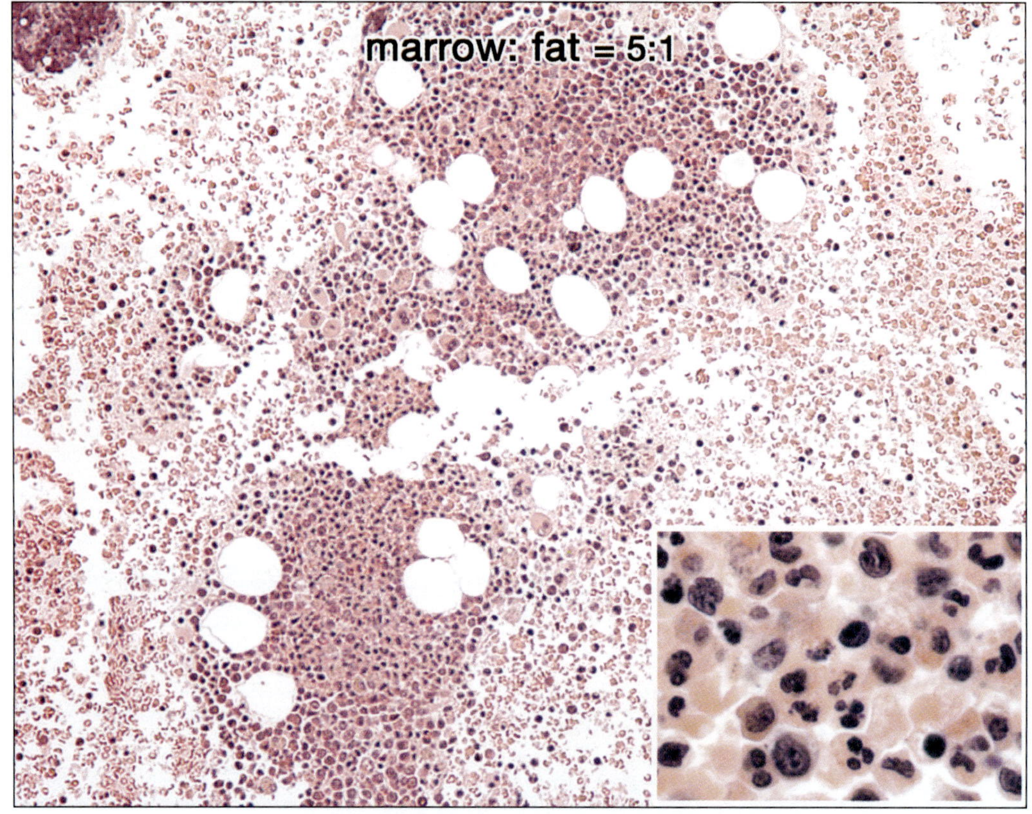

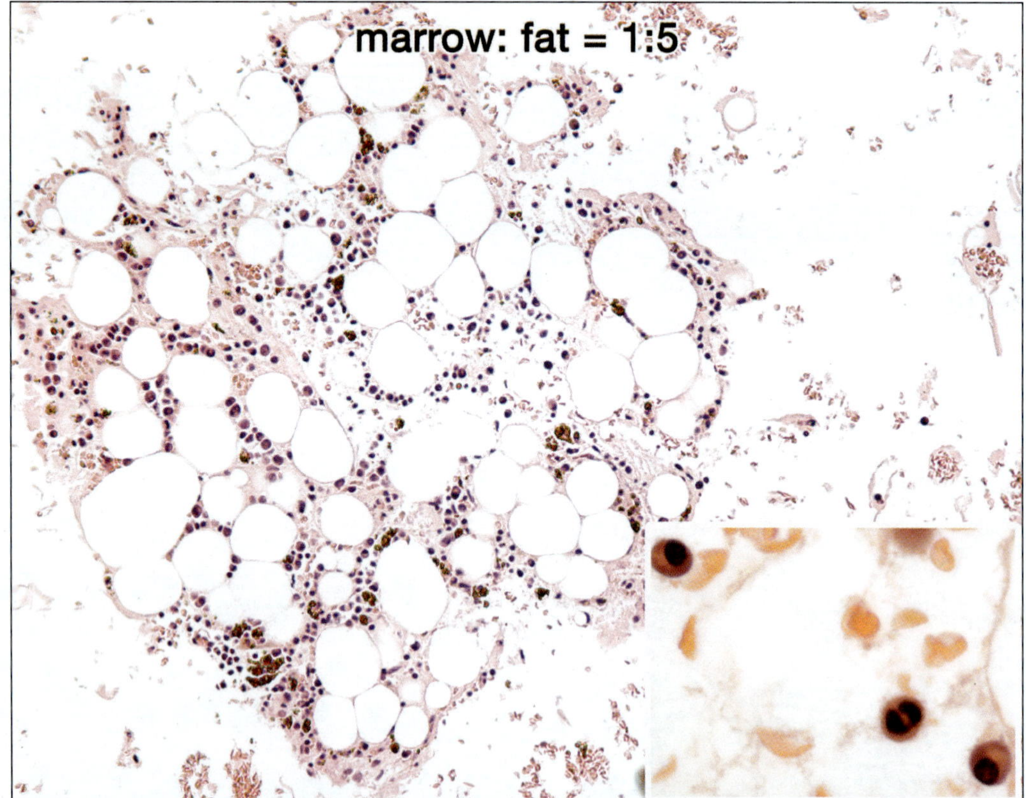

Figure 8.47. Estimating cellularity and cellular composition from the clot section. The top panel shows a clot section with granulocytic hyperplasia, and the bottom is a hypoplastic specimen. Clot sections can be valuable alternatives to biopsies. Compared with biopsies, clot sections are less invasive, require little time and few resources to prepare, and often are more amenable to antigen retrieval techniques for immunohistochemistry because decalcification is not required.

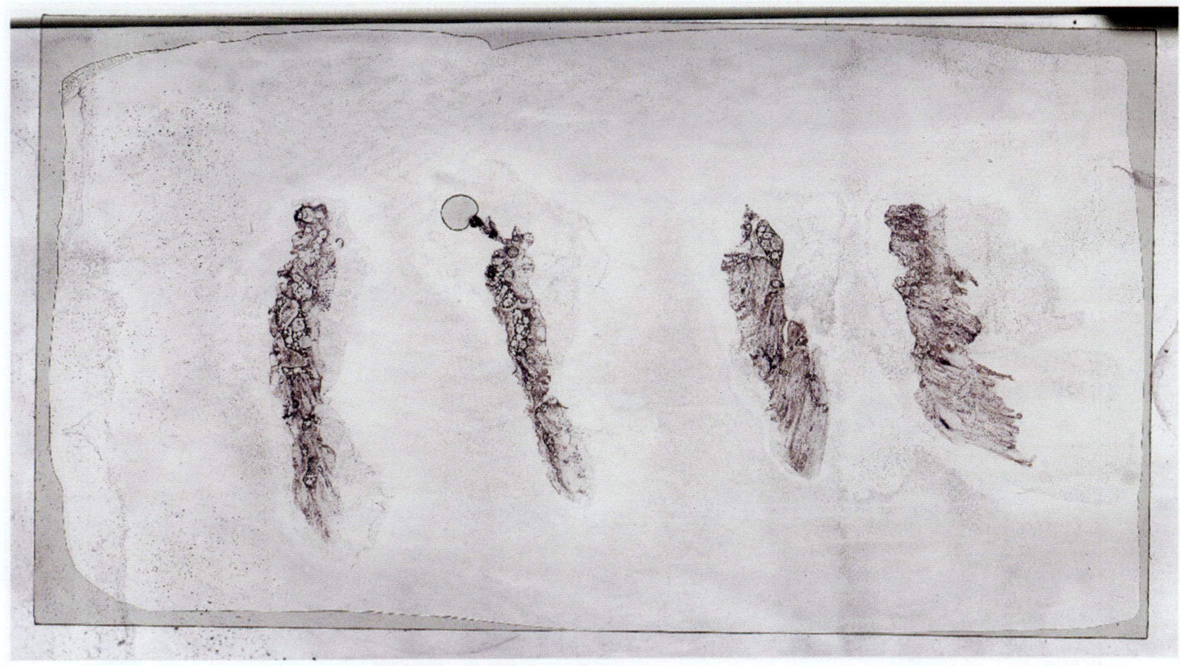

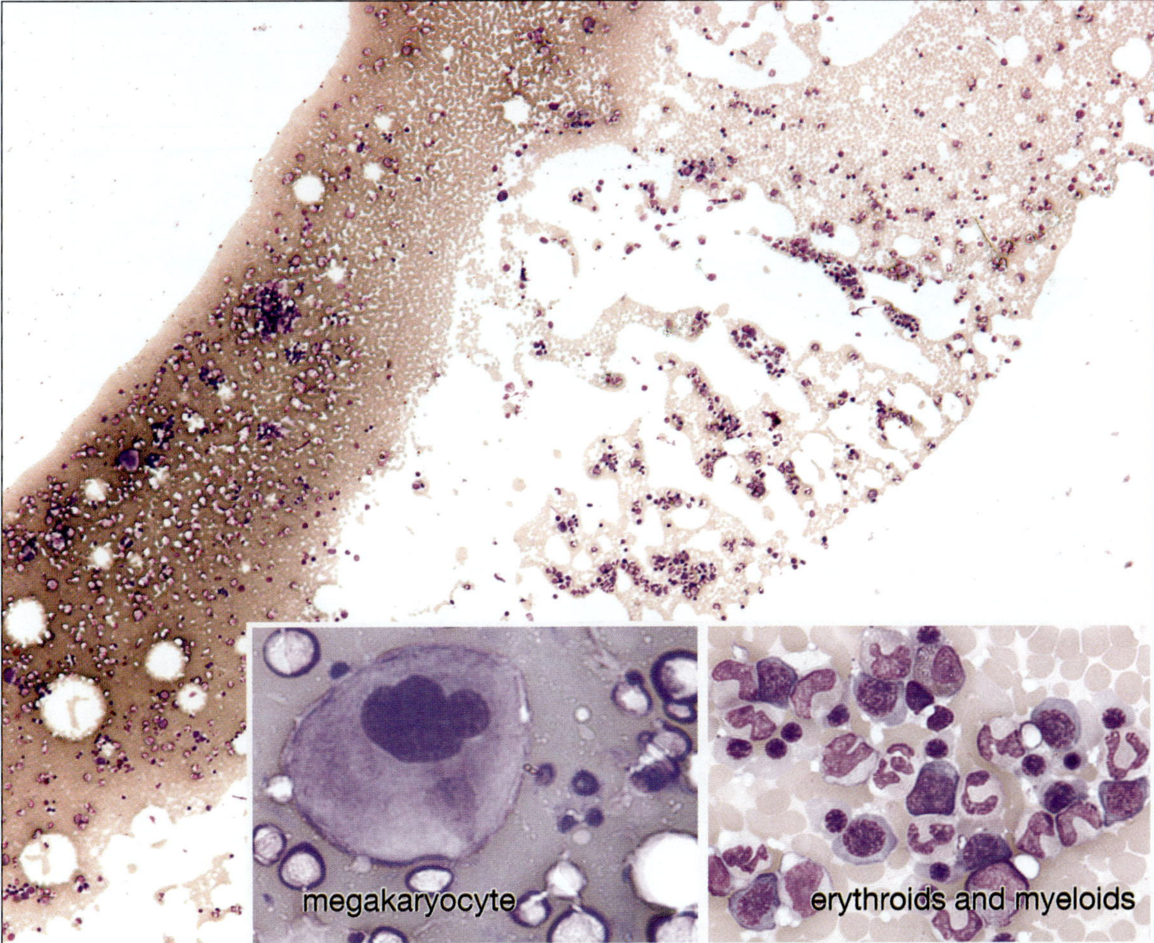

Figure 8.48 Touch preparations (touch or imprint preps). Touch preps offer a "quick look" into what the biopsy will show and sometime give better cytologic detail than the biopsy specimen. On occasion, excessive air-drying artifact and cytoplasmic stripping in touch preps can make cells appear more primitive than they actually are.

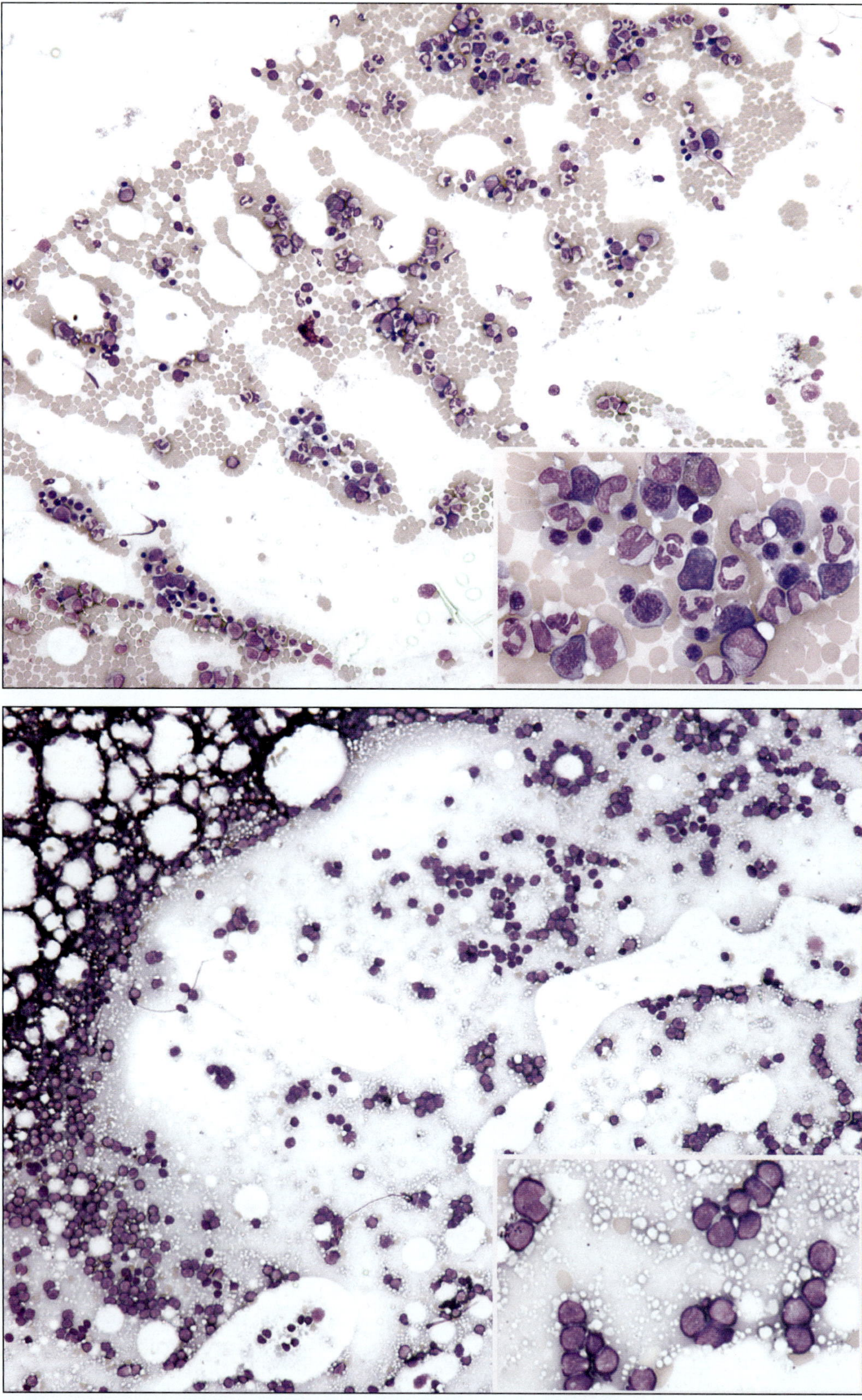

Figure 8.49.   Touch preps: A representative cytologic composition of bone marrow. The top panel is a touch prep showing a normal mixture of erythroids and maturing myeloid precursors. The bottom panel shows a marrow composed exclusively of a monotonous population of primitive cells in a case of acute myeloid leukemia.

Index

Page numbers followed by f indicate figures; page numbers followed by t indicate tables.